W

Epidemiology and

Joint Education and Training Library

This book is to be returned on or before the last date
stamped below. Overdue charges will be incurred by
the late return of books.

Renew in person, by phone (01270 612538, or
internal x2538/3172) or online at:
http://libcat.chester.ac.uk (NHS staff ask for
password)

Epidemiology and Disease Prevention
a global approach

Second edition

Edited by

John Yarnell
Centre for Public Health, Queen's University, Belfast

Dermot O'Reilly
Centre for Public Health, Queen's University, Belfast

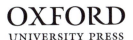

OXFORD
UNIVERSITY PRESS

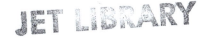

OXFORD
UNIVERSITY PRESS

Great Clarendon Street, Oxford OX2 6DP,
United Kingdom

Oxford University Press is a department of the University of Oxford.
It furthers the University's objective of excellence in research, scholarship,
and education by publishing worldwide. Oxford is a registered trade mark of
Oxford University Press in the UK and in certain other countries

First Edition published in 2007

Second Edition published in 2013

Impression: 1

British Library Cataloguing in Publication Data

Data available

ISBN 978-0-19-966053-7

Printed in Great Britain by
Ashford Colour Press Ltd, Gosport, Hampshire

Preface

Our second edition retains the main aim of the first of making disease prevention a primary concern for medical and dental undergraduates, and also for postgraduate students, particularly those in public health sciences. Prevention of disease is now a necessary concern for the global population, not only in high-income countries, but also in the growing middle-income economies, and in the poorest regions and countries of the world, which now have to contend with the rise of non-communicable diseases (cardiovascular diseases, cancers, chronic respiratory disease, and the neurodegenerative diseases of ageing) in addition to the ancient infectious diseases of tuberculosis and malaria, among others, and newly emerging epidemics such as HIV/AIDS.

For all of these reasons we have expanded this second edition to introduce these elements, while retaining the original overall structure. We have attempted to introduce and develop the core principles and global practice of epidemiology in three parts: the history and main methods of epidemiological enquiry, including chapters on screening and evidence-based practice; the epidemiology and possibilities for prevention of the major disease groups, focusing on what is already known from the extensive epidemiology of cardiovascular disease, but also attempting to highlight what is yet unknown or undiscovered in the molecular epidemiology of cancers and other chronic diseases. Maternal and child health are of critical importance for the poorest countries of the world and for infectious diseases we

welcome the contribution and experience of Professor Adriano Duse from South Africa; this chapter has been considerably extended to include the major infectious diseases which are limiting the sustainable development of some of the middle-income countries and many of the poorer countries in the world. The final chapters chronicle the slowly emerging importance of genetic and epigenetic mechanisms in population health, the critical importance of social, cultural, and behavioural factors for the development of chronic diseases, the practice of public health, and we introduce a new chapter on global health which includes contributions from the World Health Organization's Regional Directors and Dr Shanthi Mendis, Director of NCD Prevention at WHO headquarters, Geneva. In this chapter we attempt to summarize the current state of global health practice and the role of international players in an increasingly complex web of organizations which attempt to improve the health of the world's growing population.

We have written this book with a particular emphasis on self-directed learning, and we would encourage students to pursue and update the references quoted. Most journal references in this textbook are available from the bibliographical database PubMed Central in which abstracts, and often full text articles, can be obtained. Students should pose questions for themselves and for their teachers whenever possible. Only by such interaction will epidemiology become relevant to the student's future practice.

Acknowledgements

We thank several contributors from the first edition: Peter McCarron, Maureen Scott, Liam Murray, and Frank Kee, whose material has been updated in this edition, and the anonymous reviewers from Oxford University Press who made constructive suggestions for the second edition. We are very grateful to several reviewers and consultants for individual chapters or sections of the new text, particularly to Alun Evans, Christopher Patterson, Anthony Bayer, Samlee Pliambangchang, Freddie Bray, Inez Cooke, Ruari Brugha, Sean Keaveney, and KK Cheng. Enrique Loyola, Ivo Rakovac, Claudia Stein, and Natela Nadareishvili contributed to the draft report from WHO Euro. We thank Samantha Jameson for technical support and Joseph Clint for his diligent and persistent work in obtaining copyright permissions. We greatly appreciate the invaluable contribution of Oxford University Press in the preparation of this second edition, especially in obtaining the input of reviewers and for their support and craft in the production process. Particular thanks are due to Jonathan Crowe, Holly Edmundson, Geraldine Jeffers, Hannah Lloyd, Alice Emmott, Nic Williams, Beth McAllister, and Abigail Stanley. Finally, we gratefully acknowledge the forbearance and patience of our wives and families and for their support for our work.

Contents

Contributors

Dr Lesley Anderson
Centre for Public Health, Institute of Clinical Science Building, Belfast, UK

Dr Karen Bailie
Consultant in Transfusion Medicine, West of Scotland Blood Transfusion Centre, Glasgow, UK

Dr Roberto Bertollini
WHO Regional Office for Europe, Copenhagen, Denmark

Dr Shivaram Bhat
Specialty Registrar in Gastroenterology, Royal Victoria Hospital, Belfast, UK

Dr Marie Cantwell
Centre for Public Health, Institute of Clinical Science Building, Belfast, UK

Professor Ivor Chestnutt
Professor and Honorary Consultant in Dental Public Health, Cardiff University Dental School, Cardiff, UK

Professor Michael Clarke
Centre for Public Health, Institute of Clinical Science Building, Belfast, UK

Dr Sheelah Connolly
Research Fellow, Trinity College, Dublin, Ireland

Dr Gordon Cran
Centre for Public Health, Institute of Clinical Science Building, Belfast, UK

Dr Kathy Cullen
Respiratory Consultant/Clinical Academic Teaching Fellow, Centre for Medical Education, Mulhouse Building, Belfast, UK

Dr Lorraine Doherty
Director, Health Protection, Public Health Agency, Belfast, UK

Professor Helen Dolk
Institute of Nursing and Health Research, University of Ulster, Newtownabbey, Ireland

Dr Michael Donnelly
Centre for Public Health, Institute of Clinical Science Building, Belfast, UK

Professor Adriano Duse
Clinical Microbiology and Infectious Diseases, Johannesburg Hospitals Academic Complex, National Health Laboratory Service, School of Pathology, NHLS and University of Witwatersrand, Johannesburg, South Africa

Professor Emeritus Alun Evans
Centre for Public Health, Institute of Clinical Science Building, Belfast, UK

Dr Damian Fogarty
Centre for Public Health, Institute of Clinical Science Building, Belfast, UK

Professor Sharon Friel
National Centre for Epidemiology and Population Health, Australian National University, Canberra, Australia

Dr Anna Gavin
The Cancer Registry, Mulhouse Building, Belfast, UK

Dr Stanley Hawkins
Centre for Medical Education, Mulhouse Building, Belfast, UK

Zsuzsanna Jakab
WHO Regional Director for Europe, WHO Regional Office for Europe, Copenhagen, Denmark

Dr Jacqueline James
The Dental School, Queens University, Belfast, UK

Professor Brian Johnston
Honorary Professor and Consultant Gastroenterologist, Royal Victoria Hospital, Belfast, UK

Derege Kebede
Manager, African Health and Observatory and Knowledge Management Unit, World Health Organization, Regional Office for Africa, Djoue City, Brazzaville, Republic of the Congo

Professor Gerard Linden
The Dental School, Queens University, Belfast, UK

Dr Maureen McCartney
Consultant, Public Health Agency, Belfast, UK

Dr Sinead McGilloway
Director, Mental Health and Social Research Unit, Senior Lecturer, Department of Psychology, NUI Maynooth, Maynooth, Ireland

Dr Amy Jayne McKnight
Centre for Public Health, Institute of Clinical Science Building, Belfast, UK

Professor Peter Maxwell
Centre for Public Health, Institute of Clinical Science Building, Belfast, UK

Dr Shanthi Mendis
Coordinator, Chronic Diseases, Prevention and Management, Department of Chronic Diseases and Health Promotion, World Health Organization, Geneva, Switzerland

Dr William Moore
Consultant in Public Health Medicine, NHS Grampian, Aberdeen, UK

Dr James Morrow
Consultant Neurologist, Royal Hospitals Trust, Belfast, UK

Professor Liam Murray
Centre for Public Health, Institute of Clinical Science Building, Belfast, UK

Dr Tony O'Neill
Centre for Public Health, Institute of Clinical Science Building, Belfast, UK

Dr Dermot O'Reilly
Centre for Public Health, Institute of Clinical Science Building, Belfast, UK

Dr Jackie Parkes
Senior Lecturer, Cerebral Palsy Register, Mulhouse Building, Belfast, UK

Professor Christopher Patterson
Centre for Public Health, Institute of Clinical Science Building, Belfast, UK

Dr Heather Reid
Consultant, Public Health Agency, Belfast, UK

Dr Madeline Rooney
Consultant Physician, Musgrave Park Hospital, Belfast, UK

Dr Luis Gomes Sambo
Regional Director, World Health Organization, Regional Office for Africa, Djoue City, Brazzaville, Republic of the Congo

Professor W. Cairns Smith
Emeritus Professor of Public Health, School of Medicine and Dentistry, Polwarth Building, Foresterhill, Aberdeen, UK

Dr Richard Smithson
Consultant, Public Health Agency, Belfast, UK

Dr Brian Smyth
Consultant, Public Health Agency, Belfast, UK

Professor Jayne Woodside
Centre for Public Health, Institute of Clinical Science Building, Belfast, UK

Dr John Yarnell
Centre for Public Health, Institute of Clinical Science Building, Belfast, UK

Professor Shicheng Yu
Professor and Chief, Office of Health Statistics, National Centre for Public Health Surveillance and

Information Services, Chinese Centre for Disease Control and Prevention, Beijing, China

Dr Kun Zhao
Office of Health Statistics, National Centre for Public Health Surveillance and Information Services, Chinese Centre for Disease Control and Prevention, Beijing, China

1 Epidemiology: from Hippocrates to the human genome

JOHN YARNELL AND ALUN EVANS

CHAPTER CONTENTS

This chapter describes a brief history of epidemiology, some important epidemiological terms, and how epidemiology can contribute to the understanding of causes of disease and its prevention.

1.1 Epidemiology: a short history

Epidemiology (Greek: epi—upon; demos—the people) adopts a population approach to the study of the distribution and determinants of disease with the aim of controlling and preventing further disease. Its origins are perhaps nowhere better demonstrated than in Hippocrates' *On Airs, Waters, and Places* shown in Box 1.1.

According to Porter (1997), Hippocrates was a school, rather than one man, whose writings were widely disseminated in the Greek-speaking world between the 5th and 3rd centuries BC; they included treatises on **endemic** and **epidemic** diseases with descriptions of the clinical symptoms and signs of diphtheria, mumps, and malaria. These works, while pointing towards the causes of diseases, had the practical purpose of helping

Greek explorers decide whether the terrain and habitat of a new landfall in North Africa or the eastern Mediterranean would support a colony of the Greek empire. During this era the task of **hygiene** was to maintain a 'balanced constitution' to prevent disease and this was perpetuated in the prolific work of Galen in the 2nd century AD, and in Arabic medicine which continued the Greek tradition into the Middle Ages. *Airs, Waters and Places* remained the basic epidemiological text for physicians for 2000 years (Rosen 1993).

The Black Death (bubonic plague) came to Europe in the 14th century, spread from city to city, and killed about a quarter of Europe's population within a few years. It continued to wreak destruction over the next two centuries and public health developed out of the need to control the disease. Physicians recognized its **contagious** nature but failed to link it with rats and

Box 1.1 Descriptive epidemiology in 400 BC

Whoever wishes to investigate medicine properly should proceed thus: in the first place to consider the **seasons of the year**, and what effects each of them produces . . . Then the **winds**, the hot and the cold . . . then such as are peculiar to each **locality**. We must also consider the qualities of the **waters** . . . when one comes into a **city** to which he is a stranger, he ought to consider its **situation**, how it lies as to the winds and the rising of the sun. . . . These things one ought to consider most attentively, and concerning the waters which the inhabitants use, whether they be marshy and soft, or hard, and running from elevated and rocky situations, and then if saltish and unfit for cooking; and the ground, whether it be naked and deficient in water, or wooded and well watered, and whether it lies in a hollow, confined situation, or is elevated and cold; **and the mode in which the inhabitants live and what are their pursuits, whether they are fond of drinking and eating to excess, and given to indolence, or are fond of exercise and labour, and not given to excess in eating and drinking**.

Extracted from: *On Airs, Waters, and Places*. Hippocrates 400 BC. Translated by Francis Adams. Source: Internet Classics. Available at: **http://classics.mit.edu/**

fleas; the only weapons against plague was **quarantine**, isolation of patients, and burial of corpses, but *health boards* were created in many cities to initiate and regulate these public health measures to limit the spread of the disease. The first documented health board was founded in Venice in 1348 (Rosen 1993). Two centuries later, Fracastoro, working in Verona, published his seminal work *On Contagion, Contagious Diseases and Treatment* in 1546. He proposed three routes of infection: direct contact; spread from clothes and sheets (*fomites*); and through the air or water by contagious seeds which he termed *seminaria*. He described the clinical symptoms and signs of smallpox, syphilis, measles, tuberculosis, bubonic plague, rabies, leprosy, and typhus. He began the concept of the germ theory of disease proposing that there were specific *seminaria* for specific diseases. Some key advances in the understanding of the epidemiology of disease are shown in Table 1.1.

In medieval European cities overcrowding, poverty, and disease were standard for the majority of the population. Life expectancy was short, infant mortality was high; less than half of babies born survived to the age of 20 years. Population growth was slow; for example, in England the population grew from only one and a half million in the 11th century to five and a half million in the 16th. Working conditions for most were harsh and, at the turn of the 18th century, Ramazzini published *De Morbis Artificium Diatriba*, his major work

on the diseases of occupations as diverse as miners, glassblowers, painters, potters, and weavers, which remained a standard text until the Industrial Revolution a century and a half later. In England, following the Great Plague, parish registers of births, christenings, and deaths were kept from 1692 and, in the mid-17th century, Graunt published his *Natural and Political Observations upon the Bills of Mortality* which showed that residents of the city of London had a considerable excess mortality compared to those who lived in country parishes. Indeed he showed that the population of the city of London was only maintained by fresh immigration from the surrounding rural areas (Brockington 1958). Graunt constructed the first simple life tables but it was not until two centuries later that civil registration began in England (1837) and the discipline of vital statistics became more strongly established under the direction of the first appointed medical statistician for England, William Farr.

Epidemics of smallpox and syphilis were common in Europe and some medical scientists took heroic measures to investigate the causes of disease. In an attempt to understand gonorrhoea, in 1767 John Hunter took pus from an infected patient and inoculated his own penis with it in two places, and, sure enough, he contracted gonorrhoea. Unfortunately for Hunter, several weeks later the characteristic lesion of syphilis (large pox) developed. Because the original patient was harbouring both diseases Hunter ended up with one more

Table 1.1 Some landmarks in epidemiology and disease prevention up to the 20th century

Date	Author	Concept	Application
400BC	Hippocrates	Medical geography/ecology	Basic epidemiological principles of endemic and epidemic disease
1546	Frascastoro	Contagion 'particle theory' of infection	Quarantine for leprosy, plague
1662	Graunt	Mortality and fertility	Life tables
1700/1713	Ramazzini	Occupational disease (in 42/54 occupations)	Health and safety (limited)
1753	Lind	Simple experimental trial	Prevention of scurvy with citrus fruits
1798	Jenner	Inoculation/vaccination (cowpox/smallpox)	Vaccination against smallpox
1839	Farr	Death rates/causes	Vital statistics
1846	Panum	Epidemic cycles/incubation period (measles)	Infectivity
1849	Semmelweis	Particle transmission of infection (childbirth fever)	Antisepsis with chlorinated lime
1854	Snow	Waterborne disease	Sanitation reform [This was already part of the 1848 Public Health Act]
1840/1870	Henle/Koch	Criteria for disease causation	Disease classification/prevention
1888	Pasteur	Resistance to infection	Attenuation of pathogenicity/inoculation and vaccine development

disease than he had predicted. Hunter's experiment pre-dated the Henle–Koch postulates (see Box 1.2) by almost a century.

Smallpox was endemic in Europe, Asia, and Africa in the Middle Ages and was introduced to the Americas by the first explorers; this facilitated the plundering of these new lands because the colonists had immunity to these diseases, whereas the indigenous inhabitants did not. The practice of inoculation, in which infected material from a mild case of disease was injected into a healthy person, was widely practised in China and was introduced into England and France in the 18th century. Voltaire was a strong advocate for this but it was not without the risk of inducing a serious or fatal attack of smallpox instead of the intended mild case.

At the turn of the century (in 1796) the Gloucestershire general practitioner, Edward Jenner, took this concept further by inoculating individuals with matter from a related disease affecting cattle and humans, cowpox. Vaccination with cowpox appeared to be more reliable, less hazardous, and more readily available than inoculation with smallpox and the practice became widely popular in Britain, Europe, and in the USA.

As a young doctor in 1846, Peter Ludwig Panum was appointed by the Danish government to study a serious outbreak of measles on the Faroe Islands where the last case had occurred sixty-five years previously. The mortality was close to 10 per cent. His meticulous report helped establish the science of field epidemiology and outbreak investigation in infectious diseases.

Childbearing was known to be particularly hazardous and delivery (lying-in) hospitals were established in some European cities in the 19th century but mortality continued to be high. In Vienna Semmelweis noticed that mothers and children delivered by medical students were more likely to die than those delivered by midwives during a period of several years. Mortality improved when the medical students were instructed to wash their hands in limewash after working in the dissecting rooms. Such measures, however, were rejected by the medical establishment who ostracized Semmelweiss. Today Semmelweiss' contribution is recognized by a one day national holiday in Hungary. Basic hygienic and sanitary principles established by the Greeks and Romans were not maintained in most of the districts and dwellings of European cities and cholera spread from India carried by merchant ships and also overland. The first major epidemic hit London in 1832 with 7000 deaths (Porter 1997) and the London Epidemiological Society was formed in 1850 largely to combat the successive outbreaks of cholera in London and other cities in Britain. In the 1850s, John Snow, an anaesthetist practising in Soho, London, recognized from the geographic distribution of cholera cases that the disease was linked with water likely to have been contaminated by sewage. Sanitary reform, the provision of clean drinking water, and disposal of sewage became established in the major cities of Britain, Europe, and the USA. By the late 19th century, particularly in Germany, the microscope had been developed to an extent that permitted the identification of the bacteria responsible for anthrax, cholera, tuberculosis, and many others. This was only made possible by staining techniques which were facilitated by Germany's extensive chemical industry. With the development of laboratory and immunological tools by Pasteur and others, infectious disease epidemiology was able to start in earnest (Chapter 18). A myriad of bacteria were being discovered and it was clear that many of these caused no disease. Two pioneers in bacteriology and microscopy formulated the Henle–Koch postulates to assist the process of linking specific bacteria with particular diseases; these postulates are shown in Box 1.2 and are particularly relevant for bacterial infections. Although they serve as a useful yardstick for all infectious diseases, viruses and

Box 1.2 The Henle–Koch postulates

1 The organism must be found in all cases of the disease.
2 It must be isolated from patients with the disease and grown in pure culture.
3 When the pure culture is inoculated into susceptible animals or man, it must reproduce the disease.

parasites can be host-specific, and evidence of infection is more readily obtained from immunological tests of antibody formation which have been developed in the 20th century.

During the 19th century life expectancy for the general population began to improve and population growth began to accelerate rapidly. Five and a half million population in England in 1700 became nine million in 1800, and 33 million by 1900. The improvements in life expectancy have been termed the *health transition* which occurred widely in Europe during the 19th century (Riley 2001) and even more rapidly in a wider range of countries in the latter half of the 20th century. By the end of the first quarter of the 20th century with improvements in nutrition and living conditions, particularly for the poor, infectious diseases began to wane in the more advanced industrialized countries, and chronic diseases such as lung cancer and cardiovascular disease (coronary heart disease and stroke) began to emerge as important causes of death and illness. This process is known as the *epidemiological transition*. Coronary disease was not new, but had previously been confined to the better off. In England, Heberden described the disease in 1772 and in Ireland in 1777 David Macbride included this condition in the second edition of his medical textbook. Samuel Black noted in 1818 that: 'the primary and original cause of the disorder (angina pectoris) is ossification of the coronaries' (Evans 1995). Drawing on Macbride's work, he went on to describe and contrast the distribution of the disease in the Irish and in the French, and these he linked with contrasting lifestyles (Evans 2011). The concept of **risk factors** (see later) for disease clearly exercised these early researchers, although the term was not introduced into medicine until 1956.

By the 1950s the epidemics of heart attack and lung cancer, principally in men, were well advanced and widely recognized by the leading medical authorities, particularly in Britain and the USA. *Epidemiological studies* were developed to investigate the causes of these diseases, the first of these was in St Andrews in Scotland and established by Sir James Mackenzie. He was visited by a young American cardiologist, Paul Dudley White, and from this sprang the Framingham and Seven Countries Study around 1950. Other **prospective studies** such as those among British doctors clearly established the link between tobacco smoking and both lung cancer and coronary disease (Doll and Hill 1954; Doll *et al.* 1994). Epidemiologists became interested in both the prevention and treatment of disease. In the 1960s Cochrane showed that less than half of routine medical and surgical treatments were based on solid scientific evidence, and the discipline of *evidence-based medicine* was born (Cochrane 1972) (Chapter 6). To establish **causality** there is a hierarchy of different types of epidemiological studies, both **observational** and **experimental** (see Chapter 2) and often a painstaking process in mounting these steps. Sometimes it is possible to bypass a step; sometimes it is impossible to proceed at all. Often people who criticize epidemiology do not understand its strengths and weaknesses: the method applied must be appropriate to the situation. If not, to criticize is rather like blaming a carthorse for being useless at flat racing. In an otherwise excellent book, *Cancer: The Evolutionary Legacy*, Greaves (2000) draws attention to the limitations of epidemiology but praises the Linxian Study (Blot *et al.* 1993) which is a population-based nutritional interventional study in a poor region of China designed by epidemiologists in an attempt to reduce the high incidence of gastric cancer in that region. Although the first well-known recorded experiment in curative/preventive medicine was performed by James Lind, who allocated six types of treatments to twelve sailors with scurvy on HMS *Salisbury*'s return to Plymouth in 1747 (only the treatment with citrus fruits was effective), only recently has its methodology been developed and ratified with the growth of evidence-based medicine (see Chapters 4 and 6) and the '**gold standard**' of the **randomized controlled trial** (RCT) become established. The methodology was

originally applied widely in crop trials, and subsequently in medicine, but human beings proved altogether more difficult to regiment than plots of wheat. In certain circumstances, where evidence is lacking, or the studies required are just too costly or impracticable to conduct, causality may be strongly suggested by applying several criteria (see section 1.3 and Box 1.4) all of which have certain limitations: it is simply the best we can do in the circumstances until new evidence is accumulated or new techniques of investigation become available.

At the beginning of the 21st century *epidemiology is a broad-based population science* drawing on many disciplines from biological, laboratory, and clinical science and from biostatistics to sociology and philosophy of science. *Epidemiology investigates the causes of human disease* and *methods for their control.* Past and future epidemiology has been discussed by others (Davey Smith and Ebrahim 2001) but the need for scientific rigour cannot be overstated. The science of molecular biology, biomarkers, and the human genome offer many opportunities for epidemiology to contribute to the understanding of chronic diseases (Day *et al.* 2001; Khoury *et al.* 2011) whilst the broad scope of epidemiology ensures that its future evolution and development will remain at the forefront of the control of human disease. The breadth of applications for epidemiology is discussed in more detail elsewhere (Detels 2009).

1.2 Defining and measuring disease in populations

The word **disease** (literally: dis-ease) is often used rather loosely by doctors and lay persons alike. Usually it is self-limiting, but if it does not resolve and becomes an **illness** we may seek the opinion of a general practitioner, who, in turn, would try to decide if it could be a specific disease entity requiring treatment, which may warrant a full diagnostic assessment. Hospital specialists and other medical scientists such as pathologists, microbiologists, immunologists, and radiologists tend to work with disease entities where the **natural history** (the causes and unhindered clinical progression) of the disease is generally well described and

Box 1.3 Hierarchical definitions of disease and disorders in medical research

Causal research:		Disease entity			
Applied epidemiology and health services research:	Specific conditions:	Disease syndrome	Disorder	Condition	Trait
	Non-specific conditions:	Disability		Illness	Sickness

treatment options are known. The scope of epidemiology has become so broad that epidemiologists have to work at a number of different levels of diagnostic certainty which are described in Box 1.3.

A disease entity may have a single **cause** such as a bacterium or virus, or a combination of causes which have been well defined. Even for the infectious diseases there is still the issue of **host susceptibility/resistance** for most agents. For many infectious diseases a minimum of three components is required for disease: a susceptible **host**, an infectious **agent**, and an **environment** favourable for the reproduction and growth of the infectious agent. Most diseases are defined solely on the typical clinical history, symptoms, and signs with or without the assistance of laboratory or other diagnostic facilities. If the cause of a particular disease is not understood, then the disease may possibly comprise more than one disease entity and this is termed **disease heterogeneity**. **Disorder** tends to be used for malfunction of particular systems, e.g. cardiovascular disorder, endocrine disorder, etc. **Condition** is usually a state of the body or of an organ, e.g. being overweight or obesity. **Trait** indicates a predisposition to disease ranging from a specific genetic trait to a personality or psychological trait predisposing to mental illness. The term **syndrome** (a collection of symptoms and signs occurring together) is widely used (and abused) in medical practice. Some syndromes are well established as disease entities, e.g. Wernicke's syndrome (encephalopathy)—a complex of neurological signs associated with thiamine deficiency and alcoholism, whilst others are either poorly defined, e.g. chronic fatigue syndrome (myelo-encephalopathy—ME) or even artificially created by doctors, e.g. metabolic syndrome. **Disability** (formerly handicap) implies a malfunctioning of a particular body system, e.g. mental disability. **Illness** refers to the subjective state of an individual or unspecified disease state whilst **sickness** usually signifies a dysfunctional state or, in the language of sociology, as the 'sick role'—the social consequences of illness. '**Sickness absence**' is much studied by epidemiologists and other health care researchers, but it is notoriously difficult to standardize definitions of disorders, conditions, or illnesses which have been described either by the patient or by their doctor as a 'cause' of absence from work.

Measurement of disease How the epidemiologist attempts to measure the level of a disease in a population depends to a certain extent on the purpose of the measurement or the study, which is dealt with in Chapter 2; but for basic, descriptive purposes two types of measurement of disease are important:

1 *Prevalence*—this counts the *number of cases* in a given population. It can be at a particular point in time: **point prevalence** (often referred to simply as prevalence), **period prevalence**—measured over a period of time, and **cumulative prevalence** which may refer to the total number of episodes of disease accumulated during the individual lifespan of each member of the population. Although prevalence was just described as a number it is most often used in the sense of **prevalence rate, ratio, proportion,** or **percentage** where the number of cases is divided by the population size. Clearly the type of measurement used greatly depends on the natural history of the disease in question. Some diseases such as measles, for example, may occur once in an individual and confer lifelong immunity. Other diseases may be episodic in nature and recur during life, such as epilepsy and recurrent heart attacks; point **prevalence** and **attack rates** are the measurement of choice for these conditions. Yet other diseases may be chronic and long term in nature (e.g. multiple

sclerosis, diabetes mellitus). Some diseases carry a very high **case-fatality** (80–100 per cent) whilst others may be rarely life-threatening. It is helpful in the descriptive epidemiology of a new disease to be able to count the number of cases and to describe their distribution according to *who* has acquired the disease, *where* they have acquired it, and *when* (i.e. distribution of disease by *person, place,* and *time*— see Chapter 2).

2 *Incidence* The other important measure of disease is **incidence** which is the number of *new cases* of disease occurring in a specified period of time. The attack rate or **cumulative incidence** refers to the number of new episodes of disease in a given time period. Again, incidence is frequently used as shorthand for **incidence rate** which relates it to a given population (its size used as the denominator) and enables different populations to be compared. Typically incidence rates would be calculated per annum.

Incidence rate is a measurement that tends to be used in **longitudinal** studies in which people are followed up for new cases of disease over a period of years. Proxy indicators of disease (traits, diagnostic, and screening tests) are discussed in Chapter 5, but prevalence and incidence measurements of these indicators are largely identical to those for disease entities. Box 1.4 shows the main types of measures used in epidemiological studies.

1.3 Models of causation and determinants of disease

Rothman has described epidemiology as an 'embryo among the sciences such as physics and chemistry' (Rothman 1998). This 'embryo' however can claim many public health successes, such as the control of the major water-borne diseases or the identification of

Box 1.4 Measuring disease: prevalence and incidence

Prevalence		Incidence	
Point	**Period**	**Proportion**	**Rate**
Number of cases of disease in a population at a particular point of time	Number of cases in a population during a specific period of time	Proportion of people in a population developing a disease in a given time period	Rate at which new disease events occur in a population
Prevalence rate		**Attack rate or cumulative incidence**	**Incidence (density)***
Number of cases÷population at risk (often *P*%)		New cases or episodes developing in study period÷population at risk at beginning of study period	New cases developing in study period÷person–years at risk
• New and old cases included • Follow-up not required • Diseases of long duration will inflate prevalence with age • Preferred measure to assess burden of disease in population		• New cases or episodes of disease only • Follow-up of whole population required • Duration of disease will not inflate incidence • Preferred measure to assess risk of disease and cause and effect	

*Commonly referred to as incidence rate.

the links between tobacco smoking and coronary heart disease and cancer; the methodology and theoretical basis of epidemiology continue to develop. The concept of 'cause' is critical to the philosophy of scientific method and medical sciences are no exception to this. Epidemiology seeks to examine 'causes' of disease in whole populations and is fortunate today in having basic medical sciences it can draw upon, such as microbiology, biochemistry, pathology, and immunology. At first sight the 'cause' of an infectious disease is straightforward: the single infectious agent associated with the clinical manifestation of the disease. However, the reality is different: for the majority of infectious diseases infectivity rates are low, i.e. many individuals can be exposed to the agent but do not develop the clinical disease. Tuberculosis was a major cause of death

in Europe, and remains so in the developing world; but factors such as malnutrition, overcrowding, lack of sunlight, and smoking are strongly associated with the likelihood of clinical disease. These elements which contribute to the development of the disease are known as risk factors and are discussed further in Chapter 3. McKeown (1976) has shown, by simple examination of trends in mortality from major infectious diseases, the crucial role of external factors (social and environmental) entirely separate from the infectious agent itself in 'causing' their decline (see Fig. 1.1).

For an infectious disease the infectious agent is clearly a factor **necessary** for the development of a disease. Such a factor is known as a **necessary cause**. If an agent causes a clinical disease in 100 per cent of individuals exposed to it (which is rare, but

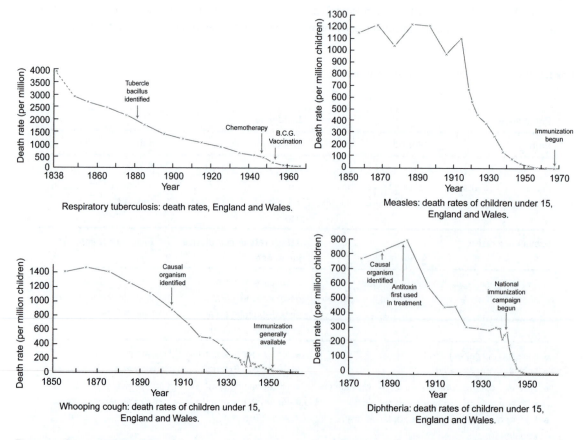

Figure 1.1 Question 1: What factors do you think are most likely to have contributed to the demise of these diseases as important causes of death? Question 2: What lessons could be inferred from these data for developing countries in the 21st century?
Source: McKeown T (1976) *The Modern Rise of Population*. London: Edward Arnold.

infectivity is high in some infectious diseases, such as anthrax, smallpox, Ebola virus, and measles) then this is said to be also a **sufficient cause**. For chronic diseases there are instances of single sufficient (and necessary) causes for **monogenic disorders** but for the majority a combination of factors act together to produce a **combined sufficient cause** (multiple causes) in the *sufficient-component model* of disease causation (Fig. 1.2). For some chronic diseases, for example, lung cancer, cigarette smoking is a necessary cause for 90 per cent of cases, but this level of attribution is rare. It is not a sufficient factor as not all smokers will develop the disease (although, for long-term smokers, their average life expectancy is seven years less than that of the general population). Similarly, for the development of premature coronary heart disease (see Chapter 7) raised plasma cholesterol may be a necessary factor in a given population but this is insufficient as a single causal factor for all cases of the disease. Different sets of multiple causes for coronary heart disease are illustrated using Rothman's pie charts as shown in Fig. 1.2. It is the task of the

epidemiologist to examine as many potentially causal factors as possible, both *proximal* and *distal*, and to quantify their likely contribution to the development of the disease. These factors can be examined by a number of different study designs, which are discussed in Chapter 3. It should be noted that 'causal' factors may be related to each other and not show truly independent effects, but it may be helpful to define all possible causes in order to create the maximum potential for prevention. Causal models, inference, and statistical approaches to testing causal hypotheses are discussed in more detail elsewhere (Davey Smith and Ebrahim 2001; Hofler 2005; Rothman and Greenland 2005).

Bradford Hill, a medical statistician, worked with Doll on the link between tobacco smoking, lung cancer, and other important diseases. He also developed the randomized controlled trial (see Chapter 3), and devised a set of principles or guidelines which he suggested could help in distinguishing causal and non-causal associations (Box 1.5) (Bradford Hill 1971).

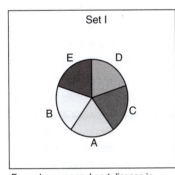
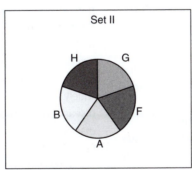
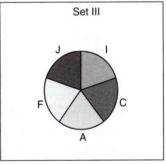

Example: coronary heart disease in
Set I: 45-year-old white man

Set II: 45-year-old Asian man

Set III: 55-year-old white woman

A, raised plasma cholesterol ≥ 5.5 mmol/l.
B, smoking 20 cigarettes a day.
C, raised blood pressure ≥ 160/95 mmHg.
D, low high-density lipoprotein cholesterol ≤ 1.0 mmol/l.
E, raised plasma homocysteine.

F, diabetes mellitus (type 2).
G, central obesity.
H, raised plasma triglyceride ≥ 3.0 mmol/l.
I, raised plasma fibrinogen.
J, severe periodontal disease.

Notes: 1. Cut-points for continuously distributed variables may be arbitrary.
   2. Some causes may be partly associated with each other and not exert an independent effect.
   3. In practice each 'cause' would not contribute equally towards the creation of the disease entity.
Modified from Rothman and Greenland (1998).

Figure 1.2 Three different sets of multiple causes sufficient to induce disease entity: coronary heart disease.
Source: Rothman, K. J. (1976). 'Reviews and Commentary: Causes'. *American Journal of Epidemiology*, **104**: 587–92.

Box 1.5 Criteria used in observational epidemiological studies to distinguish causal from non-causal associations

- **Strength**: relative risk of lung cancer in smokers is 10 times that in non-smokers.
- **Consistency**: similar results in several studies from different countries, possibly using different methodologies.
- **Specificity**: specific exposures (often occupational) may be associated with specific diseases.
- **Temporality**: did the putative cause precede the onset of the disease?
- **Biological gradient**: risk of respiratory cancers and of cardiovascular diseases increases with amount of cigarettes smoked and number of years of smoking.

- **Plausibility**: a biological mechanism should exist.
- **Coherence**: evidence from different sources provides biological 'coherence' to the overall hypothesis.
- **Experimental evidence**: from 'natural' or observed preventive experiments (without evidence from a scientifically conducted intervention study).
- **Analogy**: comparison with other diseases caused by similar biological mechanism.

Adapted from: Hill, AB (1971) *Principles of Medical Statistics*, 9th edn. London: The Lancet.

Multiple sclerosis provides another example of a complex disease which is probably the result of the interaction of several risk factors. Risk factors include: exposure to Epstein–Barr virus, limited exposure to sunlight or low vitamin D levels, cigarette smoking, genetic predisposition, and infections as a protective factor. These factors have been evaluated using the Rothman pie charts (van der Mei *et al.* 2011) and the Bradford Hill guidelines (Giovanni and Ebers 2007). Bradford Hill's parting thoughts (1965) for his readers are still worth quoting:

> **. . . All scientific work is incomplete—whether it be observed or experimental. All scientific work is likely to be upset or modified by advancing knowledge. That does not confer upon us a freedom to ignore the knowledge that we already have, or to postpone the action that it appears to demand at a given time.**

1.4 Prevention and treatment of disease

The concept of prevention is crucial in medical practice, but is frequently neglected in the pursuit of glamorous new forms of 'curative' medicine. Only by adopting a population approach can the **natural history** of a disease be established; the clinician, by studying the fully developed disease, often gets a biased picture.

Epidemiology is the core discipline in examining the natural history of diseases and, for each disease entity, the possibilities for prevention can be examined at each phase or time period of the natural progression of the disease.

Primary prevention denotes the prevention of the *onset of the disease*, before any signs of the disease have developed. In practice, the distinction between primary and secondary prevention can be problematic if the onset of the disease is uncertain or the natural history of the disease is poorly understood. Immunization with 'attenuated' live or otherwise modified micro-organisms which cause the natural disease, is widely used to prevent previously deadly infectious diseases of childhood, and also the tropical infectious diseases encountered with increasing global travel (see Chapter 18). Outbreaks of infectious disease can be controlled by well-tried public health measures which include: isolation of cases, identification and isolation, or elimination of the source of infection, and other public health and hygienic measures such as quarantine and disinfection, particularly if no vaccine is available. For chronic diseases the situation can be more complex, although some appear to have a single 'main' cause. Many nutritionally related diseases, such as iodine deficiency (Chapter 9), neural tube defects (folic acid deficiency, Chapter 16), and dental caries (water fluoridation, Chapter 10) can be largely prevented by dietary supplementation for the general population. Some *screening procedures*, in neonates, for example, such as for those with a genetic basis, e.g. phenylketonuria, prevent the clinical onset of the disease by changing the diet of the neonate, a diet free of phenylalanine, or in the case of hypothyroidism, by treatment with thyroxin for the prevention of cretinism.

As noted earlier for lung cancer, the accumulated evidence overwhelmingly suggests that tobacco smoking causes 90 per cent of cases of this disease. If tobacco smoking ceased, 90 per cent of lung cancer would be prevented. But tax revenues from tobacco products, the addictive nature of nicotine, and a powerful, apparently unscrupulous tobacco industry have impeded public health policy. In contrast, there is the case of asbestos, to which workers in several industries were exposed for decades from the beginning of the 20th century. This is closely linked with mesothelioma, which accounts for a small, but significant, percentage, and potentiates other forms, of lung cancer. Legislation has ensured that asbestos is being slowly phased out as a major ingredient of industrial products; in particular, blue and brown asbestos, which are most closely linked to mesothelioma, have been banned for several decades. Legislation was passed earlier in the USA than in the UK with the result of differing trends for this disease in these countries (see Chapter 8). The incremental adoption of ever lower limits for asbestos, illustrates the fact that when the risk is dose-dependent, the wisest course of action is to abolish it. Asbestos took years to ban because it was a cheap, efficient insulator and resistant to fire.

For chronic diseases with multiple causes, such as the major cardiovascular diseases (coronary heart disease and stroke), primary prevention may be required to target more than one major cause of the disease. Nevertheless, Rose has shown that large benefits to the whole population could result from a population 'shift' (decrease) in the average blood pressure, plasma cholesterol, and, more controversially, alcohol consumption, for example. This is illustrated in Fig. 1.3 (see also Chapter 7) (Rose 1994; Rose and Day 1990), an extreme example in which the blood pressure distribution of London civil servants is 'shifted' compared to that of Kenyan nomads who are at considerably less risk of stroke due to hypertension. Plasma cholesterol distributions also

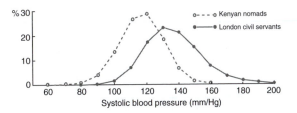

Figure 1.3 Distributions of systolic blood pressure in middle-aged men in two populations.
Reproduced from Rose G (1985) 'Sick Individuals and Sick Populations'. *International Journal of Epidemiology* **14**(1), 32–8, with permission from Oxford University Press.

provide an opportunity for public health prevention and Fig. 1.3 could be replaced by cholesterol distributions in Japan and the UK or USA. Population cholesterol levels are closely linked to dietary factors which are mainly culturally determined (see Chapter 7).

Several studies of changes in population levels of risk factors for cardiovascular diseases (CVD) by dietary policies and by pharmacological treatments show that these preventative measures account for a larger part of the decline in the incidence of these diseases than do treatments, both medical and surgical, following a heart attack or stroke (see Chapter 7). Primary prevention strategies form the bedrock of prevention of most infectious and many chronic diseases across the lifespan (particularly when the natural history is well understood) and many examples of low-cost, effective primary prevention can be found in the following chapters.

Secondary prevention of disease denotes the interruption of the full development of the natural progression of the disease and the restoration of normal health. This activity covers a broad spectrum of the natural history cycle from the beginning, in the case of pre-symptomatic disease, e.g. screening for early breast tumours or carcinoma *in situ* of the cervix, to the early treatment of myocardial infarction by thrombolytic therapy, which minimizes the area of myocardial damage. Secondary prevention is also used in the sense of preventing the recurrence of the disease. In Europe, for example, the European Society of Cardiology has formulated a series of guidelines on secondary prevention following several European-wide surveys, which showed that many patients with myocardial infarction were poorly followed up, and that many

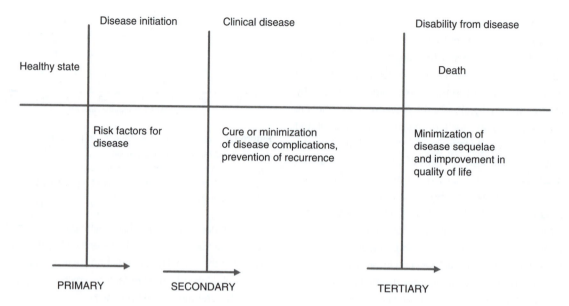

Figure 1.4 Principal features of primary, secondary, and tertiary disease prevention during the natural, uninterrupted progression of a disease.

clinicians had failed to check and modify cardiovascular risk factors on discharge from hospital (De Backer *et al.* 2003).

Tertiary prevention denotes the prevention of the major consequences of the natural history of a disease once its effects in a patient have become established. Examples in medical practice are: the rehabilitation of patients with long-term disability from coronary heart disease or stroke with exercise and psychological support; the long-term management and treatment of chronic diseases such as schizophrenia or Alzheimer's disease. Epidemiologists and biostatisticians have a role with clinicians in developing effective treatments and efficient management of these diseases and to promote primary, secondary, and tertiary prevention at all stages of disease progression, whenever the scientific information and evidence permit it. Further discussion of these topics is to be found in Chapters 5 and 21. The main features of primary, secondary, and tertiary prevention are shown in Fig. 1.4.

Consideration of the principles shown in this figure provides a framework for clinical practice and also for research questions in specific diseases. This framework is also useful in the design of screening programmes, which may be at the primary or secondary (and occasionally tertiary) level of disease prevention (see Chapter 5 and Fig. 5.1).

Further reading

Gordis L (2004) *Epidemiology*, 3rd edn. Philadelphia: Elsevier.

Fletcher RW and Fletcher SW (2005) *Clinical Epidemiology: The Essentials*. Baltimore: Lippincott, Williams and Wilkins.

Detels R, Beaglehole R, Lansang MA, and Gulliford M (eds) (2009) *Oxford Textbook of Public Health*, 5th edn. Oxford: Oxford University Press.

References

Blot WJ, Li JY, Taylor PR, Guo W, *et al.* (1993) Nutrition intervention trials in Linxian, China: supplementation with specific vitamin/mineral combinations, cancer incidence, and disease-specific mortality in the general population. *Journal of the National Cancer Institute* **85** (18), 1483–92.

Brockington WF (1958) *World Health*. Harmondsworth: Penguin.

Cochrane AL (1972) *Effectiveness and Efficiency. Random reflections on health services*. London: Nuffield Provincial Hospitals Trust.

Davey Smith G and Ebrahim S (2001) Epidemiology—is it time to call it a day? *International Journal of Epidemiology* **30** (1), 1–11.

Day IMN, Gu D, Ganderton RH, Spanakis E, and Ye S (2011) Epidemiology and the genetic basis of disease. *International Journal of Epidemiology* **30**, 661–7.

De Backer G, Ambrosioni E, Borch-Johnsen K, Brotons, C, *et al*. (2003) European guidelines on cardiovascular disease prevention in clinical practice: third joint task force of European and other societies on cardiovascular disease prevention in clinical practice (constituted by representatives of eight societies and by invited experts). *European Journal of Cardiovascular Prevention and Rehabilitation* **10** (4), S1–S10.

Detels R (2009) Epidemiology: the foundation of public health. In: Detels R, Beaglehole R, Lansang MA, and Gulliford M (eds). *Oxford Textbook of Public Health*, 5th edn; pp. 447–53. Oxford: Oxford University Press.

Doll, R and Hill, AB (1954) The mortality of doctors in relation to their smoking habits; a preliminary report. *BMJ* **1** (4877), 1451–5.

Doll R, Peto R, Wheatley K, Gray R, *et al*. (1994) Mortality in relation to smoking: 40 years' observations on male British doctors. *BMJ (Clinical Research Ed)* **309** (6959), 901–11.

Evans A (1995) Dr Black's favourite disease. *British Heart Journal* **74** (6), 696–7.

Evans A (2011) The French paradox and other ecological fallacies. *International Journal of Epidemiology* **40** (6), 1486–9.

Giovannoni G and Ebers G (2007) Multiple sclerosis: the environment and causation. *Current Opinion in Neurology* **20** (3), 261–8.

Greaves M (2000) *Cancer: The evolutionary legacy*. Oxford: Oxford University Press.

Hill AB (1965) The environment and disease: association or causation? *Proceedings of the Royal Society of Medicine*. **58**, 295–300.

Hill AB (1971) *Principles of Medical Statistics*, 9th edn. London: The Lancet.

Höfler M (2005) Causal inference based on counterfactuals. *BMC Medical Research Methodology*, **5**, 28.

Khoury MJ, Bowen MS, Burke W, Coates RJ, *et al*. (2011) Current priorities for public health practice in addressing the role of human genomics in improving population health. *American Journal of Preventive Medicine* **40** (4), 486–93.

McKeown T (1976) *The Modern Rise of Population*. London: Edward Arnold.

Porter R (1997) *The Greatest Benefit to Mankind: A Medical History of Humanity from Antiquity to the Present*, pp. 55–62. London: Harper Collins.

Riley JC (2001) *Rising Life Expectancy: A Global History*. Cambridge: Cambridge University Press.

Rose G (1985) Sick individuals and sick populations. *International Journal of Epidemiology* **14** (1), 32–8.

Rose G (1994) *The Strategy of Preventive Medicine*. New York: Oxford University Press.

Rose G and Day S (1990) The population mean predicts the number of deviant individuals. *BMJ (Clinical Research Ed)* **301** (6759), 1031–4.

Rosen G (1993) *A History of Public Health*. 2nd edn. Baltimore: Johns Hopkins University Press.

Rothman KJ and Greenland S (1998) *Modern Epidemiology*, 2nd edn. Philadelphia: Lippincott-Raven.

Rothman KJ and Greenland S (2005) Causation and causal inference in epidemiology. *American Journal of Public Health* **95** Suppl. 1, 144–50.

van der Mei IAF, Simpson S, Jr, Stankovich J, and Taylor BV (2011) Individual and joint action of environmental factors and risk of MS. *Neurologic Clinics* **29** (2), 233–55.

2 Basic epidemiological tools

DERMOT O'REILLY AND JOHN YARNELL

CHAPTER CONTENTS

This chapter introduces the basic tools of epidemiology. Sources of data, both routinely available and collected specifically for particular studies, are reviewed. Qualitative and preliminary studies are discussed.

2.1 Purpose of the study

As implied in Chapter 1, epidemiology has come to embrace a broad range of studies seeking to answer questions about disease in humans, usually by studying whole or sub-populations, but sometimes only in patient groups. Increasingly, epidemiology is described in sub-specialities, e.g. social, genetic, and clinical epidemiology, the latter emphasizing the use of epidemiological (and statistical) methods in clinical settings particularly for diagnosis and clinical decision-making (see Chapter 6). Silman (2002) has suggested that six aspects of human disease fall into the remit of epidemiology: *disease definition, occurrence, causation, outcome, management*, and *prevention*, as defined individually in Chapter 1. Epidemiologists tend to ask questions about disease occurrence, causation, definition, and prevention; clinicians often ask about diagnostic accuracy, the effectiveness of therapy, management, and outcome. Many published human studies fall under the general umbrella of epidemiology, but this is often not mentioned specifically in the abstract or text, and an epidemiologist may not be included among the authors. Increasingly, clinicians have the opportunity to undertake epidemiological training and work alongside biostatisticians. Certain journals are widely read and highly influential internationally in changing established views of disease treatment and prevention, e.g. *New England Journal of Medicine, Journal of the American Medical Association*, and *Archives of Internal Medicine* published in the USA, and *The Lancet* and *British Medical Journal* published in the UK. Articles in such journals will usually have been peer-reviewed by experts in the field to ensure, as far as possible, that the methodology is sound and the conclusions valid. An abstract published by such journals provides the busy clinician or medical student with an outline which should include: *the purpose of the study, its most important features, and why the authors feel that the findings are important*. An example of such an abstract is given in Box 2.1.

Whatever the purpose of the study, previous similar studies should be reviewed in detail as they will often indicate the choice of study design or help to refine hypotheses. A thorough electronic search using a number of key words in a major database, such as that

Box 2.1 Example of abstract structure in a medical journal

Title Central overweight and obesity in British youth aged 11–16 years: cross-sectional surveys of waist circumference.

Objective To compare changes over time in waist circumference (a measure of central fatness) and body mass index (a measure of overall obesity) in British youth.

Design Representative cross-sectional surveys in 1977, 1987, and 1997.

Setting Great Britain.

Participants Young people aged 11–16 years surveyed in 1977 (boys) and 1987 (girls) for the British Standards Institute (n = 3784) and in 1997 (both sexes) for the national diet and nutrition survey (n = 776).

Main outcome measures Waist circumference, expressed as a standard deviation score using the first survey as reference, and body mass index (weight (kg)/height (m²)), expressed as a standard deviation score against the British 1990 revised reference. Overweight and obesity were defined as the measurement exceeding the 91st and 98th centile, respectively.

Results Waist circumference increased sharply over the period between surveys (mean increases for boys and girls, 6.9 and 6.2 cm, or 0.84 and 1.02 SD score units, P < 0.0001). In centile terms, waist circumference increased more in girls than in boys. Increases in body mass index were smaller and similar by sex (means 1.5 and 1.6, or 0.47 and 0.53 SD score units, P < 0.0001). Waist circumference in 1997 exceeded the 91st centile in 28 per cent (n = 110) of boys and 38 per cent (n = 147) of girls (against 9 per cent for both sexes in 1977–1987, P < 0.0001) whereas 14 per cent (n = 54) and 17 per cent (n = 68), respectively, exceeded the 98th centile (3 per cent in 1977–1987, P < 0.0001). The corresponding rates for body mass index in 1997 were 21 per cent (n = 80) of boys and 17 per cent (n = 67) of girls exceeding the 91st centile (8 per cent and 6 per cent in 1977–1987) and 10 per cent (n = 39) and 8 per cent (n = 32) exceeding the 98th centile (3 per cent and 2 per cent in 1977–1987).

Conclusions Trends in waist circumference during the past 10–20 years have greatly exceeded those in body mass index, particularly in girls, showing that body mass index is a poor proxy for central fatness. Body mass index has therefore systematically underestimated the prevalence of obesity in young people.

Reproduced from McCarthy *et al.* 'Central overweight obesity in British youth aged 11–16 years: cross sectional surveys of waist circumference', *British Medical Journal*, **326**, (2003), with permission from BMJ Publishing Ltd

held by the American Library of Medicine (*PubMed*) and freely available to any internet user, is the minimum necessary for any epidemiological study. Techniques for searching the medical literature will be described in more detail in Chapter 6.

2.2 Sources of data and uses of routine health data

Public health activities rely on accurate population health data. Here, we provide a brief overview of the major sources of *official or routine health data* which can be used to assemble a detailed picture of population health. Fuller discussion of routine health statistics and surveys available in the UK (Kerrison and Macfarlane 2000), in the USA (Luck 2002), and internationally (World Health Organization 2012) is to be

found elsewhere. Web-based sources of routine data are shown in Box 2.2.

Vital statistics (births, deaths, and marriages)

The majority of countries record each birth and death making such registries of vital statistics an ongoing census of the population. A census is usually a prerequisite for establishing a *demographic profile* for a country, which provides a picture of the age structure of a particular country or population. In other countries the introduction of universal registration of citizens has obviated the need for a census. As *fertility rates* (number of births per thousand women aged between 15–44 years (sometimes 49 years) in a defined geographical area) are usually also available, future estimates of population growth and structure can be

Box 2.2 Web-based sources of routine data

Some of the variety and extent of datasets and research based on routine data can be found at the following web pages. Most have links to even more abundant data sources.

World Health Statistics http://www.who.int/whosis/whostat/2011/en/index.html

University of California at Berkeley http://www.lib.berkeley.edu/PUBL/internet.html

Partners in Information Access for The Public Health Workforce, US http://phpartners.org/

National Cancer Institute, US http://cis.nci.nih.gov/

Healthcare Cost and Utilization Project, Agency for Healthcare Research and Quality, US http://www.ahrq.gov/data/hcup/hcupnet.html

Centres for Disease Control, US http://www.cdc.gov

European Health Profile Tool http://www.apho.org.uk/resource/item.aspx?RID=114909

Health Statistics Quarterly http://data.gov.uk/dataset/health_statistics_quarterly

National Statistics, UK http://www.statistics.gov.uk/hub/index.html

Scottish Health Informatics Programme http://www.scot-ship.ac.uk/

UK Data Archive (University of Essex) http://www.data-archive.ac.uk/

UK Data Service http://www.census.ac.uk/

made. Some country profiles are shown in Chapter 16 (Fig. 16.4). The UK decennial census is discussed later in this chapter.

Mortality data

In most countries recording of death is a statutory requirement for all age groups and **infant mortality** (death rates in the first year of life) is commonly used as an indicator of the general health and the effectiveness of the preventive health service infrastructure which we take for granted in modern industrialized societies. Other indicators of population health include mortality in children under five years of age and mortality under 65 years of age. *Life expectancy* is a useful summary of current mortality rates and is often quoted for different ages (zero, one, and 65 years old). Life expectancy at birth incorporates the mortality rates at all later ages, whereas life expectancy at age 65 includes only the mortality experience at older ages. Most (published) life tables are constructed using current mortality rates and are called *period* life tables because they calculate the average number of years a person would live, if they experienced the particular area's *current* age-specific mortality rates for that time period throughout their life. This method makes no allowance for any projected changes in mortality. *Cohort life expectancies*

are calculated using *projected* age-specific mortality rates and are therefore regarded as a more appropriate measure of how long a person of a given age would be expected to live, on average.

In the UK, most death certificates are completed by doctors (a small percentage are also completed by coroners), according to a standardized protocols proposed by the World Health Organization (WHO). Box 2.3 shows the layout of the medical certificate of cause of death. It is divided into two parts: Part one lists the conditions that lead directly to death, with the one that started the morbid train of events (the underlying cause of death) entered last in the list. Conditions that contributed to, but did not directly cause death, are entered in Part two. These conditions are then coded according to the International Classification of Disease (ICD) (WHO 1992).

Routine mortality statistics are therefore based on identifying a single underlying cause of death. In order to derive the most useful information from the death certificates, even when it has been badly completed, ICD incorporates selection rules and modification rules, which apply to particular conditions, combinations, or circumstances.

While the accuracy of death certification is enhanced by the fact that certification is done by a doctor or coroner, in practice death certificates are usually

Box 2.3 Certifying the cause of death

CAUSE OF DEATH

The condition thought to be the 'Underlying Cause of Death' should apply in the lowest completed line of Part 1

(ICD10)*

| I (a) | Disease or condition directly leading to death† | *Cardiac arrest* | (I46.9) |

| (b) | Other disease or condition, if any, leading to: I(a) | *Congestive heart failure* | (I50.0) |

| (c) | Other disease or condition, if any, leading to: I(b) | *Acute myocardial infarction* | (I21.9) |

| II | Other significant conditions | | |

| | CONTRIBUTING TO THE DEATH but not related to the disease or condition causing it | *Diabetes mellitus, insulin dependent* | (E10.8) |

*Coded by the Office of National Statistics (ONS)
†Immediate cause of death

(From the UK death certificate)

completed in hospitals by junior doctors often without instruction. Inspection of the causes of death in Box 2.3 will indicate the potential for miscoding if the 'underlying cause' is inappropriately placed.

There have been ten versions of the ICD since its inception in 1900 and each revised classification has been developed to incorporate advances in medical knowledge and understanding of the disease process. ICD-10 now includes 8000 unique codes which comprise a letter that denotes a broad chapter or system of disease and two or three numbers which further refines the classification (e.g. 'I' represents all circulatory disease; I21 represents acute myocardial infarction).

While mortality data are very accurate in terms of the number and timing of events they are somewhat less robust when specifying cause of death. They are also subject to changes in investigation, diagnostic, and coding practices which can render comparisons between areas and across time problematical. Perhaps surprisingly, finding the exact cause of death can be difficult, even in modern medical environments and this level of uncertainty increases with age as older patients often suffer from multiple pathologies and there may be a reluctance to subject them to invasive diagnostic procedures. The most accurate way to determine the cause of death, and check the accuracy of death certificates, is to perform post-mortem examinations but this has largely fallen out of fashion and is undertaken in less than 10 per cent of hospital deaths in the UK, but other countries may have higher rates. One reason for this may be the belief that current medical technology can detect most of the important medical information about a person, including the cause of death. However, studies throughout the world have repeatedly demonstrated a worrying discrepancy between the diagnosis given on the death certificate compared with that at hospital post-mortem.

It is possible that some of the increase in deaths over the 20th century attributed, for example, to cancer has been artefactual and due to an increased clinical awareness allied to an increased availability of investigative technology. Radiological examination has become more refined (e.g. computed tomography) and is now complemented by ultrasound (Doppler) and magnetic resonance imaging. Endoscopic examination is now a common outpatient procedure allowing direct examination and biopsy of suspect areas. Analysis of blood chemistry, serology, biomarkers, and cytology are becoming increasingly sophisticated and available to a wider range of doctors. All these and other diagnostic facilities will both increase the chances of diagnosing cancer, if it is present, and the accuracy of cancer coding.

Other difficulties, particularly when comparing time (secular) trends, can be caused by changes in the way diseases are coded. In the early 20th century 'old age' was a bona fide cause of death and one of the most commonly certified cause of death for those aged 70 and over up until the 1950s. Changes in coding practices after that time required a more accurate diagnosis and deaths due to bronchopneumonia, circulatory disease, and, to some extent, cancers, increased to fill the vacuum left by the demise of 'old age' as a cause of death. The introduction of ICD-10 in the UK in 2001 further changed the coding rules used to select the underlying cause of death from the death certificate and was associated with a 20 per cent reduction in the number of deaths attributed to pneumonia and a corresponding increase in those attributed to chronic debilitating diseases, particularly the musculo-skeletal system, and various types of dementia. In order to facilitate comparisons over time, many countries have undertaken a 'bridging' exercise, where all deaths in one year are coded according to both ICD-9 and ICD-10 classifications, to produce estimates of the changes arising from the introduction of the new classification system.

There are additional difficulties in interpreting international mortality data which relate to different population structures in countries; in particular, comparisons between rich and poor countries require standardization of the age structures in each country and WHO produces mortality rates that are standardized to the European Standard populations (for advanced industrialized countries) and the World Standard population (for a global estimate which includes a large population of countries with young populations). Crude (overall) deaths rates for the UK or the US are higher than those for Egypt or Iraq (in the year 2000), which is entirely due to the high proportion of children and young adults in the latter countries. These issues are discussed further in Chapter 16.

Morbidity data

A disadvantage of mortality data is that they inadequately reflect the burden of morbidity from important diseases, e.g. mental health problems, which seldom result in death or diabetes mellitus, which places a disproportionate burden on the health services but is poorly recorded on death certificates. The International Classification of Diseases is also used by hospitals and primary care to record morbidity but additional classification systems also exist. The WHO has a classification system for cancer which is based on histological type rather than site. This classification may be more relevant to survival as different types of tumour may respond differently to therapy. Clinicians and epidemiologists may also use other classification systems, particularly in health care research, where ICD codes may be inappropriate or inadequate for the purposes of a particular study.

Morbidity data too, however, have their deficiencies: the definition of what constitutes a disease is often imprecise, no one source covers the range of illness episodes, and coverage and available information are often incomplete. Therefore, a wide range of sources is needed for any attempt at completeness.

Morbidity data from secondary care

In the UK, the first hospital survey was conducted in 1949. The Department of Health currently compiles the **hospital episode statistics** (HES) database, containing all patient-based records of finished consultant episodes (ordinary admissions and day cases) by diagnosis, operation, and specialty from National Health Service (NHS) hospitals in England. However, the confidentiality of such data is an issue under the Data Protection Act and anonymized data are usually supplied for research purposes. The greater availability of data in electronic systems aligned with the development of new methods of safely linking sensitive health (and non-health) related data and the introduction of unique identifiers in the health services have facilitated data linkage in the UK. This has lead to more efficient and innovative use of morbidity data and a greater understanding of the causes of ill health, effect of health policy, and the quality and equality of care. The Scottish Health Informatics Programme (SHIP) in Scotland, the Secure Anonymized Information Linkage (SAIL) in Wales, and the Clinical Practice Research Datalink (CPRD) in England are excellent examples of what can be achieved (CPRD 2012; Lyons *et al.* 2009; SHIP 2012). Other examples of linkage of routine data sources with other data are shown in Table 2.1.

Morbidity data from primary care

In the UK most people are registered with a general practitioner, often the first port of call for an ill patient, who deals with a wide range of health problems; information relating to these problems is often not well captured in other health care datasets. In general, data from primary care has not been easily assessable, though this is changing, again thanks to greater use of electronic records. Examples of these include the data from sentinel practices in the UK to form the General Practice Research Database (GPRD) and The Health Improvement Network (THIN) database. With longitudinal data on several million patients these are unique data sources for research into many aspects of disease risk, management, and treatment. *Prescribing data* from primary care, which are collected nationally in the UK as a statutory requirement, are frequently used as proxy indicators for diseases requiring continuous medication, for example, epilepsy, type I diabetes, and schizophrenia. Again the linkage of separate health databases has lead to new findings; for example, data from general practice morbidity records,

cashed prescriptions, hospital records, and attendance at retinopathy screening clinics have been linked to produce a register of all patients in Tayside with diabetes (Morris *et al.* 1997), and linkage of dispensed prescriptions and data on road traffic accidents from police records demonstrated the increased risk of accidents for people taking psychoactive medication such as benzodiazepines (Barbone *et al.* 1997).

Disease registers/registries

Disease registers identify individuals in a well-defined geographical area, who have some disease in common and allow disease **incidence** to be measured with precision. Such registers are particularly useful to obtain a complete perspective on diseases, both common and rare, whose diagnosis and care may be shared between several types of health professional or consultant.

Cancer registers

These were first introduced in the 1930s in England to monitor radium treatments for cancer. In the UK there are currently nine regional registers in England and one each in Wales, Scotland, and Northern Ireland. From 1993 data submission became mandatory within the NHS. Cancer registries attempt to record data on everyone with a cancer diagnosis; information was initially abstracted manually by clerks searching hospital records but, more recently, through electronic data capture. A high level of **ascertainment** (>95 per cent), has been achieved for most cancers. Data collected include personal and demographic details, and extensive information on the cancer (including morphology, pathological verification, stage, and treatment). The annual reference volume, *Cancer Statistics: Registrations*, Series MB1 (Office of National Statistics (ONS) website) presents information about cancer incidence in the UK (see also Chapter 17).

Congenital anomalies register

In the UK a national congenital anomalies notification system was initiated in 1964 following the thalidomide epidemic, in order to detect any similar hazard without delay. This has been replaced by a series of regional and disease-specific registries that feed into the British Isles

Table 2.1 Some examples of research use of routine data

Geographical area	Study topic	Data used	Design	Reference
World	Global mortality attributable	Vital statistics. Smoking surveys	Cross-sectional	Ezzati M and Lopez AD (2003) Estimates of global mortality due to smoking. *Lancet* **362**, 847–52.
Country England & Wales	Health inequality in migrants	Census and mortality statistics	Longitudinal-record linkage	Harding S and Maxwell R (1997) Differences in mortality of migrants. In: Drever F and Whitehead M (eds) *Health Inequalities*, pp. 108–21. London: HMSO.
Country England & Wales	Occupational mortality	Census and mortality statistics	Longitudinal-record linkage	Dreyer F (ed) (1995) *Occupational Health: Decennial Supplement*. London: HMSO.
Country Denmark	Familial predisposition to subarachnoid haemorrhage	Hospital data and population registries	National linkage study	Gaist D, Vaeth M, Tsiropoulos I, *et al.* (2000) Risk of subarachnoid haemorrhage in first degree relatives with subarachnoid haemorrhage: follow-up study based on national registries in Denmark. *Br Med J* **320**, 141–5.
Country England	Consequences of alcohol consumption	Health survey	Cross-sectional	Colhoun H, Ben-Shlomo Y, Dong W, Bost L, and Marmot M (1997) Ecological analysis of collectivity of alcohol consumption in England: importance of average drinker. *Br Med J* **314**, 1164–68.
Country Scotland	Epidemiology of multimorbidity	Morbidity data from GP computers	Population based	Barnett K, Mercer S, Norbury M, Watt G, *et al.* (2012) Epidemiology of multimorbidity and implications for health care, research, and medical education: a cross-sectional study. *Lancet* **380** 37–43.
Great Britain	Inequalities in health	Census data	Cross-sectional	Doran T, Drever F, and Whitehead M (2004) Is there a north-south divide in social class inequalities in health in Great Britain? Cross-sectional study using data from the 2001 census. *Br Med J* **328**, 1043–45.
Country USA	Inequalities in cancer incidence, treatment & survival	Census data, cancer registry data	Cross-sectional and longitudinal	Singh G, Miller B, Hankey B, and Edwards B (2003) *Area socio-economic variations in US cancer incidence, mortality, stage, treatment and survival 1975–1999*. NCI Cancer Surveillance Monograph Series No. 4. Bethesda: NCI.

Network of Congenital Anomaly Registers that aims 'to provide continuous monitoring of the frequency, nature, and outcomes of congenital anomalies for the population of the British Isles' (see also Chapter 16).

Other disease registers

More localized registers are also available for conditions such as stroke, diabetes, and accidents (Newton and Garner 2002). Public health observatories (see Chapter 21) are usually based, at least in part, on disease registers. Research using data from disease registers and record linkage is discussed in detail elsewhere (Goldacre *et al.* 2000).

Communicable disease surveillance

While the major killers in the developed world, and to an increasing extent in the less developed world, are chronic diseases, frequent outbreaks of 'old' and 'new' infectious diseases attest to the need for adequate information systems. Most countries collect data on infectious disease based on **notification**. Worldwide this is coordinated by WHO. In the UK notification of diseases based often only on clinical signs, and of microbiologically-confirmed outbreaks, from primary care, local authorities, and public health laboratories, are the main sources of communicable disease information. The aim of notification (which is statutory) is to speed detection of possible outbreaks and epidemics. Diseases which are notifiable are discussed further in Chapter 18. The major problems with the system are not inaccuracy of notifications (these can be altered when biological samples are read), but delays and variability of reporting, though this has been reduced through the use of 'spotter' or sentinel practices, which though not entirely representative, are known to provide more accurate and timely information. Efforts have been made to improve under-reporting by trimming the extensive main notification list, but consensus has not been reached. Aggregated data are published weekly in the *Communicable Diseases Review* (see Chapter 18).

Population estimates and population health

Perhaps the most important step in describing the health of an area is to detail the population structure; indeed it has been suggested that the relative *health needs* of a local area is determined primarily by the *numbers* and the demographic profile (age/sex/ethnic mix/level of poverty) of the population which often provide a proxy indicator for the overall level of health. Accurate population estimates are also required in epidemiology to turn the crude number of *events* from the vital statistics into the more informative *rates*, such as those for mortality and fertility.

The UK decennial census

The first thorough survey of England was in 1086 when William the Conqueror ordered the production of the Domesday Book, thus providing a remarkable picture of life in Norman Britain. In 1798, Thomas Malthus suggested that population growth would soon outstrip supplies of essential resources (Gilbert 2008). Concerned at this alarmist view, Parliament passed the Census Act in 1800 and the first official census of England and Wales took place on 10th March 1801. The Act also applied to Scotland, while in Ireland, the first modern census was in 1821. The decennial census in the UK is the only survey which provides a detailed snapshot of the entire population at the same time, and asks the same core questions, making it easy to compare different parts of the country. It is obligatory, so the completeness, accuracy, and coverage of the data are high. The last census was taken in 2011 and the data relate to household composition on a single night in March. The census provides basic demographic data, and more specific information on general health, long-term illness, and on the carers of those with long-term illness. These data are used in the strategic planning of health and social services at the level of small geographical areas, such as electoral wards. The data collected are confidential and only now can the 1911 census be searched by research workers after a hundred years of remaining confidential.

However, the decennial census is expensive and there is a delay of two to three years before the data become available. In practice this means that good data are available for only a few years after a census, and, after this period, there is increasing reliance on estimates of the population. In recent years there have also been concerns about the completeness of the census in Westernized countries, especially the enumeration of younger males in inner-city areas. As a result alternatives are being actively investigated, including the extensive linkage of routine administrative datasets including the health-card registration system. Intercensal population estimates are derived from knowledge of the three drivers of population change: births, deaths, and migration. For example, the population of an area one year after the census$_{(t+1)}$ is equal to the original population at the time (t), plus the *natural increase* (births – deaths), plus the *net migration* (immigration – emigration), i.e.:

$$Population_{t+1} = Population_t + births - deaths + immigration - emigration$$

Population movement is the main reason why it is difficult to produce accurate inter-censal estimates of the population, and especially so for small areas. International migration estimates are derived in the UK from the *International Passenger Survey* which is a continuous survey that samples a selection of persons arriving at, or departing from, the main air and seaports. Tracking population movement within a country is even more difficult, though this can be assessed from changes in other data sources such as the electoral register, uptake of social security benefits, etc.

The electoral register

This is potentially an alternative source of population estimates in the UK and elsewhere. Its strength is that it is validated and updated on an annual basis in the UK. Its weakness is that it only contains lists of people who are old enough to vote and will miss people who do not want to vote or who have not been able to register, for example, because they have recently changed address. Data protection issues have placed increasing restrictions on the use of these data.

General practitioner lists

Almost everyone in the UK is registered for free medical care and to a general practice. As these data are held centrally, they can provide descriptions of the age/sex composition of small areas throughout the country. There are two main weaknesses with these data: (i) list inflation, which arises because of the address inaccuracies, because practices may not be aware that the patient has changed address. However, the introduction of a unique NHS number in the UK and the greater use of record linkage is likely to have greatly improved the accuracy of such systems.

National insurance data

Recent years have seen an increasing use of administrative databases, such as receipt of pensions, which can be used to provide good indications of older people by age, sex, and geography. The main weakness of such systems is the variability of the uptake. Some countries such as the Netherlands and Sweden have a system of continuous population registration (in which all changes of permanent residence are registered) that are so complete as to render the census obsolete. It is possible that this will become more common in other European countries in future years. In the UK, however, there is an increasing tendency to supplement the census-based area characteristics with those based on routine administrative databases, such as those for national insurance and social security benefits, which are usually well maintained.

The General Household Survey

The General Household Survey (GHS) is a multi-purpose continuous survey carried out by the Social Survey Division of the Office of National Statistics (ONS) which collects information on a range of topics from people living in private households in Great Britain. The survey started in 1971 and has been carried out almost yearly since then. From a changing sample of approximately 13,000 addresses all adults aged 16 years and over are interviewed in each responding household. Core data comprise detailed socio-demographic and health information. More recent studies such as *Understanding Society* (ISER 2012) which, by following the lives of 100,000 individuals in 40,000 households in the UK, will provide new evidence about the wider societal determinants and consequences of ill health and health behaviours.

Health Survey for England

In 1991 this became a series of annual surveys, used to underpin and improve targeting of nationwide health policies. From a national 'representative' sample of about 20,000 individuals the survey estimates the proportion of the population with specific health conditions, including psychological health, and risk factors associated with those conditions, examines differences between population sub-groups, and monitors targets in the health strategy. Each annual survey retains core items but may focus on a particular health topic. From 1995 the height and weight of children at different ages has become an added component, monitoring overweight and obesity, replacing the earlier national study of health, and growth which was designed to evaluate trends in undernutrition. Similar surveys are performed periodically but less frequently in Scotland, Wales, and Northern Ireland. Sampling issues (how to obtain a 'representative' sample) are discussed in Chapter 4. Some of these countries have (with the respondents' permission) enhanced these cross-sectional surveys and introduced a longitudinal element by linking their survey data to health service and mortality data (see, for example, Gray *et al.* 2010). This facilitates the examination of the role of social, psychological, lifestyle, and biological factors in the development of a range of important chronic diseases in representative samples of the population. As this is achieved using routine data sources, there is no additional burden on the survey respondents, recall bias is eliminated and there is no non-responder bias to follow up.

In the USA, the National Health and Nutrition Examination Survey (NHANES) is such a programme of studies which began in the 1960s and is now conducted annually across the country.

Using routine data in health research

Routine data have several important strengths which enable them to be used to answer pertinent health questions: these include their power and efficiency and that they are often population-based. However, they remain an under-utilized source of data that could enable epidemiological studies to be undertaken and have an important role in understanding and improving the health of populations. Types of epidemiological study are discussed in Chapter 3, but some examples of the research uses of routine data both from the UK and other European countries are shown in Table 2.1. A major repository for routine data is the UK Data Archive (UKDA), which allows interested individuals or groups to register and access a wide range of data sources for research purposes (see Box 2.2).

Dedicated studies

It is increasingly clear that the formation of large dedicated studies is often needed to answer specific research questions. Some of these are multipurpose, such as the UK Biobank study that, between 2006–2010, recruited 500,000 people aged between 40–69 years; subjects have completed questionnaires, undergone physical examinations, and provided blood, urine, and saliva samples for future analysis; their health outcomes will be assessed through record linkage. The Kadoorie Biobank Study has also recruited over 500,000 men and women aged between 35–74 years from rural and urban areas throughout China. These large cohort studies will greatly enhance the understanding of the aetiology of a wide array of diseases including the interplay between genes and environment. Other studies are focused on specific diseases or age groups. For example, given the concerns related to our ageing societies, many countries have started dedicated ageing cohort studies to better understand the determinants of disease and disability as people get older; examples include ELSA (English Longitudinal Study of Aging), CLSA (in Canada), the Health and Retirement Study in the US, and TILDA (The Irish Longitudinal Study of Ageing) in Ireland. Alternatively, the realization that many diseases have their origins in early life (the life-course paradigm) has stimulated the initiation of studies such as the Millennium Cohort Study (MCS), which has tracked around 19,000 children born in the UK between 2000/2001 through their early childhood years and plans to follow them into adulthood. Publications such as the *International Journal of Epidemiology* regularly produce information in a structured format about these large cohort studies and how the data can be accessed.

2.3 Quantitative and qualitative studies

Epidemiological studies are **quantitative** in nature usually producing population estimates of disease prevalence and incidence, and, for the majority of studies, statistical tests can be applied to examine particular hypotheses. In contrast, **qualitative studies** place an emphasis on the development of concepts rather than on numbers or statistics—that is, on the meaning, views, and experiences of research participants (or subjects) which assist the formulation of research hypotheses. Qualitative studies have their origins in disciplines such as sociology and social anthropology, and are used increasingly by epidemiologists, often in collaboration with specialists in the core disciplines. One of the ways in which qualitative research methods can be used by epidemiologists and health care researchers is to develop questionnaires suitable for quantitative use, particularly in social and psychiatric epidemiology, and in the development of instruments (questionnaires) designed to evaluate physical and medical functioning (well-being). A number of different instruments have been developed on the basis of extensive qualitative studies for use as comparators of health status in different communities and even countries (e.g. SF-36, Euroquol, etc. which measure several different aspects of physical and mental health) and were an essential first step in developing the weighting (adjusting) factors used to calculate quality-adjusted life-years (QALYs) and disability-adjusted life-years (DALYs) (see Chapters 12 and 17 for examples of their use). The key terms and methods used in qualitative studies are shown in Box 2.4.

There are a number of reasons why we need qualitative research in health and health care. According to Black (1994), qualitative methods can be used

effectively to illuminate and contribute to quantitative studies, including epidemiological research by:

- Identifying the most appropriate variables that should be measured.
- Generating hypotheses for subsequent investigation by quantitative methods.
- Increasing understanding about the way quantitatively assessed variables were defined, understood, and completed.
- Explaining results, particularly unexpected findings, reported in quantitative studies.

Furthermore, qualitative methods, such as observation, interviews, and the analysis of documentary material, are more appropriate than quantitative methods when there is uncertainty and a lack of clarity about a health issue (such as waiting lists) or about the variables that may comprise the subject of a study.

Two types of preliminary study likely to have qualitative aspects may be carried out prior to large-scale quantitative investigations: **feasibility studies** can be used to examine the practical possibility of conducting a large-scale study and *pilot studies* may be carried out to develop hypotheses, establish questionnaire design or to estimate the sample size required for a main study.

References

Barbone F, McMahon AD, Davey PG, Morris AD, *et al*. (1998) Association of road-traffic accidents with benzodiazepine use. *Lancet* **352** (9137), 1331–6.

Black N (1994) Why we need qualitative research. *Journal of Epidemiology and Community Health* **48** (5), 425–6.

Clinical Practice Research Datalink (CPRD) (2012) Available at: http://www.cprd.com/home/.

Gilbert G (ed) (2008) Thomas Malthus *An Essay on the Principle of Population*. Oxford: Oxford University Press.

Goldacre M, Kurina L, Yeates D, Seagroatt V, *et al*. (2000) Use of large medical databases to study associations between diseases. *QJM* **93** (10), 669–75.

Box 2.4 Glossary of terms used in qualitative research

- **Analytic induction**—use of constant comparison specifically in developing hypotheses, which are then tested in further data collection and analysis.
- **Case studies** focus on one or a limited number of settings; used to explore contemporary phenomenon, especially where complex interrelated issues are involved. Can be exploratory, explanatory, descriptive, or a combination of these.
- **Consensus methods** include **Delphi** and **nominal group techniques** and **consensus development conferences**. They provide a way of synthesizing information and dealing with conflicting evidence, with the aim of determining extent of agreement within a selected group.
- **Constant comparison**—iterative method of content analysis where each category is searched for in the entire dataset and all instances are compared until no new categories can be identified.
- **Content analysis**—systematic examination of text (field notes) by identifying and grouping themes and coding, classifying, and developing categories.
- **Epistemology**—theory of knowledge; scientific study which deals with the nature and validity of knowledge.
- **Fieldnotes**—collective term for records of observation, talk, interview transcripts, or documentary sources. Typically includes a field diary which provides a record of the chronological events and development of research as well as the researcher's own reactions to, feeling about, and opinions of the research process.
- **Focus groups**—method of group interview which explicitly includes and uses the group interaction to generate data.
- **Hawthorne effect**—impact of the researcher on the research subjects or setting, notably in changing their behaviour.

- **In-depth interviews**—face-to-face conversation with the purpose of exploring issues or topics in detail. Does not use pre-set questions, but is shaped by a defined set of topics or issues.
- **Induction**—process of moving from observations/data towards generalizations, hypotheses, or theory; **grounded theory**—hypothesizing inductively from data, notably using subjects' own categories, concepts, etc.; opposite of **deduction**, process of data gathering to test predefined theory or hypotheses.
- **Naturalistic research**—non-experimental research in naturally occurring settings.
- **Observation**—systematic watching of behaviour and talk in naturally occurring settings.
- **Paradigm**—framework of theory in which the investigator is operating.
- **Participant observation**—observation in which the researcher also occupies a role or part in the setting in addition to observing.
- **Purposive sampling**—deliberate choice of respondents, subjects, or settings, as opposed to **statistical sampling**, concerned with the representativeness of a sample in relation to a total population. **Theoretical sampling** links this to previously developed hypotheses or theories.
- **Reliability**—extent to which a measurement yields the same answer each time it is used.
- **Social anthropology**—social scientific study of peoples, cultures, and societies; particularly associated with the study of traditional cultures.
- **Triangulation**—use of three or more different research methods in combination; principally used as a check of validity.
- **Validity**—extent to which a measurement truly reflects the phenomenon under scrutiny.

Reproduced from Mays N and Pope C *Qualitative Methods in Health Care*, 1996, with permission from Wiley.

Gray L, Batty GD, Craig P, Stewart C, *et al.* (2010) Cohort profile: the Scottish health surveys cohort: linkage of study participants to routinely collected records for mortality, hospital discharge, cancer, and offspring birth characteristics in three nationwide studies. *International Journal of Epidemiology* **39** (2), 345–50.

ISER (2012) Understanding Society. Available at: http://www.understandingsociety.org.uk/.

Kerrison S and Macfarlane A (2000) *Official Health Statistics: An Unofficial Guide*. London: Arnold.

Luck J (2002) Applications of information systems to public health: In: Detels R, McEwan J, Beaglehole R, and

Tanaka H (eds) *Oxford Textbook of Public Health*, 4th edn. Oxford: Oxford University Press.

Lyons R, Jones K, John G, Brooke C, *et al.* (2009) The SAIL databank: linking multiple health and social care datasets. *BMC Medical Informatics & Decision Making* **9**, 3. Available at: http://www.biomedcentral.com/1472-6947/9/3.

Morris AD, Boyle DI, MacAlpine R, Emslie-Smith A, *et al.* (1997) The diabetes audit and research in Tayside Scotland (DARTS) study: electronic record linkage to create a diabetes register. DARTS/MEMO Collaboration. *BMJ (Clinical Research Ed)* **315** (7107), 524–8.

Newton J and Garner S (2002) *Disease Registers in England*. Oxford: Institute of Health Sciences.

Scottish Health Informatics Programme (SHIP) (2012) Available at: http://www.scot-ship.ac.uk/.

Silman AJ (2002) *Epidemiological Studies: A Practical Guide*, 2nd edn. Cambridge: Cambridge University Press.

World Health Organization (1992) *International Statistical Classification of Diseases and Related Health Problems*. Tenth Revision, 1–3. Geneva: World Health Organization.

World Health Organization (2012) Health statistics and health information systems (HSI). Geneva: World Health Organization. Available online at: http://www.who.int/healthinfo/en/.

3 Epidemiological studies

JOHN YARNELL AND DERMOT O'REILLY

In this chapter we distinguish the descriptive from the analytical approach in epidemiology, describe the main varieties of study and what factors dictate the choice of study design. The concept of risk is developed using particular study designs and epidemiological data.

3.1 Descriptive and analytical studies

As discussed in Chapter 1, a fundamental aim of epidemiology is the description of the occurrence of a particular disease in the population, usually according to the *personal characteristics* of individuals (e.g. age, sex, occupation, etc.), *place*, and *time* of occurrence. Hence many epidemiological studies involve a description of the disease or condition in the population. Such *descriptive studies* are often quick to complete, particularly when they are based on routinely collected data, and may generate hypotheses which can be tested in analytical studies. For many diseases, particularly relatively rare diseases, this basic **descriptive epidemiology** is well known from prevalence and incidence studies in different countries; for example, the descriptive epidemiology of cancers which are rare in one country but more common in others. However, analytical studies for these cancers remain largely uninformative (Chapter 17). Similarly, multiple sclerosis has a marked female/male distribution and a north/south gradient in Europe but there are few clues as to the causal factors (Chapter 13).

Descriptive studies Several study designs are described which are particularly useful in the early stages of definition of a new disease, condition or syndrome, etc. (see Box 1.2). A **case series** is simply a series of cases of disease which can raise awareness initially of a new disease or disease variant. Conditions such as legionnaires' disease, acquired immunodeficiency disease syndrome (AIDS), and bovine spongiform encephalopathy (BSE) were initially described from the excess occurrence of cases of related rare diseases, which eventually led to new disease definitions, an essential first step in descriptive epidemiology. A **population prevalence study** counts the number of cases of a particular disease or condition in the general population, usually by means of a special survey or census (see Table 2.1 for examples of this). Such studies can be used to estimate cases in the population, to assess the health needs of the population, and to determine trends over time (secular trends). Population prevalence studies can also be used for analytical purposes, in which causal hypotheses are tested, provided that relevant data have been collected. Other examples of this type of study design are shown in Box 2.1 and Fig. 11.2 which show secular trends in childhood obesity and the international prevalence of gastric symptoms, respectively.

Ecological studies are quite widely used in preliminary descriptive epidemiology, particularly in describing differences between different geographical areas or regions, and in different ethnic and social groups. In an ecological study the outcome event (usually the disease under study) is not linked to individual subjects but to groups of subjects leading to the possibility of the **ecological fallacy** (an observed relationship in-between characteristics at an area or aggregate level that is not supported by subsequent analysis at the individual level). Data on possible individual **confounding variables** (see section 3.2) cannot be used, often leading to inappropriate and non-causal association in ecological studies. An example of a sound ecological study can be found in Table 2.1 (Colhoun *et al.* 1997).

Analytical studies These are usually inferential or hypothetico-deductive in nature and require statistical methods of analysis, i.e. the data from a sample are used to estimate characteristics or test **hypotheses** about the population from which the sample was taken (see Chapter 4). Often the hypotheses are concerned with the **associations** or relationships between exposure status and disease occurrence. An **exposure** variable may represent a risk factor or a treatment, depending on the nature of the study. In practice, there can be some overlap between descriptive and analytical studies, particularly in the case of new diseases such as AIDS, legionnaires' disease, and chronic fatigue syndrome in which the same datasets are used for the descriptive epidemiology and for analytical purposes. Analytical studies can be further subdivided into observational and experimental studies. In an **observational** study the exposure of a subject occurs naturally and is 'observed' or recorded by the epidemiologist; in an **experimental** (or **intervention**) study the exposure is 'assigned' to the 'patient' by the investigator. In passing, epidemiologists tend to term volunteers or members of the public recruited from the general population 'subjects' or 'participants' to distinguish them from patients who are recruited from patient populations under clinical care.

Observational studies are the most common type of epidemiological study and are classified by their *designs*; some common designs are displayed in Fig. 3.1. The classification of these studies is based on the *time* (past, current, future) when the exposure is measured and when the disease occurrence is ascertained this determines whether it is a **cohort** study (beginning with exposed and non-exposed groups and then studying the occurrence of the disease) or a **case-control** study (beginning with the cases, diseased subjects, and the **controls**, non-diseased subjects, and then investigating their exposure status). The term cohort is derived from the idea of a Roman troop of soldiers marching onwards together (Latin: tenth part of Roman legion). If exposure and disease status are measured concurrently, the study is said to be **cross-sectional**. If disease information is collected currently and exposure status from past records, the study is described as **retrospective**. If exposure information is collected currently and disease status in the future, the study is described as **prospective** (or **longitudinal**). Usually case-control studies collect exposure information retrospectively and cohort studies collect disease information prospectively, but there are exceptions. The **retrospective cohort study** defines a cohort and its exposure status retrospectively from existing records typically from occupational sources. The **nested case-control** study is increasingly conducted as part of a prospective cohort study, particularly when stored biological samples are available; these can be more efficiently used in a case-control rather than in a cohort setting.

In Chapter 7, Table 7.2 gives an example of a large case-control study and Table 7.3 an example of a prospective cohort study.

Experimental or intervention studies are frequently carried out to compare different treatments (e.g. drugs or surgical procedures) in which the patients (volunteers who have given **informed consent**) are receiving treatment in hospital or in primary care. Non-clinical interventions (e.g. dietary, behavioural, or public health) can also be investigated within a clinical setting or in the community. The gold standard for an experimental study is the **randomized controlled trial (RCT)** which compares interventions that are allocated to subjects by a randomization procedure; in addition the subject and the

Time of Study

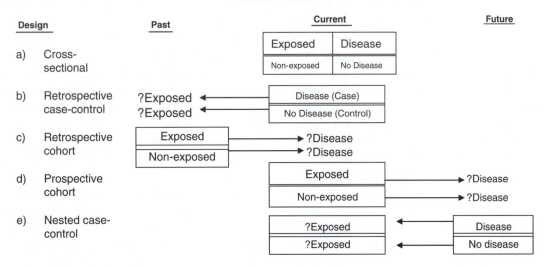

Figure 3.1 Observational studies.

?Exposed ≡ Exposure Yes or No ? Disease ≡ Disease or No Disease.

Adapted from Silman AJ (2002). *Epidemiological Studies: A Practical Guide*, 2nd edn. With permission from Cambridge University Press.

investigator should be *blinded* (unaware of the type of treatment) if possible. Examples of RCTs are to be found in Chapters 8 and 20. In community studies **cluster randomized trials** are being increasingly used: the intervention is allocated to a cluster of subjects, e.g. all patients on a general practice list, a pharmacy, or a school may provide the sampling unit rather than an individual subject or participant. Finally there are designs which involve no formal randomization in the allocation of interventions to subjects—these are referred to as **quasi-experimental**. These designs are frequently used to inform public health practice and in other situations where randomization is difficult to achieve.

3.2 Choice of study design

Observational Studies Several factors govern the choice of study design. These include the following: *the purpose of the study, previous studies, available data, and the balance between feasibility (time and costs) and validity.*

Cross-sectional and **retrospective case-control studies** are closely related and frequently overlap, as the exposure status is in practice often assessed retrospectively, based on recall by cases and controls. These studies are relatively quick and easy to undertake and are the first line of inquiry into any rare disease or newly emerging disease of uncertain aetiology. For example, BSE, legionnaires' disease (see Chapter 18), AIDS, and severe acute respiratory syndrome (SARS) were all initially investigated using such studies. Non-infectious chronic diseases are also extensively investigated by cross-sectional or retrospective case-control studies, but usually exposures are chronic and may occur over a considerable period of time; thus exposure data collected retrospectively provide a concurrent test of the hypothesis in question.

Because of the possibility of **bias** (systematic error) selection of controls is a critical issue in case-control studies. In general, controls drawn by random selection from the general population, and possibly matched with cases by age and sex and for one or two other major **confounding variables**, such as smoking habit or social class are preferred. *Confounding variables are those linked both to the disease and to the exposure under investigation.* Matching effectively eliminates such variables from the comparison of exposures in cases and controls. Hospital-based controls are particularly unlikely to be representative of the general population, as selective factors operate to put people into hospital even for apparently 'random' accidents (see Chapter 20). Population-based controls are, however, cumbersome and expensive to obtain, in addition to being less likely to volunteer than other possible comparison groups. In the example of a case-control study in Chapter 7 (Table 7.2), the smoking habits of patients admitted to hospital with a heart attack (myocardial infarction) have been compared with those of their family members. The investigators ran the risk of reducing the chance of finding an association if a higher proportion of family members had similar smoking habits to the patients than was true of the general population (which is likely!). However, because of the large number of patients and controls studied, and because of the strong association, the link between heart attack and smoking habit is supported; in reality, it may have been underestimated.

Prospective or **longitudinal cohort studies** are generally considered superior to cross-sectional and retrospective case-control studies; they may be used to confirm findings from those latter studies. One advantage is that individual exposure status is known at the commencement of the study prior to the development of the disease. Hence these studies are less likely to suffer from **recall bias** that can exist in cross-sectional and retrospective case-control studies. Another advantage of the prospective approach is that multiple **end points** (or **outcome events**) can be studied which could include fatal and non-fatal disease or the occurrence of more than one disease: This is not usually possible in retrospective and cross-sectional case-control studies. However, as cohort studies are observational studies, the exposure has not been randomly distributed and might therefore be systematically associated with subject characteristics. If these characteristics are also related to the outcome this would represent confounding and if they are not

measured and adjusted for in the analysis could lead to incorrect conclusions. The relationship between hormone replacement therapies (HRT) and subsequent disease risk is a good example of where observational and randomized studies produce different findings. Some of the largest observational studies ever undertaken suggested that HRT was cardio-protective, while RCTs found an increased risk of coronary heart disease (Hernán *et al.* 2008). Similarly, breast cancer risk was lower in RCT than in the observational studies. As RCT are held to be the gold standard, these discrepancies called into question the validity of observation studies. However, it now appears that neither study design held superior truth; recent and reanalyses of data showed that the differences were due to the timing and duration of HRT (Vandenbroucke 2009). Prospective cohort studies are also costly, difficult to carry out and time-consuming, requiring a period of follow-up ranging from about two years upwards, depending on the size of the study and the nature of the disease or diseases under study. They are unsuitable for the study of rare diseases.

Nested or prospective case-control studies increasingly form an important component of major prospective studies examining the development of relatively common chronic diseases or conditions. They are usually based on the availability of biological samples (blood, plasma, serum, DNA, urine, saliva, etc.) stored at the commencement or baseline examination of the recruited cohort members. A large number of potential physio-pathological risk factors can be examined in a cost-effective manner without requiring analysis of samples from the whole cohort. More than one end point can be examined if required. These studies are termed 'nested' since the exposure status is created and ascertained at the baseline examination (and subsequently 'incubated' until the end points are evaluated).

Retrospective cohort studies In these, the exposure status of a whole cohort (for example, an occupational cohort) is accurately known from historical or occupational records, and the disease status of individuals from the whole cohort is obtained in current time. Such studies are relatively quick and inexpensive to conduct.

Experimental (intervention) studies are widely held to be 'de rigueur' by the medical establishment prior to acceptance of a new therapy or intervention. Several types of study design are possible and all have advantages and disadvantages at both the practical and scientific level. In treatment trials in patients a comparison group is used who receive an existing treatment or a **placebo** (dummy) treatment. In the past a control group comprising patients from a previous time period was sometimes used, termed a *historical control group*; but this approach can give misleading results. A review of empirical comparisons of randomized and non-randomized clinical trials has been reported which supports this view (Kunz and Oxman 1998). Patient trials can be in *parallel* in which only one treatment is received by each patient or *crossover*, when a second treatment is given to a patient replacing the initial treatment, sometimes after a suitable 'washout' period. Crossover trials tend to measure alterations in symptoms or quality of life in chronic conditions. A *factorial* design can be used to compare two or more treatments, and combinations of treatments. The International Studies of Infarct Survival (ISIS) provide examples of large-scale factorial trials of treatment in acute myocardial infarction, e.g. ISIS-3 (Anon 1992). The process of **random allocation** of patients to treatment has been shown to be an important step in minimizing the possibility of bias in the selection of these patient groups in controlled trials. Therefore in evidence-based medicine, particularly in most patient-centred studies, the randomized controlled study is the design of choice.

When an intervention is directed at a group of individuals randomization of the sampling unit is not always possible. As noted earlier, a cluster of subjects at a school or at a general practice can be selected as the sampling unit for random allocation, but this may not always be possible. Generally, the broader the intervention strategy, particularly if mass media interventions are used, the more likely 'contamination' of control areas may occur. Two large-scale whole population studies in which **multifactorial** public-health cardiovascular interventions were used over a period of several years showed comparable net changes in each intervention area (Wales: Tudor-Smith *et al.*

1998 and Kilkenny county, Ireland: Shelley *et al.* 1995) and in the respective control area. One possibility cited by these authors is that contamination of each control area occurred in these quasi-experimental studies.

In developing countries, public health intervention trials can be particularly important to inform and direct medical care in the absence of a well-established and resourced medical infrastructure. An example of a geographically-based quasi-experimental study to reduce neonatal mortality in rural India is shown in Fig. 3.2. Cluster randomized trials may be possible in rural areas in developing countries in separate communities, which are relatively isolated from each other, so that interventions do not spread into control areas unintentionally. Two examples of well-conducted cluster randomized trials to treat common sexually transmitted diseases to reduce the spread of HIV infection in rural African communities are described elsewhere (Grosskurth *et al.* 1995; Wawer *et al.* 1999).

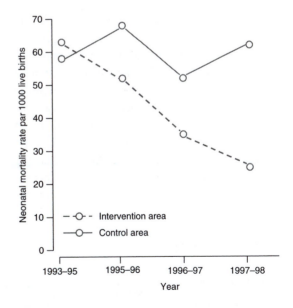

Figure 3.2 Neonatal mortality in rural Indian communities, 1993–98: a public-health intervention study using home-based neonatal care.
Source: Bang, AT, Bang, RA, Baitule, SB, Reddy, MH, and Deshmukh MD (1999). 'Effect of Home-Based Neonatal Care and Management of Sepsis on Neonatal Mortality: Field Trial in Rural India'. *The Lancet*, **354**, 1955–61.

There are now guidelines for the standardizing and clear reporting of most study designs, and collectively the links to these can be located at the Cochrane Collaboration Website (**http://www.cochrane.org/about-us/evidence-based-health-care/webliography/books/reporting**).

3.3 Risk

The concept of risk is crucial to a basic understanding of epidemiology. An overall definition of **risk** for epidemiological purposes is: *the probability of the occurrence of a future adverse event such as death, a disease, or a complication of disease*. Epidemiology employs a variety of risk indices which are based on rates so that an understanding of the construction of the **rate of an event** (see Box 3.1), and in particular the role of the **reference population**, is essential.

For example, **absolute risk** implies the overall risk for an individual in a given reference population. If the reference population is a whole country, region, or geographically-based community, the absolute risk of a future event can only be calculated from census or vital statistics data as described in section 1.2 (Box 1.3). **Life tables** for a reference population can be calculated using actuarial methods based on current life expectancies at birth and in subsequent age groups through to the most elderly members of the population (see section 16.1). Such tables enable the average number of **life-years lost** to be calculated for

a particular disease. Increasingly, life-years lost are used in public health studies to compare particular diseases, to describe and calculate mortality that may be amenable to public or health service interventions (**avoidable mortality**), and to guide future public health policies. The number of life-years lost is dependent on the average age of death for the particular disease. In order to enhance the usefulness of these estimates to compare different preventive approaches, life-years lost are usually adjusted for the quality of the life of an individual with a particular disease. Thus commonly used measures are: **quality-adjusted life-years (QALYs)** lost and **disability-adjusted life-years (DALYs)** lost which are described in more detail elsewhere (Murray and Lopez 1997; Lopez *et al.* 2006; Powles and Day 2002); see also Chapters 8, 14, 15, 20, and 22.

Absolute risk can also be calculated for the reference populations used in some types of analytical, observational, epidemiological studies (cohort and ecological studies), but not in case-control studies, unless the controls are selected randomly from the general population; nor in experimental studies, as subjects are usually selected to a small or large extent from a 'narrower' patient or general population. Usually this occurs since subjects have to meet entry and exclusion criteria and may also be restricted by the severity of their illness. However, even in cohorts drawn randomly from the **study population** and where the **response rate** (the percentage of the selected sample participating in the study) is high, the sample of participants is unlikely to be wholly representative

Box 3.1 Definition of a rate

$$\text{Rate} = \frac{\text{Numerator}}{\text{Denominator}} \times \text{Multiplier}$$

Where:

Numerator = number of events which have occurred in a given time period (e.g. one year)

Denominator = number of subjects *at risk* in the given time period

Multiplier = a convenient large number (e.g. 1000) used to avoid numerous decimal places

The rate is described as, for example, 'per 1000 per year'.

Note that: numerator and denominator must relate to the same population in terms of age-group, gender, geographical area, etc.

of the general population (healthier subjects may be more likely to volunteer to participate). Studies in which this has been examined have shown mortality in non-participants to be considerably higher than that among participants (Jousilahti *et al.* 2005).

The primary purpose of analytical, observational studies, however, is not to calculate the absolute risk of disease, but to examine the relationship between a particular exposure and the risk of the disease. Systematic examination of these risks for particular exposures are based on the risk of exposed individuals **relative** to the risk of non-exposed individuals and the epidemiological concept of **risk factor**. The term risk factor tends to be used in the epidemiological and biostatistical literature both in the widest sense as *any factor under test in a particular epidemiological study*, and also in the more specific sense of *a factor that has become established in many studies to be linked causally with the development of a particular disease*. Factors which are associated with increased risk of disease but may not be directly associated *causally* with the disease, are known as **risk markers**.

The risk index employed is dependent on the design of the study. Assuming complete follow-up, the basic information from a **cohort study** can be displayed in a 2 × 2 table. Box 3.2 details the calculations of two measures of association of exposure status and disease occurrence, **relative risk** (or **risk ratio**) and **odds ratio** (the odds of exposure). Although relative risk is more easily interpretable than the odds ratio, the latter generally has better statistical properties and is the measure used in logistic regression (see Chapter 4). The **rate ratio** is a more sophisticated measure and is based on comparing the total **person-years at risk** in the two exposure groups during the study. It is used in longitudinal studies where follow-up is incomplete or subjects are studied for varying lengths of time. The *hazard ratio* is a variant of the rate ratio based on Cox proportional hazards analysis (Chapter 4).

In a case-control study there is a group of subjects with the disease (cases) and a sample of subjects without the disease (controls); the exposure status for each subject is then determined and compared in the two groups. As the exposure status of the *whole* population is not known (see Box 3.3 and Table 3.2) it is not possible to estimate the odds of disease in the exposed and non-exposed groups, nor the risk of disease in those groups, nor the relative risk unless controls are drawn randomly from the general population (which is not usually the case). However, the odds ratio of disease can be calculated (see Box 3.3).

Box 3.2 Risk indices for cohort studies

Table 3.1 Risk indices for cohort studies

	Disease	No disease	Total
Exposed group	a (20)	b (80)	a + b (100)
Unexposed group	c (1)	d (99)	c + d (100)

Probability or **risk** or **incidence rate** (Ie) of disease in the exposed group

= a / (a+b) (20/100) = 0.20

Odds of disease in the exposed group = a / b (20/80) = 0.25

Probability or **risk** or **incidence rate** (Iu) of disease in the unexposed group

= c / (c+d) (1/100) = 0.01

Odds of disease in the unexposed group = c / d (1/99) = 0.0101

The risk ratio, rate ratio, or **relative risk** of disease (comparing the exposed group with the unexposed group) is defined by:

RR = Ie/Iu = { a / (a+b) } divided by { c / (c+d) } [20/100 divided by 1/100 = 20]

Odds ratio of disease (again comparing the exposed group with the unexposed group) is defined by:

OR = { a / b } divided by { c / d } = { a × d } / { b × c } [(20x99) divided by (80x1) = 24.75] (the **cross-product ratio**)

Box 3.3 Odds ratio of disease in a case-control study

Table 3.2 Odds ratio of disease in a case-control study

	Disease	No disease
Exposure group	a (7)	b (3)
Non-exposure group	c (2)	d (8)
Total	a + c	b + d

Although the odds on disease in the exposed or unexposed groups cannot be calculated, the ratio of the odds of disease (comparing the exposure group with the non-exposure group) is equal to the ratio of the odds of exposure (comparing the disease group with the non-disease group) and is defined by the **odds ratio** (also called the **cross-product ratio**):

$$OR = \{ a / c \} \text{ divided by } \{ b / d \} = \{ a \times d \} / \{ b \times c \}$$
$$= 7/2 \text{ divided by } 3/8 = 7 \times 8/3 \times 2 = 56/6 = 9.3$$

The odds ratio is a good approximation to the relative risk when the proportion of diseased individuals in each group is low (e.g. < 10 per cent). This would occur whenever the disease is rare in both groups, as will be described in subsequent chapters, many factors associated with our environment and culture (lifestyle) have been shown to be associated with the risk of common chronic diseases. For example, blood cholesterol levels, blood pressure, and smoking habit have become well-established (classic) risk factors for coronary heart disease (CHD); more recently, lack of exercise, overweight, and diabetes have also become established as risk factors. In order to design a strategy for intervening to reduce the incidence of CHD, for example, it is helpful to be able to estimate the relative contribution of each risk factor. For an individual risk factor this is known as the **excess risk** or the **risk difference**. It can be calculated from data obtained from a cohort study (see Box 3.4). An example using blood pressure as an example of a risk factor of subsequent heart attack is shown in Table 3.3.

Calculations of excess risk rely on the risk factor in question not being associated with another risk factor for the same disease, i.e. that the risk factor is operating **independently** of other risk factors. However this is not always the case and this will be discussed further in Chapter 20.

As already described, the **attributable risk** or **fraction** is calculated using data from a cohort study. But we have also noted that cohorts are often not entirely representative of the general population as they tend to be, firstly, from a selected age group and, secondly, to have volunteered to participate. In order to estimate the potential impact of an intervention on the general population it is necessary to have an estimate of the level of the exposure in the general population. This is frequently done using cross-sectional surveys and enables the **population attributable risk** or fraction to be calculated as shown in Box 3.5.

Box 3.4 Attributable risk in a cohort study

Using the definition of risk given in Box 3.2, the **excess risk (ER)** is defined as the **risk difference** (data from Box 3.2):

ER = risk of disease in the exposed group (20/100)
    – risk of disease in the non-exposed group (1/100)
    = 0.20 – 0.01 = 0.19

The **attributable risk** or the **attributable fraction (exposed)** or the **aetiologic fraction (exposed)** is defined as:

AR = attributable risk divided by the risk of disease in the exposed group

$I_e - I_u$ (where I_e is incidence in exposed and I_u in unexposed)

    = 20 – 1 divided by 20
    = 0.95 (95%)

often expressed as a percentage.

Table 3.3 Relative and attributable risk of heart attack in a cohort of men according to their initial blood pressure

	Systolic, mm Hg	Diastolic, mm Hg	% of men	Person years of risk (PYR)[a]	No. of men developing heart attack	Heart attack rate /1000PYR	Relative risk ratio (compared to normal BP)[b]	Excess or attributable risk /1000PYR[c]	Attributable risk per cent [d]
Normal (including optimal)	<130	<85	44	13524	110	8.1 (I_o)	1	0	
High normal	130–139	85–89	20	6307	77	12.2 (I_{e_1})	1.5	4.1	33%
Hypertension stage I	140–159	90–99	23	6695	115	17.2 (I_{e_2})	2.11	9.1	53%
Hypertension stage II–IV	≥160	≥100	13	3628	81	22.3 (I_{e_3})	2.75	14.2	64%

[a] Person years of risk calculated from sum of years of follow-up for each man at each level of blood pressure
[b] Relative risk of heart attack by blood pressure category = I_e / I_o
[c] Heart attack rate attributable to raised blood pressure = I_e – I_o
[d] Attributable risk per cent = (e / c) × 100 %

Box 3.5 Population attributable risk*

Population ER = risk of disease in the total population
(21/200)

– risk of disease in the non-exposed
population (1/100)

= 0.105 – 0.010 = 0.095

The **population attributable risk** or the **attributable fraction (population)** or the **aetiologic fraction (population)** is defined as:

Population PAR = population ER divided by the risk
of disease in the total population,

= 0.095 divided by 0.105

= 0.905 (90.5%)

often expressed as a percentage

*Data from Box 3.2

For an experimental study comparing two treatments with a binary outcome, the data can be summarized in a 2 × 2 table similar to Table 3.1; the risk difference is often used as an alternative summary measure.

Further reading

Gordis L (2004) *Epidemiology*, 3rd edn. Philadelphia: Saunders.

Porta M and Last JM (2008) *A Dictionary of Epidemiology*, 5th edn. Oxford: Oxford University Press. (This provides a comprehensive set of definitions of all technical terms which cause confusion in epidemiology, e.g. relative risk, risk ratio, rate ratio, cumulative incidence, etc.).

Silman AJ (2002) *Epidemiological Studies: A Practical Guide*, 2nd edn. Cambridge: Cambridge University Press.

References

Anon (1992) ISIS-3: a randomised comparison of streptokinase vs tissue plasminogen activator vs anistreplase and of aspirin plus heparin vs aspirin alone among 41,299 cases of suspected acute myocardial infarction. ISIS-3 (Third International Study of Infarct Survival) Collaborative Group. *Lancet* **339** (8796), 753–70.

Bang AT, Bang RA, Baitule SB, Reddy MH, *et al.* (1999) Effect of home-based neonatal care and management of sepsis on neonatal mortality: field trial in rural India. *Lancet* **354** (9194), 1955–61.

Grosskurth H, Mosha F, Todd J, Mwijarubi E, *et al.* (1995) Impact of improved treatment of sexually transmitted diseases on HIV infection in rural Tanzania: randomized controlled trial. *Lancet* **346** (8974), 530–6.

Hernán MA, Alonso A, Logan R, Grodstein F, *et al.* (2008) Observational studies analyzed like randomized experiments: an application to postmenopausal hormone therapy and coronary heart disease. *Epidemiology* **19** (6), 766–79.

Jousilahti P, Salomaa V, Kuulasmaa K, Niemelä M, *et al.* (2005) Total and cause specific mortality among participants and non-participants of population based health surveys: a comprehensive follow up of 54 372 Finnish men and women. *Journal of Epidemiology and Community Health* **59** (4), 310–15.

Kunz R and Oxman AD (1998) The unpredictability paradox: review of empirical comparisons of randomized and non-randomized clinical trials. *BMJ (Clinical Research Ed)* **317** (7167), 1185–90.

Lopez AD, Mathers CD, Ezzati M, Jamison DJ, *et al.* (eds) (2006) *Global Burden of Disease and Risk Factors*. Washington: World Bank/Oxford University Press.

Murray CJ and Lopez AD (1997) Global mortality, disability, and the contribution of risk factors: Global Burden of Disease Study. *Lancet* **349** (9063), 1436–42.

Powles J and Day N (2002) Interpreting the global burden of disease. *Lancet* **360** (9343), 1342–3.

Shelley E, Daly L, Collins C, Christie M, *et al.* (1995) Cardiovascular risk factor changes in the Kilkenny Health Project. A community health promotion programme. *European Heart Journal* **16** (6), 752–60.

Silman AJ (2002) *Epidemiological Studies: A Practical Guide*, 2nd edn. Cambridge: Cambridge University Press.

Tudor-Smith C, Nutbeam D, Moore L, and Catford J (1998) Effects of the Heartbeat Wales programme over five years on behavioural risks for cardiovascular disease: quasi-experimental comparison of results from Wales and a matched reference area. *BMJ (Clinical Research Ed)* **316** (7134), 818–22.

Vandenbroucke JP (2009) The HRT controversy: observational studies and RCTs fall in line. *Lancet* **373** (9671), 1233–5.

Wawer MJ, Sewankambo NK, Serwadda D, Quinn TC, *et al.* (1999) Control of sexually transmitted diseases for AIDS prevention in Uganda: a randomized community trial. Rakai Project Study Group. *Lancet* **353** (9152), 525–35.

4 Data analysis in epidemiology

GORDON CRAN AND CHRISTOPHER PATTERSON

CHAPTER CONTENTS

This chapter introduces the basic statistical terms and methods used in descriptive and analytical epidemiological reports. Where possible, examples are provided in subsequent chapters. Students are recommended to consult the references for additional reading, particularly for details of more advanced statistical techniques frequently used in modern epidemiological practice.

Introduction

The study of the distribution of a disease is generally **descriptive** in nature whereas the study of factors that are possibly associated with or cause the disease is usually **analytical**, and requires the gathering of data to test prior hypotheses. There is frequently an overlap between these approaches, particularly in health surveys. Some epidemiological studies use data from routinely collected sources (see section 2.2). However, most are based on data collected by **sampling** from **populations**. For such studies statistical methods of analysis are required. This chapter outlines the basic principles of statistical inference and briefly describes some multivariable methods that are increasingly being used in epidemiological studies. More detailed descriptions of statistical methods are given in the references listed at the end of the chapter.

4.1 Populations and samples

The population that is to be investigated is called the **target population**, often selected or stratified by age from the *general population*. The actual population from which data are obtained is termed the **study population** and is often defined by geographical, institutional (for example schools, factories), occupational, or disease criteria. How well conclusions from the study population can be applied to the target population is a matter of judgement. Whole or general population studies are often based on vital statistics that are routinely collected (see section 2.2). Otherwise such a population study is only feasible if the population is well-defined and the information required can be collected from every member of the population. In practice, however, collection of data from all members of the study population is often impossible (the decennial census of the population is a notable exception) so that data must be obtained from a **sample** of the study population. A sample may be selected from a **sampling frame** or list of all members of a population; however, no single sampling frame is likely to be completely representative of the study population (see Chapter 2). For example, electoral or voting registers, although compiled annually in the UK, are voluntary and in areas with high population movements may underestimate the true population by 10–30 per cent.

The use of a sample has several practical advantages:

- the number of subjects is smaller, the effort and costs are less and the information is more timely;
- the information may be more extensive and of higher quality;
- a higher response rate may be achieved resulting in a reduction in **non-response bias**, which may arise if there are differences between those who choose to respond and those who do not.

To obtain useful and valid information about a population from a sample, it is important that the sample be representative of the population. This is achieved by drawing the sample **randomly** from the population: this protects against **selection bias** (a systematic difference between those selected for the sample and those in the population), and provides a theoretical basis for the application of statistical methods.

There are a variety of sampling schemes. In *simple random sampling* each member of the population has the same chance of being selected. The sample is usually selected from a list of all members of the population by means of computer-generated random numbers. A disadvantage of this method of sampling is that it may give practical difficulties for the data collection. Provided there are no periodic features in the list, *systematic sampling* may be more convenient: subjects are selected at regular intervals from the list (for example every tenth individual). In **stratified sampling**, a heterogeneous population is divided into strata and a sample randomly selected from each stratum. The strata are defined by one or more **categorical variables** (see section 4.2), for example, gender or age group, which may have a bearing on the factors being studied. This type of sampling is recommended when the prevalence of a disease or risk factor varies across strata. Stratification then improves the precision of the analysis; it can also ensure that small subgroups of special interest (for example, ethnic minority groups) are adequately represented. In **cluster sampling** the population comprises of several first-stage sampling units or clusters (for example, schools, households, hospitals), each of which is made up of several second-stage units (for example, classes, individuals, wards, etc.). The clusters are sampled by some suitable method; for each selected cluster, all second-stage units are then investigated. Alternatively, further sampling of the second-stage units within the selected clusters can be performed; for example, within a selected school, classes are randomly selected (**multistage cluster sampling**). Although these methods lead to savings in cost, effort, and time, the statistical results are less precise than those obtained using a simple random sample. Different sampling methods can be combined into a single sampling scheme, for example, stratification and clustering.

In certain circumstances (for example, surveys of specific groups, pilot studies) non-random sampling methods such as convenience sampling, snowball sampling, and quota sampling are used. These methods are the stock-in-trade of market research companies sometimes employed to conduct health and social surveys, but they do not provide a suitable basis for the methods of statistical inference described later in this chapter.

4.2 Summarizing sample data

Epidemiological data consist of measurements or observations on the **variables** (the disease status, risk factors, exposures, demographic characteristics) collected from the subjects selected. The choice of summary measures, graphical displays, and analyses depends on the type of variable.

There are two main types of variable: **quantitative** (or *measurable*) and **qualitative** (or **categorical**).

Quantitative variables

A quantitative variable may be either **continuous** or **discrete**. A **continuous variable** is measured on a continuous scale with an associated unit of measurement; it is recorded to a certain degree of accuracy. So, for example, height is a continuous variable but is often recorded to the nearest centimetre. A **discrete variable** is one that takes a list of values; in practice, it is often a *count*, for example, the number of persons in a household.

Categorical (qualitative) variables

A characteristic of a patient may be described as belonging to one of several categories. If the categories are unordered, the variable is described as **nominal categorical**; for example, the four blood groups A, B, AB, and O. When there are only two categories, the variable is usually described as **binary** or **dichotomous**; for example, the presence or absence of a factor. When the categories have a natural ordering, for example, a variable representing some outcome with categories poor, satisfactory, good, the variable is described as **ordinal** or **ordered categorical**. Social class (see Chapter 20) and smoking habit are examples of ordinal variables: (smoking habit is grouped into categories such as never, ex-smoker, light (1–14 cigarettes per day), medium (15–24), and heavy (25+) smokers).

A quantitative variable can be converted into a binary variable or an ordered categorical variable by the application of suitable cut-points to the original variable. The cut-points may be calculated from the sample data, for example, using the three sample quartiles (see Box 4.1) to divide the sample into four approximately equal-sized groups. Alternatively, cut-points that are in widespread use can be chosen, for example, body mass index (BMI) in adults is categorized as underweight, normal weight, overweight, obese by the cut-points 18.5, 25, 30 kg/m^2 (see Section 9.3).

A large sample of observations on any type of variable can be summarized in a **frequency table**, which could include frequencies and relative frequencies (or percentages). In the case of a continuous variable or a discrete variable with many distinct values, suitable classes of equal width, usually between 10 and 20 in number, need to be defined before the calculation of the frequencies. For such variables the frequencies, relative frequencies, or the percentages of the classes can be displayed in a **histogram** (see Figs. 4.1 and 4.2). For a categorical variable or a discrete variable with few distinct values, the frequencies can be displayed in a **bar chart**, which emphasizes the discrete nature of the variable (see Fig. 7.3).

Box 4.1 Sample summary measures

Let $x_1, x_2, \ldots, x_n$ denote the observations on a quantitative variable in a sample of size n.

The **mean**, denoted by $\bar{x}$, is the arithmetic mean of the observations:

$$\bar{x} = (x_1 + x_2 + \ldots\ldots + x_n)/n = \sum x_i / n.$$

The **standard deviation**, denoted by **s**, is defined by:

$$s = \sqrt{\sum(x_i - \bar{x})^2 /(n-1)},$$

that is, the square root of the approximate mean of the squares of the deviations, $(x_i - \bar{x})$, of the observations from the sample mean.

The **coefficient of variation**, denoted by **c**, is only defined for variables taking positive values:

$$c = \frac{s}{\bar{x}} \ 100\%$$

Percentiles are calculated by sorting the observations in order of magnitude. The percentiles divide the distribution of observations into one hundred equal-sized parts.

The 50th percentile is the **median** or second quartile, Q_2; the 25th and 75th percentiles are the first and third quartiles, Q_1 and Q_3, and define the **inter-quartile range** = $Q_3 - Q_1$.

The mean and standard deviation are the most commonly used summary measures if the distribution of observations or results is roughly symmetric (Fig. 4.1). However, the median and inter-quartile range are used for heavily skewed distributions (Fig. 4.2).

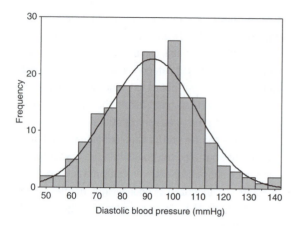

Figure 4.1 Histogram of the diastolic blood pressures of a random sample of 200 males with fitted Normal distribution curve.

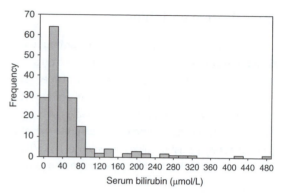

Figure 4.2 Histogram of serum bilirubin values in 200 patients with cirrhosis.

In the case of a quantitative variable, more succinct summary measures are available: the appropriate measures depend on the distribution of the observations in the sample which can be inferred from the shape of the histogram. If the histogram has a long tail to the right, as shown in Fig. 4.2, the sample is **skewed** *to the right* or *positively skewed* (if *skewed to the left* then it is *negatively skewed*).

The following sample summary measures are described in Box 4.1. The most widely used *measure of location* or the 'centre' of a sample is the **mean**. However, it is inappropriate for highly skewed data, and the **median** or 50th percentile is then preferable. The **standard deviation** is a common *measure of dispersion* (or variation) usually presented in conjunction with the sample mean. For a skewed sample, the variation is better described by the 25th percentile (or first quartile, $Q1$) and 75th percentile (or third quartile, $Q3$) or by their difference, the **inter-quartile range**. By its definition, this range contains half of the distribution. Finally, the **coefficient of variation** expresses the standard deviation as a percentage of the mean and provides a measure of relative variation that is independent of the units of measurement and hence can be used to compare the variation of variables measured in different units. The coefficient of variation is therefore widely used for quantifying measurement error in laboratory work.

The relationship between two categorical variables can be displayed in a two-way frequency table, also called a **contingency table** (see Table 5.1). For two quantitative variables, or a quantitative variable and a categorical variable, a **scatter diagram** (see Fig. 4.4) indicates the form of any association; for quantitative variables any linear association can be summarized by a **correlation coefficient**, r, ranging from -1 (perfect linear negative association) through 0 (no linear association) to $+1$ (perfect linear positive association).

A feature of some cohort studies and clinical trials is that they involve follow-up of subjects over prolonged periods until some event or end-point (such as disease recurrence or death) is observed. Such studies give rise to quantitative data in the form of 'times to events', but in some subjects (for example, patients C and D in Fig. 4.3) the event is not observed during the period of follow-up and such times are said to be *censored*. Such data require special analytical techniques which take account of this censoring.

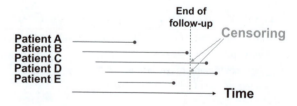

Figure 4.3 Illustration showing censored survival times in an analysis of a follow-up study.

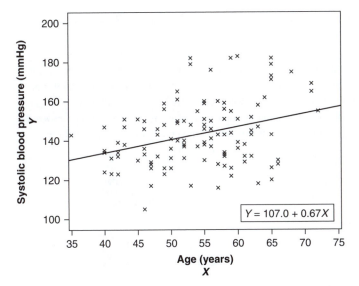

Figure 4.4 Scatter diagram and fitted simple regression line to describe the relationship between systolic blood pressure and age for 112 participants in a nutritional intervention study.

The probability of survival at any follow-up time is usually displayed graphically in a Kaplan–Meier plot (see Fig. 8.2).

It may be beneficial to transform a quantitative variable to another scale so that the assumptions for a statistical method are satisfied. How to choose an appropriate transformation is beyond the scope of this text but in medical studies the **logarithmic transformation** is very commonly used because many variables exhibit positive skewness. Having analysed the logarithmically transformed data, the results should be interpreted on the original scale. Another type of variable that is extensively used in comparison studies is the standardized version of a quantitative variable, often called a **z-score**:

$$\text{z-score} = (\text{variable value} - \text{sample mean}) / \text{sample standard deviation.}$$

An example is given in Fig. 15.3.

Finally, in some statistical methods (for example, non-parametric hypothesis tests), the ordered sample of n values of the variable is replaced by the set of **ranks** 1, 2, . . ., n.

4.3 Simple methods of statistical inference

Statistical inference is the process of drawing conclusions from sample data about the characteristics of the population or populations that have been sampled.

Because the information available is incomplete, these conclusions are subject to uncertainties, which are expressed in terms of probabilities and probability distributions. Statistical methods require the assumption that the samples obtained are random samples drawn from the populations being studied in order that inferences are valid. The possibility of biased conclusions resulting from the use of non-random samples (as is often the case in practice) must be assessed by the researcher. Generally, statistical methods only take **sampling error** into account and do not quantify biases due to non-random sampling. The two forms of statistical inference are **estimation** and **hypothesis testing**.

Suppose a characteristic of a population (the 'average' value) is represented by a single quantity (for example, the population mean). Such a quantity is called a **parameter** and is typically unknown. Given a sample from the population, a single value, often referred to as a **statistic**, is calculated as an **estimate** of the parameter. For example, the sample mean is an estimate of the population mean. The properties of the statistic or estimate are determined by its **sampling distribution**: the frequency distribution obtained by calculating the statistic for every possible sample (of the same size) from the population. When the sample size is large, the sampling distribution is often approximated by a **normal distribution** (see Fig. 4.1). The precision of a statistic is measured by its

Box 4.2 Example of calculation of a confidence interval for a population proportion from a large sample

To investigate the risk of irritable bowel syndrome after an episode of bacterial gastroenteritis, 386 patients were surveyed by questionnaire six months after bacterial gastroenteritis infection and it was found that 27 had developed irritable bowel syndrome. Assuming that these 386 patients represent a random sample from the population of all bacterial gastroenteritis patients, calculate 95 per cent confidence limits for the proportion of the population who develop irritable bowel syndrome.

$n = 386$ Proportion, $p = 27/386 = 0.070$ or 7.0%

The limits are given by:

$$p \pm 1.96 \, SE(p)$$

$$p \pm 1.96\sqrt{p(1-p)/n}$$

$$0.070 \pm 1.96\sqrt{0.070(1-0.070)/386}$$

$$0.045, 0.095$$

The 95 per cent confidence limits are 4.5 per cent and 9.5 per cent, while the 95 per cent confidence interval is from 4.5 per cent to 9.5 per cent. Then 95 per cent of intervals like this will include the actual proportion of the population of bacterial gastroenteritis patients who develop irritable bowel syndrome. A larger sample would give a narrower confidence interval.

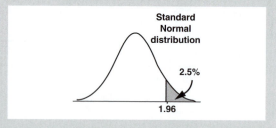

Figure 4.5 Normal distribution and upper 95% confidence limit.

Data from: Neal KR, Hebden J, and Spiller R (1997).

standard error (SE), the standard deviation of its sampling distribution, which can be reduced by increasing the sample size; standard errors are used in calculating confidence intervals and in hypothesis testing.

An alternative that provides more insight into the precision of a statistic is **confidence interval** estimation: for a chosen degree of confidence (usually 95 per cent), an interval is calculated from the sample data and is said to include the unknown parameter with the specified degree of confidence. The **confidence limits** (the lower and upper values of the interval) are generally calculated from knowledge of the sampling distribution of the statistic. For means, proportions, and their differences, approximate 95 per cent confidence limits are given by:

$$\text{statistic} \pm 1.96 \times SE(\text{statistic})$$

when samples are large. For odds ratios and relative risks (see Chapter 3) similar calculations of confidence limits are performed on a logarithmic scale. In repeated samples (of the same size) the confidence limits will change from sample to sample. However, for 95 per cent confidence intervals, it is expected that 95 per cent of these intervals will contain the unknown parameter. For

a chosen degree of confidence, the narrower the confidence interval the better is the estimation process. Using a larger sample reduces the standard error and hence narrows the confidence interval. An example of the calculation of a confidence interval for a proportion is given in Box 4.2. Fig. 4.5 shows a standard Normal distribution with the upper 95% cut point.

The second form of statistical inference is **hypothesis testing** (also called **significance testing**). The general aim of hypothesis testing is to investigate whether sample data are consistent with an assumption about the population (or populations) from which the samples were drawn (for example, two population means are equal).

A hypothesis test can be considered as a series of six steps (see Box 4.3 for a worked example). Fig. 4.6 shows the relevant t distribution and calculated t-statistic.

1 The study hypothesis is expressed in terms of two statistical hypotheses about the population distributions: the **null hypothesis**, usually representing the current state of knowledge, or expressing 'no difference' if two or more distributions are being compared; and the **alternative hypothesis**, which is often simply the negation of the null hypothesis. The null hypothesis is not rejected unless the sample evidence

Box 4.3 Has the length of the neck of the femur changed over the course of the 20th century in Scotland? A worked example of a statistical hypothesis test

A study compared femoral neck lengths (in millimetres) in the anatomy collection of a Scottish university in 43 men who had died in the early 20th century (1900–1920) with 22 men who had died in the late 20th century (1980s).

$$n_{Early} = 43 \qquad n_{Late} = 22$$
$$\bar{x}_{Early} = 34.9\,mm \quad \bar{x}_{Late} = 38.3\,mm$$
$$s_{Early} = 3.9\,mm \quad s_{Late} = 3.8\,mm$$

Is there evidence of a change in femoral neck length between the two periods?

1 The means in these samples clearly differ by 3.4 mm, but does this provide evidence that the population means differ? The null hypothesis is that the mean femoral neck length in the male population of Scotland in the early 20th century is the same as the mean in the late 20th century. The alternative hypothesis is that there has been a change in length. It is assumed that each group of men is a random sample from the Scottish male population of the time.

2 Because femoral neck length is a continuous variable and is to be compared in two independent samples of men, reference to Box 4.3 shows that the *independent samples* t-test is appropriate. Femoral neck length must be assumed to follow a normal distribution, although this assumption can be relaxed in large samples.

3 The conventional five per cent significance level is chosen for this test, and consequently it must be accepted that there will be a one in 20 chance of making a type I error (i.e., rejecting the null hypothesis when it is actually true).

4 From these two samples a *t*-statistic is calculated as 3.35 and used to derive from the *t* distribution with 63 degrees of freedom the *P*-value of 0.0014 (see inset). This represents the probability of seeing a difference in sample means as large as, or larger than, the difference actually observed in this study assuming that in reality there has been no change in femoral neck length.

The test statistic is calculated as:

$$t = (\bar{x}_{Late} - \bar{x}_{Early})/SE(\bar{x}_{Late} - \bar{x}_{Early})$$
$$= (38.3 - 34.9)/1.03$$
$$= 3.35$$

and is from the t distribution with:

$$n_{Late} + n_{Early} - 2$$
$$= 22 + 43 - 2$$
$$= 63 \text{ degrees of freedom (df).}$$

where $SE(\bar{x}_{Late} - \bar{x}_{Early})$ has been evaluated from n_{Early}, n_{Late}, s_{Early}, and s_{Late} (details omitted).

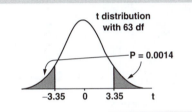

Figure 4.6 *t* distribution and *t*-statistic.

5 This *P*-value is less than the chosen significance level for the test, so the null hypothesis is rejected. A difference as large as that observed between the samples is not likely to arise often if the null hypothesis were true.

6 There is evidence of an increase in the femoral head diameter in Scottish men during the period. The risk of type I error is small (the null hypothesis would still have been rejected had we chosen to use a lower probability cut-off). However, some caution must be advised in interpreting these findings since men whose bodies were donated to the university may not necessarily have been representative of the male population of Scotland at the time.

Data from: Duthie RA, Bruce MF and Hutchison JD (1998). Changing Proximal Femoral Geometry in North East Scotland: An Osteometric Study. *British Medical Journal*, **316**: 1498.

is strongly against it, in which case it is rejected in favour of the alternative hypothesis. In the worked example, the null hypothesis is that the length of the neck of the femur has not changed over the course of the 20th century (the alternative hypothesis is that the length has changed).

2 A suitable *test* is chosen. This choice depends on the number of groups, the type of variable, and the form of its distribution; Table 4.1 lists some widely used tests. Associated with the test is a **test statistic**, which is a function of the sample data and the nature of the hypotheses.

Table 4.1 Guide to selecting the appropriate statistical test for comparisons between samples. This table covers only the more commonly used methods for making simple comparisons between samples.

Type of variable	Two samples		R samples (R > 2)	
	Independent	**Paired**	**Independent**	**Matched**
Continuous				
(Normality assumptions satisfied)	Independent samples t-test*	Paired samples t-test*	One-way analysis of variance	Randomized block analysis of variance
Discrete, Continuous				
(Normality assumptions **not** satisfied)	Mann–Whitney U-test or Wilcoxon rank sum test	Wilcoxon signed-rank test	Kruskal–Wallis analysis of variance	Friedman two-way analysis of variance
Categorical				
Two categories	X^2 test for 2 × 2 table or Fisher's exact test	McNemar's test	X^2 test for R × 2 table	Cochran's Q test
C categories (C > 2)	X^2 test for 2 × C table	–	X^2 test for R × C table	–

*Or equivalent large samples z-test.

3 The **significance level** of the test is chosen, usually 0.05 (or 5 per cent), but smaller probabilities can be used. The choice of significance level depends upon the particular problem and how serious the consequences would be if a true null hypothesis were rejected.

4 The **P-value** is calculated using a statistical computer package: it is the probability of the observed value of the test statistic, with any other equally extreme or more extreme values that might have occurred, assuming that the null hypothesis is true.

5 The P-value is compared with the significance level, say 0.05. If $P \leq 0.05$, the *test is significant at the five per cent level*, the null hypothesis is rejected, and the alternative hypothesis is accepted; if $P > 0.05$, the test is not significant at the five per cent level and the null hypothesis is not rejected. In the worked example, the P-value is calculated as 0.0014 or 0.14 per cent, a low probability leading to rejection of the null hypothesis.

6 A statistically significant result must be interpreted with regard to the aims and size of the study; a statistically significant result need not necessarily be clinically or biologically important. In certain situations (as in the worked example) there were doubts about the representativeness of the sample, and this can also cast doubt on the conclusion of the test.

Statistical significance and power

A non-significant result does not imply that the null hypothesis is true but that, on the available evidence, the null hypothesis cannot be rejected. A significant result often, but not invariably, indicates that the alternative hypothesis is true. Hence errors may occur in this decision-making process. A *type I error* occurs if the null hypothesis is rejected when in fact it is true; it has a one in twenty chance of happening when the five per cent level of significance is chosen. Accordingly, testing of numerous hypotheses in a study may result in an increased chance of type I error (a false-positive result). Adjustment for multiple testing is usually made by adopting a smaller probability cut off, for example a one per cent level of significance. A *type II error* (a false-negative result) occurs if the null hypothesis

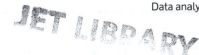

Box 4.4 Classification of errors in hypothesis testing

True situation	Result of test	
	Reject null hypothesis	Do not reject hypothesis
Null hypothesis true	Type I error	Correct decision
Alternative hypothesis true	Correct decision	Type II error

is not rejected when in fact the alternative hypothesis is true; the probability of this happening can be calculated for a specified alternative hypothesis. Box 4.4 displays the possible outcomes of a hypothesis test. The probability of not making a type II error is called the **power** of the test. The concept of power is important in designing a study to ensure that it is of adequate size to detect a clinically worthwhile difference; typically a power of at least 0.8 (80 per cent) is recommended. Many research studies are underpowered, and research protocols usually include an estimate of the necessary sample size to ensure a conclusive result.

Generally, a statistic together with its associated confidence interval is more useful than a hypothesis test, because a statistic gives information on the magnitude and direction of an effect, and the confidence interval provides a measure of the precision of the statistic. In many analyses, a confidence interval can also be used to test the null hypothesis (the null hypothesis is rejected only if the confidence interval does not include the value specified by the null hypothesis). For examples, see Table 7.2 and Fig. 7.3.

4.4 Regression modelling

The methods of section 4.3 can be used to investigate the association between the disease state (represented by a quantitative or a categorical variable) and a single exposure or treatment variable (again either quantitative or categorical), except when they are both quantitative. In this latter case, a scatter diagram of the paired values of the two variables should be constructed followed by either a **correlation analysis** or, preferably, a **linear regression** analysis (the fitting of a straight line) if appropriate.

The latter is illustrated in Fig. 4.4 which shows the association between systolic blood pressure (Y) and age (X) observed in 112 participants in a nutritional intervention trial. The relationship may be described by a line with slope (i.e. change in Y per unit change in X) of 0.67 mmHg per year and intercept (the predicted Y value when $X = 0$) of 107.0 mmHg. In keeping with many regression problems, this intercept has no biological interpretation and is of little interest since it involves *extrapolation* well beyond the range of the X variable. However, it is required to construct the prediction equation as shown in the box in Fig. 4.4.

Where there are possibly several exposure variables and other available information about the subjects being studied, multivariable **regression modelling** is a suitable approach. The general aim is to explain the variation in a response or outcome variable, sometimes representing the disease state, in terms of explanatory or predictor variables which can be quantitative or categorical; specific objectives may be the testing of hypotheses of the effect of an explanatory variable (also termed by some as an independent variable), estimation of effects, and the making of predictions.

In epidemiological studies, regression modelling is generally considered to be the best approach for estimating an exposure effect after controlling or adjusting for the effects of confounding variables. (A **confounding variable** is one that is associated with the outcome and the exposure; for example, smoking habit is associated with risk of heart attack and socio-economic status so smoking habit could confound an analysis of the association between socio-economic status and heart attack.) See, for example, Table 7.4. When a third variable modifies the relation between an exposure and the outcome, **effect modification** or **interaction** occurs; this can also be investigated in regression analysis. In Table 7.2, age is an effect modifier of smoking habit for the risk of myocardial infarction, because the relative risk associated with smoking decreases steeply with increasing age. In this text, three forms of regression modelling are now considered: multiple linear regression for a continuous outcome, binary logistic regression for a binary outcome and Cox's proportional hazards regression model for the type of censored survival data described in section 4.2.

A fitted **multiple linear regression** model takes the form:

$$Y = b_0 + b_1 X_1 + b_2 X_2 + \ldots + b_k X_k$$

where Y represents a continuous outcome, and the Xs represent the explanatory variables (or functions of these variables). The bs are estimated **regression coefficients**, b_0 representing the intercept and $b_1, \ldots, b_k$ the k slopes: an individual coefficient represents the change in the outcome variable associated with a unit change in the corresponding X variable, when the remaining X variables are kept fixed. The relative contributions that variables such as age, smoking habit, and physical activity make to the prediction of continuous variables such as weight or body mass index are typically assessed by such methods.

A fitted **binary logistic regression** model takes the form:

$$\log_e \{p/(1-p)\} = b_0 + b_1 X_1 + b_2 X_2 + \ldots + b_k X_k$$

where p represents the probability or risk of the outcome occurring, $p/(1 - p)$ is the odds of the outcome occurring, and the Xs represent the explanatory variables (or functions of these variables). The function $\exp(b_i)$ is the **odds ratio** associated with the variable X_i, that is, comparing the two odds obtained by a unit change in X_i, when the remaining X variables are kept fixed. Many risk factors have been shown to be associated with risk of coronary heart disease and the relative contributions of each risk factor is typically estimated using this approach.

A fitted *Cox's proportional hazards regression* model takes the form:

$$\log_e \{h(t)/h_0(t)\} = b_1 X_1 + b_2 X_2 + \ldots + b_k X_k$$

where the **hazard function**, $h(t)$, represents the risk of the event occurring at time t after entry to the study,

given that it has not occurred from entry to just before time t, and where $h_0(t)$, the baseline hazard function, represents this same risk when all the X variables take the value zero. The ratio of these two risks is assumed to be constant throughout time of follow-up, the proportional hazards assumption. The function $\exp(b_i)$, associated with the variable X_i, is interpreted in a similar manner to the odds ratio of the logistic regression model, except that in the Cox model it is as a *hazard ratio* (or **relative hazard**). Relative hazards may be considered as having a similar interpretation to **relative risks** which have been calculated in the example in Table 3.1.

In all three models the bs are estimated from the sample data using a suitable statistical computer package, for example, SPSS. Stata, or SAS. Not all the explanatory variables may be required to obtain an adequate fit to the data; an explanatory variable may only be associated with the outcome variable because it is highly correlated with one or more of the other explanatory variables. For this reason, before beginning any modelling it is very important first to perform preliminary analyses using independent samples t-tests, chi-squared tests (or *log rank* tests in the case of censored survival data) and examine scatter diagrams and correlation coefficients. This will help to establish which variables are likely to confound relationships with outcome variables.

Most statistical computer packages contain routines to select a subset of the explanatory variables. **Forward selection** successively adds the most significant X variable until none of the remaining variables makes a further contribution according to a predetermined significance level. In contrast, **backward elimination** starts with all X variables in the model and successively removes the least important at each stage until any further elimination would result in a significant variable being removed. **Stepwise selection** is a combination of these approaches which has the benefit that a decision to add (in the case of forward selection), or to remove (in the case of backward elimination), may be changed at a later stage. It may also be used as a generic term for these automatic selection procedures. However, the selection of variables should primarily be based on the researcher's understanding of the data and the context of the study, particularly in choosing confounders to be controlled. The further reading section gives more details about modelling strategies in the regression analysis of epidemiological studies.

Biostatistics is a core discipline of epidemiology and preventive medicine; students are encouraged to read one or more of the following texts to develop their ability to evaluate the current research literature.

Further reading

Altman DG (1997) *Practical Statistics for Medical Research*. London: Chapman & Hall.

Armitage P, Berry G, and Matthews JN (2002) *Statistical Methods in Medical Research*, 4th edn. Oxford: Blackwell.

Bland M (2000) *An Introduction to Medical Statistics*, 3rd edn. Oxford: Oxford University Press.

Campbell MJ and Machin D (1999) *Medical Statistics: A Commonsense Approach*, 3rd edn. Chichester: Wiley.

Kirkwood BR and Sterne JAC (2003) *Essential Medical Statistics*, 2nd edn. Oxford: Blackwell Science Ltd.

Pereira-Maxwell F (1998) *A–Z of Medical Statistics. A Companion for Critical Appraisal*. London: Arnold.

Woodward M (2005) *Epidemiology Study Design and Data Analysis*, 2nd edn. Boca Raton, USA: Chapman & Hall.

References

Duthie RA, Bruce MF, and Hutchison JD (1998) Changing proximal femoral geometry in north east Scotland: an osteometric study. *BMJ (Clinical Research Ed)* **316** (7143), 1498.

Neal KR, Hebden J, and Spiller R (1997) Prevalence of gastrointestinal symptoms six months after bacterial gastroenteritis and risk factors for development of the irritable bowel syndrome: postal survey of patients. *BMJ (Clinical Research Ed)* **314** (7083), 779–82.

5 Screening for diseases

SHIVARAM BHAT, ANNA GAVIN, AND HELEN DOLK

CHAPTER CONTENTS

This chapter introduces the topic of screening in public health and medical practice. The principles, purposes, and methods of screening are discussed, and concepts of validity, which are common to screening tests used in the general population and to those used for clinical diagnosis. Case studies are given for prostate cancer, colorectal cancer, and antenatal screening for Down's syndrome.

Introduction

To 'screen' is used in the general sense to mean 'to sift or investigate' and can be applied in public health or clinical medicine. **Screening** results in a classification of an individual as either 'diseased' (or 'at risk of a disease') or 'not diseased' (or 'not at risk'). Many of the concepts and cross-tabulations relating to risk, developed in Chapter 3 (section 3.3), also apply to screening tests. Borderline cases are likely to be retested but, essentially, individuals are classified dichotomously or categorically by tests that are often measured on a clinical scale. These tests, therefore, are indicators either for the disease itself, for a risk factor or for a particular trait that could affect the health of the individual or others. Issues about the **validity** of the test will be discussed later, but it is firstly necessary to discuss *why* and *how* a particular test is applied.

5.1 Types and principles of screening

Mandatory screening is usually designed for the preservation of the health or safety of others, often as a condition of employment, or before blood donation. Doctors, airline pilots, and applicants to many other occupations must expect to undergo a screening examination formulated according to medico-legal guidelines. Among blood donors, unexpected results may cause distress to individuals testing positive for human immunodeficiency virus (HIV) or hepatitis B or C, for example, and informed consent and counselling are part of the procedures used by the Blood Transfusion Service in the UK.

Prescriptive screening implies potential benefit for the individual and is usually a systematic screening programme, either delivered as an integrated component of routine practice, as in antenatal and neonatal care, or as a voluntary public health programme such as those for cervical breast and colorectal cancer screening. Screening may be: **uniphasic**, where one screening test is used, for example, a blood test for cholesterol; **multiphasic**, for example, screening for colorectal cancer where a preliminary filter test, such as the faecal occult blood test, identifies a subgroup at higher risk, and for whom further screening (colonoscopy/sigmoidoscopy) is recommended. Multiphasic is also used to indicate multiple screening tests used on the same occasion.

Opportunistic screening is also prescriptive but involves screening for a risk factor or disease when an individual presents for another reason; one example is when the opportunity to screen for raised blood pressure is taken during a routine visit to the general practitioner. Screening can be further categorized as **selective**, if confined to individuals at high risk of a particular disease, or **mass**, if offered to the general public.

A few examples of the wide range of screening tests used in preventive medical practice are shown in Box 5.1. Detailed discussion of screening services available in the USA is to be found elsewhere (Anon 2010).

Principles

Screening can be introduced at any phase of the natural history of a disease; whether this interrupts the natural progression of the disease depends on the speed of progression and other important characteristics of the natural history. Fig. 5.1 shows stages at which screening tests can be performed that relate particularly to cancers, but are relevant for all diseases. Screening is a preventive activity, as illustrated previously in Chapter 1 (Fig. 1.4), where primary, secondary, and tertiary prevention are described. Screening activities can thus be categorized depending on whether or not the disease has started (primary), become detectable by the screening test (secondary), or become clinically manifest (tertiary). In practice, screening tests usually aim either: to prevent the occurrence of detectable disease (as in the case of screening for risk factors for coronary heart disease, such as hypertension or high blood cholesterol); or to detect an asymptomatic

disease (as in the case of secondary prevention of the complications of diabetes, or of early breast cancers). In practice, it can be difficult sometimes to distinguish adequately between primary and secondary prevention in screening tests, because the natural history of diseases offer a wide spectrum of possibilities. For example, cervical cancer screening aims to detect a premalignant stage of disease and thus prevent development of a cancer. With the increased knowledge of genes, there is some scope for identification of high-risk individuals using genetic markers.

5.2 Evaluation

Screening has considerable potential for the detection of pre-symptomatic disease but it was recognized early in medical screening that new screening tests should be fully evaluated before their general introduction. This is important as the screening may be associated with more harm than benefits to patients and may not be suitable or cost-effective for all potential beneficiaries. Wilson and Jugner (1968) proposed a set of criteria to be used when evaluating screening programmes, particularly prescriptive programmes, where there is implied benefit for an individual. These have been recently modified and updated by others (Box 5.2).

The first requirement is that the condition should be a serious health problem but this may change over time. For example, in the UK, chest X-rays were introduced in the 1950s to screen the general population for tuberculosis and this helped to reduce the considerable public health burden of the disease. However, X-ray screening for TB is no longer used as the incidence of the disease in the population has diminished markedly so it is no longer a major public health problem. The same programme was then adapted to screen for lung cancer but was found to be ineffective, as lung cancers were usually too advanced when detected (see Chapter 8). But recent evidence has prompted the National Comprehensive Cancer Network, USA, to recommend low-dose CT scanning in older long-term smokers (Aberle et al. 2011) although this has sparked debate as the results of another large screening trial were negative (Oken et al. 2011).

Box 5.1 Screening tests in preventive medical practice

Mandatory	Prescriptive	Opportunistic (often in primary care)
Cardiovascular and optical examination for heavy-goods vehicle (HGV) drivers, airline pilots, train drivers, etc.	**Antenatal care** Urinalysis: glucose, protein, blood, etc.	Blood pressure Blood cholesterol Blood glucose
Donor blood tested for hepatitis B, HIV, syphilis, etc.	Blood analysis: haemoglobin, full blood count (FBC), etc.	Body weight/height (body mass index)
Occupational health monitoring in workers exposed to asbestos, X-rays, lead, carcinogens, etc.	Infectious diseases: rubella, syphilis, HIV, hepatitis B	
	Blood pressure Fetal ultrasound	
	Post-natal care Neonatal blood tests for phenylketonuria, hypothyroidism, etc.	
	Selective screening Tonometry in relatives of glaucoma patients	
	Women's health Cervical smear Mammography	

Most conditions or diseases that have important consequences for the individual or for the health of others can be viewed as eligible for consideration for preventive screening tests. As noted earlier, mandatory tests are designed to protect others and may not benefit the individual being tested. Difficulties have arisen for screening programmes for some diseases, such as prostate cancer, which demonstrates a wide range of invasiveness. It has an estimated prevalence of 55 per cent in men in their fifth decade of life and 64 per cent in the seventh; most of these malignancies remain localized and do not present clinically (Haas 2007).

The screening test should ideally be cheap, quick to administer, and acceptable. It should be *reliable*, i.e. produce the same result if repeated. It should also be **valid**, i.e. good at discriminating those who have the disease from those who do not. Similar remarks also apply to tests used for clinical diagnosis (see section 5.3) except that, for clinical diagnostic tests, whereas diagnostic power is clearly important, the issue of cost and acceptability is less important than in mass screening in public health practice.

The choice of cut-off points for continuously distributed variables such as blood pressure, or intra-ocular pressure, must be carefully considered, as all those screened must be categorized into either positive or negative for further investigation. If the cut-off is too low then too many subjects will be counted as positive and vice versa. This is critical to the issue of **sensitivity** and **specificity** in public health and clinical practice, and in laboratory medicine.

Validity, or the accuracy of a test, is measured using sensitivity and specificity. The sensitivity of a test is the measure of its ability to detect disease when present. A highly sensitive test has no or very few missed cases

Box 5.2 Requirements for a screening programe

The condition

- This should be an important health problem.
- The natural history of the disease including latent disease should be adequately understood and risk groups identified.
- There is a recognizable pre-disease or early symptomatic stage.

The test

- Should be safe, simple, effective, valid, and acceptable.
- A suitable cut-point for the test value should be agreed in the target population.

The treatment

- Should be effective and lead to better outcome and improved survival with earlier intervention.
- Facilities exist for diagnosis and treatment.

The screening programme

- Evidence should be available from RCTs that the programme is effective in reducing mortality and morbidity.
- The benefit from the screening programme should outweigh the possible physical and psychological harm caused by the test, diagnostic procedures, and treatment.
- The costs should be considered in the context of other demands for resources.

Modified from: UK National Screening Committee (2003): http://www.nsc.nhs.uk/.

(**false negatives**). Specificity measures the ability to identify healthy people as such (non-diseased), and therefore there are few **false positives**. These definitions are shown in Box 5.3.

For serious diseases, screening tests should clearly have a high sensitivity, preferably close to 100 per cent, so that few cases are missed. However, the specificity, which reflects the percentage of false positives, will only be consequential if further procedures are indicated for a screenee; for example, in the case of positive mammography, needle biopsy will be necessary, which will create anxiety during the waiting period.

In the case of **continuous variables**, such as blood pressure, plasma cholesterol, and **body mass index**, the choice of the cut-point to define hypertension, high blood cholesterol, and overweight or obesity will be critical in determining the 'sensitivity' and 'specificity' of the risk factor test for predicting future disease or non-disease (see Table 3.1 and Chapters 7 and 9). Risk factor cut-off points can only be accurately determined from large-scale observational studies, reinforced, where possible, by randomized controlled trials (RCTs), because the diseases may take years to present clinically. Hypertension provides a recent example of this, as the World Health Organization and US, European, and UK medical societies recommended that the threshold for hypertension be lowered from 160/95 mmHg to 140/90 mmHg (see Chapter 7).

Two other measures are used to evaluate screening tests. These depend on the **prevalence** of the disease in the population and use the row values rather than the column values in Box 5.3: the **positive predictive value (PPV)** measures the ability of the test to correctly diagnose the disease; and the **negative predictive value (NPV)** the ability of the test to correctly identify absence of disease. Diseases with a high prevalence will have a higher chance of correctly testing positive than those with a low prevalence for any given level of sensitivity and specificity (see Table 5.1).

Examination of the formulae in Box 5.3 and the examples in Tables 5.1 show that sensitivity and specificity are based on the test results only, whereas positive and negative predictive values are based on the numbers with disease. Predictive values of screening tests are more directly relevant to patients or screened subjects than are sensitivity and specificity, which are principally used by epidemiologists in their evaluation of screening tests.

Given a relatively high sensitivity and specificity for a particular test, PPV increases rapidly with a higher prevalence of disease. The PPV is also known as the *yield* for a particular test and, in clinical and public health practice, screening tests clearly provide a greater yield in 'high-risk' groups, which have a higher initial prevalence of disease compared with that in the general population.

Box 5.3 Indices used to evaluate accuracy of a screening or diagnostic test

Test result	Disease present	Disease absent
Positive	True positive (**TP**)	False positive (**FP**)
Negative	False negative (**FN**)	True negative (**TN**)

Sensitivity: percentage of positive results in those with disease $= \dfrac{TP}{TP+FN} \times 100\%$

Specificity: percentage of negative results in those without disease $= \dfrac{TN}{FP+TN} \times 100\%$

Positive predictive value: percentage of correct results in those with a positive test result $= \dfrac{TP}{TP+FP} \times 100\%$

Negative predictive value: percentage of true negative results in those with negative results $= \dfrac{TN}{TN+FN} \times 100\%$

Table 5.1 Positive and negative predictive values for screening tests in diseases with a high and a low prevalence

	Disease		Total
Low prevalence disease (1%)	Present	Absent	
Positive screening test	1.8 (TP)	39.6 (FP)	41.4
Negative screening test	0.2 (FN)	158.4 (TN)	158.6
Total	2	198	200

$$\text{Positive predictive value} = \frac{1.8}{41.4} \times 100\% = 4.3\%$$

$$\text{Negative predictive value} = \frac{158.4}{158.6} \times 100\% = 99.9\%$$

	Disease		Total
High prevalence disease (20%)	Present	Absent	
Positive screening test	36 (TP)	32 (FP)	68
Negative screening test	4 (FN)	128 (TN)	132
Total	40	160	200

$$\text{positive predictive value} = \frac{36}{68} \times 100\% = 52.9\%$$

$$\text{Negative predictive value} = \frac{128}{132} \times 100\% = 97.0\%$$

For both sets results sensitivity of screening test = 90%; specificity = 80%

Issue	Question
Abnormality	Is the patient sick or well?
Diagnosis	How accurate are tests used to diagnose disease?
Frequency	How often does a disease occur?
Risk	What factors are associated with an increased risk of disease?
Prognosis	What are the consequences of having a disease?
Treatment	How does treatment change the course of disease?
Prevention	Does an intervention on well people keep disease from arising? Does early detection and treatment improve the course of disease?
Cause	What conditions lead to disease? What are the pathogenic mechanisms of disease?
Cost	How much will care for an illness cost?

Reproduced from Fletcher, R. H., Fletcher, S. W. and Wagner, E. H. (1996). *Clinical Epidemiology. The Essentials* (3rd edn) with permission from Lippincott, Williams and Wilkins.

5.3 Clinical epidemiology and clinical diagnosis

One simple definition of clinical epidemiology is: *epidemiology in patient populations rather than general populations*. Fletcher *et al.* (1996) extended this definition to include all aspects of **clinical decision-making** and have formulated the main clinical questions that fall within the remit of clinical epidemiology (see Box 5.4).

All these clinical questions could be equally applied to the general population; but in this chapter we will confine the discussion to that concerning the diagnosis of disease. Firstly, in the case of simple categorical tests (that is, disease present/absent) such as radiological

detection of tumours or magnetic resonance imaging (MRI), opportunities exist for observer variation. If there are systematic differences in interpretation (inter-observer variation) this will result in **observer bias**, but even 'random' differences in interpretation will lead to lower levels of diagnostic certainty. 'Random' differences of recategorization by individual observers is known as intra-observer variation. Fletcher *et al.* (1996) describe a study of MRI assessment of prolapsed intervertebral disease, which 'blinded' radiologists as to whether or not a subject had symptoms of back pain or was a healthy volunteer. Prolapsed or protruding discs were found in about two-thirds of asymptomatic subjects, a very similar proportion to that in symptomatic patients, indicating that MRI was unhelpful, at least in the initial clinical diagnosis.

For laboratory tests in immunology and biochemistry, the results are usually computed as quantitative variables. It is clearly important for new tests to establish a **normal range** (mean ± two standard deviations) in a large, unselected population encompassing healthy subjects from both genders, a wide range of social groups, and even different ethnic groups. 'Normal ranges' often differ by age, sex, and ethnic group and are often presented accordingly. It should be noted that laboratory tests often are not normally distributed (see Chapter 3) and logarithmic or other transformations may be required to approximate 'normality'. Of critical importance is the choice of cut-point. Gerstman (1999) has provided an example from serological testing for exposure to HIV by using three different cut-off points to define positive test (Fig. 5.1a).

When the cut-point is set at position A there are no false negatives and sensitivity is 100 per cent. In position B there are both false positives and false negatives (the usual situation in practice). In position C there are no false positives and the specificity is 100 per cent.

Two-stage screening is becoming more common and Fig. 5.1b provides such an example in the case of postnatal testing for cystic fibrosis in the UK. Here again the choice of cut-points is critical to the sensitivity and specificity of the first stage test.

Receiver operator characteristic (ROC) curves can be used to define a suitable cut-point by plotting

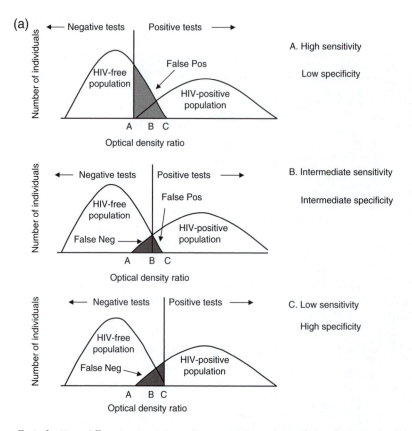

Figure 5.1 (a) The effect of setting different cut-points on the sensitivity and specificity of an enzyme-linked immunosorbent assay (ELISA) for HIV.
Adapted from Gerstmann BB (1999) *Epidemiology Kept Simple. An Introduction to Classic and Modern Epidemiology*, with permission from Wiley-Liss.

the sensitivity (the true positive rate) against the false positive rate (1-specificity). These curves are particularly useful for comparing two different laboratory tests that both attempt to diagnose the same clinical entity. Fig. 5.2 shows the level of diagnostic certainty for clinically confirmed congestive heart failure obtained using plasma levels of four different cardiac peptides (produced by cardiac endothelium in response to cardiac dilatation). The comparative standard for this test was heart size on radiography. Currently echocardiography would be more likely to provide a higher level of diagnostic certainty (see Chapter 7).

In this example, the cardiac peptide BNP performs better than other cardiac peptides in the prediction of a clinical diagnosis of congestive heart failure.

Both diagnostic testing and clinical interventions fall under the general remit of **health technology assessment**. This broad area of study can be considered an important component of evidence-based medicine (Chapter 6). The systematic quantitative use of external evidence using **Bayes' theorem** in health technology assessment is discussed in detail elsewhere (Spiegelhalter *et al.* 2000). Bayes' theorem is particularly appropriate for this area of work, and for clinical decision-making in general (see Chapter 6), as it incorporates the prevalence of the particular disease into the calculations of the predicted risk (**odds**) of a true result: the higher the prevalence of the disease, the greater the probability that a positive test result will represent true disease.

(b)

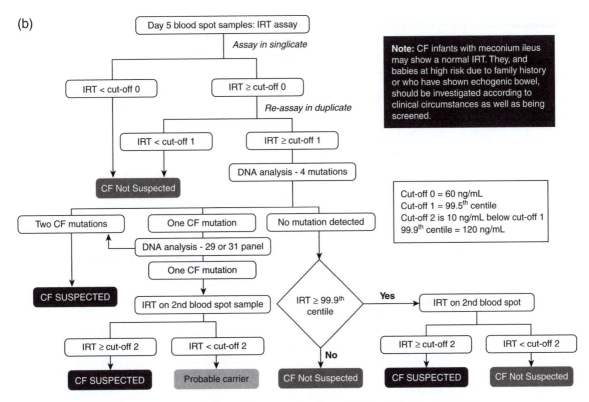

Day 5 blood spot samples: IRT assay

Assay in singlicate

Note: CF infants with meconium ileus may show a normal IRT. They, and babies at high risk due to family history or who have shown echogenic bowel, should be investigated according to clinical circumstances as well as being screened.

IRT < cut-off 0 | IRT ≥ cut-off 0

Re-assay in duplicate

IRT < cut-off 1 | IRT ≥ cut-off 1

DNA analysis - 4 mutations

CF Not Suspected

Cut-off 0 = 60 ng/mL
Cut-off 1 = 99.5th centile
Cut-off 2 is 10 ng/mL below cut-off 1
99.9th centile = 120 ng/mL

Two CF mutations | One CF mutation | No mutation detected

DNA analysis - 29 or 31 panel

One CF mutation

CF SUSPECTED

IRT on 2nd blood spot sample

IRT ≥ 99.9th centile   **Yes** →   IRT on 2nd blood spot

IRT ≥ cut-off 2 | IRT < cut-off 2 | **No** | IRT ≥ cut-off 2 | IRT < cut-off 2

CF SUSPECTED | Probable carrier | CF Not Suspected | CF SUSPECTED | CF Not Suspected

Figure 5.1 (b) Algorithm and cut points for two-stage screening for cystic fibrosis in neonates in UK. Reproduced with permission from Newborn Screening Programme Centre **www.newbornbloodspot.screening.nhs.uk.**

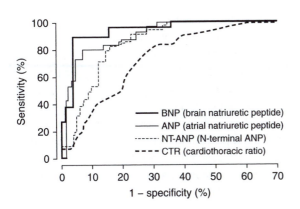

Figure 5.2 Receiver operating characteristic curves for natriuretic peptides and cardiothoracic ratio in the prediction of clinically confirmed congestive heart failure. Reproduced from Cowie MR, Struthers AD, Wood DA, *et al.* (1997) 'Value of Natriuretic Peptides in Assessment of Patients with Possible New Heart Failure in Primary Care'. *The Lancet* **350,** 1347–51 with permission from Elsevier.

(Figure 5.2 legend: BNP (brain natriuretic peptide); ANP (atrial natriuretic peptide); NT-ANP (N-terminal ANP); CTR (cardiothoracic ratio). Axes: Sensitivity (%) vs 1 – specificity (%))

5.4 Screening for cancers

Survival from cancer is linked with the stage of the cancer at diagnosis. Early detection of a tumour raises the possibility of intervention and cure, and new screening tests are being developed for this, which require full evaluation. Stages at which screening may be introduced into the natural history of cancer are shown in Fig. 5.3.

Critical time points that are invariably approximate and variable between individuals are T_0, at which the screening test is capable of detecting asymptomatic disease, T_1, the average time of clinical presentation, and T_2, the time in practice when a screening test detects preclinical disease. Definitions that stem from these time points are shown in Fig. 5.3.

Very small tumours are unlikely to be detected by conventional radiological techniques unless metabolites, which can be 'tagged', accumulate in the tumour. Biochemical tests for secretory products of tumours are often evaluated as potential markers (see Chapter 17).

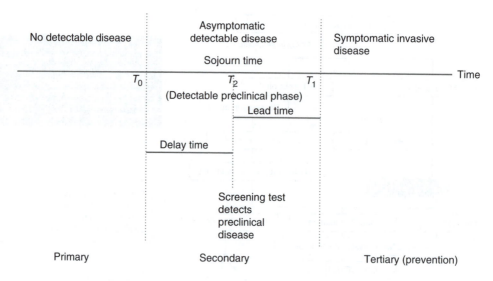

T_0 – Tumour potentially detectable by screening test
T_1 – Tumour detectable clinically
T_2 – Actual date of detection by screening test

Figure 5.3 Interval and non-interval cancer: relationship to screening examinations.
Adapted from Vainio H and Bianchini F (2002). *Breast Cancer Screening. IARC Handbook of Cancer Prevention* (vol. 7) with permission from IARC Press.

Mutations of certain genes, such as *p53*, *BRCA1*, and *BRCA2*, are associated with a high risk of cancers (Chapter 17), but have a low prevalence in the general population. Apart from tamoxifen (Cuzick *et al.* 2007) effective non-surgical interventions are currently lacking. Prophylactic mastectomy is a surgical intervention occasionally chosen by women with *BRCA1/2* to prevent development of breast cancer. Another problem is a wide variation in the natural history and invasiveness of cancers with varying rates in malignant development or conversion of pre-cancerous cells, for example, cervical and prostatic cancers.

Particular issues in the evaluation of screening tests for cancer are as follows.

Frequency of testing

If the period between tests (the screening interval) is too long, disease may develop between them. Such cancers are called *interval cancers*, and are made up of the following types of case:

● false negatives, i.e. the screening test failed to detect the cancer;

● cases in people who did not attend for follow-up investigation;

● true interval cases which appear *de novo* and usually represent fast-growing tumours.

Screening frequency has to take account of the costs and benefits of more versus less screening. For example, screening every five years for cervical cancer will reduce the incidence of disease by 84 per cent, every three years by 91 per cent and, annually by 93 per cent. But screening annually, as opposed to every three years, trebles the cost of the programme with only a two per cent reduction in disease (Eddy 1990). In Fig. 5.4 halving the screening interval would have detected one more interval cancer, but still fails to detect two interval cancers.

Lead time bias

Effective screening, by definition, leads to earlier diagnosis of disease, and consequently, a longer period between diagnosis and death, or longer survival. However, early diagnosis may not prolong the date of death,

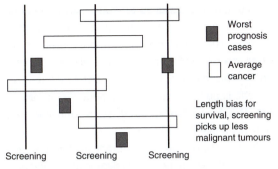

Worst prognosis cases

Average cancer

Length bias for survival, screening picks up less malignant tumours

Screening   Screening   Screening

Four non-interval, slow growing cancers detected.
One interval, rapid growing cancer detected.

Figure 5.4 Interval and non-interval cancer: relationship to screening examinations.

and it is important to consider this when comparing screened and non-screened groups for differences in outcome such early diagnosis without changing the date of death is called **lead time bias**, this cannot be measured directly except in RCTs and, therefore, adjustment for this bias is liable to error. The implication of lead time bias is that it is not possible to distinguish between bias and real benefits of screening using observed case survival data only, such as those routinely obtained from cancer registries (see Chapters 2 and 17). The difficulty in evaluating *observational* data on prostate cancer in the USA, where testing for prostate-specific antigen (PSA) has been widely used for many years, has been reported elsewhere (Shaw *et al.* 2004). Currently, there is debate on the contribution of mammographic breast cancer screening to the marked reduction in mortality from breast cancer (Autier *et al.* 2011). It is important that with improvements in treatment that the value of screening is continually monitored. The reduced cost-effectiveness of screening for TB following its reduced prevalence is a case in point and screening for testicular cancer is not advocated as there is no suitable test, but also because treatments are very successful even for late stage disease.

Length bias

Length bias, which is also influenced by the screening interval, is another major potential source of bias when examining survival rates in the context of screening. The detection of cancers by screening is generally considered

a success especially if they can be completely removed or treated. However, if these were slower growing and less malignant tumours that may never otherwise have been detected, cause symptoms, or disease, this would not represent a success and is potentially harmful to patients. It is this issue, related to the progress of ductal carcinoma *in situ*, that has sparked the recent debates over the effectiveness or otherwise of breast screening. The difference between slow and fast growing cancers may be detected by histological grading of the tumour. In contrast, those cases presenting between screens (interval cancers) tend to have a worse prognosis than those picked up at screening. The benefits and potential harms associated with breast screening have been reviewed recently in detail (Anon 2012).

Selection bias

Case-control studies of screening have problems with selection bias. In a practical example, invitations to a screening programme may result in a 70 per cent acceptance, but those who accept may have a different risk than the general population. For example, if the risk in those who accept the rest is 0.8 and the 30 per cent refusers have a higher underlying risk at 1.5. The refusers therefore will contribute 45 per cent (30 per cent × 1.5) of the cases, and the acceptors will contribute 55 per cent (0.8 × 70 per cent) of the cases. An evaluation may find that there is a reduction in disease among those who attend for screening (45 per cent of cases in 70 per cent of the population) but would fail to detect the effect of the 45 per cent of cases who were not screened.

Will Rogers phenomenon

The importance of the role of changing diagnostic tools in screening is illustrated by the 'Will Rogers phenomenon'. Will Rogers is reported to have said; 'When the Okies left Oklahoma and moved to California they raised the average intelligence level in both states'. The Will Rogers effect raises issues of reliability of stage-adjusted survival over time, and it is important to consider this in view of ongoing technological advances. In a disease with four defined stages, for example, lung cancer, patients are allocated into these four categories using chest X-ray, stage 4 being the worst disease. If a newer and better diagnostic tool is discovered, for example, scanning with computed tomography (CT), it is likely that some of the stage 1 cases will be discovered to have more widespread disease than was previously thought, and they will be moved from stage 1 to stage 2. This will result in an improved survival of stage 1 as they lose their worst cases to stage 2. Stage 2 will get some less severe cases previously categorized as stage 1, and the worst stage 2 cases will become stage 3 on CT scan, so the prognosis for stage 2 cases will improve. The same happens with stage 3, whereas stage 4 gets some of the old stage 3, which had a better prognosis. Thus each stage has improved survival but the overall survival is the same (Feinstein *et al.* 1985).

The problems encountered in evaluating the effectiveness of treatments from routinely collected cancer registration and survival data are summarized in Box 5.5.

Negative aspects of screening

Routine screening tests can also have some negative consequences as well as potential benefits. Some of these can be predicted from the list of requirements in Box 5.2. Mandatory tests may not benefit an individual;

Box 5.5 Problems in the interpretation of trends in cancer survival

Observed improvements in survival may come about for the following reasons:

- There is early detection and better cure rates reflected by changes in stage.
- It may be the result of lead time bias, length bias and/or selection bias.
- It may be the effect of improvements in treatment or a change in the disease.
- It may reflect a change in the available information, for example, new diagnostic methods.

indeed, they are designed to protect others and may prevent an individual taking up a particular occupation, or continuing to work in it, or from donating blood. The disease screened for may have no suitable treatment, and for this reason screening for several mature-onset genetic conditions, such as Huntington's disease, is not recommended except to advise on future parenting or to allow planning of care.

For prescriptive screening, problems for screenees can arise if they are tested as false-positives and have to undergo further testing and unnecessary anxiety. Test specificity is the issue here; and for some common tests, such as mammography, it is sufficiently low as to create a sizeable proportion of false-positives. For some large screening programmes, testing false-positive has been shown to affect participation in subsequent routine testing in future years.

For screening tests with continuous distributions there is the problem of the choice of cut-point. This will determine the specificity and sensitivity of a particular test and, for risk factors such as hypertension or cholesterol which are classified as 'borderline raised' on testing, such results can create a group of 'worried well' individuals. Adequate communication about the level of risk, and the significance of the results to a screenee by health professionals should reduce the possibility of this outcome, which has been investigated only to a limited extent in research studies.

In the following worked examples we have used the framework provided in Box 5.2 to evaluate screening proposals. First, we examine the case for prostate cancer, screening. The prostate-specific antigen (PSA) blood test has provided a method which in many areas has been used as a screening test. Secondly, we discuss colorectal cancer screening. Then we examine screening for Down's syndrome during the antenatal period.

5.5 Case studies

1 Should we screen for prostate cancer?

Is the disease an important health problem?

Yes, prostate cancer causes 12.6 per cent of male cancer deaths in the UK. It is a disease primarily of older men: 56 per cent are aged 70 years and over at

diagnosis. There is an increasing detection of cases, and death rates are rising. It is a disease that will assume increasing significance as the population ages.

Is the natural history known?

Post-mortem study show that latent prostate cancer is found in up to 29 per cent of males with a median age of 64 years, and it increases with age (Haas 2007). Most latent tumours do not become life threatening, but some evolve into invasive tumours.

Is there a recognizable latent early symptomatic stage?

Many cases of prostate cancer are clinically silent, the likelihood of a tumour progressing or metastasizing is highly variable, and the disease outcome is uncertain. There are two main tests for detecting prostate cancer: digital rectal examination, which is prone to inter-examiner variability, and the PSA blood test, which may also be raised in benign hypertrophy, prostate inflammation, and after prostate surgery. There is no uniform standard for this test so results between laboratories and countries are not comparable. It is recognized that using these tests risks treating non-aggressive tumours. It has been reported that 1410 men would need to be screened and 48 treated for prostate cancer in order to save one death from prostate cancer (Schröder et al. 2009).

Table 5.2 compares the validity measures of the two available screening tests for prostate cancer.

These data suggest that the sensitivity, specificity, and yield (PPV) of digital rectal examination as a screening test are low at PSA levels under 4.0 ng/mL. In this study up to 65 per cent of 'cancers' were missed by digital rectal examination and ultrasonography at PSA levels between 2.0 and 4.0 ng/mL, but these 'cancers' may have a more favourable prognosis than those in subjects with higher PSA levels. Elsewhere it has been shown that 15 per cent of men with a PSA measure < 4 ng/mL will have

a malignant prostate cancer when biopsied (Thompson et al. 2004). Men with low-grade prostate cancers have a minimal risk of dying from prostate cancer during 20 years of follow-up, and should not receive aggressive treatment (Albertson et al. 2005). However, men with high grade prostate cancer and who received no treatment had a high probability (40–80 per cent depending on age) of dying from prostate cancer within 10 years (Albertson et al. 2005). The difficulty is in predicting which men have low-grade and which high-grade disease.

Is there an effective treatment?

Treatments for prostate cancer are 'watchful waiting' with regular reviews of PSA levels, radiotherapy, surgery, and palliative hormonal therapy. It is still not clear if surgery or radiotherapy is a better treatment option for men than watchful waiting particularly when cancer is localized and has been detected through screening (Hoffman 2011). Radiotherapy and surgery are not without side effects; for example, several studies report that impotence is still present in 15–51 per cent of surgical patients, and some degree of incontinence is found in 4–72 per cent of patients at 18 months' follow-up (Selly et al. 1997). There is a 14 per cent relapse rate for early tumours seven years after surgical treatment or radiotherapy. After 15 years' follow-up, neither stage nor treatment was found to be predictive of outcome, perhaps because patients are generally old at time of diagnosis (50 per cent of cases are 70 years or over when diagnosed) (Selly et al. 1997).

Does early diagnosis improve survival?

Survival from prostate cancer is strongly related to the stage of disease at diagnosis. The five-year relative

Table 5.2 Evaluation of the digital rectal examination for prostate cancer (verified by biopsy) at two ranges of prostate-specific antigen (PSA)

PSA cut-point	Sensitivity (%)	Specificity (%)	PPV (%)	NPV (%)
<3.0 ng/mL	62	42	0.9	55
<4.0 ng/mL	50	54	16	86

Adapted from: Postma R and Schröder FH (2005) 'Screening for Prostate Cancer'. *European Journal of Cancer*, **41**, 825–33 with permission from Elsevier.
PPV: positive predictive value; NPV: negative predictive value

(continued)

survival for clinically detected cancer confined to the prostate is 77 per cent without systematic screening in the UK. If the disease is widespread, with bony metastases, five-year relative survival is about 30 per cent (South West Public Health Observatory 2008).

The UK National Screening Committee does not recommend screening for prostate cancer but there is evidence that many doctors use PSA testing as a screening tool (Gavin *et al.* 2004). A population-based randomized trial for prostate cancer screening has shown a 20% reduction in prostate cancer mortality but was associated with a high risk of over diagnosis (Schröder *et al.* 2009). A similar trial in the USA failed to demonstrate a benefit of screening (Andriole 2012).

2 Colorectal cancer screening

Colorectal cancer is the third most common cause of cancer death worldwide (Ferlay *et al.* 2008) with the incidence rising in most countries. Tackling the growing burden of this cancer has therefore become a priority for public health bodies. Patients with colorectal cancer that is detected and treated at an early stage have five-year survival rates exceeding 90 per cent, compared with survival rates of less than 10 per cent for patients with metastatic disease (Cancer Research UK 2010). The vast majority of colorectal cancer is thought to develop from adenomatous polyps within the bowel (Ballinger and Anggiansah 2007). Adenomatous polyps are thought to progress over time in size, and severity, and may eventually develop into invasive cancer. The symptoms of colorectal cancer can include altered bowel habit, rectal bleeding, and weight loss. Many patients however have no gastrointestinal symptoms and present with unexplained anaemia. Polyps that are detected during colonoscopic examination of the bowel can usually be safely removed endoscopically without the need for surgery. The detection of bowel polyps or early colorectal cancer forms the basis of colorectal cancer screening programmes. Various methods of screening for colorectal cancer have been studied although the most widely used are faecal occult blood testing, flexible sigmoidoscopy, or colonoscopy. The main screening methods are summarized in Box 5.6.

Box 5.6 Main methods of screening for colorectal cancers and advantages and disadvantages

Test	Description	Advantages	Disadvantages
Faecal occult blood testing	Tests stool for the presence of blood; colonoscopy performed in patients that initially test positive	Initial FOB test inexpensive and non-invasive Easy to perform	Uptake may be variable due to patient preference Poor sensitivity
Colonoscopy	Endoscopic examination of the entire large bowel	Less risk of missing proximal lesions High sensitivity	Relatively costly Small procedure-related morbidity
Flexible sigmoidoscopy	Endoscopic examination of the distal large bowel	Easier to perform than colonoscopy Less procedure-related morbidity than colonoscopy	Unable to identify proximal lesions
Virtual colonoscopy	Uses X-ray CT to construct 3-dimensional views of the colon	Non-invasive No sedation required	Exposes patient to ionizing radiation Unable to biopsy or remove polyps

Table 5.3 Estimated performance characteristics of different colorectal cancer screening strategies

Screening test	Sensitivity for CRC (%)	Sensitivity for advanced adenomas (%)	Specificity for CRC (%)	Specificity for advanced adenomas (%)
FOBT				
gFOBT	11–64	11–41	91–98	n.a.
iFOBT	56–89	27–56	91–97	n.a.
Flex sig	60–70	50–81	60–70	50–80
Colonoscopy	95	95	95–99	90–95

Flex sig, flexible sigmoidoscopy; advanced adenomas, adenomas with high-grade dysplasia, villous components or size <9 mm; n.a., not applicable; FOBT, faecal occult blood test; gFOBT—Guiac; IFOBT—immunochemical.
Reproduced from Bretthauer M (2011) 'Colorectal cancer screening'. *Journal of Internal Medicine* **270** (2), 87–98, with permission from John Wiley & Sons.

The best method of screening is the subject of ongoing research (Atkin *et al*. 2010). Variation in the design of screening studies has made it difficult to identify the optimum screening modality or strategy. The method used to screen for colorectal cancer varies worldwide mainly due to differences in screening costs, resource capacity, and population preferences. In the UK, the bowel cancer screening programme was phased in gradually from 2006 and the target age group varies slightly between regions. In England individuals aged between 60 and 69 years are invited for screening with a biennial faecal occult blood test followed by colonoscopy for individuals that have a positive initial screening test (NHS BCSP 2011). The faecal occult blood test is used in the knowledge that bowel polyps or colorectal cancer may bleed (Hewitson *et al*. 2007). Although there is debate about the optimal screening test, several randomized controlled trials have demonstrated that screening is effective at reducing bowel cancer incidence and mortality (Bretthauer 2011); although no single method has emerged as the most cost-effective (Lansdorp-Vogelaar *et al*. 2010). The performance of the available screening strategies is shown in Table 5.3.

Questions

1 What are the main factors that may influence the effectiveness of a colorectal cancer screening programme?

2 How would you set up a study to investigate the value of colorectal cancer screening?

3 Describe how forms of bias may influence the results of studies evaluating colorectal cancer screening?

3 Screening for Down's syndrome

Down's syndrome is caused by an extra chromosome 21 (occasionally only part of an extra chromosome 21), thus the name trisomy 21. The extra chromosome is usually of maternal origin. This syndrome is characterized by learning disability (mild to severe), developmental delay, and characteristic facial features, and is often associated with cardiac anomalies and duodenal atresia, and hearing, ophthalmic, and respiratory problems. In high-income countries, many children with Down's syndrome can expect to live semi-independent lives as adults, and to live beyond 50 years of age, but are at higher risk of developing dementia. In low-income countries, childhood survival is very low.

The risk of having a baby with Down's syndrome increases with maternal age. For mothers under 30 years of age, the risk is approximately 0.7 per 1000 births. At 30–34 years, the average risk increases to 1.5 per 1000 births, and above the age of 35 years the average risk is

(continued)

around six per 1000; at age 44 years the risk is approximately 34 per 1000, but it seems risk does not continue to increase in mothers older than 45 years (Morris *et al.* 2003). These risks are based on births; risk figures would be much higher if we included spontaneous abortions, as there is a high fetal loss rate. Very similar risks have been reported across different populations in the world. Note that the term 'risk' here is used in the epidemiological sense, whereas in everyday language, organizations representing persons with Down's syndrome and their families such as the UK Down's Syndrome Association recommend using the term 'chance' rather than 'risk'.

In many countries, prenatal diagnosis of Down's syndrome gives the mother the choice to terminate an affected pregnancy. In other countries (such as Ireland and Malta in Europe and a number of countries in South America and Africa) termination of pregnancy for fetal anomaly is illegal. Some mothers want prenatal diagnosis only so that they can be prepared before birth.

Because of the high risk associated with older maternal age, the first prenatal diagnosis programmes offered older mothers (above 35, 36, or 38 years depending on the country) a prenatal diagnostic test. Both chorionic villus sampling (first trimester) and amniocentesis (second trimester) can be used to look for the extra chromosome in a fetal sample. These are invasive methods which carry a small risk of miscarriage.

Since a large proportion of cases are born to mothers younger than 35 years (Table 5.4), prenatal screening strategies have been developed which identify higher risk mothers of any age to whom an invasive test can be offered. Screening strategies determine risk according to a combination of maternal age, multiple biochemical serum markers, and ultrasound markers (nuchal translucency). Choice of a screening test and associated risk cut-off point that categorizes mothers as higher or lower risk balances a number of different criteria: sensitivity (what proportion of cases are detected?), specificity (what proportion of unaffected pregnancies are correctly identified among the lower risk?), and how early in pregnancy the test can be carried out. Mothers may prefer earlier testing, but not if this is at the expense of sensitivity and specificity. Moreover, earlier testing means that some mothers will have actively to cope with a Down's syndrome diagnosis who would otherwise have lost this baby later as a spontaneous abortion.

Research developments in screening over the last two decades have been rapid. The other area of research has concerned the diagnostic test itself—in order to improve the speed with which a result is given, and in order to develop non-invasive methods which do not risk miscarriage and therefore lower the harm of a false-positive screening result. Rapid (1–3 day) limited karyotype analysis has become available which detects trisomy 21 and a few other major chromosomal anomalies. This test does not detect the full range of rarer chromosomal anomalies, but has the advantage of not raising the ethical and counselling dilemma of detecting chromosomal anomalies which are of unknown significance, or are compatible with a normal life (often otherwise going undetected). Recently, non-invasive testing has reached a stage where the sensitivity and specificity are not yet 100 per cent, but its use as an alternative screening method may be possible.

The UK National Screening Committee recommended in 2007 that screening programmes should provide a

Table 5.4 Proportion of births by maternal age in England and Wales 2010,[1] and standard prevalence[2] per 1000 births of Down's syndrome by maternal age

Maternal age	Births	Down's syndrome
	Number (%)	Prevalence per 1000 births
< 30	377,000 (52.2)	0.7
30–34	202,500 (28.0)	1.5
35+	143,500 (19.9)	6.0
All ages	723,000 (100.0)	2.0

[1] www.ons.gov.uk
[2] Includes: livebirths, stillbirths, and terminations of pregnancy.

detection rate for Down's syndrome of greater than 75 per cent of affected pregnancies with a false positive rate of less than 3 per cent in 2007 (Kumar and O'Brien 2004). By 2010 they recommended that this should rise to a detection rate of greater than 90 per cent of affected pregnancies with a false positive rate of less than 2 per cent. The risk cut-off point for distinguishing mothers into 'higher risk' and 'lower risk' categories associated with these recommendations is between 1 in 150 and 1 in 200 (i.e. between 6.7 per 1000 and 5 per 1000), equivalent to the risk for mothers aged 37–38 years.

There are a number of potential harms of screening to be considered. Since sensitivity is less than 100 per cent, mothers who have false negative screen results may have more difficulty coming to terms with the fact that their child is diagnosed with Down's syndrome at birth. Since specificity is less than 100 per cent, mothers who have false positive screen results run a small risk of miscarriage associated with invasive testing, and might go through a period of anxiety and uncertainty while they wait for diagnostic test results, which may affect bonding with the unborn child. Mothers may be unprepared for making decisions about termination of pregnancy after a diagnosis, and may at first be insufficiently informed about the quality of life they could expect for their child and their family. Highly trained prenatal counsellors are essential to facilitate informed decision-making by parents through non-directive counselling, both at the offer of screening and in communicating results of screening and diagnostic tests. There are also concerns regarding societal attitudes to disability and how these are reflected in the screening programme, and about the experience of mothers of children with Down's syndrome who choose not to undergo screening, or choose to continue a pregnancy despite the diagnosis. Others observe that the choices open to families depend on the level of support services they can expect, again a question of societal attitudes and priorities.

Question

4 To what extent do you think that screening for Down's syndrome fulfils the requirements for a screening programme in Box 5.2?

Web addresses

Cancer Research Campaign
http://info.cancerresearchuk.org/cancerstats/

UK National Screening Committee
www.screening.nhs.uk/

Public Health Genomics (PHG) Foundation
http://www.phgfoundation.org/

Calculation of the risk of Down's syndrome
http://www.wolfson.qmul.ac.uk/epm/screening/calcrisk.html

NHS Fetal anaomaly programme
www.fetalanomaly.screening.uk

US Preventive Services Taskforce (information on many diseases)
http://www.uspreventiveservicestaskforce.org/uspstopics.htm

Further reading

Fletcher RH, Fletcher SW, and Wagner EH (1996) *Clinical Epidemiology. The Essentials*, 3rd edn. Philadelphia: Lippincott, Williams and Wilkins.

Gerstmann BB (1999) *Epidemiology Kept Simple. An Introduction to Classic and Modern Epidemiology*. New York: Wiley-Liss.

References

Aberle DR, Adams AM, Berg CD, Black WC, *et al.* (2011) Reduced lung-cancer mortality with low-dose computed tomographic screening. *The New England Journal of Medicine* **365** (5), 395–409.

Albertsen PC, Hanley JA, and Fine J (2005) 20-year outcomes following conservative management of clinically localized prostate cancer. *JAMA* **293** (17), 2095–101.

Andriole GL, Crawford ED, Grubb RL 3rd, Buys SS, *et al.* (2012) Prostate screening in the randomized Prostate, Lung, Colorectal, and Ovarian Cancer Screening Trial: mortality results after 13 years of follow-up. *Journal of the National Cancer Institute* **104** (2), 125–32.

Anon (2012) The benefits and harms of breast cancer screening: an independent review. *Lancet* **380** (9855), 1778–86.

Anon (2010) PMID: 21850778. *The Guide to Clinical Preventive Services 2010–2011: Recommendations of the U.S. Preventive Services Task Force*. US Preventive Services Task Force Guides to Clinical Preventive Services. Rockville: Agency for Healthcare Research and Quality (US).

Atkin WS, Edwards R, Kralj-Hans I, Wooldrage K, *et al.* (2010) Once-only flexible sigmoidoscopy screening in prevention of colorectal cancer: a multicentre randomized controlled trial. *Lancet* **375** (9726), 1624–33.

Autier P, Boniol M, Gavin A, and Vatten LJ (2011) Breast cancer mortality in neighbouring European countries with different levels of screening but similar access to treatment: trend analysis of WHO mortality database. *BMJ (Clinical Research Ed)* **343** (4411).

Ballinger AB and Anggiansah C (2007) Colorectal cancer. *BMJ (Clinical Research Ed)* **335** (7622), 715–18.

Bretthauer M (2011) Colorectal cancer screening. *Journal of Internal Medicine* **270** (2), 87–98.

Cancer Research UK, 2010. Bowel cancer—survival statistics. Available at: http://info.cancerresearchuk.org/cancerstats/types/bowel/survival/#stage [Accessed: 11 November 2011].

Cowie MR, Struthers AD, Wood DA, Coats AJ, *et al.* (1997) Value of natriuretic peptides in assessment of patients with possible new heart failure in primary care. *Lancet* **350** (9088), 1349–53.

Cuzick J, Forbes JF, Sestak I, Cawthorn S, *et al.* (2007) Long-term results of tamoxifen prophylaxis for breast cancer—96-month follow-up of the randomized IBIS-I trial. *Journal of the National Cancer Institute* **99** (4), 272–82.

Eddy DM (1990) Screening for cervical cancer. *Annals of Internal Medicine* **113** (3), 214–26.

Feinstein AR, Sosin DM, and Wells CK (1985) The Will Rogers phenomenon. Stage migration and new diagnostic techniques as a source of misleading statistics for survival in cancer. *The New England Journal of Medicine* **312** (25), 1604–08.

Ferlay J, Shin HR, Bray F, Forman D, *et al.*, 2008 GLOBO-CAN 2008 v1.2, Cancer Incidence and Mortality World-wide: IARC Cancer Base No. 10 [Internet]. Lyon, France: International Agency for Research on Cancer; 2010. Available from: http://globocan.iarc.fr [Accessed: 25 January 2013]

Fletcher RH, Fletcher SW, and Wagner EH (1996). *Clinical Epidemiology. The Essentials*, 3rd edn. Philadelphia: Lippincott, Williams and Wilkins.

Gavin A, McCarron P, Middleton RJ, Savage G, *et al.* (2004) Evidence of prostate cancer screening in a UK region. *BJU International* **93** (6), 730–34.

Gerstmann BB (1999) *Epidemiology Kept Simple. An Introduction to Classic and Modern Epidemiology*. New York: Wiley-Liss.

Haas GP. Delongchamps NB, Jones RF, Chandan V, *et al.* (2007) Needle biopsies on autopsy prostates: sensitivity of cancer detection based on true prevalence. *Journal of the National Cancer Institute* **99** (19), 1484–9.

Hewitson P, Glasziou P, Irwig L, Towler B, *et al.* (2007) Screening for colorectal cancer using the faecal occult blood test, Hemoccult. *Cochrane Database of Systematic Reviews* (1), CD001216.

Hoffman RM (2011) Clinical practice. Screening for prostate cancer. *The New England Journal of Medicine* **365** (21), 2013–9.

Kumar S and O'Brien A (2004) Recent developments in fetal medicine. *BMJ (Clinical Research Ed)* **328** (7446), 1002–6.

Lansdorp-Vogelaar I, Knudsen AB and Brenner H (2010) Cost-effectiveness of colorectal cancer screening - an overview. *Best Practice & Research. Clinical Gastroenterology* **24** (4), 439–49.

Morris JK, Wald NJ, Mutton DE, and Alberman E (2003) Comparison of models of maternal age-specific risk for Down syndrome live births. *Prenatal Diagnosis* **23** (3), 252–8.

Oken MM, Hocking WG, Kvale PA, Andriole GL, *et al.* (2011) Screening by chest radiograph and lung cancer mortality: the Prostate, Lung, Colorectal, and Ovarian (PLCO) randomized trial. *JAMA* **306** (17), 1865–73.

Postma R and Schröder FH (2005) Screening for prostate cancer. *European Journal of Cancer* **41** (6), 825–33.

Selly S, Donovan J, Faulker A, Coast J, *et al.* (1997) Diagnosis, management and screening of early localized prostate cancer. *Health Technology Assessment* **1** (2), 1–96.

Shaw PA, Etzioni R, Zeliadt SB, Mariotto A, *et al.* (2004) An ecologic study of prostate-specific antigen screening and prostate cancer mortality in nine geographic areas of the United States. *American Journal of Epidemiology* **160** (11), 1059–69.

Schröder FH, Hugosson J, Roobol MJ, Tammela TLJ, *et al.* (2009) Screening and prostate-cancer mortality in a randomized European study. *The New England Journal of Medicine* **360** (13), 1320–28.

South West Public Health Observatory (2008) *Prostate Cancer Survival By Stage. Briefing 4*. Bristol: SWPHO.

Spiegelhalter DJ, Myles JP, Jones DR and Abrams KR (2000) Bayesian methods in health technology assessment: a review. *Health Technology Assessment* 4 (38), 1–130.

Thompson IM, Pauler DK, Goodman PJ, Tangen CM, *et al.* (2004) Prevalence of prostate cancer among men with a prostate-specific antigen level < or =4.0 ng per milliliter. *The New England Journal of Medicine* 350, 2239–46.

Vainio H and Bianchini F (2002) *Breast Cancer Screening. IARC Handbook of Cancer Prevention*, Vol. 7. Lyon, France: IARC Press.

Wilson JMG and Jugner G (1968) *Principles and Practice of Screening for Disease*. Geneva: WHO (Public Health Paper).

Answers to case studies questions

Question 1

Factors that may influence the effectiveness of a colorectal screening programme are:

- The uptake of the screening test within the population.
- The sensitivity of the screening test in identifying early cancers.
- The effectiveness of therapies to treat early cancer or polyps.

Question 2

- The study would aim to examine differences in clinical outcomes between colorectal cancer patients within a screened population and a similar non-screened population.

- Ethical approval and patient consent for screening would be required.
- The population would be clearly defined before the start of the study and monitored for a fixed time period in order to detect any differences in outcomes between the groups.
- There should be adequate resources for the screening test, any treatments and measurement of outcomes.
- Sufficient information should be provided to the public and health professionals about the study.

Question 3

Studies comparing survival in screened and non-screened patients may be susceptible to lead time bias and length bias. Lead time bias can occur where patients detected at screening are diagnosed at an earlier age than patients diagnosed outside of screening. When survival is calculated from age at cancer diagnosis there appears to be a survival benefit even if patients were to die at the same age.

Length bias occurs when screening detects slower growing and less aggressive tumours than those that present outside of screening. The screen detected patients have an improved survival due to the nature of their tumour rather than the effect of screening.

Question 4

The condition is an important health problem and non-invasive testing appears to be as reliable as many other similar tests. However, the only treatment options consist of counselling and possible abortion, which raises ethical issues for many parents given that the level of intellectual impairment etc. of children and adults with Down's syndrome is very variable.

6 Clinical epidemiology and evidence-based practice

MICHAEL CLARKE, KAREN BAILIE, SHEELAH CONNOLLY, AND LIAM MURRAY

CHAPTER CONTENTS

6.1 Clinical epidemiology

6.2 Evidence-based practice

6.3 Three case scenarios

6.4 Working with evidence-based health care

6.5 Economics of health care

This chapter provides a brief introduction to clinical epidemiology and an overview of the principles that guide the use of evidence in clinical and public health practice.

The elements of critical appraisal of research findings are illustrated through topical, health-related scenarios, and relevant published studies. These studies use the techniques of: (1) cross-sectional design (evaluation of a diagnostic test for venous thrombosis); (2) a randomized trial (solar disinfection of water to prevent diarrhoeal disease); and (3) systematic review (workplace smoking bans on employees' smoking habits). A practical guide including sources of evidence, critical appraisal, and the role of economic analysis is provided.

6.1 Clinical epidemiology

One simple definition of clinical epidemiology is: *epidemiology in patient populations rather than in general populations*. Fletcher *et al.* (1996), authors of a pioneering textbook in this area, stress that the discipline seeks to answer clinical questions, and to guide clinical decisions with the best available evidence. Clinical epidemiology thus utilizes most of the epidemiological tools and biostatistical methods described elsewhere in this book and is the cornerstone of evidence-based practice. Box 6.1 summarizes the main clinical questions that fall within its remit, and it is worth noting that the term 'clinical' does not restrict the scope to any particular areas of health care. The evidence-based approach to informed decision-making is relevant to all aspects of health care, many of which might not be regarded as 'clinical', covering prevention, diagnosis, treatment, and rehabilitation. The validation of diagnostic tests is reviewed in detail in Chapter 5 because such tests have much in common with those for population screening.

Box 6.1 Clinical questions in epidemiology

Issue	Question
Abnormality	Is the patient sick or well?
Diagnosis	How accurate are tests used to diagnose disease?
Frequency	How often does a disease occur?
Risk	What factors are associated with an increased risk of disease?
Prognosis	What are the consequences of having a disease?
Treatment	How does treatment change the course of disease?
Prevention	Does an intervention on well people keep disease from arising? Does early detection and treatment improve the course of disease?
Cause	What conditions lead to disease? What are the pathogenic mechanisms of disease?
Cost	How much will care for an illness cost?

Reproduced from Fletcher RH, Fletcher SE, and Wagner EH (1996) *Clinical Epidemiology. The Essentials*, with permission from Lippincott Williams and Wilkins.

Box 6.2 The five steps of evidence-based practice

1 Formulate a structured question.
2 Undertake an effective and efficient search for information.
3 Appraise the information gathered for relevance, validity, and usefulness.
4 Apply the information in practice, taking account of individual or population characteristics, preferences, and values.
5 Evaluate the impact of the information and the process on the patient, clinical practice and the service through self-appraisal and audit.

Reproduced from *Evidence-Based Medicine, 2nd Edition*, D. Sackett *et al.* with permission from the authors.

6.2 Evidence-based practice

In certain respects, the use of evidence-based practice may seem self-evident to the modern practitioner; why would we not choose the most effective treatment for our patients which fits best with our experience, their values and preferences, and what is feasible in the setting in which we work? *Patients* are entitled to receive the best possible care or advice that is appropriate to their needs. *Practitioners* wish to deliver the best possible service, and those in public health or health care more generally who are responsible for allocating funding for services expect the best possible use of scarce resources. Furthermore, *policymakers* and the *public* also wish to ensure that interventions and actions are more likely to

do good than harm (Antes and Clarke 2012). Surprisingly, however, the concept of evidence-based practice is a comparatively recent development, fuelled in part by spiralling health costs and Cochrane's seminal work in the 1960s which showed that less than half of routine medical and surgical treatments were based on solid scientific evidence (Cochrane 1972). More recent research has reinforced the ongoing need for attention to evidence when making decisions and choices in a variety of areas of health care (Ayre and Walters 2009; Khan *et al.* 2006; McAlister *et al.* 2007; Murray *et al.* 2005).

Sackett *et al.* (2000) have identified the key steps of evidence-based practice which, in essence, provide a review of current practice, with a view to its improvement (Box 6.2).

The value of asking a *structured* (and answerable) *question* is threefold: firstly, it defines the problem to be addressed; secondly, it helps to identify words and phrases that can be used in searching electronic databases for relevant information; and finally, it keeps our efforts focused on finding the best answer to the question posed.

The elements of a structured question are determined by identifying the type of patient or problem for which information is being sought; defining the intervention and possible alternatives being considered; and considering which outcomes are of particular interest. Some examples are given in Table 6.1.

Table 6.1 Examples of structured clinical questions

	Elements of the structured question			
	Patients or populations	**Problem**	**Intervention**	**Outcome**
A 58-year-old lady with a previous deep vein thrombosis requests hormone replacement therapy; you are aware of an increased risk of venous thrombo-embolism with this treatment and wish to discuss the issues with her to enable her to make an informed choice.	Post-menopausal women	History of deep vein thrombosis	Hormone replacement therapy	Risk of venous thrombo-embolism
A 75-year-old man presents with symptoms and signs of heart failure. You are considering digoxin therapy.	Elderly patients	Heart failure	Digoxin therapy	Reduction in mortality
Patients in your OP clinic with anaemia routinely have serum ferritin levels measured. You want to know if this is helpful in distinguishing those with iron deficiency.	Patients	Anaemia	Ferritin measurement	Presence of iron deficiency
Your health board is implementing a breast screening programme and want to set a target against which to audit its effectiveness.	Women	Death from breast cancer	Screening by mammography	Reduction in incidence
There has been a fall-off in uptake of the MMR vaccine in your area and you have been tasked with preparing a case to present to the local media to increase awareness of the benefits of this programme.	Children under 5	Severe complications of measles	MMR vaccination	Reduction in incidence
You are preparing a teaching session on the benefits of seat belt legislation for your local secondary school.	Car users	Death in road traffic accidents	Seat belt legislation	Reduction in traffic accident fatalities

The first two questions relate to routine clinical problems in general practice, but both may require extra research and advice tailored to individual patient needs. The third example questions routine practice in an outpatient setting, and the remaining examples are from public health practice. In seeking to answer the question, we need to appraise the available evidence base to determine if it is fit for purpose and to assess whether biases which might lead to the wrong answer have been minimized.

6.3 Three case scenarios

To provide some worked examples of critical appraisal the following three case scenarios are derived from different branches of health care. In the first, a simple, rapid screening test for deep vein thrombosis is evaluated. In the second scenario you are working as a public health physician in a resource-poor setting and need to consider the evidence for solar disinfection of water as a means of reducing diarrhoeal disease. In the third case you are asked to examine the evidence base at the time of the implementation of the workplace smoking ban, in order to examine the connection between research evidence and policy.

Abstracts have been provided but you may require the complete reports to fully work through these practical examples of the process of critical appraisal. Finally, it is worth remembering that the evidence base comes from a continuous, dynamic process, and a current search of the research literature should always be made before recommending a change in practice.

•••

Scenario 1: Evaluation of a study of a diagnostic test

You are a radiologist working in a UK hospital, with responsibility for providing duplex ultrasonography (DUS) for the investigation of patients suspected of having a deep venous thrombosis (DVT). You have noticed that the demand for this test has increased to such an extent that you are no longer able to provide a timely service to referring clinicians. You

have also noticed that less than 25 per cent of patients referred for DUS are shown to have a DVT. You recall a presentation at a conference you attended a couple of years ago where a unit, which seemed similar to yours, employed rapid fibrin D-dimer testing (a marker for clotting) before DUS. You find the paper relating to the conference presentation (Aschwanden et al. 1999) and read it to assess whether the study is robust and relevant to your practice.
•••

1 Are the results of the study valid?

(a) Was there an independent, blind comparison with a reference standard?
All patients in the study underwent structured clinical evaluation, a rapid D-dimer assay and the gold standard test, duplex ultrasonography. Operators applying each test were blind to the results of the other two tests.

(b) Did the patient sample include an appropriate spectrum of patients to whom the diagnostic tests will be applied in clinical practice?
The study investigated consecutive patients referred to the Angiology Department of a university hospital in Switzerland in a four-month period for investigation of suspected DVT. Seventeen out of 360 patients were excluded because independent D-dimer testing was unavailable. No other exclusion criteria were applied. A wide range of ages, both sexes, and inpatients and outpatients were included.

(c) Did the results of the test being evaluated influence the decision to perform the reference standard?
All patients underwent all three tests.

(d) Were the methods for performing the test described in sufficient detail to allow replication?
A commercial D-dimer assay was used, the manufacturer's details were provided, and a detailed description of how to use the test was referenced. The structured clinical evaluation used had been previously published and was referenced and its main components were listed.

Abstract 1

Purpose Large studies have shown that most cases referred for duplex sonography for suspected deep vein thrombosis (DVT) have normal scan results. For medical and economic reasons, a pre-selection procedure, which allows the detection of true negative cases before duplex scanning, is required; this procedure should be characterized by a high sensitivity and a high negative predictive value.

Methods In 343 patients (398 lower extremities) with suspected DVT, the DVT probability was clinically assessed, and a whole blood D-dimer agglutination test and a duplex scan were performed. The diagnostic sensitivities of the D-dimer test alone, a high clinical DVT probability alone, and the combination of both were evaluated.

Results The sensitivity values for the D-dimer test to diagnose proximal and distal DVTs were 88.7 per cent and 80.9 per cent, the negative predictive values (NPV) were 96.3 per cent and 97.9 per cent, and the specificity and the positive predictive value (PPV) were 54.8 per cent and 49.6 per cent and 26.6 per cent and 8.2 per cent, respectively. The sensitivities of the clinical DVT probability assessment for the diagnosis of proximal and distal DVTs were 83.9 per cent and 66.7 per cent, respectively; the corresponding NPVs were 94.9 per cent and 96.5 per cent, respectively. The specificity was 56.1 per cent and 50.8 per cent, and the PPVs were 26.1 per cent and 7.0 per cent, respectively. The combined use of the results of the clinical probability assessment and the D-dimer test resulted in sensitivities for proximal and distal DVTs of 98.4 per cent and 90.5 per cent, NPVs of 99.3 per cent and 98.6 per cent, a specificity of 43.4 per cent and 38.4 per cent, and PPVs of 24.3 per cent and 7.6 per cent, respectively.

Conclusion The combined use of a clinical DVT probability assessment scheme and the D-dimer test largely avoids false negative results, has a high sensitivity and NPV, helps to reduce the costs of DVT diagnosis, and may, in the future, be useful as a preselection procedure before duplex sonography.

Reprinted from: Aschwanden M *et al.* (1999) 'The Value of Rapid D-Dimer Testing Combined with Structured Clinical Evaluation for the Diagnosis of Deep Vein Thrombosis'. *Journal of Vascular Surgery* **30** (5), 929–35. Copyright (1999), with permission from The Society of Vascular Surgery.

2 What are the results of the study?

(a) Are likelihood ratios for the test results presented or data necessary for their calculation provided?

Likelihood ratios were not presented but sensitivities, specificities, negative, and positive predictive values (NPVs and PPVs) (for proximal and distal DVTs) were provided for the D-dimer assay alone and in combination with the result of the structured clinical evaluation (see Chapter 5 for NPVs and PPVs).

(b) What are the main findings of the study?

The combination of a structured clinical evaluation and a rapid D-dimer assay has high sensitivity (98.4 per cent) and NPV (99.3 per cent) for identifying proximal DVTs. This means that, when applied together, the patients with a low clinical evaluation score and a negative D-dimer test were very unlikely to have a DVT. There was no difference in the performance of the combined tests (clinical evaluation and assay) between inpatients and outpatients.

3 Will the results help me in providing a more timely investigative service for referring clinicians?

(a) Will the reproducibility of the test's results and their interpretation be satisfactory for my setting?

It would appear that all the tests applied in the study are reproducible within normal hospital practice.

(b) Are the results applicable to my patients?

No specific exclusion criteria were applied so the findings should be applicable to patients from a similar setting. It may have been helpful for the authors to have included more information on their hospital (for example, is it a tertiary referral centre) and the sources from which the patients were referred. This would enable you to judge how similar your setting and that of the study are.

(c) Will the result of this study change your practice? *This is only one study and your literature review has identified a similar study published around the same time from a UK hospital. You need to obtain and assess this paper also. Perhaps a systematic review of all published studies has been done. To change your practice the agreement of referring clinicians is required. The more evidence you can muster, and the more robust it is, the more likely you are to receive their agreement. You could consider implementing the procedure within your department for a trial period and auditing the results.*

(d) Will patients benefit if your department employed a structured clinical evaluation and rapid D-dimer assay before DUS? *Any benefits to patients are likely to be indirect as DUS is a non-invasive procedure although access times for screening are likely to be faster. Cost savings and reduction of pressure on investigative services may enable resources to be invested in other important areas.*

···

Scenario 2: Evaluation of a randomized trial
*You are part of the UK's humanitarian aid response and have been asked to develop a policy for use after earthquakes and other natural disasters which cause disruption to the already under strain water supplies in rural areas. There are likely to be major concerns about potential outbreaks of diarrhoeal disease and you have been asked to provide advice that could improve water quality at the household level. You are aware of the collection of resources put together by Evidence Aid (**www.EvidenceAid.org**; Clarke and Kayabu 2011) and identify the Cochrane Review of ways to improve water quality for preventing diarrhoea (Clasen et al. 2006). One of the interventions shown to be beneficial within this is solar disinfection, based on a meta-analysis of two trials, with an odds*

ratio for diarrhoea of 0.69 (95 per cent confidence interval 0.63 to 0.74). You also identify a more recently reported randomized trial (Mäusezahl et al. 2009) which has not yet been incorporated into the review and you decide to look in more detail at how this trial was done.
···

1 Are the results of the study valid?

(a) Was the assignment of children to the intervention/non-intervention group randomized? *Individual children were not randomized within this trial, rather communities were randomly allocated to intervention and non intervention groups. 'Clustered' randomized controlled trials such as this are often the most appropriate method of assessing different methods of delivering care especially in cases such as this where components of the intervention need to be delivered at the community level. The randomization was done by drawing coded balls from a sealed container at a public event to increase perceived fairness among the participating district and municipal authorities.*

(b) Were all children who entered the trial properly accounted for and attributed at its conclusion? *All twenty-two community clusters were accounted for at the end of the trial.*

(c) Was follow-up complete? *Fifty-nine households (94 children) were not available at the start of follow-up and 103 households (158 children) were lost to follow-up. This left 425 households (725 children) available for analysis. A total of 166,971 person-days of follow-up were available across the trials, representing 79.9 per cent and 78.9 per cent of the total possible person-days of child observation in the intervention and control groups, respectively.*

(d) Were patients analysed in the groups to which they were randomized? *Yes, intention to treat analysis was used and the clustered nature of the trial design was taken into consideration in the analysis.*

Abstract 2

Background Solar drinking water disinfection (SODIS) is a low-cost, point-of-use water purification method that has been disseminated globally. Laboratory studies suggest that SODIS is highly efficacious in inactivating waterborne pathogens, though previous field studies provided limited evidence for its effectiveness in reducing diarrhoea.

Methods and Findings We conducted a cluster-randomized controlled trial in twenty-two rural communities in Bolivia to evaluate the effect of SODIS in reducing diarrhoea among children under the age of five. A local non-governmental organization conducted a standardized interactive SODIS-promotion campaign in eleven communities targeting households, communities, and primary schools. Mothers completed a daily child health diary for one year. Within the intervention arm 225 households (376 children) were trained to expose water-filled polyethyleneteraphtalate bottles to sunlight. Eleven communities (200 households, 349 children) served as a control. We recorded 166,971 person-days of observation during the trial representing 79.9 per cent and 78.9 per cent of the total possible person-days of child observation in intervention and control arms, respectively. Mean compliance with SODIS was 32.1 per cent. The reported incidence rate of gastrointestinal illness in children in the intervention arm was 3.6 compared to 4.3 episodes/year at risk in the control arm. The relative rate of diarrhoea adjusted for intracluster correlation was 0.81 (95 per cent confidence interval 0.59–1.12). The median length of diarrhoea was three days in both groups.

Conclusions Despite an extensive SODIS promotion campaign we found only moderate compliance with the intervention and no strong evidence for a substantive reduction in diarrhoea among children. These results suggest that there is a need for better evidence of how the well-established laboratory efficacy of this home-based water treatment method translates into field effectiveness under various cultural settings and intervention intensities. Further global promotion of SODIS for general use should be undertaken with care until such evidence is available. Trial Registration: http://www.ClinicalTrials.gov NCT00731497

Reprinted from: Mäusezahl D *et al.* (2009) 'Solar drinking water disinfection (SODIS) to reduce childhood diarrhoea in rural Bolivia: a cluster-randomized, controlled trial'. *PLoS Medicine* **6**, e1000125.

(e) Were patients, health workers and study personnel blind to the intervention?

This was not possible, as is often the case in trials of the delivery of care.

(f) Were the groups similar at the start of the trial?

The households in the two study groups were well balanced on most factors at baseline, although storing water for longer than two days was more common among the intervention group (26.8 per cent) than the control group (13.9 per cent).

(g) Aside from the experimental intervention were the groups treated equally? *Yes.*

2 What were the results?

(a) What were the overall findings?

Children in the intervention group (SODIS) reported a total of 808 episodes of diarrhoea (mean: 3.6 per child per year-at-risk), compared to 887 episodes (mean: 4.3 per child per year) in the control group. The median length of episodes was three days in both groups. There were 891 episodes of dysentery (SODI: 431; control: 460). A multivariable model adjusting for age, sex, baseline-existing water treatment practices, and child hand washing was consistent in its estimate of effects on diarrhoea.

(b) How large was the treatment effect?

The unadjusted relative rate estimate for the number of episodes of diarrhoea was 0.81 and the odds ratios of severe diarrhoea and dysentery were 0.91 (95% CI 0.51–1.63) and 0.80 (95% CI 0.55–1.17), respectively. The multivariate analyses gave similar results.

(c) How precise was the estimate of the treatment effect?

The 95 per cent confidence interval around the unadjusted relative rate estimate was 0.59 to

1.12, and the confidence intervals for the odds ratios of severe diarrhoea and dysentery are given in part (b) of the answer.

3 Will the results help you and the others in your team in advising people affected by the earthquake?

(a) Are the results applicable in your setting?

The trial was undertaken within communities in Bolivia and although it was not done following an earthquake or other natural disaster, there were other factors that disrupted the ability to implement the intervention. The implementing NGO had global experience in disseminating SODIS and adapted their campaign to the local and cultural needs and also involved the public health and educational system in the roll-out. It would be important to do likewise in planning the response to an earthquake or other natural disaster.

(b) Were all clinically important outcomes considered?

The study concentrated on episodes of diarrhoea and dysentery, but also reported effects on vomiting, fever, cough and eye irritation; as well as compliance.

(c) Are the likely treatment benefits worth the potential harm and costs? *There was no evidence of harm occurring as a result of inclusion in the intervention group. Although the effects in the SODIS and the control groups were not statistically significantly different, there was a reduction in episodes of diarrhoea which is consistent with the meta-analysis in the earlier Cochrane Review. Therefore, in order to obtain a reliable estimate of the likely effect of a solar disinfection programme, you recognize that there is a need for an up-to-date systematic review, because there might be other studies, in addition to the trial from Bolivia (Mäusezahl et al. 2009) which should be included in this. This review might also need to include some economic analysis, but you realize that this will be difficult for setting policy because the costs might be quite different in different settings.*

(d) Will you recommend that this form of solar disinfection be used?

The case for doing so is not yet clear but it seems worthy of further work. You recommend that discussions should take place with the authors of the Cochrane Review to determine their schedule for updating the review and offer to join the team to facilitate this updating. You also initiate discussions with colleagues about the possibility of conducting a randomized trial in a disaster setting, should the intervention continue to look promising after the updated review, but with ongoing uncertainty about whether solar disinfection will, on balance, do more good than harm.

....

Scenario 3: Evaluation of a systematic review

You have been asked to prepare a report on the evidence base for public health policy in the UK over the past decade, with the specific task of showing how the findings of preceding research might have contributed to decisions. Your current assignment is on the banning of smoking in the workplace and you have conducted a search of PubMed. Although you find a recent Cochrane Review (Callinan et al. 2010), you need something from before the ban and identify an earlier systematic review (Fitchenberg and Glantz 2002). You need to assess whether the findings of this review were robust and whether they are supportive of the implementation of the smoking ban.

....

1 Are the results of the study valid?

(a) Did the review address a focused question relevant to the task you have been charged with?

The review's objective was to quantify the effect of smoke-free workplaces (total workplace bans) on smoking by employees. The authors also aimed to compare the effects to those achieved by cigarette taxation increases.

(b) Were the criteria used to select articles for inclusion appropriate?

Criteria for study selection were not clearly defined. Several types of study were included, all of which were observational in nature.

Abstract 3

Objective To quantify the effects of smoke-free workplaces on smoking in employees and compare these effects to those achieved through tax increases.

Design Systematic review with a random effects meta-analysis.

Study selection Twenty-six studies on the effects of smoke-free workplaces.

Setting Workplaces in the USA, Australia, Canada and Germany.

Participants Employees in unrestricted and totally smoke-free workplaces.

Main outcome measures Daily cigarette consumption (per smoker and per employee) and smoking prevalence.

Results Totally smoke-free workplaces are associated with reductions in prevalence of smoking of 3.8 per cent (95 per cent confidence interval 2.8–4.7 per cent) and 3.1 (2.4–3.8 per cent) fewer cigarettes smoked per day per continuing smoker. Combination of the effects of reduced prevalence and lower consumption per continuing smoker yields a mean reduction of 1.3 cigarettes per day per employee, which corresponds to a relative reduction of 29 per cent. To achieve similar reductions the tax on a pack of cigarettes would have to increase from $0.76 to $3.05 ($0.78–3.14) in the USA and from £3.44 to £6.59 (£5.32–10.20) in the UK. If all workplaces became smoke-free, consumption per capita in the entire population would drop by 4.5 per cent in the USA and 7.6 per cent in the UK, costing the tobacco industry $1.7 billion and £310 million annually in lost sales. To achieve similar reductions tax per pack would have to increase to $1.11 and £4.26.

Conclusions Smoke-free workplaces not only protect non-smokers from the dangers of passive smoking, they also encourage smokers to quit or to reduce consumption.

Reproduced from Fichtenberg CM and Glantz SA (2002) 'Effect of smoke-free workplaces on smoking behaviour: systematic review', *BMJ* **325**, 188, with permission from the BMJ Publishing Group.

(c) Is it unlikely that important relevant studies were missed?

*All relevant databases were searched, as were other reviews and the references in identified studies. The authors do not mention that all relevant conference proceedings were examined or that experts in the field were contacted to identify suitable studies. However, a **funnel plot** (the effect estimate plotted against sample size) did not show evidence of publication bias.*

(d) Was the validity of the included studies appraised?

The studies were appraised but scant details on the process used were provided.

(e) Were assessments of studies reproducible?

Details not provided.

(f) Were the results similar from study to study?

There were no significant differences between study types for smoking prevalence, cigarette consumption per employee, or relative change in consumption.

2 What were the results?

(a) What are the main findings?

Implementation of totally smoke-free workplace policies was associated with an absolute reduction (95 per cent confidence interval) in the prevalence of smoking of 3.8 (2.8, 4.7) and in daily cigarette consumption per continuing smoker of 3.1 (2.4, 3.8).

(b) How precise were the results?

Ninety-five per cent confidence intervals around the effect estimates were tight.

(c) Were all relevant outcome measures assessed?

The effect on passive smoking was not assessed but this was not an objective of the review.

(d) How do the results of the study relate to other work in the field?

The authors set the findings in context by comparing the effects of the workplace ban to those achieved by increasing taxation on cigarettes.

3 Will the results assist you in reporting to the task force?

(a) Can the results be applied to 'your' population?

The studies included in the review were from Australia, Canada, Germany, and the USA, but not the UK. However, the consistency of findings between countries indicates that they may be relevant to the UK population. Fewer workplaces in the UK than in the USA are smoke-free so countrywide legislation should be more effective in reducing cigarette consumption in the UK.

(b) Are the benefits to the population worth the costs?

The costs of introducing workplace smoking bans were not assessed. However, large increases in cigarette taxation would be required to achieve the reduction in cigarette consumption possible from total workplace smoking bans. Estimates of the costs of implementing smoke-free workplace legislation in the UK are required.

(c) Are there alternative 'treatment' options?

Legislation for smoke-free work places is one of a range of options for reducing smoking prevalence and population tobacco consumption. Other possibilities include raising taxation, advertising bans, cessation assistance, etc. The task force needs to review and compare the evidence for and costs/benefits of each approach before reporting to the Government.

4 General comment

Provision of more explicit detail on the methods used to appraise the studies reviewed would have enhanced confidence in the review's findings and enabled you to provide more definitive advice to the task force.

6.4 Working with evidence-based health care

Fig. 6.1 illustrates the major disciplines involved in the practice of health care and the multidisciplinary nature of the health service in a well-resourced country.

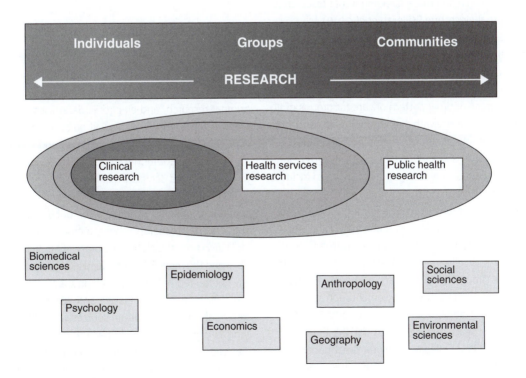

Figure 6.1 The spectrum of clinical and public-health practice.

In clinical practice, evidence-based health care has been defined as 'the conscientious, explicit and judicious use of current best evidence about the care of individual patients' (Sackett *et al.* 1996). The need is for evidence about the accuracy of diagnostic tests, the power of prognostic markers, and the comparative *effects* of interventions, considering both benefits and harms. Clinical skills and clinical judgement are vital for determining whether the evidence (or a guideline derived from it) applies to the individual patient at all and, if so, how. In addition, good practice in the care of patients requires consideration of the patient's wishes.

In *public health practice*, evidence is used to inform policy and public health interventions rather than individual patient care. Nevertheless, the same principles may be applied and there is a similar need to integrate the findings from relevant research with the particular health needs and values of the population being served. However, one of the special challenges with the design, conduct, and use of evidence in public health practice relates to the complexity of the interventions. This requires careful consideration both for those conducting research and those deciding if that research is relevant to their setting (Killoran *et al.* 2010).

Between decision-making for the individual patient and for the general population as a whole, lies the whole area of provision of health services, whose purpose is to benefit patient and population health. Here, the perspective is the optimal pattern of care for groups of ill people, such as those with diabetes or breast cancer, or groups of people at risk of developing particular conditions, such as smokers or those with hypertension. The evidence base for managed care is likely to include that used to inform both individual patient care and health service organization. The former underpins the production of evidence-based guidelines (for example, those produced by the National Institute for Health and Clinical Excellence (NICE), and the Scottish Intercollegiate Group Network (SIGN)), whereas the latter could be expected to inform implementation strategies (for example, National Service Frameworks in the UK for coronary heart disease (CHD), for the Elderly, for Diabetes, and for Epilepsy). The new practitioner, feeling daunted by the volume of research material available (Bastian *et al.* 2010) might, in fact, wish to begin by searching for potentially relevant guidelines from organizations such as NICE and SIGN, bearing in mind the need to appraise these to assess their relevance and whether they are sufficiently up to date (Brouwers *et al.* 2010; Owen-Smith *et al.* 2010).

Provision of health care is complex, and good quality evidence is unlikely to be available for all decisions, circumstances, and questions that arise. Nevertheless, there is an obligation to be explicit about current practice and its evidence-base and to be clear about uncertainties, to make more balanced, cost-effective decisions about health care, and to inform the research agenda to address the gaps in knowledge.

A practical guide

In the examples quoted earlier in this chapter we have used the framework proposed by Sackett *et al.* (2000) (Box 6.2) to guide the responses to the structured questions which were posed. In the following, we briefly review the remaining steps in achieving such outcomes in practice.

Effective and efficient searching

An overwhelming range of information sources are available within which evidence might be found. These include textbooks, guidelines, consensus statements, original research, and electronic databases of the literature. Today, much of this will be accessed through your computer. Furthermore, patients and colleagues are likely to be additional sources of the evidence vital to well-informed decision-making.

There are many electronic databases to chose from, containing millions of records for published articles and original research. These include *PubMed* and *MEDLINE* from the National Library of Medicine in the USA, and the more European-focused *Embase*. A strategy is required before approaching these databases if your efforts are to be efficient and effective. The first step might be to look within sources where the underlying evidence has already been appraised and synthesized, such as *The Cochrane Library* which contains several databases including the *Cochrane Database of Systematic Reviews* (CDSR) and the *Database of*

Abstracts of Reviews of Effects (*DARE*) from the Centre for Reviews and Dissemination at the University of York in England. As of 2012, *CDSR* contains the full text for more than 5000 full Cochrane Reviews, with protocols for 2000 more that are at earlier stages of preparation. In 2008, the 2321 full Cochrane Reviews which contained at least one meta-analysis included a total of more than 22,000 meta-analyses (Davey *et al.* 2011). Cochrane Reviews are produced by an extensive network of volunteers from around the world. They seek to tackle areas of uncertainty that have been identified by the authors and agreed with the relevant Cochrane Review Group but are not commissioned to tackle specific areas of high priority (Allen and Richmond 2011; Gøtzsche *et al.* 2011). In contrast to Cochrane Reviews, national organizations such the National Institute for Health Research's Health Technology Assessment programme in the UK commission reviews of particular relevance to local or regional interventions and actions.

Alongside Cochrane Reviews, more than 15,000 systematic reviews are available from elsewhere and the total number is growing at several thousand per year (Bastian *et al.* 2010). However, if you are unable to find an up-to-date, well-conducted systematic review, you are likely to be faced with having to tackle the original research literature, searching for relevant studies and then appraising those that you find. While each electronic database will have its own instructions for use, the technique for efficient electronic searching has some common principles: consider the terminology used to define your patient population, intervention and outcome, and consider potential alternatives, particularly spelling; use Boolean operators ('and', 'or', 'not'); use appropriate limits such as language, subject, type of article; use 'clinical query' options where available. The resources of the local health library and its librarians should not be underestimated: they can provide helpful advice and training.

The type of evidence sought should be appropriate to the question being addressed: to address a question which involved a choice between therapies, the best evidence will be derived from a systematic review of several randomized trials or, failing that, a single, well-conducted randomized trial. To address a question on prognosis, a cohort study will produce the best

information, while a diagnosis question would be best answered by information from a cross-sectional study (Chapter 3); but, again, systematic reviews of a collection of relevant studies are likely to more reliable, avoiding undue emphasis on the results of any single study. The development of search filters designed to increase the relevant yield of articles in these categories has been helpful and is discussed elsewhere (Haynes *et al.* 1994).

Critical appraisal of the literature

The evidence you have obtained from your search should be 'critically appraised' to discover whether it fully answers your question, for example, 'How good is this treatment or intervention?' or 'How good is this test?'. In evaluating the evidence presented, an assessment needs to be made of its *relevance* (generalizability) in relation to the setting in which it is to be used, whether or not it is *important* enough to implement, and whether or not it has *validity*.

Relevance

A study will be relevant if the results would help in caring for your patient or planning for your population. The assessment of relevance requires a comparison of the study subjects with your patients or population; of the study setting and intervention with yours; and of the study outcome with the desired outcome for your patients or population. In general, if your patient or population could have been included in the study, the results are likely to be applicable to your situation. If there are differences in these elements, then the findings may need to be modified; if the differences are large, the study is unlikely to be able to address your question. You should try to answer the question: 'Are there any reasons why the people, interventions or settings in this study are so different to what I am faced with, that the findings of the study will not be relevant?'.

Importance

Any assessment of importance considers the measured outcomes of the study, the size of the effect, and the level of statistical significance. Is the size of the effect likely to be important to your patients, to public health, or to clinical diagnosis? For a study addressing an intervention the effect size may be presented as a difference, a ratio, or as a 'number needed to treat' (NNT), along with the appropriate **confidence interval** (see Chapter 4). The importance of a study of the performance of a diagnostic test is assessed by asking how well the test distinguishes patients who have a specific disorder. This is summarized in measures of test performance (see Chapter 5) such as sensitivity, specificity, positive and negative predictive values, and likelihood ratios.

The study report should contain these estimates or at least present the data required for their calculation.

Validity

The validity of a study is assessed by determining to what extent study findings can be supported. **Internal validity** reflects the assessment of the adequacy of the study design and **external validity** (generalizability) places the study finding against those of other studies.

The specific criteria by which the validity of a study can be assessed will vary according to the type of question being addressed and the type of study design used. The validity of a study of therapy or prevention can be assessed by using the questions set out in Box 6.3 (Guyatt *et al.* 1993, 1994).

For diagnosis, the best evidence is derived from a cross-sectional study in which a comparison of the results of the test undergoing evaluation against a gold standard which is used to define the presence of disease. Both are applied to the same group of patients and an assessment made of the number of times the two tests agree or differ. Box 6.4 shows questions that can be used to assess such studies (Jaeschke *et al.* 1994*a*, 1994*b*).

Reviews of evidence

In general, questions about health and health care are inadequately addressed by single studies. The most robust conclusions are derived from an examination of the totality of available evidence relevant to the question being addressed. Such literature reviews may include only one type of evidence, for example, a number of RCTs of a particular intervention. Alternatively, they may derive information from a range of study designs; for example, a review examining water fluoridation contained studies with a range of designs, from ecological to cohort studies (see Chapter 10, section 10.2).

As well as summarizing large amounts of information, reviews have the following merits: they increase statistical power, improve the accuracy and precision of the estimated effect, assess the consistency and generalizability of findings, and can help to explain heterogeneity among studies. All of these attributes provide better building blocks for decision-making.

Box 6.3 Validity of a study of therapy/prevention

- Was the assignment of treatments randomized?
- Was follow-up complete and for long enough?
- Were all the patients analysed in the groups to which they were randomized (an intention to treat analysis)?
- Were patients and clinicians kept 'blinded' to the treatment?
- Were groups treated equally?
- Were groups similar at the start of the trial?

Reproduced from *Evidence-Based Medicine, 2nd Edition*, D. Sackett *et al.* with permission from the authors.

Box 6.4 Validity of a study of a diagnostic test

- Was there an independent, blind comparison with a reference 'gold standard'?
- Was the test evaluated in an appropriate spectrum of patients?
- Was the reference standard applied regardless of the diagnostic test result?
- Was the test validated in a second, independent group of patients?
- Were the methods for performance of the test described in sufficient detail to allow their replication?

Reproduced from *Evidence-Based Medicine, 2nd Edition*, D. Sackett *et al.* with permission from the authors.

Furthermore, they may prevent the unnecessary duplication of research effort, and it is now possible to prospectively register the reviews themselves so that others will know which reviews are underway (Booth *et al.* 2011a, 2011b, 2012).

The key element in producing a good quality review is that it is *systematic*—i.e. it is prepared using an explicit, systematic approach to minimize biases and random errors (Oxman *et al.* 1994). This means that its scope, evidence base, criteria for inclusion and exclusion of primary studies, studies which use original data, and data extraction, and analysis techniques, are clearly stated. In contrast to the conventional review which usually summarizes the information available from only the author's perspective a systematic approach minimizes bias arising from an incomplete selection of studies, inappropriate synthesis of data, and subjective interpretation of primary evidence (Cook *et al.* 1995).

A further requirement for a good quality review is that the primary studies selected are themselves of good quality. Therefore, the inclusion criteria for the review should include those based on an assessment of the methodological quality of the primary studies, i.e. the internal validity of the individual primary studies.

The term **meta-analysis** is used to describe a quantitative synthesis of primary data which yields an overall summary statistic. The synthesis may involve the re-analysis of individual level data collected in the primary studies, or combining the published summary statistics from individual primary studies. Fig. 6.2 shows an example of a meta-analysis of the effectiveness of intensive advice for smoking cessation. In this example three of the controlled trials eligible for inclusion showed inconclusive results, while two showed positive, statistically significant, results. The combined odds ratio was 1.46 (1.18, 1.80) indicating that the odds on success with intensive advice was nearly 50 per cent greater than with routine practice. The first test at the foot of the meta-analysis shows that this combined odds ratio differed significantly from one (P < 0.001). However, it is generally only reasonable to combine results when the primary studies show consistent effects, and

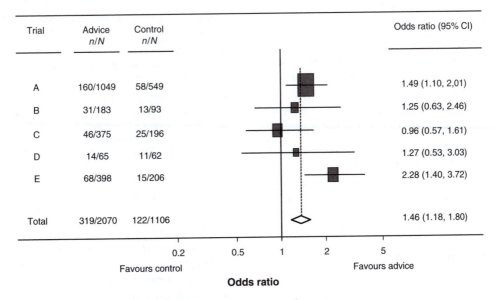

Test for difference between advice and control: $\chi^2 = 11.0$, d.f. = 1; $P < 0.001$.
Test for heterogeneity between trials: $\chi^2 = 6.71$, d.f. = 4; $P = 0.15$. $I^2 = 40\%$

Figure 6.2 Meta-analysis of quitting rates in controlled trials of intensive advice for smoking cessation.
Reproduced from Ashenden R, Silagy C, and Weller D (1997) 'A Systematic Review of the Effectiveness of Promoting Lifestyle Change in General Practice'. *Family Practice*, with permission from Oxford University Press.

an important step in any meta-analysis is therefore to perform a test for **heterogeneity** (statistical) between studies (Turner 2012). Also widely used is a measure of heterogeneity, I^2, which estimates the proportion of the variation between studies that is attributable to heterogeneity rather than chance, with values less than 30 per cent considered acceptable, and values exceeding 50 unacceptable. These findings are also shown at the foot of Fig. 6.2 and indicate that, although there was moderate heterogeneity ($I^2 = 40$ per cent), the test did not attain statistical significance ($P = 0.15$). If study results do show significant heterogeneity, an explanation for this should be sought using a **sensitivity analysis** or a meta-regression approach.

In critically appraising a systematic review, relevance and importance are assessed as for primary studies. Relevance will be determined by the similarity of your population/patient/setting to the study populations, interventions, and outcomes, which are the focus of the review. Significant heterogeneity (systematic differences in study populations, etc.) indicates that the relevance to general populations may be limited. Importance is assessed by considering how big an effect is evident, how precise the estimate of effect is, and whether the effect is clinically significant.

The assessment of validity is an evaluation of the methodology used in the review. Some of the validity criteria for the review will be the same as those presented for primary studies, and will depend on the focus of the review—therapy, diagnosis, etc. Additional questions that need to be addressed for appraisal of reviews are listed in Box 6.5.

Systematic reviews and meta-analyses, which will be increasingly available to guide medical practice and public health policies, are discussed in further detail elsewhere (Egger et al. 1997; Liberati et al. 2009).

Applying the evidence

Once relevant, valid, and important information is identified, it needs to be applied to the care of a particular patient or to the provision of a service or information for a particular population. This requires integrating the evidence with the particular circumstances and values of the patient or population concerned. An assessment of usefulness would include the questions in Box 6.6 (Sackett et al. 2000).

The evidence may point to a particular action but the individual benefit to a patient may be small enough to warrant doing nothing. Other obstacles to

Box 6.5 Appraisal of a systematic review

- Did the review address a clearly focused question in terms of the population studied, intervention applied, and outcomes considered?
- Did the studies that were sought have the appropriate design to address the issue?
- Was the search strategy used to find potentially eligible studies described and was it appropriate and comprehensive? Could important studies have been missed?
- What were the criteria for inclusion and exclusion of studies? Did this include an appraisal of the potentially eligible studies for methodological quality?
- Were the results similar from study to study or was there heterogeneity among the results of the included studies? If the results of these studies were combined in a meta-analysis, was it appropriate to do so?
- Was a sensitivity analysis presented?
- Are the author's conclusions supported by the evidence presented?
- Are recommendations linked to the strength of the evidence presented?

Reproduced from Heneghan C, Badenoch D, 2nd edn (2006). *Evidence-based Medicine Toolkit*, with permission from Wiley.

Box 6.6 Assessing the usefulness of evidence

- Do the results apply to your patient/population?
- Is the treatment feasible in your setting?
- What are your patient's/population's potential benefits and harms from the treatment?
- What are your patient's/population's values and expectations for both the outcome you are trying to prevent and for the treatment you are offering?

Reproduced from *Evidence-Based Medicine, 2nd Edition*, D. Sackett et al. with permission from the authors.

implementing the evidence include patients' values and preferences, geography, economics, administrative, or organizational characteristics, traditions, and 'expert' opinion. Ultimately, only the first of these is an acceptable reason for not applying evidence in practice. Implementing evidence may also require a change in behaviour from service providers and/or patients. This may not be achievable: all that evidence can do is to specify the recommended behaviour.

There will often be evidence to suggest change in a number of areas. In balancing the cost of applying one guideline rather than another, cost-effectiveness criteria may be useful.

Evaluating the impact of evidence on your routine practice

Just as evidence is sought for the effectiveness of health care practices, so should we assess whether this has become incorporated into our routine practice. This can be approached through the process of **health care audit**, looking at both processes and outcomes of care, and through an assessment of personal practice. The questions in Box 6.7 are useful in assessing your personal practice (Sackett *et al.* 2000).

The scheme illustrated in Fig. 6.3 sets out the dimensions of personal practice of evidence-based medicine, sources of evidence used, and level of critical appraisal skills.

Traditionally, during professional training, students tend to start at the origin of these three scales using supplied information which is not necessarily linked to specific clinical or public health problems, and followed intuitively. Increasingly, however, curricula are moving towards *problem-based learning* incorporating many of the principles discussed in this chapter. On graduating to clinical practice, clinicians move on to the clinical problem scale with information needs firmly grounded in patient and service issues. Attainment

Box 6.7 Assessing personal practice

- What is my professional approach? (Do I use or generate evidence-based guidelines or protocols?)
- How good are my generic evidence-based practice skills? (Formulating questions, searching for information, critical appraisal.)
- Do I need additional training?

Reproduced from *Evidence-Based Medicine, 2nd Edition*, D. Sackett *et al.*, with permission from the authors.

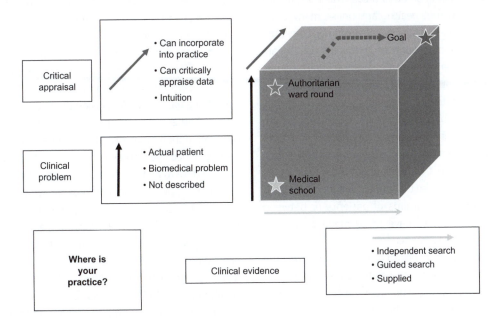

Figure 6.3 The dimensions of evidence-based practice.

of fully established evidence-based practice requires continuous development of personal skills in searching research databases and in critical appraisal. New studies are continuously added to research databases, and periodic updating of your routine practice should become an integral part of any programme of continuous professional development.

In this chapter we have briefly described the discipline of clinical epidemiology and shown how epidemiological tools can be used in routine clinical or public health practice. The development of critical appraisal skills is likely to develop during undergraduate training and in clinical practice should be incorporated into a programme of continuous professional development.

6.5 Economics of health care

Increasingly clinicians, managers, and policymakers are required to make difficult decisions about which health care interventions to provide or fund. These decisions need to balance the relative effects of the interventions with their relative costs and, in considering these costs, decision-makers also have to think about how the use of resources in one area, such as health, might impact on other areas. This is especially important given that health care, unlike many other goods and services, is heavily subsidized or free at the point of use in many countries. In the UK, health care is funded from general taxation revenue and competes for limited government income with other government departments, including education and defence. Despite significant expenditure on health care, health care resources are scarce and it is not possible to fund all potentially effective health care interventions; decisions therefore must be made about the interventions to be funded and those that remain unfunded. Choices between competing groups of patients or between treatments will always have to be made in publicly funded health care systems.

There are a variety of health economic tools to aid the decision about how scarce health care resources can be allocated; however, ultimately there is no formula or algorithm that will give the 'right answer'. *Economic evaluation* is widely used and involves comparing the costs and consequences of two or more health care interventions. The inclusion of two or more interventions is essential as economics is concerned with scarcity and recognizes that there is an *opportunity cost* to funding a particular intervention—namely that another intervention will not be funded as a consequence.

Three main types of economic evaluation are used for health care interventions: cost-benefit analysis, cost-effectiveness analysis, and cost-utility analysis.

Cost-benefit analysis involves comparing the monetary benefits of an intervention to its costs. If the monetary benefits exceed the costs, then the intervention may be considered as worthwhile. A limitation of cost-benefit analysis is the difficulty in assigning money values to improvements in health status or extensions to length of life. While a number of potential approaches have been developed, including the *human capital approach*, they all come with their own limitations and for this reason cost-benefit analysis is relatively rarely used in practice. A more common method of economic evaluation is *cost-effectiveness analysis*, where the costs of an intervention are related to some health outcome, such as lives saved or cases detected. Take, for example, two screening strategies for colorectal cancer where the outcome measure may be cases detected: if the cheaper screening strategy is also the most effective, the choice of intervention is clear; however, if the more expensive strategy is the more effective then the decision becomes more complicated. In this instance, an *incremental cost-effectiveness ratio (ICER)* is calculated which shows the additional cost to detect one more case. A decision then has to be made about whether it is worth spending scarce resources on the intervention or whether the same resources could be better deployed elsewhere. *Cost-utility analysis* is used to determine the effect of a health care intervention on both quality and length of life, which are then combined into a single summary measure such as a **quality adjusted life year (QALY)** (see Chapter 2). Cost-utility analysis has the advantage over cost-effectiveness analysis in that it can be used to compare across programmes with different health outcomes. Similarly to cost-effectiveness analysis an ICER can be calculated in a cost-utility analysis, indicating the additional cost of achieving an additional QALY.

While these health economic tools are useful in deciding how scarce health care resources could be distributed, they are not sufficient to making the final choice. Other considerations include whose opinion should be taken account of, along with the overall objectives of the health care system. For example, several different groups of people may legitimately expect to have their voice heard in any decision to allocate scarce resources. These include the users of the service (patient groups), payers (tax payers, in systems such as the NHS), the general public, health care professionals and practitioners, and managers. While health care professionals may be considered useful advocates or proxies for their patients, they may also have their own agenda or purpose. In the past, the public's voice might have been expected to be heard through locally elected representatives; however, more recently citizen juries have been employed.

Another consideration when deciding on the allocation of scarce health care resources relates to the objective of the health care system. The premise of economic evaluation is to maximize health gain for a given level of resources. Box 6.8 shows how different objectives can significantly influence how limited resources are distributed. When compared to an option which allocates resources on the basis of treatment effectiveness (option 1), or on the basis of the number of subjects affected, i.e. the burden of disease (option 2), allocating resources so as to maximize health gain (option 3) provides a different use of resources.

While maximizing health or health gain may be considered a legitimate priority for any health care system, reducing inequalities in health outcomes across socio-economic and ethnic groups, and across regions may also be an important guiding principle, and resources may be legitimately redirected towards more vulnerable groups, even if a greater level of health could be achieved by directing resources to the general population. Williams (1997) argues that the 'fair innings' principle be traded off against efficiency (or maximizing health gain) when prioritizing health care, so that everyone has some normal span of life. Considerations of this type can be incorporated into economic evaluation by assigning different weights to QALYs depending on who receives them, although this has been rarely done in practice. Taking this idea further, to maximize public welfare overall, should the needs of economically active people be valued more highly because their taxes help fund health and social services? Or, alternatively, should the QALYs (and needs) of smokers, alcoholics, or drug addicts, for example, be regarded less highly than those with exemplary health behaviours who are ill?

Economic evaluation has been used in a number of countries to decide on the appropriate allocation of scarce resources. In 1999, the National Institute for Health and Clinical Excellence (NICE) was established in the UK, to provide guidance to the National Health Services of England and Wales about the funding of selected new and existing health interventions based on their clinical and cost-effectiveness. One of the reasons for the establishment of NICE was the perceived 'postcode prescribing' operating in England, with patients receiving or denied certain treatment based on which health authority they happened to reside; NICE would surmount this by making recommendations about the funding of health interventions at the national level (Appleby et al. 2007; Owen-Smith *et al.* 2010). In 1989, the US state of Oregon launched an initiative to ration treatment under the Medicaid scheme (which provides publicly funded health care for those with low income and resources). The aim was, under a fixed budget, to provide the most efficient services to the largest number of people, in order to extend some basic level of care to all citizens who fell below the federal poverty level. The approach developed a league table which ranked healthcare interventions in terms of their gains in health-related quality of life (Wonderling *et al.* 2005).

Practitioners wishing to make decisions about health care interventions on the basis of both effects and costs, may be able draw on relevant, up-to-date guidelines, or in the absence of such guidelines may need to make their decisions by considering the types of evidence discussed in this chapter. In doing so, tools are available, including the work of the GRADE Working Group on the incorporation of resource use into the grading of recommendations (Guyatt *et al.* 2008).

Box 6.8 Illustration of total number of patients treated within purchasing unit with ten different diseases using different purchasing options

							Patient groups prioritized		
Number of patients with each treatable disease	Units of health benefit (UHB)	Total UHBs	Cost per patient (£)	Total cost (£)	CE ratio	Option 1 Based on (b)	Option 2 Based on (a)	Option 3 Based on (CE ratio)	
(a)	(b)	(a × b)	(c)	(a × c)	(a × c)/(a × b)				
A. 20	9.5	190	3000	60,000	316	1		6	
B. 15	9.0	135	3800	57,000	422	2		7	
C. 30	8.6	258	2300	69,000	267	3		5	
D. 5	8.3	42	1000	5,000	119	4		2	
E. 70	7.5	525	5200	364,000	693	5	2		
F. 40	6.8	272	950	38,000	140	6		3	
G. 84	5.4	454	3000	252,000	555		1	9	
H. 18	4.3	77	2200	39,600	512			8	
I. 65	4.0	260	875	56,875	219			4	
J. 50	3.8	190	300	15,000	80			1	
397		2403		956,475					

Notes: This illustration shows the effect of different purchasing options on the total number of patients treated within a purchasing unit (for example, hospital or trust). The available budget is £600,000 but the cost of treating **all** patients is £956,475 (total cost). Three options are available: (1) Select most effective treatments until budget exhausted, (2) Select treatments benefiting the greatest burdens until budget exhausted, and (3) Select most cost-effective treatments until budget exhausted. Based on this data, these would lead to:
Option 1: Most effective treatment: cost: £593,000; patients treated: 180; health benefit: 1422.
Option 2: Burden of disease: cost: £616,000; patients treated: 154; health benefit: 979.
Option 3: Cost-effectiveness: cost: £592,475; patients treated: 327; health benefit: 1878.

Summary

In this chapter, we have briefly described the discipline of clinical epidemiology and shown how epidemiological tools can be used in routine clinical or public health practice. The development of critical appraisal skills is likely to develop during undergraduate training, and in clinical practice should be incorporated into a programme of continuous professional development.

Web addresses

The Cochrane Library
www.thecochranelibrary.com; www.cochranejournalclub.com

Centre for Reviews and Dissemination
www.york.ac.uk/inst/crd

Evidence Aid
www.evidenceaid.org

NHS Evidence
www.evidence.nhs.uk

National Institute for Health and Clinical Excellence
www.nice.org.uk

Scottish Intercollegiate Guidelines Network
www.sign.ac.uk

Centre for Evidence-Based Medicine
www.cebm.net

Further reading

Brownson RC, Baker EA, Leet T, and Gillespie KN
(2003) *Evidence-Based Public Health*. New York: Oxford
University Press.

Egger M, Davey Smith G, and Sterne JAC (2002) Systematic
reviews and meta-analysis. In: Detels R, McEwen J, Beaglehole R, and Tanaka H (eds) *Oxford Textbook of Public Health*,
Vol 2, 4th edn; pp. 655–75 Oxford: Oxford University Press.

Muir Gray JA (2001) *Evidence-based Healthcare. How to
Make Health Policy and Management Decisions,* 2nd edn.
Edinburgh: Churchill Livingstone.

References

Allen C and Richmond K (2011) The Cochrane Collaboration: International activity within Cochrane Review
Groups in the first decade of the twenty-first century.
Journal of Evidence-based Medicine **4** (1), 2–7 [2011 Jan 27
epub ahead of print].

Antes G and Clarke M (2012) Knowledge as a key resource
for health challenges. *Lancet* **379** (9812), 195–6.

Appleby J, Devlin N, and Parkin D (2007) NICE's cost
effectiveness threshold. *BMJ (Clinical Research Ed)* **335**
(7616), 358–9.

Aschwanden M, Labs KH, Jeanneret C, Gehrig A, *et al.*
(1999) The value of rapid D-dimer testing combined with
structured clinical evaluation for the diagnosis of deep vein
thrombosis. *Journal of Vascular Surgery* **30** (5), 929–35.

Ashenden R, Silagy C and Weller D (1997) A systematic
review of the effectiveness of promoting lifestyle change
in general practice. *Family Practice* **14** (2), 160–76.

Ayre S and Walters G (2009) Are therapeutic decisions
made on the medical admissions unit any more
evidence-based than they used to be? *Journal of
Evaluation in Clinical Practice* **15** (6), 1180–6.

Bastian H, Glasziou P, and Chalmers I (2010) Seventy-five
trials and eleven systematic reviews a day: how will we
ever keep up? *PLoS Medicine* **7** (9), e1000326.

Booth A, Clarke M, Ghersi D, Moher D, *et al.* (2011a) An
international registry of systematic-review protocols.
Lancet **377** (9760), 108–9.

Booth A, Clarke M, Ghersi D, Moher D, *et al.* (2011b)
Establishing a minimum dataset for prospective registra-
tion of systematic reviews: an international consultation.
PloS One **6** (11), e27319.

Booth A, Clarke M, Dooley G, Ghersi D, *et al.* (2012) The
nuts and bolts of PROSPERO: an international prospective
register of systematic reviews. *Systematic Reviews* **1** (1), 2.

Brouwers MC, Kho ME, Browman GP, Burgers JS, *et al.*
(2010) AGREE II: advancing guideline development,
reporting and evaluation in health care. *Journal of Clinical
Epidemiology* **63** (12), 1308–11.

Callinan JE, Clarke A, Doherty K, and Kelleher C (2010)
Legislative smoking bans for reducing secondhand
smoke exposure, smoking prevalence and tobacco consumption. *Cochrane Database of Systematic Reviews* **4**,
CD005992.

Clarke M And Kayabu B (2011) Evidence for disaster risk
reduction, planning and response: design of the Evidence
Aid survey. *PLoS Currents*, **14**, RRN1270.

Clasen T, Roberts I, Rabie T, Schmidt W, *et al.* (2006)
Interventions to improve water quality for preventing
diarrhoea.*Cochrane Database of Systematic Reviews* **3**,
CD004794.

Cochrane AL (1972). *Effectiveness and Efficiency*. London:
Nuffield Provincial Hospitals Trust.

Cook DJ, Sackett DL, and Spitzer WO (1995) Methodologic
guidelines for systematic reviews of randomized control
trials in health care from the Potsdam Consultation on
Meta-Analysis. *Journal of Clinical Epidemiology* **48** (1),
167–71.

Davey J, Turner RM, Clarke MJ, and Higgins JPT (2011)
Characteristics of meta-analyses and their component
studies in the Cochrane Database of Systematic Reviews:
a cross-sectional, descriptive analysis. *BMC Medical
Research Methodology* **11**, 160.

Egger M, Smith GD, and Phillips AN (1997) Meta-analysis:
principles and procedures *BMJ (Clinical Research Ed)* **315**
(7121), 1533–7.

Fichtenberg CM and Glantz SA (2002) Effect of smoke-
free workplaces on smoking behaviour: systematic review.
BMJ (Clinical Research Ed) **325** (7357), 188.

Fletcher RH, Fletcher SE, and Wagner EH (1996). *Clinical
Epidemiology. The Essentials*. Baltimore: Williams and
Wilkins.

Gøtzsche P, Tendal B, and Clarke M (2011) Review production in The Cochrane Collaboration—where is it happening and why? *Cochrane Database of Systematic Reviews* Suppl. **1**, 16–19.

Guyatt GH, Sackett DL and Cook DJ (1993) Users' guides to the medical literature. II. How to use an article about therapy or prevention. A. Are the results of the study valid? Evidence-Based Medicine Working Group. *JAMA* **270** (21), 2598–601.

Guyatt GH, Sackett DL, and Cook DJ (1994) Users' guides to the medical literature. II. How to use an article about therapy or prevention. B. What were the results and will they help me in caring for my patients? Evidence-Based Medicine Working Group. *JAMA* **271** (1), 59–63.

Guyatt GH, Oxman AD, Kunz R, Jaeschke R, *et al.* (2008) Incorporating considerations of resources use into grading recommendations. *BMJ (Clinical Research Ed)* **336** (7654), 1170–3.

Haynes RB, Wilczynski N, McKibbon KA, Walker CJ, *et al.* (1994) Developing optimal search strategies for detecting clinically sound studies in MEDLINE. *Journal of the American Medical Informatics Association: JAMIA* **1** (6), 447–58.

Jaeschke R, Guyatt G, and Sackett DL (1994a) Users' guides to the medical literature. III. How to use an article about a diagnostic test. A. Are the results of the study valid? Evidence-Based Medicine Working Group. *JAMA* **271** (5), 389–91.

Jaeschke R, Guyatt GH, and Sackett DL (1994b) Users' guides to the medical literature. III. How to use an article about a diagnostic test. B. What are the results and will they help me in caring for my patients? The Evidence-Based Medicine Working Group. *JAMA* **271** (9), 703–7.

Killoran A and Kelly M (2010). *Evidence-based Public Health: Effectiveness and efficiency.* Oxford: Oxford University Press.

Khan AT, Mehr MN, Gaynor AM, Bowcock M, *et al.* (2006) Is general inpatient obstetrics and gynaecology evidence-based? A survey of practice with critical review of methodological issues. *BMC Women's Health* **6**, 5.

Liberati A, Altman DG, Tetzlaff J, Mulrow C, *et al.* (2009) The PRISMA statement for reporting systematic reviews and meta-analyses of studies that evaluate health care interventions: explanation and elaboration. *PLoS Medicine* **6** (7), e1000100.

McAlister FA, van Diepen S, Padwal RS, Johnson JA, *et al.* (2007) How evidence-based are the recommendations in evidence-based guidelines? *PLoS Medicine* **4** (8), e250.

Mäusezahl D, Christen A, Pacheco GD, Tellez FA, *et al.* (2009) Solar drinking water disinfection (SODIS) to reduce childhood diarrhoea in rural Bolivia: a cluster-randomized, controlled trial. *PLoS Medicine* **6** (8), e1000125.

Murray IR, Murray SA, MacKenzie K and Coleman S (2005) How evidence based is the management of two common sports injuries in a sports injury clinic? *British Journal of Sports Medicine* **39** (12), 912–16; discussion 916.

Owen-Smith A, Coast J, and Donovan J (2010) The usefulness of NICE guidance in practice: different perspectives of managers, clinicians, and patients. *International Journal of Technology Assessment in Health Care* **26** (3), 317–22.

Oxman AD, Cook DJ, and Guyatt GH (1994) Users' guides to the medical literature. VI. How to use an overview. Evidence-Based Medicine Working Group. *JAMA* **272** (17), 1367–71.

Sackett DL, Rosenberg WM, Gray JA, Haynes RB, *et al.* (1996) Evidence based medicine: what it is and what it isn't. *BMJ (Clinical Research Ed)* **312** (7023), 71–2.

Sackett DL, Straus SE, Richardson WS, Rosenberg W, and Haynes RB. (2000). *Evidence-Based Medicine. How to Practice and Teach EBM*, 2nd edn. Edinburgh: Churchill Livingstone.

Turner RM, Davey J, Clarke MJ, Thompson SG, *et al.* (2012) Predicting the extent of heterogeneity in meta-analysis, using empirical data from the Cochrane Database of Systematic Reviews. *International Journal of Epidemiology* **41** (3), 818–27.

Williams A (1997) Intergenerational equity: an exploration of the 'fair innings' argument. *Health Economics* **6** (2), 117–32.

Wonderling D, Gruen R, Black N (2005). *Introduction to Health Economics.* Maidenhead: Open University Press.

7 Circulatory diseases

JOHN YARNELL

CHAPTER CONTENTS

This chapter deals with the circulatory diseases which are the leading cause of death in high-income countries and are rapidly increasing in incidence in most middle- and low-income countries. The major cardiovascular disorders are: coronary heart disease, stroke, congestive heart failure, aortic aneurysm, and peripheral vascular disease. These diseases—and coronary heart disease in particular—are typical diseases associated with the *epidemiological transition* as countries develop, and the health, lifestyle, and environment of their populations begin to change. Epidemiological data from countries across the WHO regions are shown, as well as examples of cohort studies from China and from the USA which have been used to investigate possible causes.

Introduction

Circulatory diseases have become the major cause of death worldwide causing 17 million deaths in 2008, 31 per cent of the total (WHO 2011). In low- and middle-income countries they are burgeoning in parallel with rapid social, cultural, and economic changes and increases in life expectancy in many countries, but not in all. In some of the poorest countries of the world, in sub-Saharan Africa, where malnutrition and infectious diseases prevail for a large proportion of the population, hypertension is common, particularly in urban areas, leading to stroke and congestive heart failure as important causes of hospital admission or death in adults.

The major circulatory diseases (usually known as *cardiovascular diseases—CVD*) are those of the heart and arterial blood vessel system and involve a pathological process known as atherosclerosis. This involves lipid deposition in the arterial wall, initially known as fatty streaks, but potentially developing into raised plaque encapsulating liquid lipid material, atheroma (Greek—gruel or porridge), which can endanger the integrity of the arterial wall, and in the smaller arteries can create a significant obstacle to normal blood flow. Some organs, known as end-organs, are particularly vulnerable to anoxia caused by this reduction in blood flow (*ischaemia*) both acutely and chronically. The heart, brain, and lower limbs are especially liable to the anoxic consequences of atherosclerosis. Acute obstruction of the coronary arteries appears to be often associated with rupture of a vulnerable plaque. This releases atheromatous material which is highly thrombogenic, promoting a local cellular inflammatory/thrombotic response. In the past two decades it has become increasingly recognized that atherosclerosis is also an inflammatory process (Libby *et al.* 2011) and that blood thrombosis factors influence its

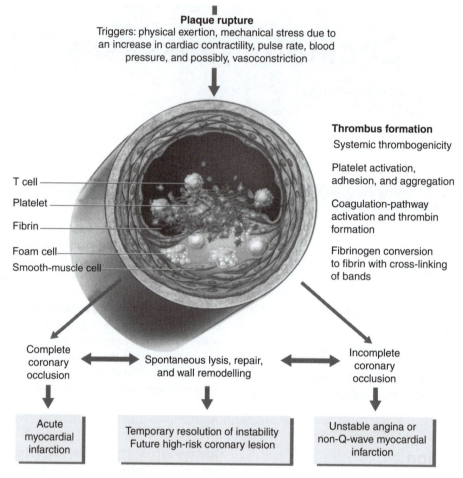

Plaque rupture
Triggers: physical exertion, mechanical stress due to
an increase in cardiac contractility, pulse rate, blood
pressure, and possibly, vasoconstriction

T cell

Platelet

Fibrin

Foam cell

Smooth-muscle cell

Thrombus formation
Systemic thrombogenicity

Platelet activation,
adhesion, and aggregation

Coagulation-pathway
activation and thrombin
formation

Fibrinogen conversion
to fibrin with cross-linking
of bands

Complete
coronary
occlusion

Spontaneous lysis, repair,
and wall remodelling

Incomplete
coronary
occlusion

Acute
myocardial
infarction

Temporary resolution of instability
Future high-risk coronary lesion

Unstable angina or
non-Q-wave myocardial
infarction

Figure 7.1 The pathogenesis of plaque rupture in atherothrombosis.
Reproduced from Yeghiazarians Y *et al*. 'Unstable angina hectoris'. *New England Journal of Medicine*, 2000, with permission from Massachusetts Medical Society.

progression (Borissof *et al*. 2011). Fig. 7.1 shows the main components of a ruptured plaque.

Both platelet and plasma factors control the extent of this response which can produce large aggregated platelet emboli and these proceed in the coronary circulation to block smaller vessels. In the larger and middle-range coronary and cerebral arteries acute obstruction will result in acute anoxia and subsequent death of heart muscle or brain cells over a substantial region, giving rise to myocardial or cerebral *infarction*. These acute events are associated with the typical clinical symptoms of *heart attack* or *stroke*; smaller emboli which may be a result of extensive plaque formation, irregularity, and erosion of the

artherial endothelium often lead to blockage of minor blood vessels and chronic anoxia. In heart muscle, chronic anoxia results in the slow death of muscle and its replacement by fibrous tissue (*ischaemic heart disease—IHD*).

Diseases of the venous blood system represent only a small proportion of the total burden of circulatory disease but *deep vein thrombosis* (DVT) and *pulmonary embolism* are of clinical importance. These diseases are thrombotic and embolic in nature and largely occur in the chronically ill or those undergoing major orthopaedic surgery (for which anticoagulant prophylaxis is usually given). Recent interest has focused on DVT and pulmonary embolism as a complication of long-haul air flights, and preventive measures have been introduced by most airlines, although risk is low.

The major circulatory diseases are shown in Box 7.1 and in Fig. 7.2.

As shown in Fig. 7.2, ischaemic heart disease accounts for the major portion of deaths from CVD but other cardiovascular deaths include: cardiomyopathies, conduction disorders, cardiac arrest, and congestive heart failure. According to WHO guidelines for coders of causes of death, IHD should be used, when applicable, as the underlying cause when cardiac arrest or congestive heart failure have been given as immediate causes of death (see Chapter 2). In some countries this advice is not always rigorously followed leading to an underestimate of IHD deaths and inflating the deaths from other CVD.

Box 7.1 Cardiovascular diseases

Major causes of mortality	Major causes of morbidity
Acute myocardial infarction	Angina: (stable) (unstable)
Ventricular fibrillation	Congestive heart failure
Chronic ischaemic heart disease	Chronic cerebrovascular disease
Congestive heart failure	Peripheral vascular disease
Stroke (cerebrovascular disease)	
Aortic aneurysm	

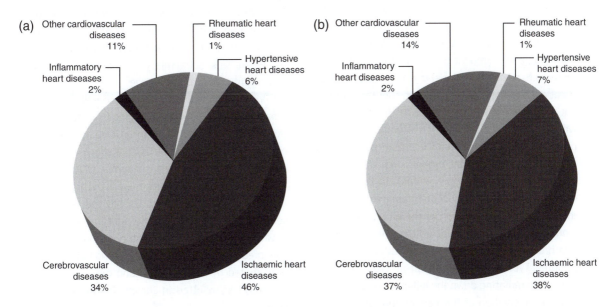

Figure 7.2 Worldwide distribution of types of cardiovascular disease in men (a) and in women (b).
Reproduced from *Global Atlas on Cardiovascular Disease Prevention and Control*. Mendis S, Puska P, Norrving B with permission from the World Health Organization.

7.1 Coronary heart disease

As shown in Box 7.1, coronary heart disease (isch-aemic heart disease) (CHD or IHD) has a variety of clinical manifestations. Acutely, these are now often termed *acute coronary syndromes* by clinicians and include: *ventricular fibrillation* (which induces cardiac arrest), *acute myocardial infarction* (MI), and *unstable angina*. In turn, acute MI can be extensive enough to cause pump failure, usually of the left side of the heart, resulting in acute *congestive heart failure* (CHF); in the elderly MI is frequently free of significant chest pain and often presents with congestive heart failure. *Acute CHF* carries a five-year mortality rate of about 80 per cent in a recent review of hospital admissions in the USA (Park *et al.* 2011).

The bundle of His and other electrical conducting fibres of the heart are particularly vulnerable to sudden ischaemia; if the blood supply to these conducting tissues is restricted then arrhythmias may develop. *Atrial* arrhythmias such as *atrial fibrillation* result in irregular ventricular contractions but are of near normal rate, which are not usually life threatening, and are a common feature of chronic ischaemia. At the *ventricular* level, arrhythmias such as *fibrillation*, which are common in acute coronary obstruction, result in stasis of the arterial blood supply to the brain, and imminent death, but the heart can be restored to *sino-atrial (sinus)* rhythm by prompt electrical defibrillation. *Asystole*, when there is no residual electrical activity detectable in the heart tissue, will not respond to defibrillation attempts, but cardio-pulmonary resuscitation can maintain blood supply and oxygenation of vital organs such as the brain in the short term (30–60 minutes). In the absence of this brain death will occur in approximately four minutes. Acute obstruction of the blood supply to a significant area of the myocardium will result in the death of the muscle in this region within a matter of minutes. Typically this will result in 'crushing' chest pain often radiating down the left arm due to the anatomical innervation of the pericardium and is often associated with sweating. Ischaemia of the ventricular myocardium, detectable by an absence of normal depolarization in the affected area of myocardium, causes typical abnormalities of electrocardiographs (ECGs), which record the electrical activity associated with each cardiac cycle. These can be read according to a standard protocol by experienced clinicians. Although computerized programmes do exist for the classification of these abnormalities, they still require refinement before being used routinely on their own. Important confirmatory evidence of myocardial damage is obtained by measurement of cardiac enzymes such as lactic dehydrogenase (LDH) or creatinine kinase (CK) which are released from dying myocardial muscle. Until recently, a level of twice the upper limit of the normal range of LDH was considered diagnostic of acute MI. But, the increasing use of troponins for diagnostic purposes, which are released at very low levels of tissue damage have blurred the distinction between myocardial infarction and *unstable angina* in which there is only minor tissue death. Studies have shown that this leads to different case definitions for epidemiologists interested in monitoring trends in incidence of CHD over time (Salomaa *et al.* 2005). Clearly, the *acute coronary syndromes* constitute a broad spectrum of clinical disorders ranging from acute MI, with or without chest pain, and with or without acute congestive heart failure, to unstable angina in which chest pain may be severe due to ischaemia, but where this ischaemia is insufficient to result in significant myocardial damage.

Chronic ischaemic heart disease constitutes another broad spectrum of diseases ranging from *stable angina* (formerly termed angina pectoris), through the various conduction defects (e.g. atrial fibrillation), and valvular disorders due to localized ischaemia, to *chronic congestive heart failure*, in which there is the gradual onset of pump failure of the heart. Usually this is of the left ventricle but sometimes of the right in *cor pulmonale* in which progressive inflammatory change to lung tissue (predominantly caused by smoking but sometimes exacerbated by occupational lung disease or chronic asthma) has resulted in chronic failure of the right ventricle.

Atrial fibrillation (AF) is found in only 0.5 per cent of the general population but its prevalence is over

10 per cent in men and women aged more than 75 years of age. With the ageing of populations this is set to increase due to chronic IHD. In low-income countries where rheumatic heart disease persists, AF is associated with mitral valve disease. Atrial fibrillation is estimated to account for a quarter of all strokes in high-income countries and prophylactic anticoagulants such as warfarin are recommended for most cases (Ahmad and Lip 2012).

Epidemiology and risk factors for acute and chronic CHD: as noted in Chapter 1, CHD is not a new disease but it became increasingly prominent during the 20th century. Clinicians in the US and in some European countries, particularly the UK and Finland, noticed increasing numbers of patients with heart attack admitted to their hospitals; these patients, who were often men, could be relatively young, perhaps only in their 30s or 40s. Many such patients never reached hospital, dying relatively suddenly at home or at work due to the rapid onset of myocardial ischaemia, often resulting in ventricular fibrillation or asystole. Community studies in the UK based on deaths and hospital admissions estimated that about 70 per cent of patients died before reaching hospital (Norris 1998). Some large-scale cohort studies were established in the 1950s and 1960s to examine possible causes of the coronary epidemic. In the US the National Institutes of Health funded a cohort study based on the inhabitants of a small town in Massachusetts called *Framingham*, and Ancel Keys established cohorts in *Seven Countries* with contrasting death rates from coronary disease. In Britain the Department of Health funded a study of male civil servants (*Whitehall Study*); many of the epidemiological methods required for standardization and validation of clinical diagnoses were developed by cardiologists who had become epidemiologists, such as Geoffrey Rose, on behalf of the World Health Organization.

A rapidly increasing trend in mortality due to IHD was observed in the 1950s and 1960s in high-income countries such as the US, Canada, Britain, and other western European countries. This was followed by a slow decline beginning in the 1970s in North America but, in Eastern Europe and latterly in Asia and Africa, there has been a rapid rise in CVD mortality such that

worldwide eight out of the nine million deaths before the age of 60 years due to non-communicable diseases such as CVD occurred in low- and mid-income countries. Table 7.1 shows the age standardized mortality from IHD and stroke in selected countries from the WHO regions for 2008.

Table 7.1 Age-standardized ischaemic heart disease (IHD) and stroke rates in selected countries in world regions (2008)

	IHD	Stroke
Africa		
Ghana	120	126
Nigeria	122	149
South Africa	71	83
Americas		
Argentina	71	44
Cuba	113	59
United States	81	25
Europe		
France	29	22
Russia	297	196
United Kingdom	69	37
Eastern Mediterranean		
Afghanistan	329	110
Egypt	174	110
Iran	195	97
South East Asia		
Bangladesh	204	108
India	166	116
Thailand	87	123
Western Pacific		
Australia	60	28
China	80	162
Japan	31	37

··
Questions

1 **The rates shown in Table 7.1 have been standardized according to the age distributions found in each country. What pattern might you expect in the crude mortality rates?**

2 **Afghanistan, Russia, and Bangladesh show the highest mortality from IHD while Russia, China, and Nigeria show the highest mortality from stroke. What are the possible explanations for these differences?**

3 **What additional age-standardized mortality data would you like to examine to determine whether there are any artifactual reasons for differences in IHD mortality between countries?**
··

The search for causes of the coronary heart disease epidemic: in the 1950s in a series of metabolic experiments with human volunteers, Ancel Keys and others established that plasma cholesterol levels could be influenced by the proportion of saturated (mainly from dairy and meat products) and polyunsaturated fatty acids (mainly from vegetable products) in the diet: the more saturated fat, the higher the cholesterol, and the more polyunsaturated fat, the lower the cholesterol. Monounsaturated fatty acids had a neutral effect. Convinced of the need for population studies he moved from hospital-based studies into international epidemiological studies, having noted that countries with high consumption of saturated fats tended to have high mortality from coronary disease. Countries such as Finland, the US, and the UK had the highest rates in the world and Mediterranean countries like Spain, Italy, France, and Greece had much lower rates, but not as low as those in countries such as Japan and China. In the Seven Countries study led by Keys, population groups of men were examined, their risk factors measured, and then followed over a number of years to determine which risk factors predicted future coronary events. This study and other cohort studies conducted in single populations, such as Framingham and Whitehall, helped establish the major classic risk factors of coronary disease—high plasma cholesterol, hypertension, and cigarette smoking (Luepker *et al.* 2004). Case-control studies also helped establish the relative contributions of the individual risk factors in different age groups and Table 7.2 shows an example of a study of smoking habit in hospitalized cases of acute myocardial infarction and in controls.

In this table the association between smoking habit is much stronger at the younger ages than in the more elderly. The high levels of cigarette smoking in the

Table 7.2 Smoking habit in cases of myocardial infarction admitted to hospital and in controls

| Age (years) | Current smoker of manufactured cigarettes only | | Non-smoker with no regular cigarette use in past 10 years | | Ratio of smoking rates* in cases compared to that in controls |
	Cases (n)	Controls (n)	Cases (n)	Controls (n)	Risk ratio (95% CI)
30–39	78	1784	35	4873	6.3 (4.2–9.5)
40–49	293	1497	190	4306	4.7 (3.8–5.7)
50–59	435	861	508	2701	3.1 (2.6–3.7)
60–69	416	653	707	2299	2.5 (2.2–3.0)
70–79	111	163	369	942	1.9 (1.5–2.5)

*Smoker vs nonsmoker rates standardized for age and sex
Reproduced from Parish S *et al.*, Cigarette smoking, tar yields, and non-fatal myocardial infarction: 14000 cases and 32000 controls in the United Kingdom, *British Medical Journal*, 1995, with permission from BMJ Publishing Ltd.

general population almost certainly contributed to the early epidemics of acute MI in Western populations and are likely to be an important factor in the emerging epidemics of CVD in low- and middle-income countries.

. . . .

Question

4 In technical terms how would you describe the influence of age on the association between smoking habit and MI? (see Chapter 4)

. . . .

These factors operate largely independently of each other, although excess weight is a major determinant of hypertension and its contribution towards the risk of CVD is largely subsumed into the risk from hypertension (see Chapter 9). Official mortality data also show that there is a strongly increasing (exponential) relationship with age in both sexes; mortality rates are much lower in middle-aged women than in men, but are almost equal in men and women over 85 years of age. With the possible exception of age, none of these risk factors is in itself *sufficient* to predict CHD, although hypercholesterolaemia may be a *necessary* factor in that, in countries where the average population levels of plasma cholesterol are low, CHD is relatively uncommon. An example of a large prospective study conducted in such a country is shown in Table 7.3.

Plasma cholesterol was the first major risk factor identified for CHD and its role was further strengthened with the identification of a deficiency in the receptor for low-density lipoprotein (LDL) cholesterol in autosomal recessive genetic disorder of familial hypercholesterolaemia. In homozygotes, which occur rarely, premature CHD often leads to death in young adulthood. Heterozygotes tend to have hypercholoesterolaemia, but this typically occurs in middle age and the prevalence of heterozygotes has been estimated to be about one in 400 in the general population, which cannot account for the global epidemics of CHD. In the late 1960s high-density lipoprotein (HDL) cholesterol was found to be protective against the development of CHD, and its contribution was independent of that from total or from LDL cholesterol.

However, all these risk factors predict future risk of CHD in individuals rather poorly and, since CHD is still such a major cause of premature death, there has been an intensive search for additional risk factors. Some studies have shown that thrombosis factors predict future IHD as well as lipids (Yarnell *et al.* 2004), but it is possible that background lipid levels may have to be above a threshold level for this to occur. Over 200 'new' risk factors have been investigated including many biomarkers that have been investigated for diagnostic clinical studies. Although several biomarkers have provided evidence on new pathways involved in the pathogenesis of IHD and stroke, none has added predictive value to existing sets of risk factors (Wang 2011). Others have suggested that age alone is as cost-effective as screening for other risk factors for IHD in Caucasian populations (Wald *et al.* 2011).

Table 7.3 Number of deaths from coronary heart disease and from stroke during 8 to 13 years of follow-up in 9021 men and women aged 35–64 years from Shanghai according to their initial cholesterol level

	Number of deaths (relative risk*)					
	Cholesterol level (mmol/L)					
Deaths from:	≤3.53	3.54–4.10	4.11–4.62	≥4.63	All subjects	χ^2 for trend
Coronary heart disease	4 (**0.38**)	9 (**0.88**)	12 (**1.07**)	18 (**1.63**)	43 (**1.00**)	8.35**
Stroke	34 (**1.01**)	35 (**1.00**)	34 (**0.87**)	43 (**1.11**)	146 (**1.00**)	

*Relative risk adjusted for age, sex (and cohort)
**p < 0.01
Reproduced from Chen Z et al, 'Serum cholesterol concentration and coronary heart disease in population with low cholesterol concentrations', *British Medical Journal*, 1991, with permission from BMJ Publishing Ltd.

All the classic risk factors show a graded relationship (**dose–response**) with risk of subsequent CHD. Such a relationship is important in indicating a **causal** link with the disease in question but a link established in an intervention study is considered to be the highest level or 'gold standard' of evidence. Within the last decade, large multicentre trials have established the **efficacy** of statins, which are powerful lipid-lowering drugs, in reducing the incidence of CHD. Similarly, large-scale multicentre studies have demonstrated the efficacy of anti-hypertensive treatments against cardiovascular disease, and a trial of smoking cessation in civil servants has indicated a reduced risk of CHD (Rose and Colwell 1992). As the global epidemic continues the search for potentially modifiable risk factors becomes even more pressing. In a large case-control study of acute myocardial infarction in 52 countries across the globe, Yusuf *et al.* (2004) found that nine such factors were related to risk of IHD: smoking history, diabetes, hypertension, abdominal obesity, ApoB/ApoA1 ratio, fruit and vegetable intake, psychosocial stress factors, exercise, and regular alcohol consumption. Abdominal obesity was measured by waist/hip ratio and ApoB/ApoA1 is equivalent to the total/HDL-cholesterol ratio. Lower levels of education (primary level education only) were associated with higher levels of these *lifestyle* risk factors (Rosengren *et al.* 2009). Recently, a detailed analysis of work and leisure physical activity in this study found that leisure-time exercise and walking at work were associated with reduced risk of IHD; but ownership of a car or television was associated with an increased risk in low- middle- and high-income countries (Held *et al.* 2012). Table 7.4 shows the main results from a cohort study of 77,782 nurses recruited nationally in the USA in 1984, re-questioned every two years and followed up for 24 years.

A combination of all four risk factors (smoking, overweight, sedentary lifestyle, and low diet quality) from Table 7.4 produced a relative risk of 7.0 (95% CI 4.5–10.6) for cardiovascular and 2.7 (95% CI 2.1–3.3) for cancer mortality. Fifty-five per cent of deaths could be attributed to this combination of risk factors (van Dam *et al.* 2008).

....

Questions

5 **What is the main advantage in scientific terms of choosing nurses as the study group? And similarly the main disadvantage?**

6 **If the resources had been available what other measurements (in order of priority) could the authors have included in their study?**

....

7.2 Congestive heart failure

This disorder is the result of pump failure of the heart and its presentation and causes are very different in high-income and low-income countries. In high-income countries, where the epidemiological transition has progressed to reach a further stage where degenerative diseases predominate, a steady and perhaps, unexpectedly sustained decline in mortality due to CHD and stroke has been witnessed during the past 25–35 years together with a marked increase in adult life expectancy. Modelling studies suggest that this is largely due to a decline in the population prevalence of risk factors but also in part to improvements in treatment (Unal *et al.* 2005). Inspection of Table 7.1 shows that age-standardized stroke and IHD rates are low in high-income countries and substantially higher in low- and middle-income countries, particularly for stroke (IHD mortality may be more variable due to coding variability between countries).

In consequence of lengthening life expectancy hospitalization rates for CHF and some other end-stage diseases of the elderly have increased in all high-income countries. In Germany, the number of hospitalizations for CHF increased by 52 per cent between the years 2000 and 2009, and the proportion estimated to be due to population ageing was 22 per cent (Nowossadeck 2012). However, treatments for CHF may have improved as a study over 20 years in seven European countries found that age standardized mortality from CHF as the underlying cause of death had declined by 40 per cent and the mean age at death increased from 80.0 to 82.7 years (Laribi *et al.* 2012).

Table 7.4 Relative risk of sudden cardiac death in nurses by degree of healthy lifestyle

Lifestyle factor	Person-years × 10^5	Cardiovascular deaths Adjusted RR (95% CI)	Cancer deaths Adjusted RR (95% CI)
Smoking (cig/day)			
15 +	2.0	3.3 (2.9–3.9)	2.1 (1.9–2.3)
1–14	1.0	2.6 (2.2–3.1)	1.8 (1.4–2.1)
Past	6.7	1.5 (1.3–1.7)	1.5 (1.4–1.6)
Never	7.9	1.0	1.0
Exercise (hrs/wk)			
0.0–0.4	1.2	1.0	1.0
0.5–1.9	6.0	0.9 (0.8–1.1)	0.9 (0.8–1.0)
2.0–3.4	3.7	0.9 (0.7–1.0)	0.8 (0.8–0.9)
3.5–5.4	2.0	0.7 (0.6–0.9)	0.8 (0.7–0.9)
≥ 5.5	2.5	0.6 (0.5–0.7)	0.7 (0.6–0.8)
BMI (kg/m²)			
≥ 30.0	1.8	2.8 (2.5–3.2)	1.3 (1.2–1.5)
25–29.9	4.0	1.5 (1.3–1.6)	1.1 (1.1–1.2)
18.5–24.9	11.7	1.0	1.0
Healthy diet score			
Least healthy fifth	3.4	1.0	1.0
	3.5	1.0 (0.8–1.1)	0.8 (0.8–0.9)
	3.6	0.8 (0.7–0.9)	0.8 (0.7–0.9)
	3.6	0.8 (0.7–0.9)	0.8 (0.7–0.9)
Most healthy fifth	3.6	0.6 (0.5–0.7)	0.7 (0.4–0.8)

Adjusted for age, time period, and other risk factors in table.
Reproduced from van Dam RM *et al.*, 'Combined impact of lifestyle factors on mortality: prospective cohort study in US women', *British Medical Journal*, 2008, with permission from BMJ Publishing Ltd.

Risk factors: in a 19-year follow-up of a national sample of US adults, new cases of CHF were attributed to IHD (62 per cent), smoking (16 per cent), hypertension (10 per cent), obesity (8 per cent), diabetes (3 per cent), and valvular disease (2 per cent) (He *et al.* 2001).

In the Copenhagen Heart Study in almost 14,000 men and women free of CHD or CHF at entry, male sex, hypertension, high body mass index, smoking, family history, and low socio-economic status were associated with risk of hospital admission for CHF (Christensen *et al.* 2011). Several prospective studies suggest a role for inflammatory markers in the prediction of incident heart failure (Pfister *et al.* 2012).

Non-IHD CHF: in low-income countries there is a continuing legacy of rheumatic valve disease estimated to affect about 16 million people worldwide, particularly in sub-Saharan Africa and in indigenous peoples in Australia and New Zealand. In South America, Chagas disease due to *Trypanosoma cruzi* is endemic, with an estimated 10 million people worldwide with the disease and 25 million at risk (Mendis *et al.* 2011). In middle- and low-income countries there is a rapid increase in hypertension, obesity, and diabetes; these disorders are often poorly treated and culminate in CHF, stroke, or renal failure.

Cardiomyopathies, in which there is primary myocardial disease, are a heterogeneous group of diseases which have many possible causes that often remain unidentified in clinical practice. In high-income countries hypertrophic cardiomyopathy, which occurs in an estimated 0.2–0.5 per cent of the population in all racial groups, can lead to sudden death in young athletes, and is reported to be predominantly an autosomal dominant trait (Stroumpoulis *et al.* 2010). Many toxic substances such as alcohol, addictive drugs, chemotherapeutic agents, and deficiency diseases (for example, selenium deficiency) can lead to myocardial damage and failure. In the US alcohol abuse is the leading cause of non-ischaemic dilated cardiomyopathy (Piano 2002).

7.3 Stroke

Stroke (cerebrovascular accident) is a sudden neurological deficit or malfunction from a vascular cause which could range from loss of consciousness to partial loss of motor or sensory function. To be classified as stroke these symptoms must persist for 24 hours or more and shorter periods of deficit are termed *transient ischaemic attack* (*TIA*). However, improved diagnostic techniques have shown that a proportion of these result in focal areas of brain infarction and would be better termed *mini-strokes*. Clinical examination cannot usually distinguish between stroke due to *ischaemia* or

that due to rupture of a blood vessel (*haemorrhagic stroke*), but neurological examination can often point to the particular part of the brain affected.

Subarachnoid haemorrhage is clinically and epidemiologically distinct, as the blood vessels are those of the subarachnoid space surrounding the brain.

Intracerebral haemorrhage is the most common type of haemorraghic stroke and occurs more commonly in the elderly population. In high-income countries, computed tomography (CT), which produces radiological, cross-sectional images sequentially of the whole brain, is frequently used to distinguish haemorrhagic from ischaemic stroke, but in the developing world these expensive diagnostic facilities are not available. Globally, 70 per cent of strokes are due to ischaemia and up to 30 per cent to haemorrhage (intracerebral 20 per cent, subarachnoid 10 per cent) (Chandra *et al.* 2006). In the INTERSTROKE study, a case-control study of 3000 stroke survivors with first events and 3000 controls in 22 countries, 78 per cent of strokes were ischaemic and 22 per cent were intracerebral confirmed by neuroimaging, but strokes due to subarachnoid haemorrhage, which are clinically and therapeutically distinct, were excluded (O'Donnell *et al.* 2010). Countries such as China and Japan are reported to have a particularly high occurrence of haemorrhagic stroke with up to 40 per cent of strokes of this type (Chandra *et al.* 2006), but in INTERSTROKE 22 per cent of strokes were classified as due to intracerebral haemorrhage in South East Asia (China, Malaysia and Philippines) compared to 34 per cent in Africa and nine per cent in high-income countries included in the study. Further studies using stroke registers may be helpful in establishing the incidence of stroke subtypes in lower- and middle-income countries.

For both clinical and epidemiological purposes it is useful to distinguish ischaemic from haemorrhagic stroke. Antiplatelet or thrombolytic drugs should be withheld from patients with haemorrhagic strokes and those with subarachnoid haemorrhage should be referred for neurosurgical opinion. Haemorrhagic strokes may have different epidemiological risk factors to those for ischaemic stroke. Ischaemic stroke can be due to local occlusion of an artery supplying the brain (the bifurcation of the internal carotid is a common site for atherothrombosis) but *thrombi* can also originate either from the left atrium in atrial fibrillation or from the left ventricle in acute myocardial infarction or congestive heart failure. Various classification systems have been developed to classify ischaemic strokes (Marnane *et al.* 2010) and, in general, large vessel disease carries a higher risk of recurrence than small vessel disease. Haemorrhagic strokes, and particularly, subarachnoid haemorrhage, are frequently associated with aneurysm (berry aneurysm) and need to be fully investigated for possible surgical repair.

In Fig. 7.3 the principal results of a survey carried out in urban and rural Tanzania are compared with data from England and Wales. Regular censuses and prospective monitoring of all deaths in three defined populations in Tanzania were carried out between 1992 and 1995. *Verbal autopsies* (witness statements of the symptoms and signs preceding death) were obtained from relatives, or carers of those who died. Mortality in men and women in three areas of Tanzania and in England and Wales are shown in Fig. 7.3.

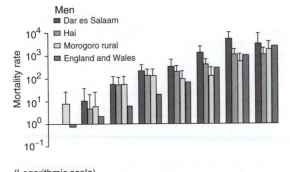

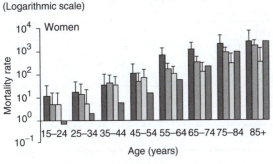

Figure 7.3 Mortality from stroke in three districts in sub-Saharan Africa and in England and Wales by age group.
Adapted from Walker R *et al.* (2000) 'Stroke mortality in urban and rural Tanzania', *The Lancet* **355**, 9216, with permission from Elsevier.

The scale used for the mortality rate is logarithmic and the results indicate that the stroke death rates rise exponentially with age. The mortality from stroke is highest in the urban area of Dar es Salaam (the largest city and commercial capital), intermediate in Hai (a well-developed rural area), and lower in Morogoro (a poorly-developed rural area), but lowest of all in England and Wales (except in men and women aged 75 or more years). Death rates from most other causes were, of course, much higher in Tanzania than in England and Wales. The authors noted that atheroma was rare in Africa and ischaemic strokes may have been mainly due to cardiac emboli, possibly from *rheumatic heart disease*; haemorrhagic strokes probably contributed disproportionately to the total as other studies indicate that this group contribute 28–33 per cent of the total burden of stroke in Africa. The high level of stroke mortality in Tanzania was attributed to untreated hypertension (Walker *et al.* 2000). A recent epidemiological survey of urban and rural populations in sub-Saharan Africa confirms the high prevalence of untreated hypertension establishing this as the commonest risk factor for CVD in the region (Hendriks *et al.* 2012).

Risk factors: as already noted, the mortality from stroke (and also the incidence) rises exponentially with age. Subarachnoid haemorrhage is the most common category in men and women under 45 years of age in Western countries but rises only linearly with age. Most studies on stroke epidemiology treat subarachnoid haemorrhage separately, although the major risk factors—hypertension and smoking habit—are shared with both ischaemic and haemorrhagic stroke. In a recent study in Europe the proportion of strokes that were haemorrhagic varied between eight and 29 per cent and subarachnoid haemorrhage accounted for between one and six per cent of all registered strokes (Heuschmann *et al.* 2009).

In comparison with CHD the epidemiology of stroke is in its infancy. A major review for the Stroke Council of the American Heart Association (Goldstein *et al.* 2001) concluded that potentially modifiable risk factors were: hypertension, smoking, diabetes mellitus, carotid stenosis, hyperlipidaemia, and atrial fibrillation. Although other risk factors have been established in observational studies (such as obesity, sedentary lifestyle, alcohol consumption, hyperhomocysteinaemia, hypercoagulability, hormone replacement therapy, and inflammatory markers), the evidence that modification of these factors was beneficial or achievable was less convincing. Smoking is a major risk factor for both ischaemic and haemorrhagic stroke, but is a particularly strong risk factor for subarachnoid haemorrhage, whose epidemiology is less well explored (as the population incidence is low in comparison with that of other types of stroke). Table 7.5 shows the risk factors reported as showing significant associations with non-fatal first strokes in the INTERSTROKE study.

The mean age of stroke patients in this study was 66 years in the high-income countries and in South America, but less than 60 years in the low- and middle income countries. Hypertension was a strongest individual risk factor for stroke overall but was several times higher for intracerebral haemorrhage than for ischaemic stroke. Moderate alcohol consumption was marginally protective for ischaemic stroke but it was significantly associated with risk of haemorrhagic

stroke. Heavier alcohol consumption and binge drinking was associated with increased risk of any stroke.

Fig. 7.4 shows the major impact of blood pressure on the risk of stroke taken from a meta-analysis of 61 observational studies among one million men and women with a combined total of 12.7 million person-years at risk. It illustrates an important point in epidemiology that it is vital to establish the nature of the association between a risk factor and the incidence or mortality from a disease. If it begins at the lowest point of the distribution then the cut-point for intervention to reduce the level of the risk factor is arbitrary and depends on cost-benefit or cost-effectiveness considerations; and the lowest possible level of the risk factor is the ideal. Within the past 10–15 years major multicentre trials have shown clear benefit in treatment of hypertension in the elderly whose blood pressure tends to be high (blood pressure increases with age in the general population) and who are at high risk of stroke. Until these trials published their results in

Table 7.5 Risk factors for stroke in the INTERSTROKE study (multivariable analysis)

	Ischaemic stroke (n = 2337)	Intracerebral haemorrhage (n = 663)
	Odds ratio (95% CI)	Odds ratio (95% CI)
Self-report hypertension or BP 160/90+	2.4 (2.0–2.8)	9.2 (6.8–12.4)
Current smoker	2.3 (1.9–2.8)	1.5 (1.1–2.0)
Waist–hip ratio (tertile 1 vs 3)	1.7 (1.4–2.1)	1.4 (1.0–1.9)
Diet risk score (tertile 1 vs 3)	1.3 (1.1–1.7)	1.4 (1.0–2.0)
Regular physical activity	0.7 (0.5–0.9)	0.7 (0.4–1.1)
Diabetes mellitus	1.6 (1.3–2.0)	NI
Alcohol 1–30 drinks per month	0.8 (0.6–1.0)	1.5 (1.1–2.2)
More than 30 or binge drinker	1.4 (1.1–1.8)	2.0 (1.4–3.0)
Psychosocial stress	1.3 (1.0–1.6)	1.2 (0.9–1.7)
Depression	1.5 (1.2–1.8)	NI
Cardiac causes	2.7 (1.8–3.2)	NI
ApoB/ApoA1 ratio	2.4 (1.9–3.1)	NI

NI = not included in multivariable analysis.

Reproduced from O'Donnell M et al., 'Risk factors for ischaemic and intracerebral haemorrhagic stroke in 22 countries (the INTERSTROKE study): a case-control study', *The Lancet*, 2010, with permission from Elsevier.

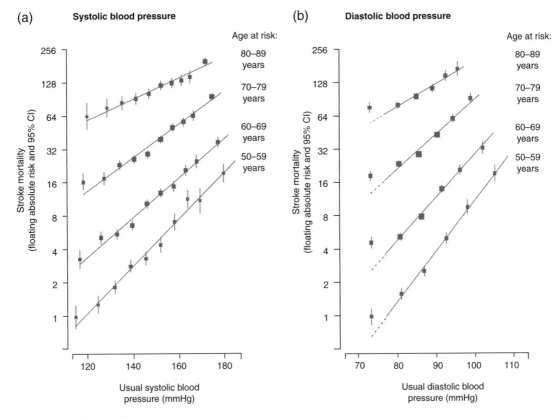

Figure 7.4 Risk of fatal stroke by usual blood pressure and age group.

Reproduced from Lewington S *et al.*, 'Age-specific relevance of usual blood pressure to vascular mortality: a meta-analysis of individual data for one million adults in 61 prospective studies', *The Lancet* **360**, 9349, 2002, with permission from Elsevier.

the late 1980s, blood pressure in the elderly was rarely treated. Now the weight of observational and experimental evidence has resulted in the recommendation that 140/90mm Hg in all age groups should be used as the new threshold for initiation of preventive treatment (both non-pharmacological and pharmacological), replacing the previous threshold of 160/95mmHg (Anon 1999).

7.4 Peripheral arterial disease and aortic aneurysm

Atherosclerosis can affect many arteries including the carotid, renal, and mesenteric arteries, the thoracic and abdominal aorta, and the arteries distal to these. Peripheral vascular disease is defined as atherosclerosis

of the major vessels supplying the lower limbs resulting in ischaemia which can produce the symptoms of calf pain on exertion (claudication) or, in more severe cases, chronic anoxia to the lower limbs resulting in gangrene. The prevalence is high in the elderly and 12–20 per cent of Americans aged 65 years or more have this disorder in national surveys (Ostchega *et al.* 2007). Cigarette smoking is a strong risk factor for this disease and coexistence with other manifestations of atherosclerotic disease is common. Surveys suggest that peripheral arterial disease is underdiagnosed and undertreated (Shanmugasundaram *et al.* 2011).

Aortic aneurysm is presumptively atherosclerotic in nature and is also closely associated with cigarette smoking. Dissection and rupture of the aorta is a potentially preventable cause of death, particularly in the case of the abdominal aorta. Small aneurysms are asymptomatic and may not progress. The incidence of both symptomatic (large) and asymptomatic aneurysms increased in most high-income countries until the 1990s but the incidence now appears to be decreasing. Screening for this condition has been suggested since elective surgical repair carries a five to eight per cent 30-day mortality in comparison with up to 90 per cent mortality for ruptured aneurysm; a trial of screening conducted in the south of England has shown encouraging results (Ashton et al. 2002), but recent declines in the prevalence of aortic aneurysm reported in Sweden, New Zealand, and in England and Wales have suggested that screening strategies may be modified to screen men older than 65 years or to routinely repeat screening. A combination of factors such as a decline in the prevalence of cigarette smoking, earlier detection, and more aggressive medical treatment with statins and antihypertensive medication may account for the changing epidemiology of this condition (Choke et al. 2012).

7.5 Prevention of cardiovascular disease

Many of the established risk factors for IHD and stroke are potentially modifiable and provide the opportunity for primary prevention in the general population. Modelling studies in several high-income countries in Europe and North America indicate that population changes in major risk factors account for over half of the population decline in IHD and modern treatments for a further third (Capewell and O'Flaherty 2011). In a recent report from Poland for the period 1991 to 2005, 41 per cent and 33 per cent of the fall in IHD mortality in men and in women, respectively, could be attributed to declines in plasma cholesterol level from changes in the diet in the general population (Bandosz et al. 2012).

A recent national survey in the USA reported that 50 per cent of adults aged 20 or more years had at least one of the major risk factors for IHD (smoking, hypercholesterolaemia, or hypertension) (Anon 2011), and a third of adults were obese (Roger et al. 2012), and it is increasingly recognized that major policy initiatives are required (Pearson 2011).

But the majority of CVD deaths occur in low- and middle-income countries where age-standardized rates are already higher than in high-income countries and the burden of risk factors is often higher (Gersh et al. 2010). Low-cost initiatives have been proposed (WHO 2011) and it has been estimated that worldwide initiatives by the United Nations to influence dietary policies along the general lines of the healthy diets consumed by a small proportion of the American nurses in the study reported in Table 7.4 could reduce the CVD deaths worldwide by up to 50 per cent. Non-pharmacological treatments and preventive strategies for the general population to lower the 'population mean' of a particular risk factor remain the public health strategy of choice but require major cultural and policy changes that may be difficult to achieve in practice (see also Fig. 1.3 and Chapter 9).

International policy initiatives in early development by agencies such as WHO designed to counter the rise of the epidemic of CVD in low- and middle-income countries are discussed further in Chapter 22.

References

Ahmad Y and Lip GYH (2012) Stroke prevention in atrial fibrillation: where are we now? *Clinical Medicine Insights. Cardiology* **6**, 65–78.

Anon (1999) 1999 World Health Organization International Society of Hypertension Guidelines for the Management of Hypertension. Guidelines Subcommittee. *Journal of Hypertension* **17**(2), 151–83.

Anon (2011) Million hearts: strategies to reduce the prevalence of leading cardiovascular disease risk factors—United States, 2011. *MMRW* **60** (36), 1248–51.

Ashton HA, Buxton MJ, Day NE, Kim LG, et al. (2002) The Multicentre Aneurysm Screening Study (MASS) into the effect of abdominal aortic aneurysm screening on mortality in men: a randomized controlled trial. *Lancet* **360** (9345), 1531–9.

Bandosz P, O'Flaherty M, Drygas W, Rutkowski M, et al. (2012) Decline in mortality from coronary heart disease in Poland after socioeconomic transformation: modelling study. *BMJ (Clinical Research Ed)* **344**, d8136.

Borissoff JI, Spronk HMH, and ten Cate, H (2011) The hemostatic system as a modulator of atherosclerosis. *The New England Journal of Medicine* **364** (18), 1746–60.

Blood Pressure Lowering Treatment Trialists' Collaboration (2000) Effects of ACEe inhibitors, calcium antagonists, and other blood-pressure-lowering drugs: results of prospectively designed overviews of randomized trials. *Lancet* **355**, 1955–64.

Capewell S and O'Flaherty M (2011) Rapid mortality falls after risk-factor changes in populations. *Lancet* **378** (9793), 752–3.

Chandra V, Pandav R, Laxminarayan R, *et al.* (2006) Neurological disorders. In: Jamison DT, Breman JG, Measham AR, *et al.* (eds) Disease Control Priorities in Developing Countries, 2nd edn; pp. 627–44. Washington, DC: World Bank.

Chen Z, Peto R, Collins R, MacMahon S, *et al.* (1991) Serum cholesterol concentration and coronary heart disease in population with low cholesterol concentrations. *BMJ (Clinical Research Ed)* **303** (6797), 276–82.

Choke E, Vijaynagar B, Thompson J, Nasim A, *et al.* (2012) Changing epidemiology of abdominal aortic aneurysms in England and Wales: older and more benign? *Circulation* **125** (13), 1617–25.

Christensen S, Mogelvang R, Heitmann M, and Prescott E (2011) Level of Education and Risk of Heart Failure: A Prospective Cohort Study with Echocardiography Evaluation. *European Heart Journal* **32** (4), 450–8.

Gersh BJ, Sliwa K, Mayosi BM, and Yusuf S (2010) Novel therapeutic concepts: the epidemic of cardiovascular disease in the developing world: global implications. *European Heart Journal* **31** (6), 642–8.

Goldstein LB, Adams R, Becker K, Furberg CD, *et al.* (2001) Primary prevention of ischemic stroke: A statement for healthcare professionals from the Stroke Council of the American Heart Association. *Circulation* **103** (1), 163–82.

He J, Ogden LG, Bazzano LA, Vupputuri S, *et al.* (2001) Risk factors for congestive heart failure in US men and women: NHANES I epidemiologic follow-up study. *Archives of Internal Medicine* **161** (7), 996–1002.

Held C, Iqbal R, Lear SA, Rosengren A, *et al.* (2012) Physical activity levels, ownership of goods promoting sedentary behaviour and risk of myocardial infarction: results of the INTERHEART study. *European Heart Journal* **33** (4), 452–66.

Hendriks ME, Wit FWNM, Roos MTL, Brewster LM, *et al.* (2012) Hypertension in sub-Saharan Africa: cross-sectional surveys in four rural and urban communities. *PloS One* **7** (3), e32638.

Heuschmann PU, Di Carlo A, Bejot Y, Rastenyte D, *et al.* (2009) Incidence of stroke in Europe at the beginning of the 21st century. *Stroke; a Journal of Cerebral Circulation* **40** (5), 1557–63.

Laribi S, Aouba A, Nikolaou M, Lassus J, *et al.* (2012) Trends in death attributed to heart failure over the past two decades in Europe. *European Journal of Heart Failure* **14** (3), 234–9.

Lewington S, Clarke R, Qizilbash N, Peto R, *et al.* (2002) Age-specific relevance of usual blood pressure to vascular mortality: a meta-analysis of individual data for one million adults in 61 prospective studies. *Lancet* **360** (9349), 1903–13.

Libby P, Ridker PM, and Hansson GK (2011) Progress and challenges in translating the biology of atherosclerosis. *Nature* **473** (7347), 317–25.

Luepker RV, Evans A, McKeigue P and Reddy KS (2004) *Cardiovascular Survey Methods,* 3rd edn. Geneva: WHO.

Marnane M, Duggan CA, Sheehan OC, Merwick A, *et al.* (2010) Stroke Subtype Classification to Mechanism-Specific and Undetermined Categories by TOAST, A-S-C-O, and Causative Classification System Direct Comparison in the North Dublin Population Stroke Study. *Stroke.* **41** (8), 1579–86.

Mendis S, Puska P, Norrving B (eds) (2011) *Global Atlas on Cardiovascular Disease Prevention and Control.* Geneva: World Health Organization.

Norris RM (1998) Fatality outside hospital from acute coronary events in three British health districts, 1994–5. United Kingdom Heart Attack Study Collaborative Group. *BMJ (Clinical Research Ed)* **316** (7137), 1065–70.

Nowossadeck E (2012) Population aging and hospitalization for chronic disease in Germany. *DeutschesÄrzteblatt International* **109** (9), 151–7.

O'Donnell MJ, Xavier D, Liu L, Zhang H, *et al.* (2010) Risk factors for ischaemic and intracerebral haemorrhagic stroke in 22 countries (the INTERSTROKE study): a case-control study. *Lancet* **376** (9735), 112–23.

Ostchega Y, Paulose-Ram R, Dillon CF, Gu Q, *et al.* (2007) Prevalence of peripheral arterial disease and risk factors in persons aged 60 and older: data from the National Health and Nutrition Examination Survey 1999–2004. *Journal of the American Geriatrics Society* **55** (4), 583–9.

Parish S, Collins R, Peto R, Youngman L, *et al.* (1995) Cigarette smoking, tar yields, and non-fatal myocardial infarction: 14,000 cases and 32,000 controls in the United Kingdom. The International Studies of Infarct Survival (ISIS) Collaborators. *BMJ (Clinical Research Ed)* **311** (7003), 471–7.

Park D, McManus D, Darling C, Goldberg JH, *et al.* (2011) Recent trends in the characteristics and prognosis of patients hospitalized with acute heart failure. *Clinical Epidemiology* **3**, 295–303.

Pearson TA (2011) Public policy approaches to the prevention of heart disease and stroke. *Circulation* **124** (23), 2560–71.

Pfister R, Sharp SJ, Luben R, Wareham NJ, *et al.* (2012) Differential white blood cell count and incident heart failure in men and women in the EPIC-Norfolk study. *European Heart Journal* **33** (4), 523–30.

Piano MR (2002) Alcoholic cardiomyopathy. *Chest* **121** (5), 1638–50.

Roger VL, Go AS, Lloyd-Jones DM, Benjamin EJ, *et al.* (2012) Executive summary: heart disease and stroke statistics—2012 update: a report from the American Heart Association. *Circulation* **125** (1), 188–97.

Rose G and Colwell L (1992) Randomized controlled trial of anti-smoking advice: final (20 year) results. *Journal of Epidemiology and Community Health* **46** (1), 75–7.

Rosengren A, Subramanian SV, Islam S, Chow CK, *et al.* (2009) Education and risk for acute myocardial infarction in 52 high, middle and low-income countries: INTER-HEART case-control study. *Heart (British Cardiac Society)* **95** (24), 2014–22.

Salomaa V, Koukkunen H, Ketonen M, Immonen-Räihä P, *et al.* (2005) A new definition for myocardial infarction: what difference does it make? *European Heart Journal* **26** (17), 1719–25.

Shanmugasundaram M, Ram VK, Luft UC, Szerlip M, *et al.* (2011) Peripheral arterial disease—what do we need to know? *Clinical Cardiology* **34** (8), 478–82.

Stroumpoulis KI, Pantazopoulos IN and Xanthos TT (2010) Hypertrophic cardiomyopathy and sudden cardiac death. *World Journal of Cardiology* **2** (9), 289–98.

Unal B, Critchley JA and Capewell S (2005) Modelling the decline in coronary heart disease deaths in England and Wales, 1981–2000: comparing contributions from primary prevention and secondary prevention. *BMJ (Clinical Research Ed)* **331** (7517), 614.

Wald NJ, Simmonds M, and Morris JK (2011) Screening for future cardiovascular disease using age alone compared with multiple risk factors and age. *PloS One* **6** (5), e18742.

Walker RW, McLarty DG, Kitange HM, Whiting D, *et al.* (2000) Stroke mortality in urban and rural Tanzania. Adult Morbidity and Mortality Project. *Lancet* **355** (9216), 1684–7.

Wang TJ (2011) Assessing the role of circulating, genetic, and imaging biomarkers in cardiovascular risk prediction. *Circulation* **123** (5), 551–65.

van Dam RM, Li T, Spiegelman D, Franco OH, *et al.* (2008) Combined impact of lifestyle factors on mortality: prospective cohort study in US women. *BMJ (Clinical Research Ed)* **337**, a1440.

Yarnell JWG, Patterson CC, Sweetnam PM and Lowe GDO (2004) Haemostatic/inflammatory markers predict 10-year risk of IHD at least as well as lipids: the Caerphilly collaborative studies. *European Heart Journal* **25** (12), 1049–56.

Yeghiazarians Y, Braunstein JB, Askari A and Stone PH (2000) Unstable angina pectoris. *The New England Journal of Medicine* **342** (2), 101–14.

Yusuf S, Hawken S, Ounpuu S, Dans T, *et al.* (2004) Effect of potentially modifiable risk factors associated with myocardial infarction in 52 countries (the INTER-HEART study): case-control study. *Lancet* **364** (9438), 937–52.

Model answers

Question 1

Crude death rates are likely to show higher mortality from IHD in high-income countries as most IHD deaths occur in the older age groups. In low-income countries there is a higher level of premature IHD.

Question 2

The differences may be artifactual due to differences in diagnostic fashion among doctors in different countries or real due to different combinations of risk factors.

Question 3

IHD is one category of heart disease. Other categories should also be checked as other heart disease often contains important non-rheumatic heart disease related to major CVD risk factors such as hypertension or diabetes.

Question 4

Age is an effect-modifier of smoking on the risk of IHD as the relative risk is substantially higher in the younger age groups than in older groups.

Question 5

They represent a well-educated and probably well-motivated group who should supply reliable data. A disadvantage is that they are unlikely to be representative of the general population.

Question 6

Biological CVD risk factors could have been measured, e.g. blood pressure, more accurate measures of weight, height, waist circumference (rather than self-reported measures), serum biomarkers such as lipids, etc.

8 Respiratory system

KATHY CULLEN AND JOHN YARNELL

CHAPTER CONTENTS

This chapter describes the main causes of respiratory morbidity and mortality worldwide. Respiratory infection is a leading worldwide cause of death in infancy and a major cause of death in the elderly. The role of cigarette smoking, air pollution, occupational, and domestic exposures as a cause of lung disease is also reviewed.

Introduction

At birth there are around 64,000 terminal bronchioles and 20 million alveoli, which increase to about 300 million during the first year of life. The delicate ciliated bronchial epithelium has several highly efficient defence mechanisms against particulate and microbiological invasion but is particularly vulnerable to pathological damage at the extremes of age. Even *in utero*, fetal lungs may be affected by the nutritional health and lifestyle of the mother. A prospective study in Dutch mothers suggested that consumption of apples during pregnancy may have a protective effect against the development of childhood asthma and fish consumption is negatively associated with eczema (Willers *et al.* 2007). Exposure to maternal tobacco smoking during pregnancy and lactation adversely affects lung development principally acting through the effects of nicotine (Maritz and Harding 2011).

Respiratory infections are an important cause of **infant mortality** (*deaths during the first year of life*), particularly in the **post-neonatal period** (*after 28 days*). This mortality occurs more frequently in developing countries, often with tropical climates, than in industrialized, well-developed countries. There is often a problem with host resistance or immunological competence, which can be due to sub-optimal nutrition. For example, in developing countries, measles and many other viral infections can leave children vulnerable to a deadly secondary bacterial pneumonia. Similarly, in old age *hypostatic pneumonia* is often the cause of death in a body incapacitated by other major diseases such as cancer or stroke. Pneumonia is the consequence of a sustained infection of the lower (or distal) part of the respiratory tract. Alveoli are party filled with fluid, and gas exchange is severely restricted. The generic term *bronchopneumonia* tends to be used for non-specific pneumonias but can be made more specific, for example, *lobar* pneumonia or *aspiration* pneumonia.

Acute upper respiratory tract infections (infections above the level of the bronchi) are circulating in populations continuously and cause significant symptoms in children and adults usually several times a year. They are the leading cause of sickness absence but are usually self-limiting. In susceptible subjects they can precede the development of lower respiratory infections and bacterial pneumonias. Influenza is epidemic in nature and new strains of influenza virus can be charted across the globe (see Chapter 18).

Besides being vulnerable to micro-organisms, lungs are prone to damage from exposure to inhaled chemical or physical agents such as tobacco smoke and atmospheric and workplace pollutants. *Pneumoconioses* are a group of diseases of the lung which are the result of occupational exposure to dusts such as silica (silicosis), beryllium (beryllosis), asbestos (asbestosis), and fungi such as *Aspergillus* (aspergillosis: farmer's lung). The terms *chronic bronchitis, emphysema,* and *chronic obstructive pulmonary disease (COPD)* are terms which reflect different aspects of the same disease: chronic bronchitis describes the inflammatory nature of the disease (productive cough for three or more months per year); emphysema is the result of over-inflation of the alveoli (destruction of their structure and functional capacity), and COPD describes the overall condition. This is characterized by airflow obstruction that is not fully reversible and is usually progressive in the long term. Chronic obstructive pulmonary disease is predominantly caused by chronic inflammation secondary to cigarette smoke and leads to airway and parenchymal damage.

Another important group of respiratory diseases are believed to have a mainly allergic basis. These include *asthma*, which is showing a rising prevalence worldwide along with other atopic diseases such as hay fever, and occupational asthma, which is highly prevalent in certain industrial environments. *Pulmonary tuberculosis* is the most important cause of mortality in adults in many parts of the developing regions of the world and is closely associated with HIV infection. Antibiotic resistance and malnutrition are responsible for the high mortality in many areas. This disease is discussed further in Chapter 18.

8.1 Acute respiratory tract infections

Upper respiratory tract infections are the commonest presenting illness in primary care and a large range of viruses are responsible which include: influenza A and B, parainfluenza, rhinovirus, adenovirus, enterovirus,

and respiratory syncytial virus (RSV); RSV is associated with the largest burden of disease in infancy (Nair *et al.* 2011). These viruses are passed easily from person to person by droplet spread from coughing or sneezing, by touch, and from household or office objects. Many patients seek treatment from their general practitioner, but a systematic review suggests that antibiotic therapy is usually unnecessary except for some bacterial infections, for example, haemolytic streptococcal infection of throat with local complications (Fahey *et al.* 1998).

Vaccines are not available for most respiratory viruses, but a review of cohort studies and trials suggests that yearly influenza vaccination significantly reduces the risk of death associated with the complications of influenza in the elderly (Gross *et al.* 1995). In the UK and elsewhere this has been adopted as public health policy and the annual influenza vaccination is offered to those older than 65, pregnant women, those with a serious medical condition (e.g. diabetes, asthma) and frontline health and social care workers. In the UK, it is now recommended that all children aged between two and 17 should have an annual influenza vaccination, offered as a nasal spray. It is estimated that this will save over a thousand deaths and tens of thousands of hospital admissions. The most common strain of influenza mutates slightly each year and these seasonal changes are monitored by the World Health Organization (WHO) so that the most appropriate vaccine can be produced every year. Further public health measures to curtail the spread of influenza include general advice regarding frequent hand washing, using disposable tissues for sneezing and coughing, and remaining at home if unwell (Fidler and Gostin 2011). Pandemic influenza is further discussed in Chapter 18. In children, *bronchiolitis*, or inflammation of the small airways of the lungs (bronchioles) is caused by RSV in over half of the cases. Infections with strains of RSV tend to occur annually in children (see Fig. 8.1) and have been associated with the onset of wheezy bronchitis and subsequent asthma in susceptible children. Parainfluenza 3 is the next most common cause. Household tobacco smoke and low admission weight have been shown to be important risk factors (Semple *et al.* 2011). Several viruses predispose to pneumonia (RSV, influenza, chickenpox, parainfluenza, measles,

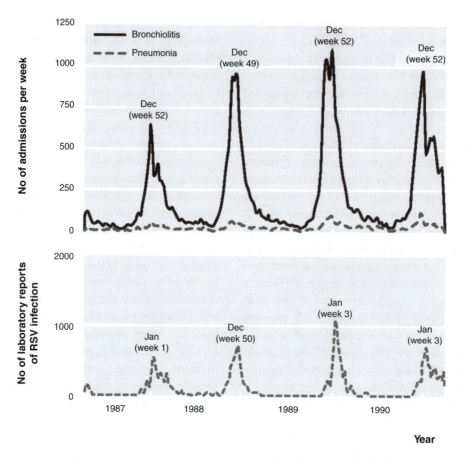

Figure 8.1 Season association between respiratory syncytial virus (RSV) infections and hospital admissions for bronchiolitis.

Reproduced from Bush A and Thomson A, 'Acute bronchiolitis', *British Medical Journal*, 2007, with permission from BMJ Publishing Ltd.

and adenoviruses). RSV is a major cause of mortality in pneumonia in infancy after pneumococcal and *H. influenza type B* infections (Nair *et al.* 2010).

Pneumonia is most simply classified into two distinct epidemiological types: community-acquired and hospital-acquired (or nosocomial; Greek: hospital). In developing countries, mortality from respiratory infections is second only to 'perinatal causes' as the leading cause of death in infancy and childhood. *Community-acquired pneumonia* causes over one million hospital admissions per year in the UK. The British Thoracic Society define community-acquired pneumonia as symptoms of an acute lower respiratory tract illness (cough and at least one other lower respiratory tract symptom), new focal chest

signs on examination, and at least one systemic feature (either a symptom complex of sweating, fevers, shivers, aches, and pains and/or temperature of 38°C or more) (Lim *et al.* 2009). In the UK, the annual incidence is 5–11 per 1000 adult population and between 22 per cent and 44 per cent of adults with this are admitted to hospital. In Europe, the most common bacterial pathogens responsible are *Streptococcus* (> 30 per cent), *Haemophilus influenzae* (10 per cent), *Moraxella catarhalis*, *Chlamydia*, *Mycoplasma*, and *Legionella*. Viruses cause another 13 per cent of these pneumonias. Studies in the USA show a similar pattern (Ruiz *et al.* 1999). It has been estimated that 40 per cent of hospitalized patients with pneumonia do not receive a microbiological diagnosis. In middle-aged adults, cigarette smoking is a major risk factor. Alcohol and corticosteroid therapy can also impair ciliary and immune function. In the elderly, general debility, recent influenza, other upper respiratory tract infections or major co-morbidities predispose to pneumonia (Lim *et al.* 2009).

Hospital-acquired pneumonia is defined as a pneumonia that develops a minimum of 48 hours after admission to hospital and which was not incubating at admission. Some two to five per cent of hospital admissions are complicated by the development of this condition and it increases the length of stay by seven to nine days per patient (Anon 2005). It is more common in those with a major co-morbidity such as COPD, or in the elderly. It may also occur as a consequence of surgery (post-operative and aspiration pneumonia). The spectrum of micro-organisms responsible for hospital-acquired pneumonia are different to those found in community-acquired pneumonia. Gram-negative organisms predominate: *Escherichia coli, Pseudomonas*, and *Klebsiella*. Methicillin-resistant *Staphylococcus aureus* (MRSA), widely found in hospitals, may also cause this condition.

8.2 Chronic respiratory disease

Chronic obstructive pulmonary disease (COPD) is the 5th leading cause of death in the UK and the 4th worldwide (Rabe *et al.* 2007); it is characterized by airflow obstruction which is usually progressive and not fully reversible. Symptoms include exertional breathlessness, chronic cough, regular sputum production, wheeze, and frequent 'winter bronchitis'. The condition can occur as early as the late 30s but it often remains undiagnosed until the individual is in their fifties and has lost a significant amount of their respiratory reserve. Rates of COPD are higher in more deprived communities.

Lung function measurement by spirometry is essential for diagnosis and may be used to classify the severity of COPD which can be helpful when developing a management plan and providing an estimate of prognosis. Forced expiratory volume in one second (FEV_1) is the most widely used and quoted lung function test in clinical practice. It is easily measured and

has very good reproducibility. During childhood and adolescence, FEV_1 gradually increases until it reaches a plateau phase in early adulthood before starting to decline, around the age of 25 years. Peak FEV_1 for each individual is influenced by multiple factors including genotype (Barton *et al.* 2009), prematurity (Halvorsen *et al.* 2006), nutrition (including breastfeeding (Guilbert *et al.* 2007)), childhood illness (Guilbert *et al.* 2007), environmental insults (e.g. smoking and pollution) height, and sex. From this peak, lung function deteriorates gradually throughout adult life, the rate of decline differing among individuals. Lung function decline may be accelerated by environmental factors such as pollution and behavioural factors such as smoking. FEV_1 is an independent predictor of all-cause mortality (Schünemann *et al.* 2000).

The internationally adopted classification for the severity of COPD is shown in Table 8.1 and the Kaplan-Meier survival curves for men with and without COPD from the general populations of four American cities are shown in Fig. 8.2.

About 90 per cent of men with GOLD (Global strategy for the diagnosis, management, and prevention of chronic pulmonary disease, 2010) category 0 or 1 disease are alive at ten years compared with only 65 per cent of men with GOLD 4. Chronic obstructive pulmonary disease characteristically leads to several years of ill health in most individuals and this is reflected in the global burden of this disease. In the developed world, COPD is the leading cause of disability-adjusted life-years (DALYs) lost and in the developing world this ranking is surpassed only by tuberculosis (Lopez *et al.* 2006). In Table 8.2, which shows mortality and the estimated burden of the disease in the 25 most populated countries in the world, the disproportionate overall burden compared to the mortality can be seen for some countries (see Chapter 20 and the Glossary).

There are several major risk factors for COPD but their relative importance varies by country and environment. Worldwide it has been estimated that 73 per cent of deaths due to COPD are caused by smoking, but the proportion is greater in high-income countries and around 40 per cent in low- and middle-income countries (Lopez *et al.* 2006). Lifetime risk of COPD in smokers has been estimated to be 15–50 per

Table 8.1 Spirometric classification of chronic obstructive pulmonary disease (COPD) severity based on post-bronchodilator FEV_1

Stage	Lung function	Clinical symptoms
1 Mild COPD	• $FEV_1/FVC < 0.7$ • $FEV_1 \geq 80\%$ predicted	At this stage, the patient may not be aware that their lung function is abnormal
2 Moderate COPD	• $FEV_1/FVC < 0.7$ • $50\% \leq FEV_1 < 80\%$ predicted	Symptoms usually progress at this stage, with shortness of breath typically developing on exertion
3 Severe COPD	• $FEV_1/FVC < 0.7$ • $30\% \leq FEV_1 < 50\%$ predicted	Shortness of breath typically worsens at this stage and often limits patients' daily activities. Exacerbations are especially seen beginning at this stage
4 Very severe COPD	• $FEV_1/FVC < 0.7$ • $FEV_1 < 30\%$ predicted *or* $FEV_1 < 50\%$ predicted plus chronic respiratory failure	At this stage, quality of life is very appreciably impaired and exacerbations may be life threatening

FEV_1—forced expiratory capacity in one second
FVC—forced vital capacity

cent (Mannino and Buist 2007). Occupational dusts, vapours, and fumes have been reported to account for 19 per cent of COPD in the USA with a third of these cases in never-smokers (Hnizdo *et al.* 2002). In mainly low-income countries WHO estimated that 35 per cent of COPD is caused by indoor smoke from wood or coal. This compares to two per cent of COPD deaths in these countries from air pollution and one per cent of deaths in high-income countries (Lopez *et al.* 2006). In older adults, COPD and asthma can occur together and, in a follow-up study of a national sample of adults from the USA, 2.7 per cent reported both conditions (5.3 per cent for COPD and also 5.3 per cent for asthma alone). Mortality was highest in those with combined COPD and asthma (Diaz-Guzman *et al.* 2011).

Alpha-1 antitrypsin (AAT) deficiency is a genetic disease which causes COPD symptoms often before the age of 40 years. The condition is most common among Europeans and North Americans of European descent and estimated to account for one to three per cent of COPD.

Asthma (Greek: panting) is characterized by variable airflow obstruction and increased airway hyperresponsiveness. Symptoms include wheeze, breathlessness, chest tightness, and cough. In contrast to COPD the airflow obstruction is usually reversible.

Some 300 million people worldwide were estimated to have clinical asthma and the prevalence appears to be increasing at up to 50 per cent per decade mainly in the developing economies (Braman 2006). Asthma is the most common chronic disease of childhood which frequently persists into adulthood. In the UK it was estimated that 14 per cent of children aged 2–15 years and four per cent of adults had symptoms requiring treatment (Braman 2006), although prevalence figures based on symptoms from the International Study of Asthma and Allergies in Childhood (ISAAC) suggest much higher prevalence rates. This study, established in 1991 to investigate asthma, rhinitis, and eczema in children due to concern that these conditions were increasing in both Western and developing countries,

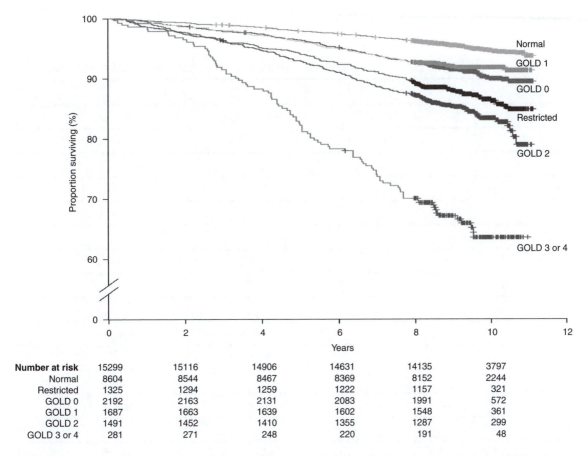

Number at risk	15299	15116	14906	14631	14135	3797
Normal	8604	8544	8467	8369	8152	2244
Restricted	1325	1294	1259	1222	1157	321
GOLD 0	2192	2163	2131	2083	1991	572
GOLD 1	1687	1663	1639	1602	1548	361
GOLD 2	1491	1452	1410	1355	1287	299
GOLD 3 or 4	281	271	248	220	191	48

Figure 8.2 Survival of patients with chronic obstructive pulmonary disease (COPD) by severity classified by GOLD criteria. Reproduced from Mannino DM and Buist S 'Global burden of COPD: risk factors, prevalence, and future trends', *Lancet* 2007, with permission from Elsevier.

used a standardized questionnaire, often with the assistance of clinical videos showing symptoms. In phase 3 based on cross-sectional surveys in 2002–2003, the investigators found a prevalence of asthma symptoms (wheeze) ranging from three per cent in Albania, 10 per cent in Spain, 18 per cent in Germany, and 26 per cent in the UK, to 22 per cent in the USA and 20 per cent in Brazil, and six per cent in China and five per cent in Indonesia in schoolchildren aged 13–14 years (Asher *et al.* 2006).

Prevalence figures can be difficult to compare between studies as different definitions of asthma may have been used. Peak expiratory flow before and after exercise has been used by some investigators to define asthma in epidemiological surveys, particularly

in children (Burr *et al.* 1994). Bronchial challenge testing is a more invasive approach which has been used in young adults with asthma symptoms drawn from the general population in the European Community Respiratory Health Survey (Janson *et al.* 2001). Questionnaires are also useful for monitoring asthma control. The asthma control questionnaire is well validated in adults and in children (Juniper *et al.* 2006).

Despite the high prevalence, the mortality from asthma is relatively low. There were 1131 deaths from asthma in the UK in 2009 but many of these may have been preventable. Despite the high incidence of asthma in children the majority of deaths occur in adults over 45 years of age and in the elderly where there may be co-morbidity from COPD or cardiovascular disease.

Table 8.2 Mortality from and burden of chronic obstructive pulmonary disorder (COPD) in the 25 most populated countries

	Age-adjusted deaths/100,000	Age-adjusted DALYs/100,000
Japan	4.4	120
France	12.0	270
Germany	12.5	291
Italy	13.7	191
Russian Federation	16.2	242
UK	23.1	442
Iran (Islamic Republic of)	26.3	395
Philippines	26.7	282
Mexico	26.8	247
USA	27.2	426
Ukraine	31.6	477
Egypt	35.9	302
Turkey	40.3	521
Brazil	42.2	504
Thailand	48.0	245
Congo	49.4	297
Nigeria	49.4	296
Ethiopia	55.4	330
Myanmar	56.4	570
Indonesia	58.4	613
Bangladesh	66.4	559
Pakistan	77.1	584
India	73.2	667
Vietnam	86.4	488
China	130.5	622

Reproduced from Mannino D and Buist S 'Global burden of COPD: risk factors, prevalence, and future trends', *Lancet* 2007, with permission from Elsevier.

A review of mortality in asthma in 20 countries found that mortality in the population aged 5–45 years declined by an average of 63 per cent since the 1980s and this has been attributed to the introduction of inhaled corticosteroids (Wijesinghe *et al.* 2009). Severe asthma, which cannot be adequately controlled by inhaled corticosteroids and bronchodilators, requires systemic steroids and occurs in up to 10 per cent of asthma cases. Because of the large prevalence of the disorder in children and in adults, and the high incidence of hospital admissions, the economic costs of asthma have been estimated to be among the highest for chronic disease (Bahadori *et al.* 2009).

Risk factors for asthma have been investigated in numerous cross-sectional and somewhat fewer cohort studies. Asthma and *atopy* (a predisposition to hypersensitivity reactions) are diseases believed to result from gene–environment interactions and both are believed to be polygenic disorders and clearly interact with environmental factors such as biological allergens (particularly with respiratory viruses early in life), tobacco smoke, atmospheric pollution, and domestic atmospheric pollutants. However, environmental changes, rather than genetic, must account for the rapid rise in the prevalence of these disorders and the 'hygiene hypothesis', which suggests that the lack of antigenic stimulation in our modern, relatively sterile environment is responsible for the development of an inappropriate chronic, allergenic, inflammatory response in many individuals, has been developed to account for this. Although there is some epidemiological evidence to support this (Matricardi *et al.* 2000; Strachan 2000) recent experimental evidence suggests that some infections can protect can protect against atopy while others can promote it (Fishbein and Fuleihan 2012). Several large cross-sectional epidemiological studies have suggested that administration of paracetamol in infancy may be a risk factor for asthma (Beasley *et al.* 2011) and a nested case-control study reported an association between maternal antibiotic consumption and an increased risk of asthma in the offspring (Martel *et al.* 2009). Large scale genetic studies have identified several loci consistently related to asthma (Zhang *et al.* 2012) but epigenetic mechanisms may also be important (Kumar *et al.* 2009).

Table 8.3 shows the results of the study by Matricardi *et al.* 2001 in which past exposure to infectious agents was investigated in 240 atopic and 240 non-atopic Italian military cadets.

Significantly fewer atopic cadets had evidence of past exposure to *Toxoplasma gondii* and to hepatitis A virus than had non-atopic cadets.

....

Question 1

What additional analyses would strengthen the case of the investigators that past exposure to orofaecal and food-borne infections protects against the development of atopy?

Question 2

The investigators also measured immunoglobulin E (IgE) levels in their sample. What additional biological measurements might be useful to establish the causal mechanisms in asthma?
....

Treatment and prevention of asthma attacks are aimed at symptom control and trigger avoidance. Triggers include pollens, house dust mite, tobacco smoke, chemical irritants, cold air, emotional distress, and drugs such as beta blockers and aspirin. There is a stepwise treatment approach using short- and long-acting beta 2 agonists and inhaled corticosteroids. Severe cases may require drugs such as anti IgE monoclonal antibodies and immunosuppressants. House dust mite control measures in the domestic environment have been common practice but a Cochrane review concluded that this did not significantly reduce symptomatology (Gotzsche and Johansen 2008).

Sleep-disordered breathing has been estimated to occur in 24 per cent of men and nine per cent of women (Prisant *et al.* 2006); obstructive sleep apnoea is the most clinically important of these and occurs in approximately two to five per cent of women and three to seven per cent of men in different ethnic world populations (Punjabi 2008). This syndrome is clinically linked with daytime sleepiness, impaired cognitive function, and as a risk factor for motor vehicle accidents (Caples *et al.* 2005). Different definitions have been used to

Table 8.3 Prevalence of antibodies against selected infectious agents in 240 atopic and 240 non-atopic Italian military cadets. Values are numbers (percentages) of participants unless stated otherwise

Infectious agent	Non-atopic group	Atopic group	Crude odds ratio (95% CI)
Orofaecal and food-borne infections			
Toxoplasma gondii	63(26)	42(18)*	0.60(0.38–0.93)
Helicobacter pylori	44(18)	35(15)	0.76(0.47–1.24)
Hepatitis A virus	73(30)	39(16)†	0.44(0.29–0.69)
Infections transmitted by other routes			
Measles	233(97)	231(96)	0.77(0.28–2.11)
Mumps	92(38)	112(47)	1.41(0.98–2.03)
Rubella	211(88)	198(83)	0.65(0.39–1.08)
Chickenpox	157(65)	157(65)	1.00(0.69–1.46)
Cytomegalovirus	112(47)	132(55)	1.40(0.97–2.00)
Herpes simplex virus type 1	181(75)	168(70)	0.76(0.51–1.14)

*$p = 0.027$
†$p = 0.004$

Reproduced from Matricardi P *et al*, Exposure to foodborne and orofecal microbes versus airborne viruses in relation to atopy and allergic asthma: epidemiological study, *British Medical Journal*, 2000, with permission from BMJ Publishing Ltd.

define the severity of the disorder but these generally use the apnoea-hypopnoea index in which apnoea is defined as cessation of breathing for 10 seconds or more and hypopnoea as a 50 per cent reduction in tidal volume and reduced oxygen saturation (Prisant *et al.* 2006). Overnight monitoring of breathing is required for diagnosis. Early epidemiological data suggested that these subjects are at greater risk of hypertension, stroke, and other cardiovascular diseases (McClean *et al.* 2008). Recent data from a large multi-centre prospective study in several American cohorts reported a modest increase in all-cause mortality (46 per cent) in men and women aged 40 or more years with the most severe level of apnoea/hyponoea; this group formed 5.4 per cent of the total cohort population. Breathing was monitored overnight using home polysomnography. Obesity, neck circumference, and age were the major risk factors (Punjabi *et al.* 2009). In the same study, apnoea/hyponoea was linked to incident stroke in a graded relationship but was associated in women with only the most severe level of the disorder (Redline *et al.* 2010). In a smaller cohort from this study severe apnoea was linked with increased risk of heart failure in men but not in women, and increased risk of incident coronary heart disease was found only in men under the age of 70 years at entry (Gottlieb *et al.* 2010).

Weight loss, avoidance of alcohol, and sedatives at night and use of the semi-prone posture at night are first-line treatments but continuous positive airway pressure (CPAP) is used in severe cases. A Cochrane review of 36 trials found that CPAP effectively reduced daytime sleepiness in severe cases but noted that longer term data were required to evaluate possible benefit for cardiovascular outcomes (Giles *et al.* 2006). A prospective observational study of stroke patients given CPAP treatment suggested a reduced mortality in the treated group (Martinez-Garcia *et al.* 2011), but trial data are needed.

Cystic fibrosis (CF) is an autosomal recessive disorder which primarily affects the mucus secretions of the respiratory and digestive systems. In the UK, one in 25 of the general population are carriers and one CF infant is born in 2300 births. In Europe it is the most common life-shortening, inherited disorder and the estimated incidence in 2004 varied from one in 1353 in Ireland to one in 25,000 in Finland (Farrell 2008). The 'cystic fibrosis transmembrane conductance regulator' or *CTFR* gene was discovered in 1989 and mutations cause abnormalities in chloride ion transport leading to abnormally thick secretions. The most common mutation is known as ΔF508 and is responsible for about 80 per cent of CF cases in Caucasian populations. The phenotype of cystic fibrosis patients depends on the mutation (Comer *et al.* 2009) and over 1700 different mutations have been described, although only about 23 mutations appear to be associated with significant disease. Cystic fibrosis patients tend to have chronic respiratory infections, pancreatic enzyme insufficiency, and associated complications; end-stage lung disease is the principal cause of death. In the UK the median age of survival was less than 10 years until the 1970s rising to 27 years by 2007. This has been attributed to several causes including early diagnosis and treatment, improved nutrition, and access to health care. Most studies show poorer survival in women compared to men and in those with lower socio-economic status (Barr *et al.* 2011).

Two different approaches to screening exist: (1) prenatal population-based carrier screening, recommended in the USA since 2001 using an array of up to 23 mutations, achieves detection rates of about 90 per cent in Caucasians but less in other ethnic groups, and only 50 per cent in those of Asian origin (Committee on Genetics 2011; Levenson 2011). In certain groups in the USA (Orthodox Jews) premarital genetic matching is practised, which has resulted in a very low incidence of CF in this group. A consensus document has recently proposed benchmarks for screening practice in Europe (Castellani *et al.* 2010). Post-natal or newborn screening is widely practised and sweat testing has been used for decades and may continue to have a role in patients with clinical symptoms (Kirk 2011). Blood spot testing as part of routine newborn screening was recommended from 2001 in the UK by the National Screening Committee using a primary screen with immunoreactive trypsinogen (IRT), raised in newborns with CF, which is a highly sensitive test but with low specificity. In babies with IRT levels above the 99.5th centile a two-stage mutation analysis of the *CFTR* gene is conducted. In regions where newborn screening has been practised for 20 years a decline in the number of CF cases has been reported due to prenatal testing in subsequent pregnancies with the option of termination (Massie *et al.* 2009).

Evidence that newborn screening and earlier diagnosis leads to improved survival and quality of life is incomplete although some trial data (Southern *et al.* 2009) and recent observational studies (Dijk *et al.* 2011) support this.

8.3 Cancers of the respiratory tract

Although this group of cancers includes those of the upper respiratory tract—lip, mouth, and oropharynx—the group is dominated by lung cancer, which is the commonest non-skin cancer worldwide.

Lung cancer is now the leading cause of cancer-related death in men *and* women worldwide (Ferlay *et al.* 2010). A histological diagnosis is required to ensure the most appropriate treatment regimen. However, more than 30 per cent of patients do not receive a histological or 'tissue' diagnosis, often due to difficulties in retrieving an adequate sample. The National Lung Cancer Audit in England and Wales (2006–2008) reported that of histologically proven cancers, 78 per cent are non-small cell (32 per cent squamous cell, 26 per cent adenocarcinoma, 4 per cent large cell, and 2 per cent bronchoalveolar), and 18 per cent are small cell tumours (the diagnosis and treatment of lung cancer: update of NICE clinical guideline 24, 2011). The different histological types have different epidemiological characteristics and respond differently to treatment, e.g. chemotherapy is the mainstay of treatment for small cell tumours (often along with radiotherapy). Computed tomography (CT) and positron emisstion tomography (PET)-CT scanning are used to determine the stage of lung cancer at diagnosis. This information,

Table 8.4   Mortality by smoking habits from respiratory disease by 40 years of follow-up in British doctors

Type of disease (number of deaths, 1951–91)	Non-smokers (never smoked regularly)	Former cigarette smokers	Current cigarette smokers (number per day)			Relative risk ≥ 25 daily versus non-smokers
			1–14	15–24	≥ 25	
Pulmonary tuberculosis (66)	4	8	7	9	20	5.0
Chronic obstructive lung disease (542)	10	57	86	112	225	2.3
Pneumonia (864)	71	90	113	154	169	2.4
Asthma (70)	4	11	6	8	6	1.5
Other respiratory disease (216)	19	28	26	31	33	1.7
All respiratory disease	107	192	237	310	471	4.4
(Number of deaths 1758)	(131)	(455)	(161)	(170)	(159)	
Cancers						
Upper respiratory sites (98)	1	3	12	18	48	48.0
Lung (893)	14	58	105	208	355	25.4

Annual mortality per 100,000 men

Reproduced from Doll R *et al*, 'Mortality in relation to smoking: 40 years' observations on male British doctors', *British Medical Journal* 1994, with permission from BMJ Publishing Ltd.

along with performance status, is crucially important in determining which patients are potentially curable.

Epidemiology and risk factors for respiratory cancers It is estimated that by 2015 there will be 6.4 million deaths worldwide each year due to tobacco-related diseases (WHO Framework Convention on Tobacco Control). At the beginning of the 20th century lung cancer was rare, accounting for less than one per cent of cancer deaths, but by the end of the century it had emerged in the developed world to be the leading cause of cancer deaths in men and, in most of these countries, either the first or second cause of cancer deaths in women. By the midpoint of the 20th century the scale of the lung cancer epidemic was recognized by physicians and epidemiologists. The search for causes launched the first major epidemiological investigations into non-infectious

or chronic diseases and stimulated a major debate among medical scientists. Undoubtedly this paved the way for improved methodological rigour in epidemiology, and the link between smoking and lung cancer provides a model for the causal guidelines proposed by Bradford Hill (see Chapter 1, Box 1.5). The strong association between cigarette smoking and the risk of respiratory cancer was tested in many longitudinal epidemiological studies. One of the best-known British studies is summarized in Table 8.4 (see also Doll *et al*. 2004). Although randomized trials of smoking cessation have been attempted (Rose and Colwell 1992), most epidemiological evidence on risk reduction after smoking cessation comes from observational studies. Table 8.5 illustrates data available from two case-control studies from Britain conducted in 1950 and 1990.

Table 8.5 Smoking status versus cumulative risk of death from lung cancer by age 75, from 1950 and 1990 studies

	Men				Women			
	Percentage of cases/controls		Cumulative risk (%)*		Percentage of cases/controls		Cumulative risk (%)*	
Smoking status	1950	1990	1950	1990	1950	1990	1950	1990
Lifelong non-smoker	0.5/4.5	0.5/19.0	~0.4	~0.4	37.0/54.6	7.6/50.3	~0.4	~0.4
Former smokers	5.2/9.1	42.7/52.5	2.9	5.5	9.3/7.4	29.8/29.4	0.9	2.6
Current pipe or cigar only	3.9/7.2	8.5[†]/7.1	2.8	8.1[†]	0/0	0.6/0.1	—	—
Current cigarette smokers	90.4/79.2	48.3/21.5	5.9	15.9	53.7/38.0	61.9/20.1	1.0	9.5
Amount smoked (% of smokers)								
<5/day	3.6/7.0	6.2/9.5	2.8	10.4	20.6/36.7	4.1/10.1	0.6	3.4
5–14/day	38.2/47.5	33.5/39.7	4.4	12.8	44.1/44.9	32.3/37.8	1.0	7.7
15–24/day	33.0/31.5	39.1/37.3	5.7	16.7		44.1/42.4		10.4
≥25/day	25.2/14.0	21.1/13.5	9.8	24.4	35.3/18.4	19.5/9.7	2.0	18.5
Total	100/100	100/100			100/100	100/100		
Number of cases	1357/1357	667/2108	—	—	108/108	315/1077	—	—

*Calculated from published relative risk estimates
[†]In 1990 88 per cent of these subjects were also former cigarette smokers
Reproduced from Peto R et al. 'Smoking, smoking cessation, and lung cancer in the UK since 1950: combination of national statistics with two case-control studies', *British Medical Journal*, 2000, with permission from BMJ Publishing Ltd.

In developed countries over 90 per cent of lung cancers can be attributed to cigarette smoking in men (Ezzati and Lopez 2003) whereas there is less epidemiological certainty in the estimates for women (approximately 71 per cent). Similarly, in developing countries other factors may also be important as 65 per cent of lung cancer in men under 70 years of age can be attributed to smoking, and in women the figure is only 26 per cent (Ezzati and Lopez 2003). Unfortunately, this pattern is likely to change to the pattern in developed countries unless global action on smoking cessation and tobacco consumption is initiated effectively in the developing world.

The pattern of histological tumour types appears to be changing over time with an increasing prevalence of adenocarcinomas in Western countries (Tyczynski *et al.* 2003). This seems to be due to the introduction of low-tar and low-nicotine cigarettes, which may be inhaled more deeply and more often than cigarettes with higher nicotine levels, resulting in the distribution of carcinogens to the peripheral regions of the lungs which predisposes this tissue to adenocarcinoma. Small cell lung cancer is believed to be most closely linked to smoking pack history, and the proportion of all lung cancers due to small cell has decreased from 20 to 10 per cent (Stephens and Johnson 2000).

Other risk factors for lung cancer include occupational causes such as exposure to asbestos, metals (for example nickel, arsenic, and cadmium), ionizing radiation, radon gas (which may be found either in the workplace or in the domestic environment in

Table 8.6 Health effects of atmospheric (mainly vehicle) pollution

Pollutant	Source	Health effect
Nitrogen dioxide (NO$_2$)	Vehicle exhaust	May exacerbate asthma and possibly increase susceptibility to infections
Particulates PM10 Total suspended particulates, black smoke	Those less than 10 pm in diameter (PM10) penetrate the lung fairly efficiently and are most hazardous. Diesel produces more particulates than petrol	Associated with respiratory symptoms. Long-term exposure is associated with death from heart and lung disease. Particulates can carry carcinogenic materials into the lungs
Acid aerosols	Airborne acid formed from common pollutants including sulphur and nitrogen oxides	May exacerbate asthma and increase susceptibility to respiratory infection. May reduce lung function in asthma
Carbon monoxide (CO)	Comes mainly from petrol car exhausts	Lethal at high doses. At low doses can impair concentration. May present a risk to the fetus
Ozone (O$_3$)	Secondary pollutant produced from nitrogen oxides and volatile organic compounds in the air	Irritates the eyes and air passages. Exacerbates asthma. May increase susceptibility to infection.
Lead	Compound present in leaded petrol to help the engine run smoothly	Impairs brain development of children
Volatile organic compounds (VOCs)	A group of chemical solvents from petrol fuel. Also present in vehicle exhaust	Benzene has given cause for concern in this group of chemicals. It is a cancer causing agent and can cause leukaemia at high doses
Polycyclic aromatic hydrocarbons (PAHs)	Produced by incomplete combustion of fuel. PAHs become attached to particulates	Includes a range of chemicals and carcinogens. PAHs in traffic exhaust poses a low cancer risk to the general population
Asbestos	May be present in brake pads and clutch linings especially in heavy-duty vehicles Asbestos fibres and dust are released into the atmosphere when vehicles brake	Asbestos can cause lung cancer and mesothelioma. The consequences of low exposure from braking vehicles are not known

association with regions of natural granite formation), and passive smoking of the cigarette smoke of others.

Prevention The scientific case for primary prevention of lung cancer and other respiratory cancers by the elimination of tobacco smoking is overwhelming. Secondary preventive measures in the form of screening programmes to detect early cancers have been evaluated. Several major trials of radiological screening for the early detection of lung cancers have indicated no overall benefit despite improved survival for asymptomatic tumours. The usual epidemiological problems associated with the evaluation of cancer-screening initiatives impede the complete evaluation of these programmes (lead-time bias, length bias, and over-diagnosis).

8.4 Environmental factors in respiratory disease

Environmental tobacco smoke (ETS) or *second-hand smoke* comes both from exhaled tobacco smoke and directly from the burning end of the cigarette in which the concentration of some carcinogens is higher than in smoke inhaled by the smoker. A recent review of the health burden on those exposed to such smoke in 192 countries (40 per cent children and 35 per cent non-smoking women) estimated that this was linked with over 600,000 deaths worldwide in 2004 (Oberg *et al.* 2011). In this study, population attributable fractions were used from extensive epidemiological data from the Global Burden of Disease Project (Lopez *et al.* 2006). These data found that ETS contributes to deaths from ischaemic heart disease, pneumonia, asthma, and lung cancer. Maternal smoking and household smoking have been linked to several illnesses in infancy and childhood including pneumonia, wheeze and asthma, middle ear disease, bacterial meningitis, and sudden infant death in many epidemiological studies. Passive smoke exposure is about three times higher if the father smokes, over six times higher if the mother smokes, and nearly nine times higher if both parents smoke. In the UK, passive smoking by infants and children has been estimated to lead to 300,000 GP consultations and 9,500 hospital admissions each year (Tobacco Advisory Group of the Royal College of Physicians 2010).

Such data fully support international and national measures to limit exposure of non-smokers and children to ETS but commercial interests and weak governmental initiatives limited public health progress in the latter part of the 20th century. However, some cities in the US did begin to ban smoking in restaurants as early as 1985 (Minnesota Clean Indoor Air Act). Since 2007, smoking in virtually all enclosed public places and workplaces is now prohibited by law throughout the UK. The latest legislation in the UK, Ireland, and in many European countries seeks to protect workers in bars and restaurants, and studies indicate reduced symptoms and improved lung health among bar workers (Ayres *et al.* 2009), reduced hospital admissions for heart attacks and, in Scotland, a reduction in preterm births and in the proportion of babies that were small for gestational age. As part of general measures to improve tobacco control in the UK and elsewhere in Europe and in North America, the sale of tobacco products to children or adolescents, or to sell via vending machines, is restricted or banned and it is unlawful to advertise or promote tobacco products.

The World Health Organization initiated a global health treaty known as the Framework Convention on Tobacco Control in 2003. The treaty aims to set international, agreed minimum standards on tobacco control and to ensure co-operation on matters such as the illegal tobacco trade. Progress in achieving these goals is more advanced in high income countries but is much slower in developing countries which are forming new markets for the powerful international tobacco industry. Tobacco control is reviewed in more detail in Chapters 20 and 22.

Air pollution is a complex mixture of thousands of pollutants (Perez *et al.* 2010), which include gases such as carbon monoxide, ozone, volatile organic carbons and nitrogen oxides, and particulate matter (solid and liquid particles suspended in air). The combustion of fossil fuels used in transport, industry, and household heating systems is an important source of air pollutants (see Table 8.6).

In the UK, public health concern was raised when an unusual London smog was associated with about three times the number of deaths normally expected in one week in the winter of 1952; many of the deaths were attributed to bronchitis and pneumonia, and also to ischaemic heart disease (IHD). Smog was caused largely by carbon particles suspended in a moist atmosphere and associated with high levels of sulphur dioxide. Regional research in a longitudinal study of children born in 1946 found that heavily polluted areas were associated with a higher incidence of childhood bronchitis and pneumonia. Accumulated evidence suggested that most of the elements producing smog were caused by domestic coal consumption; the Clean Air Act 1956 required the use of smokeless coal in British cities. Since then smogs caused by coal have declined but have been partly replaced by pollution due to vehicle exhaust gases. The main pollutants are shown in Table 8.6. Most pollutants are more highly concentrated in winter months; ozone is produced by sunlight, however, and significant health effects can occur in dry, hot conditions in association with vehicle pollution. In many developing countries pollution levels are similar or worse than in European cities when domestic coal was used but with additional pollutants from vehicle exhaust gases.

A large number of epidemiological studies have shown that the daily number of deaths, mainly from cardiovascular and respiratory diseases, follows the daily fluctuation of air pollution (Samoli et al. 2008). Patients with asthma, especially children without anti-inflammatory or bronchodilator therapy, suffer more on or after days with higher pollution levels. Long-term or lifetime exposure to ambient pollutants may also contribute to pathologies that ultimately result in chronic respiratory diseases (Perez et al. 2010).

Some attempts have been made by epidemiologists to monitor the contribution of air pollution to mortality during a longer period of time. In one such study in the US, Dockery et al. (1993) followed a cohort of 8000 adults in six cities with a range of pollution levels during the period from 1974 to 1989. After adjustment for confounding factors such as smoking, occupational exposure, etc., the excess mortality associated with air pollution was 26 per cent. During a second period (1990–1998) mortality levels, adjusted for all confounders, fell and this was accompanied by a significant fall in overall mortality (Laden et al. 2006). Future studies such as these would appear to be essential in monitoring the health effects of atmospheric pollutants.

Housing environment

Attempts have been made to investigate housing factors and health in observational studies, but problems of confounding render the interpretation of such studies problematic. One study, designed after an extensive pilot study, conducted in Edinburgh, Glasgow, and London, showed that damp and mould growth were associated with a higher prevalence of reported respiratory symptoms, particularly in children, unexplained by confounding factors and study design (Platt et al. 1989). Although fungal exposure has been strongly associated with hospitalization

and increased mortality in asthma, no controlled trials have addressed the efficacy of reduction of fungal exposure in relation to control of asthma (BTS/SIGN asthma guidelines).

Although many aspects of the housing environment such as overcrowding, inadequate and contaminated water suppliers, damp, and ambient pollution clearly have had important effects in the UK and other developed countries in the past, these problems are particularly relevant today in developing countries owing to rapid, poorly controlled urbanization. In developing countries in both urban and rural areas combustion of biomass fuels such as wood, coal, animal dung, and straw in poorly ventilated conditions are estimated to account for 35 per cent of COPD with a higher burden in women (Lopez et al. 2006). Specific environmental effects can be difficult to quantify directly, but are likely to be a major factor in determining sub-optimal health status in the developing world.

8.5 Occupational exposures

Occupational lung diseases are caused by the inhalation of specific particles in the workplace and are associated with both acute and chronic respiratory disease. Pneumoconiosis is the general term for lung disease caused by the inhalation of mineral dusts such as asbestos, silica, and coal dust. Hypersensitivity pneumonitis (or extrinsic allergic alveolitis) is caused by the inhalation of organic materials such as animal dander, avian proteins or thermophilic actinomycetes or aspergillus species from mouldy hay.

In the developed world, the pattern of occupational lung disease has changed markedly over the past 100 years. In the first half of the 20th century, heavy manufacturing industries and agriculture predominated. Fibrotic lung diseases, such as silicosis, asbestosis, and coal miner's pneumoconiosis were important causes of morbidity. During the same industrial period, COPD also contributed to poor health among workers. In the developing world, these occupational diseases persist because of poor environmental control of working conditions.

It is estimated that occupational exposures account for about five per cent of lung cancers. Neoplasms of the lung may be associated with specific industries. Smelters working with nickel, coke oven workers engaged in steel production, and insulation workers in the shipbuilding and construction industries working with asbestos, all have a higher incidence of bronchial carcinoma. The decline of these industries and the improvement of controls have led to a switch in emphasis to public-health issues such as air pollution or passive smoking.

However, one important occupational neoplasm has had an increasing incidence. Mesothelioma is a malignant tumour of the pleura which has a long latent period of 35–40 years. It is associated with asbestos exposure, in particular blue asbestos or crocidolite. Although blue asbestos was banned at the beginning of the 1970s, the incidence of mesothelioma in the UK is still increasing, and is expected to peak between 2011 and 2015 (Hodgson *et al.* 2005). The importance of early regulatory action based on good epidemiological evidence is demonstrated by a different experience in the USA, where the incidence of mesothelioma is now falling (Treasure *et al.* 2004). Industrial diseases are notified to the coroner's office in the UK to facilitate epidemiological monitoring and legal redress for workers when environmental controls have been poorly implemented.

The progressive shift from heavy manufacturing industry to service and high-tech manufacturing has been matched by a change in the pattern of occupational lung disease although it has been estimated that 19 per cent of COPD in the USA has an occupational cause (Hnizdo 2002). Occupational asthma is now the most frequently reported cause of occupational lung disease. Chemicals such as isocyanates, which are used in paint spraying, and soldering flux (used in the electronics industry), are important examples of respiratory sensitizers; biological agents are also important: for example, laboratory technicians may become allergic to inhaled animal proteins (such as rabbit fur) and bakers to flour. A large number of substances used in industry have the potential to sensitize the skin or airways of workers and health and safety measures need to be fully implemented and monitored when risk exposures have been detected (Beckett 2000). Data from a systematic review indicate that 16 per cent of adult onset asthma has an occupational origin (Torén and Blanc 2009).

The pattern of occupationally acquired respiratory infections has also changed. Diseases such as anthrax, in wool sorters, are now very rare. Tuberculosis (TB) has always been an important occupational disease, particularly among health care workers. Tuberculosis is a major cause of adult mortality in developing countries and is discussed in more detail in Chapter 18. The changing working environment has led to the emergence of new infections, such as legionnaires' disease. Old and new viral illnesses such as influenza and severe acute respiratory syndrome (SARS), which can evolve in working environments, present continuing challenges.

References

Anon (2005) Guidelines for the management of adults with hospital-acquired, ventilator-associated, and healthcare-associated pneumonia. *American Journal of Respiratory and Critical Care Medicine* **171** (4), 388–416.

Asher MI, Montefort S, Björkstén B, Lai CKW, *et al.* (2006) Worldwide time trends in the prevalence of symptoms of asthma, allergic rhinoconjunctivitis, and eczema in childhood: ISAAC Phases One and Three repeat multicountry cross-sectional surveys. *Lancet* **368** (9537), 733–43.

Ayres JG, Semple S, MacCalman L, Dempsey S, *et al.* (2009) Bar workers' health and environmental tobacco smoke exposure (BHETSE): symptomatic improvement in bar staff following smoke-free legislation in Scotland. *Occupational and Environmental Medicine* **66** (5), 339–46.

Bahadori K, Doyle-Waters MM, Marra C, Lynd L, *et al.* (2009) Economic burden of asthma: a systematic review. *BMC Pulmonary Medicine* **9**, 24.

Barr HL, Britton J, Smyth AR, and Fogarty AW (2011) Association between socioeconomic status, sex, and age at death from cystic fibrosis in England and Wales (1959 to 2008): cross sectional study. *BMJ (Clinical Research Ed)* **343**, d4662.

Barton SJ, Koppelman GH, Vonk JM, Browning CA, *et al.* (2009) PLAUR polymorphisms are associated with asthma, PLAUR levels, and lung function decline. *The Journal of Allergy and Clinical Immunology* **123** (6), 1391–1400.e17.

Beasley RW, Clayton TO, Crane J, Lai CKW, *et al.* (2011) Acetaminophen Use and Risk of Asthma, Rhinoconjunctivitis, and Eczema in Adolescents. *American Journal of Respiratory and Critical Care Medicine* **183** (2), 171–8.

Beckett WS (2000) Occupational respiratory diseases. *The New England Journal of Medicine* **342** (6), 406–13.

Braman SS (2006) The global burden of asthma. *Chest* **130** (1 Suppl.), 4S–12S.

Burr, M.L., Limb, E.S., Andrae, S., Barry, D.M., *et al.* (1994) Childhood asthma in four countries: a comparative survey. *International Journal of Epidemiology* **23** (2), 341–7.

Caples SM, Gami AS, and Somers VK (2005) Obstructive sleep apnoea. *Annals of Internal Medicine* **142** (3), 187–97.

Castellani C, Macek M, Jr, Cassiman J-J, Duff A, *et al.* (2010) Benchmarks for cystic fibrosis carrier screening: a European consensus document. *Journal of Cystic Fibrosis* **9** (3), 165–78.

Comer DM, Ennis M, McDowell C, Beattie D, *et al.* (2009) Clinical phenotype of cystic fibrosis patients with the G551D mutation. *QJM: Monthly Journal of the Association of Physicians* **102** (11), 793–8.

Committee on Genetics (2011) Committee Opinion No. 486: Update on Carrier Screening for Cystic Fibrosis. *Obstetrics & Gynecology* **117** (4), 1028–31.

Diaz-Guzman E, Khosravi M and Mannino DM (2011) Asthma, chronic obstructive pulmonary disease, and mortality in the U.S. population. *COPD* **8** (6), 400–7.

Dijk FN, McKay K, Barzi F, Gaskin KJ, *et al.* (2011) Improved survival in cystic fibrosis patients diagnosed by newborn screening compared to a historical cohort from the same centre. *Archives of Disease in Childhood* **96** (12), 1118–23.

Dockery DW, Pope CA, 3rd, Xu X, Spengler JD, *et al.* (1993) An association between air pollution and mortality in six U.S. cities. *The New England Journal of Medicine* **329** (24), 1753–9.

Doll R, Peto R, Boreham J and Sutherland I (2004) Mortality in relation to smoking: 50 years' observations on male British doctors. *BMJ (Clinical Research Ed)* **328** (7455), 1519.

Ezzati M and Lopez AD (2003) Estimates of global mortality attributable to smoking in 2000. *Lancet* **362** (9387), 847–52.

Fahey T, Stocks N and Thomas T (1998) Systematic review of the treatment of upper respiratory tract infection. *Archives of Disease in Childhood* **79** (3), 225–30.

Farrell PM (2008) The prevalence of cystic fibrosis in the European Union. *Journal of Cystic Fibrosis* **7** (5), 450–3.

Ferlay, J., Shin, H.-R., Bray, F., Forman, D., *et al.* (2010) Estimates of worldwide burden of cancer in 2008:

GLOBOCAN 2008. *International Journal of Cancer* **127** (12), 2893–917.

Fidler DP and Gostin LO (2011) The WHO pandemic influenza preparedness framework: a milestone in global governance for health. *JAMA* **306** (2), 200–1.

Fishbein, A.B. & Fuleihan, R.L. (2012) The hygiene hypothesis revisited: does exposure to infectious agents protect us from allergy? *Current Opinion in Pediatrics* **24** (1), 98–102.

Giles TL, Lasserson TJ, Smith BJ, White J, *et al.* (2006) Continuous positive airways pressure for obstructive sleep apnoea in adults. *Cochrane Database of Systematic Reviews* **1**, CD001106.

Global strategy for the diagnosis, management, and prevention of chronic obstructive pulmonary disease. (Updated 2010) Available at: http://www.goldcopd.org.

Gottlieb DJ, Yenokyan G, Newman AB, O'Connor GT, *et al.* (2010) Prospective study of obstructive sleep apnoea and incident coronary heart disease and heart failure: the sleep heart health study. *Circulation* **122** (4), 352–60.

Gotzsche PC and Johansen HK (2008) House dust mite control measures for asthma. *Cochrane Database of Systematic Reviews* **2**, CD001187.

Gross, P.A., Hermogenes, A.W., Sacks, H.S., Lau, J., *et al.* (1995) The efficacy of influenza vaccine in elderly persons. A meta-analysis and review of the literature. *Annals of Internal Medicine* **123** (7), 518–27.

Guilbert TW, Stern DA, Morgan WJ, Martinez FD, *et al.* (2007) Effect of breastfeeding on lung function in childhood and modulation by maternal asthma and atopy. *American Journal of Respiratory and Critical Care Medicine* **176** (9), 843–8.

Halvorsen T, Skadberg BT, Eide GE, Røksund OD, *et al.* (2006) Better care of immature infants; has it influenced long-term pulmonary outcome? *Acta Paediatrica (Oslo, Norway: 1992)* **95** (5), 547–54.

Hnizdo E, Sullivan PA, Bang KM and Wagner G (2002) Association between chronic obstructive pulmonary disease and employment by industry and occupation in the US population: a study of data from the Third National Health and Nutrition Examination Survey. *American Journal of Epidemiology* **156** (8), 738–46.

Hodgson JT, McElvenny DM, Darnton AJ, Price MJ, *et al.* (2005) The expected burden of mesothelioma mortality in Great Britain from 2002 to 2050. *British Journal of Cancer* **92** (3), 587–93.

Janson C, Chinn S, Jarvis D, Zock JP, *et al.* (2001) Effect of passive smoking on respiratory symptoms, bronchial responsiveness, lung function, and total serum IgE in the European Community Respiratory Health Survey: a cross-sectional study. *Lancet* **358** (9299), 2103–9.

Juniper E, Bousquet J, Abetz L, and Bateman ED (2006) Identifying 'well-controlled' and 'not well-controlled' asthma using the Asthma Control Questionnaire. *Respiratory Medicine* **100** (4), 616–21.

Kirk JM (2011) A continuing role for sweat testing in an era of newborn screening for cystic fibrosis. *Clinical Biochemistry* **44** (7), 487–8.

Kumar RK, Hitchins MP and Foster PS (2009) Epigenetic changes in childhood asthma. *Disease Models & Mechanisms* **2** (11-12), 549–53.

Laden, F., Schwartz, J., Speizer, F.E. & Dockery, D.W. (2006) Reduction in fine particulate air pollution and mortality: Extended follow-up of the Harvard Six Cities study. *American Journal of Respiratory and Critical Care Medicine* **173** (6), 667–72.

Levenson, D. (2011) Cystic fibrosis screening recommended for all women. *American Journal of Medical Genetics. Part A.* **155A** (7), ix–x.

Lim WS, Baudouin SV, George RC, Hill AT, *et al.* (2009) BTS guidelines for the management of community acquired pneumonia in adults: update 2009. *Thorax* **64** Suppl. 3iii1–55.

Lopez AD, Mathers CD, Ezzati M, *et al.* (eds) (2006) *Global Burden of Disease and Risk Factors.* Washington, DC: World Bank.

McClean KM, Kee F, Young IS, and Elborn JS (2008) Obesity and the lung: 1. Epidemiology. *Thorax* **63** (7), 649–54.

Mannino DM and Buist AS (2007) Global burden of COPD: risk factors, prevalence, and future trends. *Lancet* **370** (9589), 765–773.

Maritz GS and Harding R (2011) Life-long programming implications of exposure to tobacco smoking and nicotine before and soon after birth: evidence for altered lung development. *International Journal of Environmental Research and Public Health* **8** (3), 875–98.

Martel M-J, Rey É, Malo J-L, Perreault S, *et al.* (2009) Determinants of the Incidence of Childhood Asthma: A Two-Stage Case-Control Study. *American Journal of Epidemiology* **169** (2), 195–205.

Martinez-García, M.-A., Campos-Rodríguez, F., Soler-Cataluña, J.-J., Catalán-Serra, P., *et al.* (2011) Increased incidence of non-fatal cardiovascular events in stroke patients with sleep apnoea. Effect of CPAP treatment. *The European Respiratory Journal* **39** (4), 906–12.

Massie J (2009) Carrier screening for cystic fibrosis. *Lancet* **374** (9694), 978.

Matricardi, PM, Rosmini F, Riondino S, *et al.* (2000) Exposure to Foodborne and Orofecal Microbes versus Airborne Viruses in Relation to Atopy and Allergic Asthma: Epidemiological Study. *British Medical Journal* **320**, 412–17.

Nair H, Nokes DJ, Gessner BD, Dherani M, *et al.* (2010) Global burden of acute lower respiratory infections due to respiratory syncytial virus in young children: a systematic review and meta-analysis. *Lancet* **375** (9725), 1545–55.

Oberg M, Jaakkola MS, Woodward A, Peruga A, *et al.* (2011) Worldwide burden of disease from exposure to second-hand smoke: a retrospective analysis of data from 192 countries. *Lancet* **377** (9760), 139–46.

Perez L, Rapp R, and Künzli N (2010) The year of the lung: outdoor air pollution and lung health. *Swiss Medical Weekly* **140**, w13129.

Peto R, Darby S, Deo H, Silcocks P, *et al.* (2000) Smoking, smoking cessation, and lung cancer in the UK since 1950: combination of national statistics with two case-control studies. *BMJ (Clinical Research Ed)* **321** (7257), 323–9.

Platt SD, Martin CJ, Hunt SM, and Lewis CW (1989) Damp housing, mould growth, and symptomatic health state. *BMJ (Clinical Research Ed)* **298** (6689), 1673–8.

Punjabi NM (2008) The epidemiology of adult obstructive sleep apnoea. *Proceedings of the American Thoracic Society* **5** (2), 136–43.

Punjabi NM, Caffo BS, Goodwin JL, Gottlieb DJ, *et al.* (2009) Sleep-disordered breathing and mortality: a prospective cohort study. *PLoS Medicine* **6** (8), e1000132.

Prisant LM, Dillard TA and Blanchard AR (2006) Obstructive sleep apnoea syndrome. *Journal of Clinical Hypertension (Greenwich, Conn.)* **8** (10), 746–50.

Rabe KF, Hurd S, Anzueto A, Barnes PJ, *et al.* (2007) Global strategy for the diagnosis, management, and prevention of chronic obstructive pulmonary disease: GOLD executive summary. *American Journal of Respiratory and Critical Care Medicine* **176** (6), 532–55.

Redline S, Yenokyan G, Gottlieb DJ, Shahar E, *et al.* (2010) Obstructive sleep apnea-hypopnea and incident stroke: the sleep heart health study. *American Journal of Respiratory and Critical Care Medicine* **182** (2), 269–77.

Rose G and Colwell L (1992) Randomized controlled trial of anti-smoking advice: final (20 year) results. *Journal of Epidemiology and Community Health* **46** (1), 75–7.

Ruiz M, Ewig S, Torres A, Arancibia F, *et al.* (1999) Severe community-acquired pneumonia. Risk factors and follow-up epidemiology. *American Journal of Respiratory and Critical Care Medicine* **160** (3), 923–9.

Samoli E, Peng R, Ramsay T, Pipikou M, *et al.* (2008) Acute effects of ambient particulate matter on mortality in Europe and North America: results from the APHENA study. *Environmental Health Perspectives* **116** (11), 1480–6.

Schünemann HJ, Dorn J, Grant BJ, Winkelstein W, Jr, *et al.* (2000) Pulmonary function is a long-term predictor of mortality in the general population: 29-year follow-up of the Buffalo Health Study. *Chest* **118** (3), 656–64.

Semple MG, Taylor-Robinson, DC, Lane S and Smyth RL (2011) Household tobacco smoke and admission weight predict severe bronchiolitis in infants independent of deprivation: prospective cohort study. *PloS One* **6** (7), e22425.

Southern KW, Mérelle MME, Dankert-Roelse JE and Nagelkerke AD (2009) Newborn screening for cystic fibrosis. *Cochrane Database of Systematic Reviews* **1**, CD001402.

Stephens RJ and Johnson DH (2000) Treatment and outcomes for elderly patients with small cell lung cancer. *Drugs & Aging* **17** (3), 229–47.

Strachan DP (2000) Family size, infection and atopy: the first decade of the 'hygiene hypothesis'. *Thorax* **55** Suppl. 1 S2–10.

Tobacco Advisory Group of the Royal College of Physicians (2010). *Passive Smoking in Children*. London: Royal College of Physicians.

Torén K and Blanc PD (2009) Asthma caused by occupational exposures is common - a systematic analysis of estimates of the population-attributable fraction. *BMC Pulmonary Medicine* Jan 29 **9**, 7

Treasure T, Waller D, Swift S and Peto J (2004) Radical surgery for mesothelioma. *BMJ (Clinical Research Ed)* **328** (7434), 237–8.

Tyczynski JE, Bray F and Parkin DM (2003) Lung cancer in Europe in 2000: epidemiology, prevention, and early detection. *The Lancet Oncology* **4** (1), 45–55.

Wijesinghe, M., Weatherall, M., Perrin, K., Harwood, M., *et al.* (2009) Risk of mortality associated with formoterol: a systematic review and meta-analysis. *The European Respiratory Journal* **34** (4), 803–11.

Willers SM, Devereux G, Craig LCA, McNeill G, *et al.* (2007) Maternal food consumption during pregnancy and asthma, respiratory and atopic symptoms in 5-year-old children. *Thorax* **62** (9), 773–9.

Zhang Y, Moffatt MF and Cookson WOC (2012) Genetic and genomic approaches to asthma: new insights for the origins. *Current Opinion in Pulmonary Medicine* **18** (1), 6–13.

Model answers

Question 1

In Table 8.3 only data for the crude (unadjusted) odds ratio for each of the infectious agents are presented. It would be helpful to know whether the cases and controls had been adequately matched for potential confounding factors. If this was not the case then some attempt should be made to adjust for possible confounders in subsequent analyses.

Question 2

Investigators may also measure genetic polymorphisms which may predispose to asthma in subjects with and without atopy.

9 Nutritional, endocrine, and metabolic diseases

JAYNE WOODSIDE AND MARIE CANTWELL

CHAPTER CONTENTS

This chapter deals with the major nutritionally related diseases that are of public health importance internationally. In the developing world, malnutrition and suboptimal nutrition are endemic, whereas an epidemic of overweight and obesity has occurred in the developed world. Three examples of epidemiological studies are given: a major cohort study on mortality in American nurses according to the amount of body fat; a landmark multicentre clinical trial on the prevention of complications of insulin-dependent diabetes; and a community-based trial of iodine supplementation to fertile women in Papua New Guinea to reduce the likelihood of cretinism in their offspring.

Introduction

Several nutritionally related diseases are of major public health importance and include both diseases of *deficiency* and of *excess*. Deficiency of calories or food energy, tragically experienced to some degree by well over half of the world's population, is *malnutrition*; the diseases of calorie excess have led to an epidemic of *overweight* and *obesity*, even paradoxically among low-income groups in affluent countries. The epidemics of coronary heart disease preceded those of overweight and obesity in such countries and have been closely linked with high consumption of foods containing saturated fatty acids (particularly dairy and meat products) which raise blood cholesterol levels (see Chapter 7). There is also much epidemiological evidence linking diet with many cancers on a worldwide basis (see Chapter 17).

Former micronutrient deficiency diseases such as *beri-beri* (thiamine deficiency), *pellagra* (niacin deficiency), and *scurvy* (vitamin C deficiency) lie beyond the scope of this book but are important for a more complete understanding of the development of nutritional epidemiology (see Truswell 1999). *Vitamin A deficiency* is often associated with protein–calorie malnutrition and remains a major preventable cause of blindness in developing countries. *Rickets* and *osteomalacia* (vitamin D deficiency), once a major blight on children's skeletal development in large, industrialized cities, can still be problematic in Asian communities in the UK for whom vitamin D supplementation in childhood is recommended. *Maternal folate deficiency*, which has been closely associated with risk of neural tube defects (spina bifida) and for which preconceptual supplementary folate is advocated in the UK, is discussed in more detail in Chapter 16. Truswell notes that half of the vitamins are required in daily amounts of 1 mg or less, and with a balanced varied diet supplementation should be rarely necessary. Furthermore, in pregnant women excess levels of vitamin A have been linked with developmental abnormalities, and multivitamins containing vitamin A are not recommended in early pregnancy.

The term *metabolic disease* is used rather loosely in medical practice. Hormones play an essential role in many metabolic processes and endocrine diseases are essentially metabolic in nature. *Maturity-onset diabetes mellitus* is characterized by increasing resistance to the effects of insulin and a marked increase in insulin requirements. A rising trend in the incidence of this disorder is closely linked with the rising trend in overweight and obesity. *Iodine* is an essential micronutrient for normal thyroid function, and maternal iodine deficiency remains an important public health problem worldwide, as a cause of *endemic cretinism*; it may also cause a major proportion of cases of mental retardation in the developing world. However, the major public health and sociopolitical problems that require remedies are the problems of deficiency of food energy, protein, and micronutrients in the developing world, and of excess elsewhere.

9.1 Malnutrition

Malnutrition was common in both urban and rural populations in Europe during the 19th and early 20th centuries, particularly in children. Specific deficiency diseases such as rickets were very common, particularly in urban environments, and rickets was known as 'a disease of poverty and darkness'. Dairy products (milk, butter, eggs, etc.) were not generally available to the poor, and up to 75 per cent of poorer children showed some evidence of the disease in some large European cities. Nutritional science blossomed at the beginning of the 20th century with the demonstration of the almost total absorption and energy balance of the primary nutrients (protein, carbohydrate, and fats) in humans by Atwater (1902), and the gradual discovery that vitamins, originally recognized by Hopkins (1912), are 'accessory food factors'. This new knowledge led to new initiatives in public health and

nutritional surveillance to monitor the changes in the level of attainment of full, healthy growth potential in childhood, as it was increasingly recognized that inadequate growth in children was related to susceptibility to frequently fatal infectious diseases such as tuberculosis, diphtheria, whooping cough, measles, and influenzal or bacterial pneumonia, which accounted for large proportion of infant and childhood mortality at that time. **Growth standards** in childhood were then developed. It was shown that in Glasgow the average height of 13-year-old schoolchildren increased by 4.5 inches (11.43 cm) between 1915 and 1959 and a further 8–10 cm by the early 1990s. Nutrition in childhood in Europe and in industrialized countries in general has become adequate for almost all, but unfortunately excessive for some, partly because of an increasing cultural tendency towards sedentary activities such as watching television or playing computer games, and also to widespread availability of high-calorie fast foods. It is instructive to inquire of our grandparents their daily way of life, now termed *lifestyle*, to discover how radically this has changed during the past 50 years.

Maternal and child under-nutrition is the underlying cause of 3.5 million deaths and 35 per cent of the disease burden is in children younger than five years of age. It is also responsible for 11 per cent of total global disability-adjusted life-years (DALYs) (Black *et al.* 2008). *Marasmus* (Greek: wasting) is hard to misdiagnose but milder forms of *protein–calorie malnutrition* can have major developmental and health consequences in children. *Kwashiorkor* (originally a local name in Ghana), another form of protein–calorie malnutrition, presents without gross wasting when carbohydrate intakes are sufficient to maintain insulin secretion (averting the need for gluconeogenesis from body protein), but is also life threatening if untreated. Underweight children have a low weight compared with that expected for a well-nourished child of the same age and sex. This anthropometric variable can indicate wasting (i.e. low weight for height indicating acute weight loss) or more commonly stunting (i.e. low height for age indicating chronic restriction of a child's potential growth). These two conditions have different determinants and as a result respond differently to interventions. The devastating effects of malnutrition on intellectual ability, economic productivity, health, reproductive performance, and survival are well established (Victora *et al.* 2008). Indeed, indices of maternal and child under-nutrition are related to several other adult outcomes including height, schooling, income, offspring birth weight, glucose concentrations, and blood pressure (Victora *et al.* 2008). As a result we now have internationally set goals, such as the Millennium Development Goals (United Nations) to reduce levels of child malnutrition by half between 1990 and 2015. Several **reference standards** have been devised for children, which relate to *achieved weight or height for a given age*, although some indices have standardized for height, which is done for adults. In children, skeletal vertical growth varies at different ages; periods of accelerated growth, even in younger children, and the problem of stunting (reduced height but normal body shape) make a universal index difficult to achieve. The World Health Organization (WHO) introduced new child growth standards for use in the determination of stunting, wasting, and underweight and a recent study has shown that the WHO standards are better predictors of mortality than those determined by the previously recommended international growth references devised by the National Center for Health Statistics (NCHS) (Vesel *et al.* 2010). Box 9.1 shows two commonly used childhood indices to assess significant malnutrition.

Mid-upper arm circumference (MUAC) is particularly simple to use under field and famine conditions in young children as no scales are needed, and it is normally constant (greater than 13.5 cm) between one and five years of age. This has the advantage that simple tape-measures marked appropriately in colour can be produced in bulk and are easy to use by front-line staff. Adults can also be malnourished and here **Quetelet's index** (weight (kg)/height² (m)) has become universally used as a standard index for assessing under- and overweight in both men and women. Unless otherwise stated, the term **body mass index** (BMI) usually refers to this definition, although other indices have also been used by some investigators (see Box 9.2).

In 1992, the United Nations World Declaration on Nutrition reported 20 per cent of the population of developing countries were malnourished in terms of energy and growth requirements, and 2000 million people (about 60 per cent of the developing population), mainly children and women, had deficiencies in one or more micronutrients. These levels of malnutrition have been recently reported to have declined only slightly, and a WHO Global Database on child growth and malnutrition has now been established (de Onis and Blossner 2003). These statistics relate to *endemic malnutrition* rather than *epidemic malnutrition* induced by famine conditions, often precipitated by social disruption such as civil war. Endemic malnutrition is associated with reduced immune response and resistance to infection, particularly in infants and young children; countries in which endemic malnutrition is common experience high infant and child mortality, particularly from respiratory and gastrointestinal infections. Malnutrition particularly affects the cellular immune system, T-cell counts can be reduced and phagocytosis is impaired. Nevertheless, immunization programmes in developing countries, supported by the WHO, have had a major impact on infant and childhood mortality, and should be developed in parallel with programmes designed to improve the nutritional status of infants and children. Several other interventions have been initiated to address maternal and child under-nutrition including promotion of breastfeeding, strategies to promote complementary feeding with or without provision of food supplements; micronutrient interventions, general supportive strategies to improve family and community nutrition, and reduction of disease burden through promotion of hand-washing and strategies to reduce the burden of malaria in pregnancy (Bhutta *et al.* 2008). Of the available interventions, counselling about breastfeeding and fortification or supplementation with vitamin A and zinc (Fischer-Walker *et al.* 2009) have the greatest potential to reduce the burden of child morbidity and mortality (Bhutta *et al.* 2008).

9.2 Eating disorders

Anorexia nervosa is a behavioural disorder mainly affecting teenage girls and young women in affluent societies. The lifetime prevalence in adults of Western

Box 9.1 Assessment of malnutrition: commonly used indices

	Per cent reference[1] population	No oedema	Oedema
Weight for age[2]	60–79	Under-nourished	Kwashiorkor
	< 60	Marasmus	Marasmic kwashiorkor
Mid-upper arm circumference[3] (cm)	> 14	Normal	
	12.5–14.0	Suboptimal nutrition	
	< 12.5	Definite malnutrition	

[1] National Child Health Surveys (USA) are preferred reference population (National Centre for Health Statistics 1987).
[2] Height for age and weight for height have also been used as common indices.
[3] Constant between ages of 1–5 years, but can also be used on older age groups of children against reference standards.

Truswell AS (1999). *ABC of Nutrition*, 3rd edn. London: BMJ Books. Golden MHN and Golden BE (2000) 'Severe Malnutrition', in JS Garrow, WPT James and A Ralph (eds.), *Human Nutrition and Dietetics*, 10th edn. Edinburgh: Churchill Livingstone.

countries is about 0.7 per cent. In anorexia there is usually a disturbance of the body image (the patient evaluates their self-worth primarily in terms of their shape and weight and believes she or he looks fat), the body mass index is maintained at less than 17.5 kg/m² (normal 20–25), or 15 per cent below the patient's expected weight for their age, height, and sex, and commonly there is amenorrhoea.

Bulimia nervosa is a related condition in which there are recurrent episodes of binge eating, often in private, accompanied by compensatory behaviour such as self-induced vomiting or other purging, fasting, or excessive exercise to control body shape and weight. Usually, there is the similar psychological problem to anorexia of self-evaluation largely in terms of shape and weight. The combined prevalence of bulimia and anorexia nervosa is about two to three per cent in women aged 15–35 years. The natural history and prognosis of the conditions imply that many patients eventually improve, although established anorexia is reported to have a relatively high risk of eventual death due to eating disorder-related medical complications or suicide. A review of outcome studies based on clinic attenders for anorexia nervosa among a total patient population of 5334 indicated that five per cent died, 47 per cent recovered, 34 per cent improved, and 21 per cent

remained chronically ill. In community studies, standardized questionnaires such as the Eating Attitude Test (EAT) and (SCOFF: Sick, Control, One (stone), Fat, Food) have been examined as potential screening tools. A series of case-control community studies has investigated risk factors for anorexia nervosa and bulimia nervosa (Fairburn and Harrison 2003), but population-based cohort studies are lacking. A summary of the descriptive epidemiology of eating disorders is shown in Table 9.1.

9.3 Overweight and obesity

In some ancient cultures being fat carried with it the mark of wealth and high social status, but in most modern cultures the converse is the case; in addition, overweight and obesity carry a considerable health burden. As noted by Astrup (2005), obesity is the most important nutrition-related disease in industrialized countries and in many parts of the developing world; it is a major risk factor for cardiovascular disease, maturity-onset diabetes mellitus (also known as non-insulin-dependent diabetes mellitus (NIDDM) or type 2 diabetes), some cancers, and several other major chronic diseases.

Box 9.2 Measurement of body fat

Gold standards	Comment
Measurement of total body water, bone mineral and body density using underwater weighing and isotopic measures	Technically demanding, used for research purposes only in specialized laboratories
Proxy measures	
Overall body fat	
Quetelet's index/BMI (weight/height^2) (kg/m^2)	Best overall index for men and women; only method to have internationally accepted criteria for classification of degree of obesity
Skinfold thickness at various sites (mm)	Requires careful standardization and training
Bioelectrical impedance (electrical conductance through body tissues)	Widely used but lacking universal standardization
Central obesity	
Waist/hip ratio	Differs for men and women
Waist circumference (cm)	Little epidemiological information
Abdominal/subscapular skinfold (mm)	As above (overall body fat)

Source: Garrow JS (2005). 'Body Size and Composition' in C Geissler and H Powers (eds), *Human Nutrition*, 11th edn. Edinburgh: Elsevier Churchill Livingstone.

Table 9.1 Epidemiology of eating disorders

	Anorexia nervosa	Bulimia nervosa
Worldwide distribution	Predominantly Western societies	Predominantly Western societies
Ethnic origin	Mainly white people	Mainly white people
Sex	Most female (about 90%)	Most female (uncertain proportion)
Age	Adolescents (some young adults)	Young adults (some adolescents)
Social class	Possible excess in higher social class	Even distribution
Prevalence	0.7% (in teenage girls)	1–2% (in 16–35-year-old females)
Incidence (per 100,000 per year)	19 in females, 2 in males	29 in females, 1 in males
Secular change	Possible increase	Likely increase

Reproduced from Fairburn G and Harrison P, 'Eating disorders', *Lancet* **361**, 9355, 407–416, 2003, with permission from Elsevier.

Assessment and trends in adults

As noted earlier, Quetelet's index (weight/height^2 (kg/m^2)) or BMI has been almost universally adopted as a standard measure of relative weight for men, women, and more recently for children. This provides a proxy measure of the amount of body fat. Technically precise, accurate 'gold standard' methods have been used to validate this simple measurement and these and other proxy indices are shown in Box 9.2.

As in the case of all continuously distributed variables, the cut-point at which the balance shifts to a significant future health risk in an individual has to be defined with a degree of precision from epidemiological studies; typically these are prospective studies with health outcome data. Such studies have placed 30 kg/m² as a suitable cut-point for a definition of *obesity*, above which there is clearly increased health risk to an individual, if not currently, then in the short- to middle-term (five to 20 years), and in the long term in young adults (20 years +) (Fontaine *et al.* 2003).The WHO has also adopted the standard definition of overweight as 25–29 kg/m² in adults, although the level of evidence is not as substantial as that for obesity.

Accurate measurement and assessment in populations is particularly important to monitor the steep rise in the prevalence of overweight and obesity. This has been described as pandemic in the USA, where two out of three adults are overweight or obese compared with one in four in the 1960s (Manson and Bassuk 2003). These authors also suggest that obesity will soon overtake smoking as the primary preventable cause of death should the current rise in obesity continue. European countries show similar trends, but with slightly lower levels of overweight and obesity. In a recent Department of Health survey for England (2009), the prevalence of overweight and obesity was: 66 per cent in men and 57 per cent in women; for obesity alone it was 24 per cent in women and 22 per cent in men. This growing prevalence of overweight and obesity is likely to significant health care costs (Wang *et al.* 2011). Obesity is also a growing challenge in the developing world; rates have tripled in the last 20 years in countries adopting a Western lifestyle, with the Middle East, South East Asia, Pacific Islands, and China experiencing the largest increases (Hossain *et al.* 2007).

Assessment and trends in children

In childhood, because vertical growth is accelerated at intervals, a fixed cut-point suitable for all ages cannot be used. Cole *et al.* (2000) have proposed international standards that correspond to the cut-points of overweight and obesity in adulthood for children of a specific age to the nearest six-month interval. As for most population standards, these are gender-specific (Fig. 9.1).

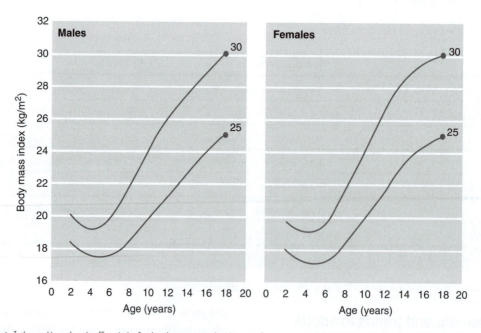

Figure 9.1 International cut-off points for body mass index by sex for overweight and obesity, passing through body mass index 25 and 30 kg/m² (data from Brazil, Britain, Hong Kong, The Netherlands, Singapore, and USA).
Reproduced from Cole TJ, Bellizzi MC, Flegal KM, Dietz WH (2000). 'Establishing a Standard Definition for Child Overweight and Obesity Worldwide: International Survey'. *British Medical Journal* **320**: 1240–3 with permission from BMJ Publishing Group Ltd.

Until recently, suitable standards were unavailable to reliably monitor trends in childhood obesity, but available data suggest that this has increased in most developed countries, with the exception of Russia and Poland, and in several developing countries, particularly in urban areas (Wang and Lobstein, 2006). Type 2 diabetes ('maturity onset' diabetes), one of the most significant complications of obesity, which is discussed in the following section, now accounts for 50 per cent of new cases of diabetes in adolescents in parts of North America, compared with almost no cases a generation previously. Although not all overweight or obese children **track** this into adulthood most do, which contributes further to the adult epidemic.

What are the complications of overweight and obesity?

There is a positive linear relation between BMI and cardiovascular mortality in prospective studies, but the relation is U-shaped for all-cause mortality (see Figure 9.2).

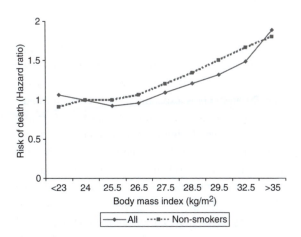

Figure 9.2 Risk of death during 16 years of follow-up in American nurses by category of body mass (relative to lowest risk category).

Source: Data from Allison DB, Fontaine KR, Manson JE, Stevens J, and VanItallie TB (1999). 'Annual Deaths Attributable to Obesity in the United States'. *Journal of the American Medical Association* **282**, 1530–8.

As an example, the Nurses' Health Study report was based on over 100,000 mainly white American nurses aged 30–55 years followed for 16 years. Most studies examining the relation between body mass and all-cause mortality show this pattern. An association between abdominal adiposity and all-cause mortality has also been shown, independent of BMI (Pischon *et al.* 2008).

··

Question 1

(a) What is the most likely explanation for the pattern of risk shown in Fig. 9.2?

(b) How could you check this explanation?

(c) Why is the relation different in non-smokers?

··

Health consequences are related to the degree of excess weight, and this has been clearly demonstrated in epidemiological studies to be associated with the risk of hypertension, diabetes mellitus, and an overall increased risk of cardiovascular disease in general. These data are largely from observational studies, but a recent meta-analysis of intervention studies indicate that systolic blood pressure can be reduced by 10 mmHg for every 10 kg of weight loss irrespective of the initial BMI (Neter *et al.* 2003). Perhaps underestimated, except by overweight or obese individuals, are the social consequences of obesity, which frequently result in prejudice in others, even in their family doctor, and may lead to low self-esteem, anxiety, and depression. Two eating disorders have been linked to depression and obesity: binge eating disorder and night eating syndrome. Many other clinical consequences of overweight and obesity are well established and are listed in Box 9.3.

Direct and indirect costs of obesity are estimated at seven per cent of the total healthcare costs in the USA and one to five per cent in Europe, and the increased health care costs due to obesity could overwhelm the health care budgets of developing countries who are also struggling to cope with communicable diseases (Wang *et al.* 2011).

Box 9.3 Complications of overweight and obesity

Mortality	Life expectancy
Overweight	Reduced 3.1 years in men/ 3.3 years in women
Obese	Reduced 6.7 years in men/ 7.1 years in women
Morbidity	
Cardiovascular diseases	(Coronary disease, stroke, congestive heart failure, hypertension)
Metabolic diseases	Type 2 diabetes, insulin resistance, or metabolic syndrome
Cancers	Colorectal, endometrial, post-menopausal breast cancer
Reproductive health	In women: infertility, menstrual disorders, gestational diabetes, pregnancy complications
Mental health	Depression, social isolation

Box 9.4 Energy expenditure by occupation and in different leisure activities

	MET level*
Occupation	
Office work (sitting tasks, light effort)	1.5
Bartending (standing tasks, light effort)	3.0
Garbage collector	4.0
Firefighting	8.0
Activity	
Sleeping	0.95
Very brisk walking (4 mph)	5.0
Badminton (social)	5.5
Squash (general)	7.3

*Metabolic equivalent of task: 1 = energy consumed sitting at rest
Reproduced from: Ainsworth BE, Haskell WL, Herrmann SD, Meckes N, Bassett DR Jr, Tudor-Locke C, Greer JL, Vezina J, Whitt-Glover MC, and Leon AS (2011) 'Compendium of Physical Activities: A Second Update of Codes and MET Values'. *Med Sci Sports Exerc*. 2011 Aug; **43**(8), 1575–1581 with permission from Wolters Kluwer Health.

What are the main causes of overweight and obesity, and are these preventable?

In the early 1900s, Atwater showed that humans absorb, metabolize, and store over 90 per cent of food energy nutrients: protein, carbohydrate, fat, and alcohol. The law of conservation of energy applies, and 1 g protein and carbohydrate each contribute four calories of food energy, 1 g alcohol contributes seven calories, and 1 g of fat contributes nine calories. Animals and humans can survive without carbohydrate and alcohol in their diet (non-essential nutrients) but protein, fat, and a very long list of micronutrients are essential to life. Dietary Reference Values (DRVs) have been published for macro- and micronutrients. Surveys conducted in the UK suggest that most of the population, both adults and children, have an adequate intake of essential micronutrients. In affluent countries and among the better-off in developing countries, a wide choice of foods is available, including *energy-dense foods* high in calories. Conversely, the need for physical activity and energy expenditure has declined rapidly in industrialized and urbanized societies. A recent cohort study conducted in US children over a 10-year period reported that the decline in physical activity during adolescence was more closely associated with the development of overweight and obesity than were changes in energy intake (Kimm *et al.* 2005).Typical energy expenditures at different levels of physical activity, nowadays mainly during leisure, and in different occupations are shown in Box 9.4. Labourers in poorer countries in comparison with most workers in developed countries, work long hours and have high energy expenditure. In times of civil disturbance or war, negative energy balance is common.

Environmental causes of overweight and obesity have been reviewed by Ebbeling *et al.* (2002) who notes that many factors conspire to increase energy intake and limit physical activity, particularly in children. Increased availability of energy dense foods, increased portion sizes, increased sugar-sweetened beverage consumption, along with more frequent eating out, fast food consumption, and more frequent snacking are all likely to contribute. Ebbeling estimates that excess calorie consumption of only 120 kcal per day (one sugar-sweetened soft drink) would produce a 50 kg increase in body weight over 10 years. A widely available and typical fast food meal—a double cheeseburger, French fries, soft drink, and dessert—may contain 2200 kcal and is unlikely to be the only meal of the day. The composition of foods, independent of their energy density, may also be important. Foods with a high proportion of refined carbohydrate—breads, many breakfast cereals, potatoes, soft drinks, cakes, and biscuits—cause a large post-prandial insulin response. Foods with a high 'glycaemic index' (the level of insulin response) have been linked with the development of type 2 diabetes in prospective studies, although long-term clinical trials have yet to be conducted.

Psychosocial and family factors are also likely to play a role in childhood and adult obesity. Television viewing and solitary playing of computer games are linked with inappropriate snacking and lack of parental interaction; these and other adversities are associated with the risk of early overweight (Ebbeling *et al.* 2002). In adults, a report from the Nurses' Health Study (50,000 nurses, non-obese and non-diabetic at baseline followed up for six years) indicated that a sedentary lifestyle and high television viewing hours were closely related to the development of both obesity and diabetes mellitus (Hu *et al.* 2003). They estimated that 30 per cent (95% CI, 24–36 per cent) of new cases of obesity and 43 per cent (95% CI, 32–52 per cent) cases of diabetes could be prevented by the adoption of a relatively active lifestyle (less than 10 hours per week television watching and at least 30 minutes of brisk walking per day). This cohort study was observational, but interventional studies in children (largely school-based), which have used single or multiple interventions on physical activity or on diet have shown some positive results,

although long-term maintenance of these behaviour changes will be a challenge. Twin studies suggest that obesity is partly genetic in origin but, with the exception of very rare genetic disorders, the usual mode of inheritance appears to be polygenic (see Chapter 19).

Prevention or limiting the size of the epidemic of overweight and obesity has become an international concern of the WHO, which has established the International Obesity Task Force to devise strategies for public health programmes. Implementation of these programmes may take considerable international effort and political will (suggested recently by Gortmaker *et al.* (2011)), such as that finally being attempted in tobacco control, some 40 years on from establishing the link between cigarette smoking and major chronic diseases (see Chapters 8 and 20).

9.4 Diabetes mellitus

This disorder is the result of failure of insulin to regulate blood glucose levels after meals and, particularly in its acute form, is characterized by excess urine production (polyuria) and the presence of glucose in the urine (glycosuria). Hyperglycemia (high blood glucose) is diagnostic of diabetes mellitus and this metabolic defect appears to be the main factor in producing the serious *microvascular*, and possibly also the *macrovascular*, complications of diabetes. There are two distinct types: *insulin-dependent diabetes mellitus* (IDDM) or *type I* in which there is a failure to produce insulin owing to progressive destruction of the β-cells of the islets of Langerhans in the pancreas. This is considered by many to be an autoimmune inflammatory disorder, and islet cell antibodies can be detected in blood before the onset of the disease. In *non-insulin-dependent diabetes mellitus* (NIDDM) or *type 2* there is progressive metabolic resistance to the effects of insulin which can also progress to insulin deficiency, but without islet cell antibodies. Type I commonly occurs in childhood, but can occur at any age although there is no increase in incidence with age in adults. Type 2 accounts for most (about 75 per cent) cases of diabetes, shows a steeply rising trend with age, and is closely associated with obesity. Owing to the rapid rise in the prevalence of obesity in some populations, particularly in North America, type 2 diabetes now accounts for about half of the newly diagnosed cases of diabetes in children and adolescents. This trend is particularly pronounced in minority racial and ethnic groups (Alberti *et al.* 2004) and the increase in the prevalence of NIDDM is closely linked to the upsurge in obesity and 90 per cent is attributable to excess weight (Hossain *et al.* 2007).

Insulin-dependent diabetes mellitus

The epidemiology of IDDM is most accurately studied in countries with advanced health care systems and specially created disease registers for children. Data for adults are less widely available as type 2 diabetics may also progress to insulin dependence; prevalence and incidence data are therefore likely to be more accurate in childhood registries. It has been estimated that 10–15 per cent of childhood cases present as diabetic ketoacidotic coma, although fewer than one per cent die at the time of diagnosis.

Insulin-dependent diabetes mellitus is a relatively common major chronic disease of childhood with an overall prevalence of 0.25 per cent (one case per 400 children aged 0–14 years), and in UK registries a standardized incidence rate of 16.4 new cases per 100,000 person years (95 % CI, 15.6–17.3) has been reported. In Europe the standardized incidence rate varies 10-fold between countries and is rising in most of these at the rate of 3.9 per cent per annum (95 % CI, 3.6–4.2 per cent) (Patterson *et al.* 2009). Reasons for the major differences in incidence between countries and the north-south gradient within Europe are poorly understood. There is a seasonal pattern coinciding with an increase in autumn and winter infections in children, but studies on viral aetiology have proved inconclusive. About 90 per cent of cases occur in children from families without a family history of IDDM, and studies investigating risk markers such as lack of breastfeeding and socio-economic conditions have proved inconclusive to date. There is also some evidence of a lower risk of childhood onset type 1 diabetes with increasing birth order, particularly in children aged less than five years of age (Cardwell *et al.* 2011). Although the

obscure aetiology does not currently provide opportunities for primary prevention, secondary prevention and, at the least, delay in the appearance of complications, appears to be achievable in many cases by maintenance of tight glycaemic control. The Environmental Determinants of Diabetes in the Young (TEDDY) study seeks to identify environmental factors influencing the development of type 1 diabetes using intensive follow-up of 421,000 infants at elevated genetic risk (Hagopian *et al.* 2011). Rasmussen *et al.* (2009) has also shown that maternal weight may predict risk of islet autoimmunity in offspring with a high genetic susceptibility for type 1 diabetes but further research in larger studies is required. The Diabetes Autoimmunity Study in the Young (DAISY) has followed 1972 children for autoimmunity and diabetes to try to predict progression to type 1 diabetes (Barker *et al.* 2004). Short-term breastfeeding has been implicated as a risk factor for beta-cell autoimmunity, clinical diabetes or both. In a double-blind randomized controlled trial 230 infants with HLA-conferred susceptibility to type 1 diabetes were randomized to receive a casein hydrolysate formula or a conventional cow's milk-based formula. Positivity for one or more auto-antibodies in the hydrolysate formula group was significantly lower compared to the control group. This study has shown that dietary intervention during infancy appears to have a long-lasting effect on markers of beta-cell autoimmunity—markers that may reflect an autoimmune process leading to type 1 diabetes (Knip *et al.* 2010; Knip *et al.* 2011).

Non-insulin-dependent diabetes mellitus

This type of diabetes mellitus is more insidious in onset than IDDM and frequently presents asymptomatically on routine urine or blood testing. Blood sugar levels, taken after an overnight fast, of 7.8 mmol/L and above were formerly used by the WHO as an internationally agreed cut-point for the diagnosis of NIDDM, but the American Diabetic Association recently endorsed a cut-point of 7.0 mmol/L (Anon 2012). This cut-point has not been formally agreed in Europe, although prospective studies support the American proposal. Such problems contribute to the difficulty of accurately defining the prevalence of this disorder, which results in similar microvascular and macrovascular disease to that arising from IDDM.

Since the disease is defined by asymptomatic glycaemia it may be present for some years in many individuals before detection; such individuals are therefore at high risk of early development of complications. Thus there is a strong case for screening for diabetes, particularly in high-risk individuals, which is frequently done opportunistically in the UK using a paper strip dipped in urine (glycosuria test). Screening tests were recently discussed by the American Diabetes Association, which recommends fasting plasma glucose as a first-line screening test used opportunistically, based on the current level of evidence from screening intervention studies (American Diabetes Association 2004) (see also Chapter 5). However, in a 2008 Consensus Statement glycated haemoglobin or haemoglobin A1c (HbA$_{1c}$) was proposed as a screening/diagnostic test for diabetes using a threshold HbA$_{1c}$ value of 6.0 per cent and during the following year an International Expert Panel (Gillett 2009) published a similar recommendation using a threshold HbA$_{1c}$ of 6.5 per cent, later advocated by the American Diabetes Association. HbA$_{1c}$ is a marker of average blood glucose levels over the previous months and high HbA$_{1c}$ represents poor glucose control. However, an acceptable HbA$_{1c}$ result does not automatically rule out poor diabetic control, as it is possible to have an acceptable HbA$_{1c}$ result even with a history of recent hypoglycaemia or even spikes of hyperglycaemia. Echouffo-Tcheugui et al. (2011) in a critical review of the literature concluded that while economic modelling suggested that screening for type 2 diabetes may be cost-effective, empirical data on tangible benefits in preventing complications or death are lacking.

Owing to the rapid rise in the prevalence of obesity, type 2 diabetes now accounts for about half of the newly diagnosed cases of diabetes in children and adolescents. The major risk factors for type 2 diabetes in children or adolescents include obesity and inactivity, which are important contributors to insulin resistance, family history of type 2 diabetes in first- and second-degree relatives, low birth weight and high birth weight (Wei et al. 2003), maternal gestational diabetes or type 2 diabetes (Young et al. 2002), and not being breastfed during infancy.

Prevalence and incidence

The overall prevalence in the British population is about five per cent in men and seven per cent in women. There is a steep rise with age (about one per cent in 20–44 year olds rising to up to 20 per cent in 65–74 year olds), which probably accounts for the higher overall prevalence in women who form a greater part of the elderly population. The incidence among middle-aged men is about two per 1000 person-years (Perry et al. 1995), but in this cohort study the incidence was increased 11-fold in the top fifth of the distribution of BMI. Clearly the pandemic of overweight and obesity in both the advanced industrialized countries and in some developing countries is set to cause a major increase in the worldwide prevalence of NIDDM (an estimated doubling in prevalence from 1994 to 2010) (Zimmet et al. 2001). A pre-diabetic state categorized as the metabolic or insulin resistance syndrome has been proposed by the WHO and other bodies, but its clinical and epidemiological validity seem questionable.

In the UK, ethnic Indians from the Indian subcontinent show a large excess prevalence of NIDDM not accounted for by overweight or obesity alone; and in North America the prevalence of diabetes in Pima Indians is about 40 per cent in adults. Twin studies indicate a significant genetic contribution. Similar findings in minority populations in other parts of the world are likely to be due to the combined effects of a genetic predisposition and change in the diet and lifestyle of such populations (gene–environment interaction), although the rapidly increasing trend in incidence of both types of diabetes points to environmental causes as the major factor.

Prevention and control of complications of diabetes

The complications of diabetes are broadly classified into microvascular and macrovascular. Microvascular changes are at the capillary level and can cause significant renal damage and failure (nephropathy), retinal damage, and blindness (*retinopathy*), and sensory impairment, particularly to the lower limbs (*peripheral neuropathy*). The latter is closely associated with vascular impairment and diabetic gangrene. Macrovascular complications are those of increased risk of cardiovascular diseases, which can be explained only in part by elevations in well-established risk factors. Both IDDM and NIDDM are associated with premature mortality and risk of complications in the medium- to long-term.

Two recent major trials demonstrated the importance of careful control of hyperglycaemia (the major risk factor for microvascular complications) by randomizing diabetics to intensive and normal control regimens. The development of complications was significantly reduced in those patients randomized to the intensive treatment group. These results have major implications for the treatment of both IDDM and NIDDM. The trial in patients with IDDM is described next.

One thousand four hundred and forty-one patients (mean age 27 years) with IDDM, 726 with no retinopathy at baseline (primary prevention cohort), and 715 with mild retinopathy (secondary prevention cohort) were randomly assigned to intensive therapy (insulin pump or three or more daily insulin injections)

or conventional therapy with one or two daily insulin injections. Patients were followed for an average of 6.5 years, and the appearance and progression of retinopathy and other complications of diabetes were assessed at intervals by 'blinded' observers. Results were calculated per 100 person-years of follow-up but are summarized graphically in Fig. 9.3 as the percentage of patients developing significant complications: retinopathy (left panel) and nephropathy (right panel) according to the mode of treatment.

....

Question 2

(a) The results indicate significant reductions in the development of complications in young diabetics for intensive insulin treatment rather than conventional treatment. What is likely to be the main side effect of intensive insulin treatment and how would you evaluate its impact?

(b) Why would it be important to 'blind' the observers who examined patients for complications of diabetes to the treatment regimen?

(c) In a multicentre trial what prerequisites are required for clinical and quantitative outcome measures?

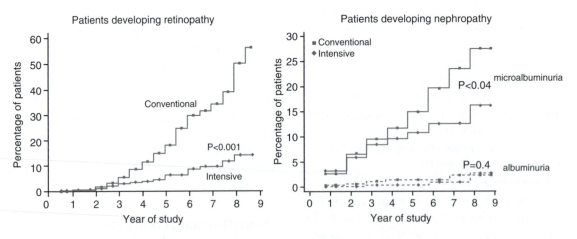

Figure 9.3 Cumulative incidence of sustained change in retinopathy (left panel) assessed by six-monthly fundus photography and of nephropathy (right panel) defined by development of albuminuria or microalbuminuria in patients with type 1 diabetes receiving intensive or conventional therapy for diabetes mellitus.

Data from Diabetes Control and Complications Trial Research Group (1993). 'The Effect of Intensive Treatment of Diabetes on the Development and Progression of Long-Term Complications in Insulin-Dependent Diabetes Mellitus'. *New England Journal of Medicine* **329**, 977–86, with permission from Massachusetts Medical Society.

(d) Why might the comparison of albuminuria rates between treatments not have attained significance although the comparison of microalbuminuria rates did attain significance?

(e) What other parameters should be evaluated following the results of this major trial?

∙∙

Such studies have led to the development in the UK of National (Health) Service Frameworks for the prevention and treatment of major chronic diseases such as diabetes, which provide guidance and clinical standards to specialist physicians, primary care trusts, and other health care workers involved in the prevention and treatment of these conditions. National Service Frameworks for coronary heart disease (CHD), the elderly, and for diabetes have been produced so far. However, for the primary prevention of NIDDM, intervention studies combining weight loss with increased exercise have shown encouraging results (Tuomilehto *et al.* 2001).

9.5 Endocrine disorders

Numerous endocrine disorders have been described clinically and are usually manifested by over-production or under-production of specific hormones. Examples are: hyperpituitarism, which includes Cushing's syndrome (over-production of adrenocorticotropic hormone (ACTH)), and acromegaly (over-production of growth hormone); diabetes insipidus (deficiency of antidiuretic hormone (ADH)); and thyrotoxicosis (over-production of thyroid hormone). None of these is as common worldwide, or as readily preventable, as deficiency of thyroid hormone, most commonly caused by lack of dietary iodine.

Iodine deficiency

Iodine is an essential constituent of the thyroid hormones thyroxine (T4) and tri-iodothyroine (T3). Iodine deficiency leads to a range of disorders at different stages of life, and this is shown in Table 9.2. The size of the thyroid gland changes inversely in response to alterations in iodine intake, with enlargement of the thyroid gland

(goitre) occurring in response to reduced intake. Severe iodine deficiency during pregnancy causes maternal and fetal hypothyroxinaemia, and this can lead to mental retardation, neurological abnormalities and cretinism in the fetus (Table 9.2). Whether mild to moderate maternal iodine deficiency produces more subtle changes in cognitive and neurological function in offspring has not yet been established (Zimmermann 2009).

Iodine deficiency is believed to be the most common preventable cause of mental defect at the world level, with some 1000 million people (20 per cent of the world's population) living in iodine-deficient regions. The ocean

Table 9.2 Range of disorders arising from iodine deficiency at different stages of life

Life stage	Iodine-deficiency disorders
Fetus	Abortions, stillbirths, congenital anomalies Increased perinatal and infant mortality Neurological cretinism (mental deficiency, deaf-mutism, spastic diplegia, squint) Myxedematous cretinism (dwarfism, mental deficiency) Psychomotor defects
Neonate	Neonatal goitre Neonatal hypothyroidism Increased susceptibility to nuclear radiation
Child and adolescent	Goitre Juvenile hypothyroidism Impaired mental function Retarded physical development Increased susceptibility to nuclear radiation
Adult	Goitre with complications such as impaired breathing and swallowing Hypothyroidism Impaired mental function Iodine-induced hyperthyroidism Increased susceptibility to nuclear radiation

Souce: West CE, Jooste PL, Pandav CS. Iodine and iodine-deficiency disorders. *Public Health Nutrition*, Blackwell Science, Oxford, 2004.

is the main source of iodine, and, if seafood is not consumed, intake will depend on iodine content of the soil. Iodine deficiency is therefore traditionally prevalent in mountainous regions where leaching of the soil occurs, as well as inland areas far from the sea. Many of these are in the developing world, for example central Africa.

Iodine deficiency can be detected by measuring urinary iodine, thyroid size, or thyroid hormone levels (thyroid stimulating hormone and thyroglobulin). *Goitre* is a sign of dietary iodine deficiency. In the 1990s some 200 million people worldwide were estimated to have goitre, which the WHO has classified into grade 1 (palpable goitre only) and grade 2 (visible goitre) to standardize definitions used in epidemiological surveys.

Prevention and control

It was in Switzerland in the late 19th century that the link between endemic goitre and cretinism was first made in extensive epidemiological surveys. Switzerland had a major problem with both, and several trials were done in school-children, which demonstrated that iodized salt or milk effectively shrunk goitres to a normal size. In 1922, the Swiss Goitre Commission recommended the use of salt with added potassium iodide on a voluntary basis and the distribution of additional weekly iodine tablets to school-children. The public health situation was monitored closely during the next

40 years, and the prevalence of goitre and cretinism was reduced 10-fold.

In the 1990s, a campaign to promote iodized salt in developing countries at risk of iodine deficiency was made by the WHO with UNICEF. It has been estimated that the number of children born with cretinism has been halved in less than a decade since the programme began (Truswell 1999), while the number of people at risk of iodine deficiency has been reduced to 500 million.

For nearly all countries, the main strategy to prevent iodine deficiency remains universal salt iodization. However, full implementation of this programme is not always possible, and this may result in insufficient access to iodized salt, which is particularly important in women who are of childbearing age or pregnant. In these situations, for example in more remote areas, iodinated oil in depot injections or iodine tablets can be used. A double-blind controlled trial in fertile young women was performed by Pharoah *et al.* between 1966 and 1972 in the remote Jimi valley of the Papua New Guinea highlands. Endemic cretinism was known to be high in this region. In collaboration with the local administrators, a census of families in the district was made; alternate families were given either intramuscular iodized oil or saline. Women of childbearing age were asked if they were pregnant. Follow-up surveys were done until children of mothers enrolled into this community study were between 10 and 16 years of

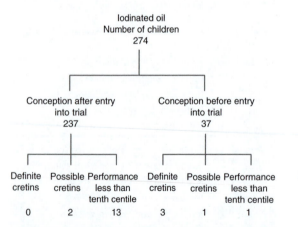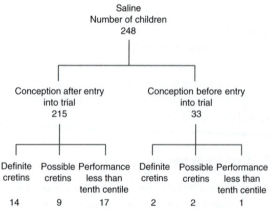

Figure 9.4 Controlled trial of depot iodine injection (versus saline) in Papua New Guinea.

Reproduced from Pharoah POD and Connolly KJ (1987). 'A Controlled Trial of Iodinated Oil for the Prevention of Endemic Cretinism: A Long-Term Follow-Up'. *International Journal of Epidemiology* **16**, 68–73 with permission from Oxford University Press.

age (Pharoah and Connolly 1987). The study results are shown in Figure 9.4. WHO/UNICEF recommends that countries assess their salt iodization programmes and then decide whether such supplementation is indicated.

An area of recent potential public health concern is that publications from the UK, which has no salt iodination policy, and Germany have suggested that, even in the developed world and close to oceans, iodine levels are low in school-children. Given the association with neuro-development, more widespread salt iodination or supplementation may be required (Johner *et al*. 2011; Vanderpump *et al*. 2011).

....

Question 3

(a) Why was a double-blinded controlled trial the ideal choice of study design?

(b) What other data would be helpful to provide an overall assessment of the effectiveness of this procedure?

(c) This trial was performed in 1966 when few trials of this type had been carried out. Under what circumstances would it be ethical to perform similar trials to extend this work?

....

Web addresses

International Obesity Task Force
www.iotf.org.

Department of Health
http://www.dh.gov.uk/en/Publichealth/Nutrition/index.htm.

Further reading

Geissler C and Powers H (2005) *Human Nutrition*, 11th edn. Edinburgh: Churchill Livingstone.

Gibney MJ, Lanham-New SA, Cassidy A, Vorster HH (2009) *Introduction to Human Nutrition*, 2nd edn. Oxford: Wiley Blackwell.

Lichtenstein AH, Appel LJ, Brands M, *et al*. (2006). Diet and Lifestyle Recommendations Revision 2006. A Scientific Statement from the American Heart Association Nutrition Committee. *Circulation* **114**, 82– 96.

Truswell AS (2003) *ABC of Nutrition*, 4th edn. London: BMJ Books.

Willett W (1998) *Nutritional Epidemiology*, 2nd edn. New York: Oxford University Press.

WHO Technical Report Series (2003) Diet, Nutrition and the Prevention of Chronic Diseases. Report of a Joint WHO/FAO Expert Consultation, No. 916. Geneva, Switzerland. http://www.who.int/hpr/NPH/docs/who_fao_expert_report.pdf.

References

Ainsworth BE, Haskell WL, Herrmann SD, Meckes N, *et al*. (2011) 2011 Compendium of physical activities: a second update of codes and MET values. *Medicine and Science in Sports and Exercise*. **43** (8):1575–81.

Alberti G, Zimmet P, Shaw J, Bloomgarden Z, *et al*. (2004) Type 2 diabetes in the young: the evolving epidemic: the international diabetes federation consensus workshop. *Diabetes Care* **27** (7), 1798–811.

Allison D B, Fontaine KR, Manson JE, Stevens J, *et al*. (1999) Annual deaths attributable to obesity in the United States. *JAMA* **282** (16), 1530–8.

American Diabetes Association (2004) Screening for type 2 diabetes. *Diabetes Care* **27**, Suppl 1, S11–S14.

Anon (2004) Screening for type 2 diabetes. *Diabetes Care*, **27** Suppl. 1 S11–14.

Anon (2012) Diagnosis and classification of diabetes mellitus. *Diabetes Care* **35** Suppl. 1S64–71.

Astrup, A (2005) Obesity. In: Geissler C and Powers H *Human Nutrition*, 11th edn; 379–99. Edinburgh: Churchill Livingstone.

Atwater, WO (1902) Principles of Nutrition and Nutritive Value of Food. *USDA Farmer's Bulletin* No. 142.

Barker JM, Barriga KJ, Yu L, Miao D, *et al*. (2004) Prediction of autoantibody positivity and progression to type 1 diabetes: Diabetes Autoimmunity Study in the Young (DAISY). *The Journal of Clinical Endocrinology and Metabolism* **89** (8), 3896–902.

Bhutta ZA, Ahmed T, Black RE, Cousens S, *et al*. (2008) What works? Interventions for maternal and child undernutrition and survival. *Lancet* **371** (9610), 417–40.

Black RE, Allen LH, Bhutta ZA, Caulfield LE, *et al*. (2008) Maternal and child undernutrition: global and regional exposures and health consequences. *Lancet* **371** (9608), 243–60.

Cardwell CR, Stene LC, Joner G, Bulsara MK, *et al.* (2011) Birth order and childhood type 1 diabetes risk: a pooled analysis of 31 observational studies. *International Journal of Epidemiology* **40** (2), 363–74.

Cole TJ, Bellizzi MC, Flegal KM and Dietz WH (2000) Establishing a standard definition for child overweight and obesity worldwide: international survey. *BMJ (Clinical Research Ed)* **320** (7244), 1240–3.

Ebbeling CB, Pawlak DB and Ludwig DS (2002) Childhood obesity: public health crisis, common sense cure. *Lancet* **360** (9331), 473–82.

Echouffo-Tcheugui JB, Ali MK, Griffin SJ and Narayan KMV (2011) Screening for type 2 diabetes and dysglycemia. *Epidemiologic Reviews* **33** (1), 63–87.

Fairburn CG and Harrison PJ (2003) Eating disorders. *Lancet* **361** (9355), 407–16.

Fischer-Walker CL, Ezzati M, and Black RE (2009) Global and regional child mortality and burden of disease attributable to zinc deficiency. *European Journal of Clinical Nutrition* **63** (5), 591–7.

Fontaine KR, Redden DT, Wang C, Westfall AO, *et al.* (2003) Years of life lost due to obesity. *JAMA* **289** (2), 187–93.

Garrow JS (2005) Body size and composition. In: Geissler C and Powers H (eds) *Human Nutrition and Dietetics*, 11th edn, pp. 65–82. Edinburgh: Elsevier Churchill Livingstone.

Gillett MJ (2009) International Expert Committee report on the role of the A1c assay in the diagnosis of diabetes: *Diabetes Care* **32** (7): 1327–34.

Golden MHN and Golden BE (2000) Severe malnutrition. In: Garrow JS James WPT, and Ralph A (eds) *Human Nutrition and Dietetics*, 10th edn, pp. 515–26. Edinburgh: Churchill Livingstone.

Gortmaker SL, Swinburn BA, Levy D, Carter R, *et al.* (2011) Changing the future of obesity: science, policy, and action. *Lancet* **378** (9793), 838–47.

Hagopian WA, Erlich H, Lernmark A, Rewers M, *et al.* (2011) The Environmental Determinants of Diabetes in the Young (TEDDY): genetic criteria and international diabetes risk screening of 421 000 infants. *Pediatric Diabetes* **12** (8), 733–43.

Hopkins FG (1912) Feeding experiments illustrating the importance of accessory factors in normal dietaries. *Journal of Physiology* **44** (5–6), 425–60.

Hossain P, Kawar B and El Nahas M (2007) Obesity and diabetes in the developing world—a growing challenge. *The New England Journal of Medicine* **356** (3), 213–15.

Hu FB, Li TY, Colditz, GA, Willett WC, *et al.* (2003) Television watching and other sedentary behaviors in relation to risk of obesity and type 2 diabetes mellitus in women. *JAMA* **289** (14), 1785–91.

Johner SA, Günther ALB and Remer T (2011) Current trends of 24-h urinary iodine excretion in German schoolchildren and the importance of iodised salt in processed foods. *The British Journal of Nutrition* **106** (11), 1749–56.

Kimm SYS, Glynn NW, Obarzanek E, Kriska AM, *et al.* (2005) Relation between the changes in physical activity and body-mass index during adolescence: a multicentre longitudinal study. *Lancet* **366** (9482), 301–7.

Knip M, Virtanen SM, Seppä K, Ilonen J, *et al.* (2010) Dietary intervention in infancy and later signs of beta-cell autoimmunity. *The New England Journal of Medicine* **363** (20), 1900–8.

Knip M, Virtanen SM, Becker D, Dupré J, *et al.* (2011) Early feeding and risk of type 1 diabetes: experiences from the Trial to Reduce Insulin-dependent diabetes mellitus in the Genetically at Risk (TRIGR). *The American Journal of Clinical Nutrition* **94** (6 Suppl.), 1814S–1820S.

Manson JE and Bassuk SS (2003) Obesity in the United States: a fresh look at its high toll. *JAMA: The Journal of the American Medical Association* **289** (2), 229–30.

Najjar MF and Rowland M (1987) Anthropometric reference data and prevalence of overweight, United States, 1976-80. *Vital and Health Statistics. Series 11, Data from the National Health Survey* (238), 1–73.

Neter JE, Stam BE, Kok FJ, Grobbee DE, *et al.* (2003) Influence of weight reduction on blood pressure: a meta-analysis of randomized controlled trials. *Hypertension* **42** (5), 878–84.

de Onis M and Blössner M (2003) The World Health Organization Global Database on Child Growth and Malnutrition: methodology and applications. *International Journal of Epidemiology* **32** (4), 518–26.

Patterson CC, Dahlquist GG, Gyürüs E, Green A, *et al.* (2009) Incidence trends for childhood type 1 diabetes in Europe during 1989–2003 and predicted new cases 2005-20: a multicentre prospective registration study. *Lancet* **373** (9680), 2027–33.

Perry IJ, Wannamethee SG, Walker MK, Thomson AG, *et al.* (1995) Prospective study of risk factors for development of non-insulin dependent diabetes in middle aged British men. *BMJ (Clinical Research Ed)* **310** (6979), 560–4.

Pharoah PO and Connolly KJ (1987) A controlled trial of iodinated oil for the prevention of endemic cretinism: a long-term follow-up. *International Journal of Epidemiology* **16** (1), 68–73.

Pischon T, Boeing H, Hoffmann K, Bergmann M, *et al.* (2008) General and abdominal adiposity and risk of death in Europe. *The New England Journal of Medicine* **359** (20), 2105–20.

Rasmussen T, Stene LC, Samuelsen SO, Cinek O, *et al.* (2009) Maternal BMI before pregnancy, maternal weight gain during pregnancy, and risk of persistent positivity for multiple diabetes-associated autoantibodies in children with the high-risk HLA genotype: the MIDIA study. *Diabetes Care* **32** (10), 1904–6.

Truswell AS (1999) *ABC of Nutrition*, 3rd edn. London: BMJ Books.

Tuomilehto J, Lindström J, Eriksson JG, Valle TT, *et al.* (2001) Prevention of type 2 diabetes mellitus by changes in lifestyle among subjects with impaired glucose tolerance. *The New England Journal of Medicine* **344** (18), 1343–50.

Vanderpump MPJ, Lazarus JH, Smyth PP, Laurberg P, *et al.* (2011) Iodine status of UK schoolgirls: a cross-sectional survey. *Lancet* **377** (9782), 2007–12.

Vesel L, Bahl R, Martines J, Penny M, *et al.* (2010) Use of new World Health Organization child growth standards to assess how infant malnutrition relates to breastfeeding and mortality. *Bulletin of the World Health Organization* **88** (1), 39–48.

Victora CG, Adair L, Fall C, Hallal PC, *et al.* (2008) Maternal and child undernutrition: consequences for adult health and human capital. *Lancet* **371** (9609), 340–57.

Wang Y and Lobstein T (2006) Worldwide trends in childhood overweight and obesity. *International Journal of Pediatric Obesity: IJPO* **1** (1), 11–25.

Wang YC, McPherson K, Marsh T, Gortmaker SL, *et al.* (2011) Health and economic burden of the projected obesity trends in the USA and the UK. *Lancet* **378** (9793), 815–25.

Wei J-N, Sung F-C, Li C-Y, Chang C-H, *et al.* (2003) Low birth weight and high birth weight infants are both at an increased risk to have type 2 diabetes among schoolchildren in Taiwan. *Diabetes Care* **26** (2), 343–8.

West CE, Jooste PL and Pandav CS. (2004) Iodine and iodine-deficiency disorders. *Public Health Nutrition*. Oxford: Blackwell Science.

Young TK, Martens PJ, Taback SP, Sellers EAC, *et al.* (2002) Type 2 diabetes mellitus in children: prenatal and early infancy risk factors among native Canadians. *Archives of Pediatrics & Adolescent Medicine* **156** (7), 651–5.

Zimmermann MB (2009) Iodine deficiency in pregnancy and the effects of maternal iodine supplementation on the offspring: a review. *The American Journal of Clinical Nutrition* **89** (2), 668S–72S.

Zimmet P, Alberti, KG, and Shaw J (2001) Global and societal implications of the diabetes epidemic. *Nature* **414** (6865), 782–7.

Model answers

Question 1

(a) On average, people who are ill, particularly those with terminal illness, tend to be lighter than average and hence experience a higher mortality than those who are not relatively undernourished.

(b) It is usual to exclude deaths within the first one to five years of a follow-up study to reduce the possibility that the seriously ill individuals may be responsible for this or similar phenomena.

(c) Tobacco smoking is associated with reduced appetite and smokers tend to be substantially lighter in weight than their non-smoking counterparts. Smokers are more likely to suffer from premature mortality and may contribute to the U-shape of the curve by causing increased mortality among lighter individuals. Smoking and BMI are therefore set to interact with each other in their association with mortality. However, in non-smokers a dose–response relation is evident between increasing body mass index and mortality.

Question 2

(a) Intensive insulin treatment should produce a stabilization of the high glucose peaks likely to be experienced after food in conventionally treated young diabetics. The main side effect is hypoglycaemia, which can lead to disorientation and unconsciousness. The frequency of these episodes should be compared in those intensively treated and those treated under the conventional regimens.

(b) Foreknowledge of the treatment given to the patient under examination may influence the observer's assessment of the clinical sign that is being observed.

(c) Outcome measures should be carefully standardized to reduce the possibility of observer variation and to be as accurate and reproducible as possible to reduce random variation.

(d) Albuminuria is much less frequent than microalbuminuria, which is a more sensitive test of renal function. Consequently, the power of the statistical analysis comparing the albuminuria end-point between treatments is lower. Possibly the test of the albuminuria end-point has produced a type II error (section 4.3), and in reality there is also a difference in the albuminuria end-point between treatments, but a much larger trial would be required to detect it.

(e) An attempt should be made to measure peripheral neuropathy, which is the other main complication of diabetes. Significant episodes of hypoglycaemia should

also be evaluated, hospital admissions, and in the longer term, mortality.

Question 3

(a) Rendering both the mother and the observer unaware of the treatment allocation should ensure an objective assessment of each infant's clinical status.

(b) Mortality experience in the first year of life would also be a useful measure of the overall effectiveness of this procedure.

(c) Because this trial provides good evidence that depot iodine considerably reduces the likelihood of cretinism provided that the iodine is given pre-conceptually, then it is unethical to repeat the experiment using a placebo. However, different doses of iodine or different modes of delivery could be tested in randomized controlled trials (RCTs) (a new treatment or mode of delivery is compared with the standard treatment).

10 Oral health

GERARD LINDEN, JACQUELINE JAMES, AND
IVOR CHESTNUTT

CHAPTER CONTENTS

This chapter describes the impact of oral disease in a global context and discusses how oral health is impacted by socio-economic determinants. The epidemiology, aetiology, and primary prevention of the three most common dental diseases—dental caries, periodontal disease, and mouth cancer—are described.

Introduction

Oral diseases pose a global health burden. They are a significant public health problem in high-income countries and their impact is continually increasing in low- and middle-income countries (Willliams 2011).

Dental caries (commonly known as tooth decay) is one of the most common chronic diseases worldwide. Moderate to severe periodontitis (gum disease) affects five to 20 per cent of most adult populations, accounting for major tooth loss in both developed and developing nations. Oral cancer, also termed mouth cancer, is the eighth most common cancer worldwide, and is the most common cancer in men in South East Asia.

In common with the majority of chronic non-communicable diseases, the major oral diseases are to a large degree related to lifestyles and life circumstances. Frequent consumption of sugars and lack of exposure to fluoride results in dental caries. Inadequate oral hygiene predisposes to periodontal disease, while tobacco use and heavy intake of alcohol are important causative factors in mouth cancer. The determinants of oral diseases are therefore the same as other major public health concerns such as heart disease, cancer, diabetes, and obesity. A common risk factor approach, which emphasizes changes to diet, tobacco, and alcohol consumption is therefore as applicable to the prevention of the major oral diseases as to wider health issues (Sheiham and Watt 2000).

10.1 Oral disease worldwide

In a global context, infectious diseases also impact to a marked degree on oral health. Human immunodeficiency virus (HIV) and its concomitant viral, fungal, and bacterial infections constitutes a major oral health problem. Noma, a polymicrobial opportunistic infection, affects those with compromised immune function and results in destruction of oral and facial tissues. Rare in the developed world, it is most commonly seen in malnourished children in sub-Saharan Africa. In the World Health Organization (WHO) African Region, noma occurs in 39 out of 46 countries. The annual incidence is 20 cases per 100,000 with a mortality rate of approximately 70 to 90 per cent in the absence of treatment (WHO 2011).

Major inequalities in oral health exist, both within and between countries, whether considered in terms of disease severity or prevalence. These inequalities are largely determined by social factors. The WHO recognizes that the greatest burden of oral disease lies on disadvantaged and poor populations. Oral disease impacts on individuals and communities in terms of pain, days lost from school or work either as a result of the symptoms or in seeking dental care. It impacts on nutrition, particularly in the elderly. It also affects quality of life, when individuals are unable to eat, speak, or function socially due to embarrassment caused by the appearance or condition of their teeth.

Years of research have provided detailed scientific information on the aetiology of oral diseases and knowledge on how to prevent them is good. The major issue is how to deliver such preventive knowledge, and in particular encourage preventive behaviours in groups and populations at greatest risk of disease.

In developed nations considerable resources are devoted to the provision of dental care with Germany and the UK having one dentist per 1000 people. Globally, however, access to oral care is a major problem with many low- and middle-income countries having one dentist per 50,000 people while in some sub-Saharan African countries the ratio is only one per 900,000 people.

Throughout the industrialized world, dental care has been focused on the treatment of the outcomes of dental disease, with insufficient focus on prevention. A system focused primarily on the treatment of disease in individuals, is not economically sustainable, and does nothing to narrow oral health inequalities or prevent oral disease in those at greatest risk. In a study of 18 industrialized countries, dental services were shown to explain only three per cent of the variation in caries levels in 12-year-olds, whereas broad socio-economic factors explained 65 per cent (Nadanovsky and Sheiham 1995).

Efforts to change personal behaviours, the so-called 'downstream' approach, have limited potential to improve oral health. Such approaches fail to address the wider social determinants that cause people to suffer disease. 'Upstream' actions that seek to address larger environmental issues are more likely to prevent the population or more specifically subgroups of the population from becoming ill. Thus, while encouraging people to brush their teeth with a fluoride-containing toothpaste (a 'downstream' action) is likely to have some degree of success in preventing tooth decay, those from disadvantaged communities, may not be able to afford toothpaste and a toothbrush and may not see toothbrushing as a priority in their daily activities. Legislating for and adding fluoride to the local water supply (an 'upstream' action), is likely to be more effective. Similarly, banning confectionary vending machines in schools (Wales Assembly Government 2009), is more effective than encouraging children not to eat sweets to avoid tooth decay sometime in the future.

10.2 Dental caries

Definition and aetiology of dental caries

Dental caries is a multifactorial disease process. It results in the destruction of tooth tissue due to the effect of acids produced by oral micro-organisms, following the fermentation of sugars derived from the diet. These bacteria-derived acids act to demineralize the tooth tissue and cause the release of calcium and phosphate ions. In the early stages of the disease, this is a dynamic reversible process, and remineralization of the tooth structure is possible. The loss and gain of calcium and phosphate ions at the tooth surface is moderated by a large range of oral environmental and personal factors (Table 10.1).

However, beyond a certain stage, the degree of tooth structure lost is such that a cavity forms (Fig. 10.1).

Cavity formation necessitates secondary prevention in the form of a restoration to halt the disease process. If left untreated the caries process advances and eventually the tooth pulp becomes infected, inflamed, and eventually loses vitality. The resulting necrotic tissue can lead to abscess formation, with consequent pain and suffering for the affected individual.

The flow of saliva is protective as it buffers the acids produced from the fermentation of sugars. Lack of saliva, as a result of head and neck irradiation or as a

Table 10.1. The factors involved in caries development

Factors that directly contribute to caries development	Oral environmental factors that influence caries development	Personal factors that influence caries development
Tooth	Fluoride	Socio-demographic status
Diet • Amount • Composition • Frequency	Saliva • Buffer capacity • Composition • Flow rate	Education
Bacteria in biofilm • *Streptoccoccus mutans* • *Lactobacillus* spp.	Antibacterial agents	Behaviour • Oral hygiene • Snacking • Chewing gum
Time	Dental sealants	Oral health literacy
	Plaque pH	Attitudes
	Ca^{2+}, PO_4^{3-}	Knowledge
	Sugars • Clearance rate • Frequency	Dental insurance coverage
	Protein	Income

Reproduced from Selwitz R *et al*, 'Dental caries', *Lancet* **369**, 9555 51–9, 2007, with permission from Elsevier.

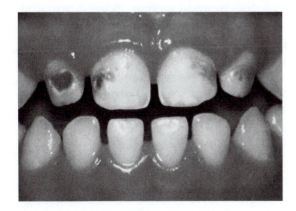

Figure 10.1 Dental caries on the labial surfaces of the upper anterior deciduous teeth.
Reproduced from Kidd et al, *Pickard's Manual of Operative Dentistry*, 8th edition, 2003, with permission from Oxford University Press.

side effect of medication or salivary gland disease (e.g. Sjögrens syndrome), can result in widespread caries lesions, particularly if patients resort to sucking sugared candies to ameliorate the effects of saliva loss.

Epidemiology of dental caries

The WHO maintains a database of caries prevalence in countries around the world (WHO 2003) and Fig. 10.2 shows the prevalence of decayed, missing or filled teeth in the WHO world regions.

In a number of developed countries, such as the UK, exposure to preventive regimens over recent decades has resulted in a reduced prevalence of dental caries, particularly in the permanent dentition and reduced tooth loss in adults. Between 1973 and 2003, the mean number of

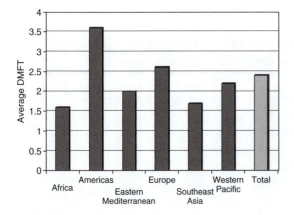

Figure 10.2 The prevalence of decayed, missing, or filled teeth in the WHO World Regions.

Reproduced from Petersen P, 'The world oral health report 2003: continuous improvement of oral health in the 21st century - the approach of the WHO global oral health programme', *Community Dentistry and Oral Epidemiology*, 2008, with permission from John Wiley and Sons.

decayed, missing, or filled teeth in 15-year-olds fell from just 8.4 in 1973 to 1.6 in 2003, whilst the proportion of adults who had lost all of their natural teeth decreased from 30 per cent in 1978 to 6 per cent in 2009.

The effect of social disadvantage on oral health is shown in Fig. 10.3. This clearly demonstrates the direct association between the mean number of decayed missing or filled teeth in Welsh five-year-olds and social and economic deprivation.

The prevention of dental caries

Dental caries can be prevented by reducing the amount and in particular the frequency of sugar consumption. The presence of sugar in the oral cavity for extended periods, as occurs when young children are fed sugared drinks in a feeding bottle, results in the maintenance of a low pH in the dental plaque biofilm, favouring demineralization of the tooth. Preventive efforts should therefore focus on encouraging both individual actions that encourage a sugar restricted diet and higher level actions such as legislation covering the advertising and marketing of sweets and carbonated drinks to children. This is in accord with general health messages aimed at the prevention of

obesity and diabetes. However, the challenges in getting the appropriate messages and desired behaviour change in those at greatest risk are the same.

Possibly the greatest advance in the battle against dental caries has been the recognition of the benefits of fluoride as a preventive agent. Fluoride works by incorporation into the tooth enamel, either during tooth development or after tooth eruption (into the mouth) as part of the remineralization process (Featherstone 2009). The substitution of a hydroxyl ion, by a fluoride ion, in the hydroxyapatite crystals that make up the tooth enamel, results in a structure that is more resistant to bacterial acid attack. In addition, the presence of fluoride ions in the plaque biofilm fluid encourages the re-uptake of calcium and phosphate ions into the tooth structure. As a result, any action that increases the bioavailability of fluoride ions in the oral cavity acts to reduce caries-risk.

The benefits of fluoride were first recognized in observational studies in the early 20th century where it was noted that individuals exposed to fluoride that was naturally present in the public water supply, had a reduced number of decayed teeth, compared with those resident in similar communities which did not have fluoride in the water. Subsequent clinical trials demonstrated the benefits of adding fluoride to the water supply at a concentration of one part per million. Fluoridation has therefore been used since the 1950s as a caries preventive measure. Its use is most widespread in the USA. In the UK about 10 per cent of the population benefit from water fluoridation, mainly in the east Midlands and the North East of England.

Throughout its history, there has been a small, but vocal minority of individuals who object to fluoridation. Adverse health effects, infringement of personal choice, mass medication, and legal arguments have been put forward by anti-fluoridationists as reasons why water supplies should not have fluoride levels adjusted. Systematic reviews have confirmed that fluoridation reduces caries prevalence as measured both by increases in the proportion of children who are caries free and by reductions in the numbers of decayed, missing, or filled teeth. The same reviews were unable to demonstrate any adverse health effects as a result of fluoridation, but did demonstrate that the prevalence of dental *fluorosis*

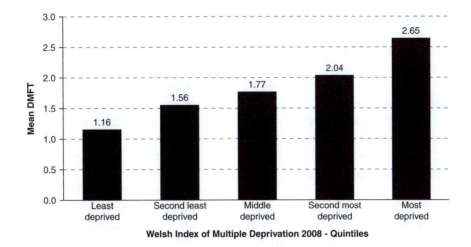

Welsh Index of Multiple Deprivation 2008 - Quintiles

Figure 10.3 Mean number of decayed missing and filled teeth in five-year-olds in Wales by quintile of social and economic deprivation.
From: Wales Oral Health Information Unit. (2003): **http://www.cardiff.ac.uk/dentl/research/themes/appliedclinicalresearch/ epidemiology/oralhealth/index.html** (author's copyright).

increases in fluoridated communities (McDonagh *et al.* 2000; NHMRC 2007).

In the absence of water fluoridation, the twice daily use of fluoridated toothpaste has been shown to be a highly effective caries prevention measure. A recent Cochrane review reported significant benefits of using fluoride toothpaste in preventing caries in children and adolescents when compared to placebo, when the concentrations of fluoride in the paste were at least 1000 ppm. It was also concluded that the relative caries preventive effects of fluoride toothpastes increase with higher fluoride concentration (Walsh *et al.* 2010). The widespread use of fluoridated toothpaste since the early 1970s is believed to have played a major role in the significant improvements in oral health in the UK since that time. Encouragement in toothbrushing should not only be the preserve of members of the dental team. All health care providers, particularly those who have contact with poor children and their families have a duty to encourage appropriate oral hygiene procedures.

Fluoride is also available in other formats such as mouthwashes for personal use or gels, varnishes, and foams for professional application. These are required only for those deemed at particular risk. Fluoride tablets and drops are no longer widely used,

as those children at greatest risk of dental caries are least likely to be given these on an ongoing basis.

10.3 Periodontal disease

Definition

The periodontium (Greek: peri, around; odontos, tooth) comprises the tissues that support the teeth and includes the gum, the periodontal ligament, and the alveolar bone. The main functions of the periodontal tissues are to attach the teeth to the bone of the jaws and to maintain the integrity of the surface of the masticatory mucosa of the mouth. Diseases of the periodontal tissues are among the most common to affect mankind.

Gingivitis represents the inflammatory response of the gum to the accumulation of dental plaque on the surface of the teeth. Those affected will often complain of bleeding gums, particularly while toothbrushing and after eating hard foods, but the condition is not usually painful. Gingivitis is a reversible disease process and removal of dental plaque and calculus (calcified plaque) will result in a return to gingival health. Gingivitis is a very common inflammatory process and is evident to some degree in virtually all adolescents at puberty. There is a reduction in the prevalence of gingivitis during teenage years before a gradual increase in adulthood.

Periodontitis is a chronic inflammatory condition which results in irreversible destruction of the periodontal ligament and the alveolar bone which supports the teeth. It is not usually painful and often does not become evident to affected individuals until they notice loosening, or a change in the position, of one or more of their teeth. Ultimately periodontitis can result in the loss of some, or all, the teeth.

There is currently no universally accepted 'gold standard' for the extent of changes in the tissues that should be present before an individual is classified as having periodontal disease. The situation is further complicated because, in individuals, different teeth may be affected to varying degrees. In the local lesion of periodontitis, as tissue damage progresses, gaps are formed between the gum tissue and the root surfaces of the teeth, termed periodontal pockets. In severe disease these pockets are several millimetres deep. There is also recession of the gum margin on to the root surface of teeth with increasing age; this complicates the assessment of periodontal disease, for example by leading to a reduction in the depth of periodontal pockets. However, where there is advanced disease the diagnosis is unequivocal. There is considerable variation between different populations with five to twenty per cent of adults suffering from periodontal disease at a level that requires some treatment.

In recent years there have been an increasing number of studies which have investigated possible associations between periodontal disease and other systemic diseases and conditions including respiratory disease, chronic renal disease, rheumatoid arthritis, Alzheimer's disease, diabetes, and premature birth. In particular there has been a strong focus on periodontitis as an independent risk factor for atherosclerosis with a possible role in coronary heart disease and stroke. These hypotheses were framed following the identification of a possible causal role for infections in the pathophysiology of other chronic diseases. Systematic reviews of studies to date support a moderate positive association between periodontal disease and atheorosclerotic vascular disease (Kebschull et al. 2010). The presence of large numbers of bacteria in the local lesions (pockets) of periodontitis

with ready access to the bloodstream underpins the possible links between oral and systemic diseases.

Hundreds of different bacterial species flourish in the oral cavity and many are present in biofilms which grow on the tooth surface (dental plaque). Because of the large number of species in dental plaque it has been difficult to identify specific bacteria which cause periodontal disease. Tissue changes which occur as periodontal disease progresses provide environmental niches which encourage the development of complex biofilms. Therefore, the identification of specific bacterial species in disease may represent an association but may not be the cause of periodontitis.

Aggressive periodontitis represents a rare type of periodontal disease, affecting less than one per cent of adolescents, in which there is rapid destruction of the tissues supporting the teeth. The bacterial species *Aggregatibacter actinomycetemcomitans* has for many years been recovered from samples taken from affected individuals. In the 1990s a specific clone of *A. actinomycetemcomitans*, the JP2 clone, was identified in some cases of aggressive periodontitis. Further investigation found that all such cases originated from North West Africa, an area with a significantly increased prevalence of aggressive periodontitis. Even when there were isolated reports of JP2 being found in sporadic cases of aggressive periodontitis worldwide, the affected individuals were always of North African descent. The JP2 clone shows a remarkably restricted host range and seems to be limited to populations whose lineage can be traced to Mediterranean Africa (Haubek et al. 2001). This provided the opportunity for a prospective population based longitudinal study aimed at testing the hypothesis that the JP2 clone of *A. actinomycetemcomitans* was a causative micro-organism for aggressive periodontitis. The researchers who had initially characterized this micro-organism studied a sample of 12-year-old schoolchildren in Rabat, Morocco. In total, 428 children who had healthy periodontal tissues at baseline presented for re-examination two years later. Children who carried the JP2 clone of *A. actinomycetemcomitans* alone at baseline had a relative risk of 18.0 (CI 7.8-41.2) of developing periodontitis (Haubek et al. 2008). The results provided important information on the temporal relationship between

A. *actinomycetemcomitans* infection and aggressive periodontitis in these adolescents. The study was the first clear demonstration that a specific bacterial species caused periodontal disease, albeit a rare form of the condition. At an individual level there was a high risk of the initiation of disease which occurred in 70 per cent of those with only the JP2 clone at baseline. At a population level the outcome explained the unusually high level of aggressive periodontitis in Moroccan adolescents.

Epidemiology

Various studies have used different clinical definitions of periodontal disease. The earliest epidemiological studies of periodontal disease in the 1950s and 1960s suggested that periodontal disease was a major global health problem with severe disease affecting most of the adult population. These studies used a scoring system known as the Periodontal Index (Russell 1956), which is now acknowledged to be flawed and to have overestimated the extent and severity of periodontal disease. Nevertheless, the early studies showed that, on a population basis, dental plaque and calculus were strongly correlated with the severity of periodontal disease. A classical longitudinal investigation of the natural history of periodontal disease was performed by Löe and his co-workers in the 1970s and 1980s. A group of Sri Lankan workers in two tea plantations was examined over a 15-year period between 1970 and 1985 (Löe *et al.* 1986). Three subpopulations were identified: a small high-risk group (eight per cent) with rapid progression of periodontal disease who had lost virtually all their teeth by the age of 45 years; a large group (81 per cent) with moderate progression, who had lost on average seven teeth by the age of 45 years; and a group (11 per cent) with no progression beyond gingivitis and no tooth loss. All these individuals were free from dental decay and had no dental treatment; therefore, it was argued that tooth loss was due to terminal periodontal disease. This study provided a significant contribution to our understanding of the natural history of periodontal disease in man. It was acknowledged that this represented a unique population

without dental intervention and, therefore, was very different from the situation in developed countries. However, the finding that sizeable variations in the progression of periodontal disease occurred in these circumstances was important. The concept of the existence of a high-risk group for severe periodontitis has been generally accepted.

There is an increase in the severity and extent of periodontal disease with increasing age. In the third National Health and Nutrition Examination Survey (NHANES III) in the USA, 13 per cent of those aged 30 years or older had moderate or severe periodontal disease (Albandar *et al.* 1999) rising to 68 per cent of those aged 65 years or over. Males had a higher prevalence of periodontal disease than females regardless of age; this has been confirmed in other studies worldwide. There were racial differences in disease; for example, in NHANES III non-Hispanic black participants had the highest, and the non-Hispanic white participants the lowest, prevalence. It is not clear whether this represents a true difference in susceptibility or is related to other factors that could promote the disease, such as poorer education, nutrition, and socio-economic circumstances. There is general agreement that smoking is the principal environmental risk factor for periodontitis and it has been shown that over 50 per cent of all periodontitis can be attributed to cigarette smoking (Tomar and Asma 2000). Other risk factors include nutritional deficiency, drug complications, psychological stress, acquired immune defects, and acquired endocrine diseases and disturbances.

Cross-sectional epidemiological studies of periodontal disease in the UK have been performed as integral parts of the national surveys of adult dental health which occur at ten-year intervals. In 2009, in the fifth Adult Dental Survey, 6500 adults had a dental examination completed in their home (UKADHS 2009). Periodontitis was widespread in the UK population and low grade, slowly destructive, periodontal disease was the norm. Only 17 per cent of dentate adults had very healthy periodontal tissues. The prevalence of at least mild disease increased with age from 19 per cent of 16 to 24-year-olds to 61 per cent of adults aged 75 to 84. Compared with the previous survey completed in 1998 there was reduction in mild disease but an increase in the prevalence of moderate and severe disease to nine per cent from six per cent in 1998.

The extent of periodontal disease is affected by the pattern of loss or retention of teeth; with the extraction of periodontally involved teeth the periodontal condition, as measured by any index, will improve. More people are retaining more teeth into later life. In the UK there has been a decrease in the proportion of the population who had no teeth from 37 per cent in 1968 to 13 per cent in 1998 with a further fall to six per cent in 2009. This improvement is expected to continue with only four per cent projected to have no teeth in 2028 (Steele *et al.* 2000). In future years, therefore, more teeth will be placed at risk of developing periodontitis and this, coupled with increased numbers of older people in society, is likely to lead to higher levels of periodontal disease and an increasing treatment burden. This probably explains the increase in the prevalence of severe periodontal disease identified in the 2009 UK Adult Dental Health Survey.

Prevention of periodontal disease

Periodontal disease consists of two major diseases: (1) gingivitis and (2) periodontitis, in which there is destruction of the periodontal ligament and supporting bone. Whereas gingivitis is very common, and can be easily prevented, periodontitis which results in irreversible changes to the supporting structures of the teeth affects 10 per cent of the adult dentate population in the UK (Kelly *et al.* 2000). The prevention of periodontitis through screening programmes is difficult because the natural history of the disease is poorly understood. Although gingivitis is probably the natural precursor of periodontitis, the evidence remains inconclusive. Davies *et al.* (2003) suggest that people must be assisted:

> **to maintain a level of plaque control which ensures that the rate of tissue destruction is reduced sufficiently to ensure . . . a comfortable and functional dentition.**

Equity in access to preventive dental care is required to help reduce the future population burden of periodontal disease. The cornerstone of primary prevention of periodontal disease is the provision and acquisition of oral hygiene skills. Regular toothbrushing is recommended to remove plaque. Dental floss or inter-dental brushes should be used on a daily basis to remove plaque from between the teeth. Toothpastes containing 'chemical plaque-suppressing agents' such as triclosan and zinc citrate and antimicrobial mouthwashes may also be useful. Smoking is a major environmental risk factor for periodontitis and efforts should be made to prevent young people from starting to smoke and to support smokers to quit the habit.

10.4 Oral cancer

Definition

Oral cancers are predominantly squamous cell carcinomas occurring at most sites in the mouth, including the lip, tongue, or any mucosal surface. Pharyngeal and laryngeal cancers may also present in dental practice. A squamous cell carcinoma may be seen with the typical appearance of an ulcerated mass with raised, rolled, everted edges, and an indurated base, or a non-healing ulcer; but, in the early stages, it may also present as a swelling or as a red or white patch(es). The latter are termed leukoplakia and are well-established as precursors of oral cancer, particularly of the tongue and cheeks.

Epidemiology

Oral cancer is one of the ten commonest cancers and is a major health problem in many parts of the world. On the Indian subcontinent, and in other parts of Asia, it remains one of the most common forms of cancer, particularly in men. In the UK, oral cancer constitutes one to four per cent of all malignant tumours, and approximately 3500 individuals are diagnosed each year with the disease. It is more common in men and this seems to be independent of tobacco use.

Oral squamous-cell carcinomas metastasize early to regional lymph nodes in the neck. Detection of early, localized lesions has not improved significantly during the past three decades and, despite the ease with which the oral cavity can be examined, it is disappointing to note that the death rate for oral cancers is comparable to that for the cervix (Sasieni *et al.* 1995).

In recent years there has been no marked improvement in the five-year survival rates, particularly for those with metastases, which remain steady at about 50 per cent.

However, in those cases that have been successfully treated, there seems to be an increase in second primary tumours. It has been estimated that 20 years from the time of the first head and neck cancer, which include oral cancers, approximately 30 per cent of male patients and 20 per cent of female patients will have developed a second primary (Warnakulasuriya *et al.* 2003). Furthermore, the relative risk for multiple primary cancer is higher in younger subjects.

Risk factors

Tobacco and alcohol

The major risk factors for oral cancer are tobacco use and alcohol consumption (Macfarlane *et al.* 1995). Most individuals who develop oral cancer smoke cigarettes, but smoking cigars, pipes, and using smokeless tobacco also poses significant risks (Rodu and Jansson 2004). As shown in Chapter 8, the relative risk for laryngopharyngeal cancers of smoking 25 cigarettes a day or more in British doctors recruited into a cohort study in the 1950s was 48, with an attributable risk of 98 per cent (see Table 8.2).

It is difficult to find evidence that alcohol is an independent risk factor for oral cancer as heavy users of alcohol also tend to be heavy smokers, and may have a poor diet. Among heavy drinkers, self-reported drinking levels may be unreliable, which may contribute to under-estimation. There is a synergistic effect between smoking and alcohol which substantially increases the risk. For people who habitually smoke and drink, it has been estimated that their relative risk of oral cancer may be 30 times greater than that for non-smokers who drink occasionally (Boffetta and Hashibe 2006). Other tobacco habits such as reverse smoking, seen in some developing countries (the lit end of a cigarette—usually hand rolled—smoked from inside the mouth), and the common practice for both sexes in Asian communities of chewing tobacco in 'betel nut quid', 'paan', or 'ghukta' significantly increases the risk of oral cancer (Balaram *et al.* 2002).

Nutrition

Diet also influences incidence rates of oral cancer. A diet that is poor in fresh fruit and vegetables may account for 10 to 15 per cent of cases of oral cancer in Europe (Edefonti *et al.* 2010). Evidence is mainly from case-control studies, but is inconsistent; the evidence generally supports the view that fruit and vegetable consumption protects against oral cancer, but individual foods that appear protective in some studies are not in others. The effects of diet appear to be modest when compared with those of smoking and alcohol consumption.

Infection

Human papillomavirus (HPV), a sexually transmitted virus, is established as a necessary cause for more than 95 per cent of cervical carcinomas; however, its association with squamous cell carcinoma in the oral cavity is less well established. Early studies revealed the presence of HPV in a significant number of normal mucosal samples as well as cases of oral cancer, indicating that the virus may not be causal. However, HPV has been identified in 15 per cent of oral cancer cases compared with less than five per cent of controls; and it has also been shown that the risk of oral cancer associated with HPV infection is independent of tobacco and alcohol use. Recent studies have shown that oropharyngeal cancer is highly associated with 'high risk' HPVs, particularly HPV 16, however, this is only associated with a minority of oral cavity cancers (Hennessey *et al.* 2009).

Age

Oral cancer increases with age and those most affected are men in their sixth or seventh decade. Despite overall reductions for oral cancer in England and Wales during the 20th century, significant increases in mortality and incidence have occurred in younger males during the past 30 years, possibly because of increased alcohol consumption, although some cases have never smoked or consumed alcohol. Recent work suggests that although oral cancer incidence continues to rise alarmingly, these increases have not been translated into higher mortality rates. This may indicate a changing natural history of oral cancers or a lower case-fatality rate due to improved treatments (Robinson and Macfarlane 2003). It may also reflect in part a rise in oropharyngeal cancer, specifically of the tonsillar regions, in young men associated with HPV 16 infection (Marur *et al.* 2010).

Lip cancer

Lip cancer is a form of oral cancer with a distinctive global epidemiology, which supports the idea that the lip should be considered as a distinct cancer site rather than its inclusion with other forms of oral cancer. High rates of lip cancer in men (between 12.0 and 13.5 new cancers per 100,000 per annum) are reported for regions of Europe, North America, and Oceania whereas it is virtually unknown in much of Asia. Factors important in the aetiology of lip cancer include solar radiation, tobacco smoking, and viruses. Incidence rates of lip cancer are generally stable or falling among males worldwide; however, they are rising in many female populations (Moore *et al.* 1999).

Health promotion and prevention

Screening for oral cancer by visual examination is simple, inexpensive, and causes little discomfort, although there is insufficient evidence to recommend population screening for oral cancer in the UK (Rodrigues *et al.* 1998). Measures aimed at primary prevention of the disease may be a more feasible form of disease control at present, although opportunistic screening is routinely conducted in dental practice.

Efforts designed to encourage smoking cessation in conjunction with programmes to discourage children from starting smoking could have a major impact in the future. There is a need also to provide information to people about the causes of oral cancer, as knowledge of risk factors is low. A lack of awareness of the signs and symptoms of oral cancer has been shown to be a factor in people who do not present early. Patient information leaflets have been shown to reduce patient anxiety while improving knowledge and willingness to be examined. The results from one randomized controlled trial suggest that people who benefit most from such campaigns are those at higher risk, especially smokers; smokers were 16 times more likely to believe that they are at risk from oral cancer (Humphris *et al.* 2004).

Smoking cessation is clearly an essential part of oral cancer prevention and people should be encouraged to adopt a healthier lifestyle with less alcohol, to increase their intake of fresh fruit and vegetables, and to attend for regular dental check-ups.

This chapter has reviewed the epidemiology and prevention of oral disease and suggests that many opportunities exist for further prevention in clinical and public health dental practice. One priority may be to improve the evidence-base for these purposes in parallel with those that have occurred in medical practice.

Further reading

Levine RS and Stillman-Lowe CR (2004) *The Scientific Basis of Oral Health Education*. London: BDJ Books.

World Health Organization (2003) *Diet, Nutrition and the Prevention of Chronic Diseases*. Geneva: World Health Organization.

References

Albandar JM, Brunelle JA and Kingman A (1999) Destructive periodontal disease in adults 30 years of age and older in the United States, 1988, 1994. *Journal of Periodontology* **70** (1), 13–29.

Balaram P, Sridhar H, Rajkumar T, Vaccarella S, *et al.* (2002) Oral cancer in southern India: the influence of smoking, drinking, paan-chewing and oral hygiene. *International Journal of Cancer* **98** (3), 440–5.

Boffetta P and Hashibe M (2006) Alcohol and cancer. *The Lancet Oncology* **7** (2), 149–56.

Davies RM, Davies GM, and Ellwood RP (2003) Prevention. Part 4: Toothbrushing: what advice should be given to patients? *British Dental Journal* **195** (3), 135–41.

Edefonti V, Bravi F, La Vecchia C, Randi G, *et al.* (2010) Nutrient-based dietary patterns and the risk of oral and pharyngeal cancer. *Oral Oncology* **46** (5), 343–8.

Featherstone JDB (2009) Remineralization, the natural caries repair process—the need for new approaches. *Advances in Dental Research* **21** (1), 4–7.

Haubek D, Ennibi OK, Poulsen K, Poulsen S, *et al.* (2001) Early-onset periodontitis in Morocco is associated with the highly leukotoxic clone of Actinobacillus actino-mycetemcomitans. *Journal of Dental Research* **80** (6), 1580–3.

Haubek D, Ennibi O-K, Poulsen K, Vaeth M, *et al.* (2008) Risk of aggressive periodontitis in adolescent carriers of the JP2 clone of Aggregatibacter (Actinobacillus) actinomycetemcomitans in Morocco: a prospective longitudinal cohort study. *Lancet* 371 (9608), 237–42.

Hennessey PT, Westra WH, and Califano JA (2009) Human papillomavirus and head and neck squamous cell carcinoma: recent evidence and clinical implications. *Journal of Dental Research* **88** (4), 300–6.

Humphris GM, Freeman R, and Clarke HMM (2004) Risk perception of oral cancer in smokers attending primary care: a randomised controlled trial. *Oral Oncology* **40** (9), 916–24.

Kelly M, Steele J, Nuttall N, *et al.* (2000) Adult dental health survey. *Oral health in the United Kingdom*. London. HMSO 1998.

Kebschull M, Demmer RT, and Papapanou PN (2010) 'Gum bug, leave my heart alone!'—epidemiologic and mechanistic evidence linking periodontal infections and atherosclerosis. *Journal of Dental Research* **89** (9), 879–902.

Löe H, Anerud A, Boysen H, and Morrison E (1986) Natural history of periodontal disease in man. Rapid, moderate and no loss of attachment in Sri Lankan laborers 14 to 46 years of age. *Journal of Clinical Periodontology* **13** (5), 431–45.

McDonagh MS, Whiting PF, Wilson PM, Sutton AJ, *et al.* (2000) Systematic review of water fluoridation. *BMJ (Clinical Research Ed)* **321** (7265), 855–9.

Macfarlane GJ, Zheng T, Marshall JR, Boffetta P, *et al.* (1995) Alcohol, tobacco, diet and the risk of oral cancer: a pooled analysis of three case-control studies. *European Journal of Cancer. Part B, Oral Oncology* **31B** (3), 181–7.

Marur S, D'Souza G, Westra WH, and Forastiere AA (2010) HPV-associated head and neck cancer: a virus-related cancer epidemic. *The Lancet Oncology* **11** (8), 781–9.

Moore S, Johnson N, Pierce A, and Wilson D (1999) The epidemiology of lip cancer: a review of global incidence and aetiology. *Oral Diseases* **5** (3), 185–95.

Nadanovsky P and Sheiham A (1995) Relative contribution of dental services to the changes in caries levels of 12-year-old children in 18 industrialized countries in the 1970s and early 1980s. *Community Dentistry and Oral Epidemiology* **23** (6), 331–9.

NHMRC—National Health and Medical Research Council (2007) *A Systematic Review of the Efficacy and Safety of Fluoridation*. Canberra: Government of Australia.

Petersen PE (2009) Global policy for improvement of oral health in the 21st century—implications to oral health research of World Health Assembly 2007, World Health Organization. *Community Dentistry and Oral Epidemiology* **37** (1), 1–8.

Robinson KL and Macfarlane GJ (2003) Oropharyngeal cancer incidence and mortality in Scotland: are rates still increasing? *Oral Oncology* **39** (1), 31–6.

Rodrigues VC, Moss SM, and Tuomainen H (1998) Oral cancer in the UK: to screen or not to screen. *Oral Oncology* **34** (6), 454–65.

Rodu B and Jansson C (2004) Smokeless tobacco and oral cancer: a review of the risks and determinants. *Critical Reviews in Oral Biology and Medicine* **15** (5), 252–63.

Russell AL (1956) A system of classification and scoring for prevalence surveys of periodontal disease. *Journal of Dental Research* **35** (3), 350–9.

Sasieni P, Cuzick J, and Farmery E (1995) Accelerated decline in cervical cancer mortality in England and Wales. *Lancet* **346** (8989), 1566–7.

Selwitz RH, Ismail AI, and Pitts NB (2007) Dental caries. *Lancet* **369** (9555), 51–9.

Sheiham A and Watt RG (2000) The common risk factor approach: a rational basis for promoting oral health. *Community Dentistry and Oral Epidemiology* **28** (6), 399–406.

Steele JG, Treasure E, Pitts NB, Morris J, *et al.* (2000) Total tooth loss in the United Kingdom in 1998 and implications for the future. *British Dental Journal* **189** (11), 598–603.

Tomar SL and Asma S (2000) Smoking-attributable periodontitis in the United States: findings from NHANES III. National Health and Nutrition Examination Survey. *Journal of Periodontology* **71** (5), 743–51.

United Kingdom Adult Dental Health Survey (2009) Summary results. http://www.ic.nhs.uk/statistics-and-data-collections/primary-care/dentistry/adult-dental-health-survey-2009--summary-report-and-thematic-series.

Wales Assembly Government (2009) Hospital vending machines to dispense their last choc bar. http://www.wales.nhs.uk/documents/W080302-Hlt.pdf.

Wales Oral Health Information Unit. (2003) http://www.cardiff.ac.uk/dentl/research/themes/appliedclinical-research/epidemiology/oralhealth/index.html

Walsh T, Worthington HV, Glenny A-M, Appelbe P, *et al.* (2010) Fluoride toothpastes of different concentrations for preventing dental caries in children and adolescents. *Cochrane Database of Systematic Reviews* 1, CD007868.

Warnakulasuriya KAAS, Robinson D, and Evans H (2003) Multiple primary tumours following head and neck cancer in southern England during 1961–98. *Journal of Oral Pathology & Medicine* 32 (8), 443–9.

Williams DM (2011) Global oral health inequalities: the research agenda. *Journal of Dental Research* 90 (5), 549–51.

World Health Organization (2003) *The World Oral Health Report 2003*. Geneva: World Health Organization. http://www.who.int/oral_health/media/en/orh_report03_en.pdf.

World Health Organization (2011) Regional Office for Africa. http://www.afro.who.int/en/clusters-a-programmes/dpc/non-communicable-diseases-managementndm/programme-components/oral-health.html.

11 Digestive system

SHIVARAM BHAT, BRIAN JOHNSTON, AND LIAM MURRAY

CHAPTER CONTENTS

This chapter discusses one of the medical complications of alcohol abuse, liver cirrhosis, and dyspepsia, one of the commonest gastrointestinal problems presenting in primary care, together with diseases associated with **Helicobacter pylori** infection. Finally, diseases mainly of the large bowel, including inflammatory bowel disease and colorectal cancer, are discussed.

Introduction

It is beyond the scope of this textbook to discuss the epidemiology of all chronic gastrointestinal diseases. Instead, several important topics have been chosen, which include liver cirrhosis, usually associated with excessive alcohol intake and of growing concern in some high-income countries, and dyspepsia, because of the substantial health costs associated with this group of symptoms. *Helicobacter pylori* is the most common bacterial infection known to man, and its association with diseases has only recently become known through epidemiological and clinical studies. The inflammatory bowel diseases ulcerative colitis and Crohn's disease are discussed as examples of disorders that are pathologically distinct, but sometimes difficult to distinguish clinically, and whose causes are largely unknown. The epidemiology of colorectal cancer, as the major alimentary cancer, will be reviewed. Basic immunological, epidemiological, and genetic research will be required for progress to be made in the understanding, treatment, and prevention of these disorders.

11.1 Cirrhosis of the liver

Cirrhosis is the end result of long-term liver damage. It results from the necrosis of liver cells and is characterized by formation of fibrous tissue, nodules, and scarring, which interfere with liver blood flow and liver cell function. Cirrhosis may lead to chronic liver failure and death. Some causes of cirrhosis are listed in Table 11.1.

Alcohol and hepatitis C infection are the most common causes of cirrhosis in the UK but hepatitis B is the most common cause worldwide. Liver cirrhosis was estimated to account for over 800,000 deaths worldwide in 2004 (WHO 2011b). In most of the developed world mortality from cirrhosis has remained relatively stable or fallen, but in the UK cirrhosis-related mortality has steadily increased over the past few decades, especially among middle-aged males (Bosetti *et al.* 2007). Binge drinking and drug use, with a risk of hepatitis, have been proposed to account for this.

Mortality data from the West Midlands for the 1990s suggested that the upward trend in cirrhosis mortality during this period resulted almost entirely from

Table 11.1 Some causes of cirrhosis

Common causes	Other causes
Alcohol toxicity	Biliary cirrhosis (primary or secondary)
Chronic hepatitis due to:	Autoimmune hepatitis
Hepatitis C	Drugs, for example, methotrexate
Hepatitis B	Non-alcoholic steatohepatitis (NASH)
	Chronic heart failure
	Haemachromatosis
	Wilson's disease
	Alpha-1-antitrypsin deficiency
	Glycogen storage disease
	Idiopathic (cryptogenic)

a threefold increase in alcoholic liver disease (Fisher *et al.* 2002). Rates of increase in deaths from alcoholic liver disease were similar for men and women. A well-conducted case-control study in France found that women who drank heavily were more at risk of cirrhosis than men, and that they also developed cirrhosis at an earlier age (Tuyns and Pequingnot 1984). There is also a genetic difference between the sexes in the levels of the enzyme alcohol dehydrogenase. This has implications for current and future trends in cirrhosis among women, as heavy drinking is increasing at a faster rate among women than men. In the UK there has been an overall increase in average weekly consumption in both men and women, although the increase is more marked in women (Smith and Foxcroft 2009). The pattern of alcohol consumption is very different among middle-aged men from France and Northern Ireland; most men from France tend to drink regular amounts each day in contrast to the smaller overall proportion of drinkers in Northern Ireland who tend to drink large amounts at weekends (Ruidavets *et al.* 2010). In younger adults trends may be tending to converge in Europe.

Hepatitis C is the second most common cause of cirrhosis in the UK. Around 216,000 people in the UK are thought to be chronically infected by hepatitis C (Health Protection Agency 2011). Many of these people are unaware that they have the infection and will have a normal lifespan. However, in about 20 per cent, persistent chronic hepatitis will lead to the development of cirrhosis over 20 to 30 years. Consumption of alcohol is an important determinant of progression of hepatitis C infection to cirrhosis; high consumption of alcohol appears to confer more than a 10-fold increased risk of cirrhosis among infected persons.

Prevention of cirrhosis in the UK hinges on several separate strategies: tackling excessive alcohol consumption, especially among young people; reducing intravenous drug abuse; ensuring the safety of blood products; and instigating treatment to reduce the progression to cirrhosis among people infected with viral hepatitis. This disorder represents a considerable challenge to current and future clinical and public health practitioners if trends are to be reversed (Fig. 11.1).

11.2 Dyspepsia

The term 'dyspepsia' covers a variety of symptoms affecting the upper gastrointestinal tract which include: epigastric pain or discomfort, heartburn, acid regurgitation, excessive burping or belching, a feeling of slow

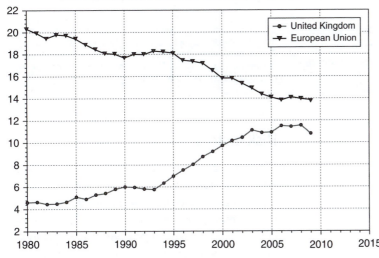

SDR*, chronic liver disease and cirrhosis, all ages per 100000

Figure 11.1 Trends in deaths from cirrhosis of the liver in the European Region and in the UK.

Data from Health for All Database (WHO 2011a)

*Standardized death rate.

digestion, early satiety, nausea, and bloating. Standardization of the definition of dyspepsia has proven difficult, as there is considerable variation in the symptom pattern between patients. The UK National Institute for Health and Clinical Excellence (NICE) includes heartburn and acid regurgitation in its spectrum of dyspepsia symptoms (NICE 2004). However, the American Gastroenterology association specifically excludes patients with predominant heartburn from the definition of dyspepsia; these patients are considered to have gastro-oesophageal reflux disease (Talley 2005).

Causes of dyspepsia

The most common underlying conditions in patients presenting with dyspeptic symptoms in primary care are oesophagitis (15 per cent), gastric (four per cent) or duodenal ulceration (nine per cent), gallstone disease (two per cent), and malignancy (two per cent). However, more than 50 per cent of patients have no underlying pathology and are considered to have functional dyspepsia. This proportion may vary between countries, and increase over time as the incidence of pathology associated with H. pylori (peptic ulceration and gastric cancer) decreases. Prospective studies following patients with functional dyspepsia show that

the symptoms improve or remit in 30–70 per cent of cases. Patients who have had symptoms for more than two years, have lower educational attainment, higher psychological vulnerability scores, or are infected with H. pylori, are less likely to experience remission of symptoms.

Prevalence

Population-based studies of dyspepsia in developed countries have shown substantial variation in the reported prevalence of dyspeptic symptoms, ranging from 13 per cent to 48 per cent of adults (NICE 2004). This could reflect major differences in the occurrence of these symptoms, but probably results from the use of different definitions of dyspepsia, and the evaluation of the symptoms in differing age-groups or time periods. The utility of these data is therefore questionable, highlighting the importance in epidemiological research of using standardized, internationally agreed definitions of diseases, syndromes, or symptom complexes (see Chapter 2). The Domestic/International Gastroenterology Surveillance Study (DIGEST) (Stanghellini 1999) examined the three month prevalence of upper gastrointestinal symptoms (Box 11.1) in random population samples from 10 countries using, as far as possible, the same

Box 11.1 Upper GI symptoms investigated in the DIGEST Study

Postprandial fullness, early satiety, localized epigastric pain, diffuse epigastric pain, heartburn, regurgitation, belching, nocturnal/fasting pain, abdominal distension.

Source: Stanghellini V (1999). 'Three-Month Prevalence Rates of Gastrointestinal Symptoms and the Influence of Demographic Factors: Results from the Domestic/International Gastroenterology Surveillance Study (DIGEST)'. *Scandinavian Journal of Gastroenterology, Supplement* **231**, 20–8.

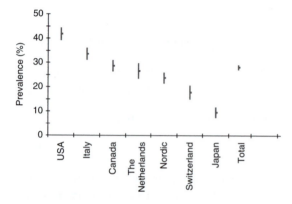

Figure 11.2 Three-month prevalence (95% CI) of moderate/severe upper GI symptoms among 5581 DIGEST respondents, by country or region.
Source: Stanghellini (1999) 'Three-Month Prevalence Rates of Gastrointestinal Symptoms and The Influence of Demographic Factors: Results from the Domestic/International Gastroenterology Surveillance Study (DIGEST)'. *Scandinavian Journal of Gastroenterology, Supplement* **231**, 20–8.

methods. Symptoms were considered clinically significant if they were moderate in intensity and occurred at least once a week (Fig. 11.2).

This study confirmed a high overall prevalence of these symptoms: 28.1 per cent of the subjects studied reported having symptoms in the three months before interview. However, symptom prevalence differed between the countries, ranging from 9.4 per cent in Japan to 41.8 per cent in the USA (Stanghellini 1999). These country-specific differences in the prevalence of dyspepsia are less likely to be artefactual than estimates from previous studies, although slight differences in methodology and response rates between countries may contribute to part of the differences seen. The incidence of dyspepsia is more difficult to assess as symptoms are relapsing and remittent in most subjects.

Risk factors

Dyspepsia does not appear to have a clear association with age. Population-based epidemiological studies have found the peak age for dyspepsia varies by country and underlying cause (ulcer-related or functional dyspepsia) (Mahadeva and Goh 2006). In a UK population the prevalence of ulcer dyspepsia was found to decrease with advanced age (Jones *et al.* 1990); in contrast, a study in an Indian population found that dyspepsia was more common in subjects over the age of 40 years (Shah *et al.* 2001). Variation has also been observed when examining gender associations and dyspepsia; in most studies functional dyspepsia has a female preponderance, whereas ulcer dyspepsia appears to have an equal sex distribution. Few studies have examined differences in the prevalence of dyspepsia based on ethnicity. A study examining a US population found that ulcer dyspepsia was more common in a black American population (Shaib and El-Serag 2004). Smoking has been shown to be a risk factor for ulcer dyspepsia but not conclusively linked with functional dyspepsia. Alcohol has not been linked with dyspepsia regardless of underlying cause. Psychological factors play an important role both in reporting dyspeptic symptoms and seeking medical attention for these symptoms. Obese people are approximately three times more likely to suffer from heartburn and regurgitation (Murray *et al.* 2003), but being overweight is less clearly related to other dyspeptic symptoms. There is a link between some medications and dyspepsia. A meta-analysis of randomized controlled trials has confirmed that users of non-steroidal anti-inflammatory drugs (NSAIDs) are three times more likely to experience dyspepsia than non-users. NSAIDs and aspirin are known risk factors for peptic ulcer disease. The relation between infection with *H. pylori* and dyspepsia is discussed later in this chapter.

Time trends

The interpretation of trends in dyspepsia is difficult for reasons related to the problems of definition, and because of a paucity of population-based studies before the 1980s. It is clear though, that dyspeptic symptoms have been very common for many years in people living in high income countries. Indeed, milk of magnesia was invented as a treatment for dyspepsia by Sir James Murray in Belfast in 1812. However, it is unclear whether dyspeptic symptoms in general, or subgroups of symptoms, have become more common. The incidence of oesophageal adeno-carcinoma has increased markedly in high-income countries since the 1970s (Vial *et al.* 2010).Gastro-oesophageal reflux is a risk factor for this cancer, and reflux disease has been increasingly diagnosed in recent decades. Greater use of endoscopy has contributed to the trend in diagnosis of reflux oesophagitis, and data are not available to confirm whether this reflects an increase in heartburn and regurgitation in the general population.

Costs associated with dyspepsia

Although only one in four patients with dyspepsia consults a physician, dyspepsia accounts for three to four per cent of general practitioner consultations and between 20 and 40 per cent of all gastrointestinal consultations. Symptom severity, fear of serious disease, and family history of gastrointestinal malignancy influence the decision to consult a medical practitioner, but psychosocial factors such as anxiety, depression, and lack of family/social support are also important. Proton pump inhibitors such as omeprazole are the most common medications prescribed to treat dyspepsia. The cost of these drugs has fallen in recent years but the costs of prescribing for dyspepsia remain high due to increased prescribing for dyspepsia and the chronic nature of the condition in the majority of patients. Medication costs form only part of the UK National Health Service (NHS) costs of dyspepsia and, because

so many patients manage dyspepsia without medical intervention, the true cost of dyspepsia to the community is much greater. The non-NHS costs of dyspepsia (over-the-counter treatments and time off work) have been estimated at £21 per person per year in the UK, totalling in excess of £1 billion, with the total NHS costs (consultations, investigations, and medication) estimated at £500 million.

11.3 *Helicobacter pylori*

Helicobacter pylori is a Gram-negative spiral bacterium that infects human gastric mucosa. Approximately 50 per cent of the world's population is infected by *H. pylori*, making it the commonest chronic infection worldwide. However, infection rates vary substantially according to geographic region (see Fig. 11.3) age, and birth cohort (Helicobacter Foundation 2006).

In low- and middle-income countries, *H. pylori* is largely acquired in childhood and is almost universally present in adults. By contrast, the rate of childhood acquisition is much lower in high-income countries (Fig. 11.4) and increases gradually by approximately one per cent per year into adulthood (Lehours and Yilmaz 2007). The prevalence of infection declines with subsequent birth cohorts: in a study of *H. pylori* prevalence in Russian children, the overall prevalence declined from 44 per cent in 1995 to 13 per cent in 2005. Similar downward trends in the prevalence of *H. pylori* have been observed in both the developing and the developed world and can probably be attributed to improved sanitation and living conditions (for example, less overcrowding), which reduces the risk of infection during childhood.

Aetiology/risk factors

Helicobacter pylori infection is believed to be spread from human to human by the faeco-oral route, and, in some countries, spread may also be by contaminated water. The prevalence of infection increases with age but this mainly reflects a declining prevalence with successive birth cohorts (the birth cohort effect). There is no clear sex difference in the prevalence of infection.

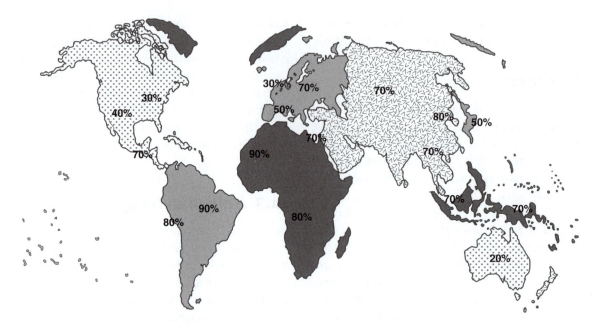

Figure 11.3 Prevalence of *Helicobacter pylori* infection by world region.
Source: Helicobacter Foundation (2006).

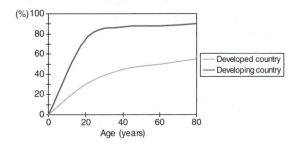

Figure 11.4 Prevalence of *Helicobacter pylori* infection according to age of population in developed and developing countries.
Adapted from Pounder RE and Ng D (1995). 'The Prevalence of Helicobacter Pylori Infection in Different Countries'. *Alimentary Pharmacology and Therapeutics* **9**, 33–9, with permission from John Wiley and Sons.

In the USA, Hispanics and African-Americans are three to four times more likely to be infected than white people. Low socio-economic status and poor living conditions during childhood are the most important risk factors for infection (Go 2002).

Clinical significance

Although it had been known for more than 100 years that spiral organisms existed in the human stomach,

their importance only became apparent in the early 1980s through the pioneering work of Warren and Marshall (Marshall and Warren 1984). Not only were they able to identify and culture the organism, Marshall also ingested the organism, giving himself acute gastroenteritis. At gastroscopy, gastritis was seen and the organism was re-isolated from biopsies of his stomach. This experiment fulfilled Koch's postulates (see Chapter 1) indicating that *H. pylori* causes acute gastritis. Marshall and Warren were eventually awarded the Nobel Prize in Physiology or Medicine for their work on *H. pylori*. It has since been shown that infection with the organism causes chronic gastritis that may progress to gastric atrophy.

Duodenal and gastric ulceration

There is strong evidence that infection with *H. pylori* is an important causative agent in peptic ulceration that is unrelated to the use of aspirin or NSAIDs. *Helicobacter pylori* infection can be diagnosed in 90–100 per cent of patients with duodenal ulcers and in 60–100 per cent of patients with gastric ulcers; infected individuals have an estimated lifetime risk of 10–20 per cent for the development of peptic ulcer disease, which is at least three- to fourfold higher than in uninfected subjects. Nested case-control studies have confirmed that infection precedes ulceration. In a Hawaiian study, individuals who were seropositive in blood samples collected during the 1960s were four times more likely to develop a duodenal ulcer over the next 20 years than subjects who were seronegative. Experimental studies have also shown that *H. pylori* eradication cures peptic ulceration (not caused by NSAIDs) and prevents its recurrence. Antibiotic resistance in *H. pylori* is common, and treatment usually involves triple or quadruple multidrug regimens. These consist of a proton pump inhibitor and a combination of antibiotics, achieving 90–95 per cent eradication in most studies. Risk of reinfection following successful eradication is low in high-income countries, estimated at three per cent per year. In low- and middle-income countries, however, risk of reinfection is much greater, at nine per cent per year (Gisbert 2005). Clearly, many people with *H. pylori* infection do not develop peptic ulceration, and, although it may be a *necessary* cause, it is not a *sufficient* cause (see Chapter 1) for ulceration, in common with most environmental risk factors for chronic diseases. Other factors such as genetic susceptibility or environmental/lifestyle factors, such as smoking, interact with *H. pylori* infection to cause peptic ulceration.

Helicobacter pylori is also an important risk factor for gastric adenocarcinoma and gastric lymphoma. The link between *H. pylori* and gastric cancer is so important that the International Agency for Research on Cancer (IARC), identified *H. pylori* as a 'group 1 (definite carcinogen)' in 1994. Its role as an important carcinogen may explain the higher incidence of gastric cancer observed in developing countries; 70 per cent of gastric cancer cases worldwide occur in the developing world (Ferlay *et al.* 2010). Other factors are clearly important in the pathogenesis of gastric cancer, as all patients with *H. pylori* do not develop cancer. It is thought that lifestyle factors, such as tobacco and alcohol, may act together with *H. pylori* (Perez-Perez *et al.* 2004). This may explain why, paradoxically, some low- and middle-income countries with a high prevalence of *H. pylori* which discourage alcohol and tobacco, have a low incidence of gastric cancer. In contrast to the association with gastric cancer, *H. pylori*

has been associated with a reduced risk of oesophageal adenocarcinoma but the mechanism underlying this is poorly understood (Islami and Kamangar 2008).

....

Question 1

Suggest possible study methods that could be used to investigate the relationship between *H. pylori* infection and gastric cancer. Discuss the strengths and weaknesses of the various options, and see Table 11.2 for a model answer.

....

Helicobacter pylori and dyspepsia

For several reasons, it has proven difficult to determine whether there is a causal link between dyspepsia and infection with *H. pylori*. In addition to the definition and measurement problems associated with dyspepsia, dyspepsia and *H. pylori* infection are both common and, therefore, frequently co-exist in the same person. Also, some patients with dyspepsia have peptic ulceration that is caused by *H. pylori* and is responsive to eradication of the organism. Studies designed to compare the benefit of *H. pylori* eradication against therapy with acid suppression alone for dyspepsia are the most robust studies examining this issue. Results are conflicting, but a meta-analysis concluded that there may be some benefit in testing for, and treating, *H. pylori* in dyspeptic patients (see Moayyedi *et al.* 2005). The authors of this meta-analysis calculated that the **number needed to treat** to cure one patient of dyspepsia was 15. This has to be balanced against the costs of the treatment and the disadvantages of widespread use of antibiotics in *H. pylori* eradication regimens, given that both dyspepsia and *H. pylori* are common.

11.4 Inflammatory bowel disease

Inflammatory bowel disease (IBD) includes ulcerative colitis (UC) and Crohn's disease (CD). Unlike the distinctive pathological features of UC and CD (see Box 11.2), the clinical features of the diseases are not sufficiently distinct to allow them to be separated

Box 11.2 Pathological definitions of major varieties of inflammatory bowel disease

Ulcerative colitis is a chronic inflammatory disease of unknown cause which primarily affects the colonic mucosa. Inflammation is limited to the superficial layers and lack of extension to the muscularis and serosal structures is typical.	Crohn's disease is a chronic, granulatomatous, inflammatory disorder of unknown cause which may involve any segment of the gastrointestinal tract from mouth to anus. Transmural inflammation is characteristic.

with reliability. The main symptoms of both conditions include diarrhoea (which may be bloody and/or contain mucus), abdominal pain, weight loss, malaise, anorexia, fever, and lethargy. Both conditions tend to follow a relapsing and remittent course.

Prevalence/incidence

Measuring the prevalence or incidence of UC and CD presents some problems. Accurate diagnosis requires access to endoscopic and laboratory facilities to enable differentiation of these conditions from each other and from other disorders causing similar symptoms, for example infective gastrointestinal diseases. This has implications for comparing the incidence of these diseases between countries, particularly between developed and developing countries. Also, mild UC may go undetected, and will lead to underestimates of UC incidence. Mortality directly related to IBD is also a poor measure of the incidence of these conditions, and outpatient management (especially in patients with mild UC) and repeated admissions to hospital (in CD patients) complicate the use of hospital admissions as measures of frequency of IBD. Population-based registers of IBD are uncommon (Rubin *et al.* 2000).

Time trends and geographic distribution

There is substantial geographic variation in the incidence of IBD. These diseases appear to be uncommon in developing countries but this may be due to under-ascertainment. In the developed world there is a north-south gradient in the incidence of IBD, both in Europe and the USA; the highest rates are seen in Scandinavia and in Scotland. A higher incidence of UC compared with

CD is a fairly consistent finding in different populations. Inflammatory bowel disease most commonly presents in people in their late teens and twenties, with the peak age of presentation of CD being earlier than UC. The incidence of CD is higher in females, especially when presentation is at an early age (Fig. 11.5). Inflammatory bowel disease, and, in particular CD, is more common in urban than rural populations but there are no clear relations with socio-economic status. The time trends

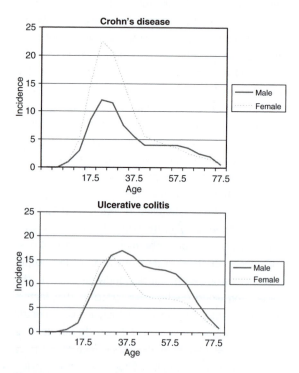

Figure 11.5 Mean annual age and gender-specific incidence rates (per 100,000 inhabitants per year) of Crohn's disease and ulcerative colitis in Northern France. Reproduced from Molinié F *et al*, 'Opposite evolution in incidence of Crohn's disease and ulcerative colitis in Northern France (1988–1999)', *Gut* **53**, 6, 2004, with permission from BMJ Publishing Group Ltd.

in IBD are difficult to interpret because of changing diagnostic practices and the possibility of diagnostic transfer between the UC and CD categories. In Europe and the USA there appears to have been a sharp rise in the incidence of UC and CD after the Second World War, with the increase in the incidence of UC preceding that in CD by about 15–20 years. In most Western countries, the incidence of IBD appears to have levelled off towards the end of the 20th century.

Aetiology and risk factors

The aetiology of IBD is unknown but there is evidence that genetic susceptibility, environmental exposures, and host immune responses all contribute to development of these conditions. There is a high IBD concordance rate among monozygotic twins, especially for CD. Inflammatory bowel disease exhibits familial aggregation: the relative risk to a sibling is estimated to be between 15 and 35 per cent for CD and between seven and 17 per cent for UC. Familial aggregation may reflect not only shared genes but shared environment, including exposure to infectious or other noxious agents. Other evidence of a genetic predisposition to IBD is provided by association with several well-defined genetic syndromes, such as Turner's syndrome. Genome-wide studies have identified several genetic sites potentially associated with UC or CD. It is clear from the available evidence that IBD is genetically complex and cannot be explained by a single-gene model (Hanauer 2006).

Ethnic and racial differences in IBD have been observed. The incidence in white and African American populations is similar, but there appears to be a reduced incidence in Asian Americans and Americans of Hispanic origin. Studies in migrant populations have highlighted the potential importance of lifestyle and environmental factors. Although IBD is thought to be rare in the Indian subcontinent, both first- and second-generations of South Asian migrants are at increased risk of UC compared to the white population (Montgomery et al. 1999).

Infection, or response to infection, may play a role in the aetiology of IBD. Crohn's disease has been shown to be more common in people who, during infancy, live in houses with running hot water and separate bathrooms (Duggan et al. 1998). Improved living conditions in childhood and altered immune modulation resulting from later exposure to infections has been proposed to explain the rise in CD in industrialized countries, as has been suggested also in the case of asthma (Chapter 8). Some studies, but not all, have suggested that breast-feeding may protect against IBD. Numerous studies have examined dietary factors in IBD, but no consensus has emerged. Observational studies examining the association between diet and disease are difficult to perform due to poor recall of diet and the possibility that diet was altered due to gastrointestinal symptoms before a formal diagnosis was made. Of particular note are studies demonstrating that smokers have more than twice the risk of CD compared with non-smokers, and patients with CD who continue to smoke follow a more aggressive clinical course than non-smokers. In contrast, smokers have half the risk of UC compared with non-smokers, and UC patients who smoke have a better clinical prognosis than non-smokers. This unusual finding has been observed in a number of studies. Trials of trans-dermal nicotine therapy for UC have had mixed results with some studies demonstrating a clinical improvement with nicotine, and others showing no significant benefit. Several studies have suggested an association between oral contraceptive use and IBD, but the mechanism of this association remains unknown. Another poorly understood association is the apparent protective effect of appendicectomy on the risk of UC shown in several studies. Contrast studies in CD have suggested an increased risk of CD following appendicectomy, although the evidence for a significant association is less strong.

11.5 Colorectal cancer

Incidence/prevalence

Excluding non-melanoma skin cancer (see Chapter 17), colorectal cancer is the third most common cancer in men and the second most common cancer in women in the UK. Survival from colorectal cancer depends on the stage of cancer at diagnosis. Early stage disease has five-year survival rates of over 90 per cent whereas

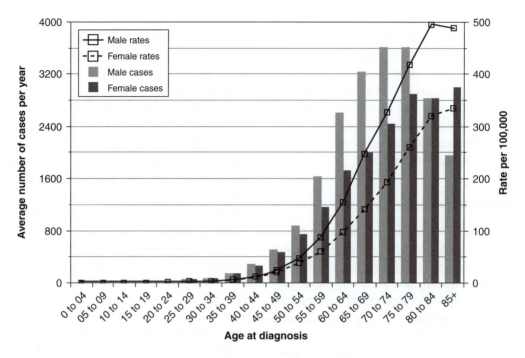

Figure 11.6 Age-specific incidence of colorectal cancer, England 2000.

Source: Office for National Statistics (2001). *Mortality Statistics – Cause. Review of the Registrar General on Deaths by Cause, Sex and Age, in England and Wales, 2000.* Mortality Data Series DH2 No. 27. London: ONS.

less than 10 per cent of patients with distant metastases will survive five years. Studies have found that mortality rates vary worldwide. Reasons include differences in incidence, stage of presentation, availability of screening, and quality of medical care. In the year 2008, an estimated 610,000 people died from colorectal cancer worldwide, making it the fourth most common cause of cancer death worldwide. The incidence of colorectal cancer is almost 50 per cent higher in men than women. Incidence in both sexes increases with age, most markedly after 50 years (Fig. 11.6).

Time trends and geographic distribution

Following a steady rise in the incidence between 1971 and 1997, the incidence of colorectal cancer has remained relatively stable over the past 15 years in the UK. However, mortality from colorectal cancer has been steadily falling in both men and women since the early 1990s and there has been a 13 per cent fall in the age standardized mortality rate in the UK between 1999 and 2008 (CRUK 2012). Similar patterns have been seen in many high income populations, although the extent and timing of the increases in incidence vary between countries. The reasons for this are not fully understood although they may, in part, result from better detection of the cancer, for example after the introduction of colonoscopy. There is a 10- to 20-fold variation in the incidence of colorectal cancer across the world. The highest rates are seen in North America, Western Europe, and Australasia (age-standardized (world) incidence rates of 30–50 in men and 20–40 in women per 100,000), whereas the lowest rates occur in Africa and India (age-standardized (world) incidence rates of three to seven per 100,000) in both sexes. Substantial variation is seen between different ethnic groups: in the USA the highest rates are seen in Japanese and in black people, and the lowest in American Indians; Jews have much higher rates of colorectal cancer than Arabs living within the same region in Israel. Studies of Japanese migrants to the USA show that colorectal cancer rates in US-born

Japanese are up to twice those of native Japanese; these rates also exceed those of white people born in the USA. The widespread variation in the geographic distribution of colorectal cancer, the recent secular trends, ethnic differences, and changes in the risk in migrants indicate the importance of environmental and lifestyle influences on risk of this cancer and suggest that the risk is modifiable, at least in part. However, genetic factors also predispose individuals to this cancer.

Aetiology

Genetics

Seventy-five per cent of colorectal cancers occur sporadically. Eighteen per cent of patients have a family history of colorectal cancer, but have no identified genetic predisposition, and five per cent of colorectal cancer patients have hereditary non-polyposis colorectal cancer (HNPCC, also called Lynch syndrome). In families with HNPCC, cancer usually occurs on the right side of the colon and at a younger age than sporadic colorectal cancer. Other cancers occur in these families, including cancers of the uterus, ovaries, stomach, urinary tract, small bowel, and bile duct. Hereditary non-polyposis colorectal cancer is caused by germ-line mutation of one of the mismatch repair genes (Calvert and Frucht 2002). One per cent of colorectal cancers occur in patients with familial adenomatous polyposis (FAP), who carry germ-line mutations of the *APC* gene (a tumour suppressor gene). In approximately 25 per cent of these patients the mutations are spontaneous. Affected individuals have multiple colonic adenomas which, if untreated, inevitably undergo malignant change. Patients may also develop thyroid and other cancers, adenomas in other parts of the gastrointestinal tract, and benign lesions of many organs. Prophylactic colectomy and routine endoscopic surveillance of the rectum are usually performed in patients with FAP to prevent the development of colorectal cancer.

Environmental/lifestyle risk factors

Most colorectal cancers occur in individuals without any known genetic predisposition, and several environmental/lifestyle risk factors have been identified.

Intake of animal fat and meat has been consistently, positively related to the risk of colorectal cancer; for example data from the US Nurses' Health Study showed that women in the highest quintile of intake of animal fat had approximately twice the risk of colorectal cancer compared with those whose intake was in the lowest quintile. Also, women who ate meat every day were 2.5 times more likely to develop this cancer than women who ate meat less than once a month.

Data from the same study did not show any protective effect of dietary fibre on colorectal cancer but a recent meta-analysis found that a high dietary intake of fibre was associated with a reduced risk of colorectal cancer (Aune *et al.* 2011). This report showed a 10 per cent reduction in risk of colorectal cancer with every 10 g of fibre taken daily. Data on the intake of fruit and vegetables and risk of colorectal cancer are inconsistent, although generally a low intake of fruit and vegetables appears to increase the risk of colorectal cancer. Systematic reviews have found that high folate intake is associated with a small protective effect against colorectal cancer, but confounding by other dietary factors is possible. High intake of calcium is also associated with reduced risk of colorectal cancer, and intervention studies have shown that calcium supplementation can reduce the occurrence of colorectal adenomas (Weingarten *et al.* 2008).

Obesity is also a risk factor for colorectal cancer, obese individuals having about twice the risk of their lean counterparts. This seems to be particularly the case in men with central adiposity, and this may be mediated through insulin resistance. There is strong evidence from epidemiological studies that physically active men and women (taking 30–60 minutes per day of moderate to vigorous intensity activity) have a 30–40 per cent reduced risk of developing colon cancer, compared with inactive persons (Lee 2003). Evidence is also accumulating that smoking is a risk factor for colorectal cancer. Epidemiological studies conducted before the 1970s in males, and before the 1990s in females, did not show this association, probably because an induction period of three to four decades is required between genotoxic exposure (from smoking) and the development of colorectal cancer.

Epidemiological studies have also shown that individuals reporting a regular intake of aspirin and other NSAIDs have a 40–50 per cent reduced risk of developing colorectal polyps and cancer. There is now growing evidence from interventional studies (primarily against CVD) that regular aspirin use reduces the incidence and mortality from colorectal cancer (Rothwell *et al.* 2010).

Prevention

There is sufficient evidence to recommend that people should reduce their intake of meat and animal fat, increase their intake of fibre, fruit, and vegetables, maintain normal weight, and take regular physical activity of at least moderate intensity, to reduce their risk of colorectal cancer. Data at present are insufficient to recommend calcium or folate supplementation to prevent colorectal cancer, but these approaches show promise for the future. The growing evidence linking smoking with colorectal cancer adds to the numerous reasons to promote smoking cessation where possible. Too much controversy exists about the safety, efficacy, and optimal treatment regimen of NSAIDs to promote them as long-term chemopreventive agents in the general population, but their use may be appropriate in high-risk groups. Randomized controlled trials have confirmed that population screening of middle-aged men and women over the age of 50 years for non-visible (occult) blood in the faeces can reduce the mortality rate for colorectal cancer (Towler *et al.* 2000), and many countries including the UK have instituted colorectal cancer screening programmes (see Chapter 5).

11.6 Other gastrointestinal diseases

In this textbook lack of space prevents discussion of the epidemiology of other important diseases of the digestive tract. The epidemiological methods used to investigate gallstone disease, appendicitis, diverticular disease, coeliac disease, and pancreatitis are described elsewhere (Logan *et al.* 2002).

References

Aune D, Chan DSM, Lau R, Vieira R, *et al.* (2011) Dietary fibre, whole grains, and risk of colorectal cancer: systematic review and dose-response meta-analysis of prospective studies. *BMJ (Clinical Research Ed)* **343**, d6617.

Bosetti C, Levi F, Lucchini F, Zatonski WA, *et al.* (2007) Worldwide mortality from cirrhosis: an update to 2002. *Journal of Hepatology* **46** (5), 827–39.

Calvert PM and Frucht H (2002) The genetics of colorectal cancer. *Annals of Internal Medicine* **137** (7), 603–12.

CRUK (2012) Cancer Research UK. Available at: http://science.cancerresearchuk.org/.

Duggan AE, Usmani I, Neal KR, and Logan RF (1998) Appendicectomy, childhood hygiene, Helicobacter pylori status, and risk of inflammatory bowel disease: a case control study. *Gut* **43** (4), 494–8.

Ferlay J, Shin HR, Bray F, et al. (2010) Estimates of worldwide burden of cancer in 2008: GLOBOCAN 2008. *International Journal of Cancer* **127** (12), 2893–917.

Fisher NC, Hanson J, Phillips A, *et al.* (2002) Mortality from liver disease in the West Midlands, 1993–2000: observational study. *BMJ (Clinical Research Ed)* **325** (7359), 312–13.

Gisbert JP (2005) The recurrence of Helicobacter pylori infection: incidence and variables influencing it. A critical review. *The American Journal of Gastroenterology* **100** (9), 2083–99.

Go MF (2002) Review article: natural history and epidemiology of Helicobacter pylori infection. *Alimentary Pharmacology & Therapeutics* **16** Suppl. 13–15.

Hanauer SB (2006) Inflammatory bowel disease: epidemiology, pathogenesis, and therapeutic opportunities. *Inflammatory Bowel Diseases* **12** Suppl. 1S3–9.

Helicobacter foundation (2006) The Helicobacter Foundation: Experts give Infomation about Helicobacter pylori, its Diseases, and Treatment. [Online] http://www.helico.com/; [Accessed 7 December 2011].

Health Protection Agency (2011) Hepatitis C in the UK: 2011 report. [Online] http://www.hpa.org.uk/web/HPAweb&HPAwebStandard/HPAweb_C/1309969907625; [Accessed 28 November 2011].

Islami F and Kamangar F (2008) Helicobacter pylori and esophageal cancer risk: a meta-analysis. *Cancer Prevention Research (Philadelphia, Pa.)*. **1** (5), 329–38.

Jones RH, Lydeard SE, Hobbs FD, Kenkre JE, *et al.* (1990) Dyspepsia in England and Scotland. *Gut* **31** (4), 401–5.

Lee I-M (2003) Physical activity and cancer prevention—data from epidemiologic studies. *Medicine and Science in Sports and Exercise* **35** (11), 1823–7.

Lehours P and Yilmaz O (2007) Epidemiology of Helicobacter pylori infection. *Helicobacter* **12** Suppl. 11–3.

Logan RFA, Farthing MJG, and Langman MJS (2002) Gastrointestinal disease: public health aspects. In: Detels R, McEwen J, Beaglehole R and Tanaka H (eds). *Oxford Textbook of Public Health*, pp. 1773–90. Oxford: Oxford University Press.

Mahadeva S and Goh K-L (2006) Epidemiology of functional dyspepsia: a global perspective. *World Journal of Gastroenterology: WJG* **12** (17), 2661–6.

Marshall BJ and Warren JR (1984) Unidentified curved bacilli in the stomach of patients with gastritis and peptic ulceration. *Lancet* **1** (8390), 1311–15.

Moayyedi P, Soo S, Deeks J, Delaney B, *et al.* (2005) Eradication of Helicobacter pylori for non-ulcer dyspepsia. *Cochrane Database of Systematic Reviews* **1**, CD002096.

Molinié F, *et al.* (2004) Opposite evolution in incidence of Crohn's disease and ulcerative colitis in Northern France (1988–1999). *Gut* **53** (6), 843–8.

Montgomery SM, Morris DL, Pounder RE and Wakefield AJ (1999) Asian ethnic origin and the risk of inflammatory bowel disease. *European Journal of Gastroenterology & Hepatology* **11** (5), 543–6.

Murray L, Johnston B, Lane A, Harvey I, *et al.* (2003) Relationship between body mass and gastro-oesophageal reflux symptoms: The Bristol Helicobacter Project. *International Journal of Epidemiology* **32** (4), 645–50.

National Institute for Clinical Excellence (Great Britain) (2004). *Dyspepsia: management of dyspepsia in adults in primary care*. London: National Institute for Clinical Excellence.

Office for National Statistics (2001) *Mortality Statistics—Cause. Review of the Registrar General on Deaths by Cause, Sex and Age, in England and Wales, 2000*. Mortality Data Series DH2 No. 27. London: ONS.

Perez-Perez GI, Rothenbacher D and Brenner H (2004) Epidemiology of Helicobacter pylori infection. *Helicobacter* **9** Suppl. 11–16.

Pounder RE and Ng D (1995) The prevalence of Helicobacter pylori infection in different countries. *Alimentary Pharmacology & Therapeutics* **9** Suppl. 233–9.

Rothwell PM, Wilson M, Elwin C-E, Norrving B, *et al.* (2010) Long-term effect of aspirin on colorectal cancer incidence and mortality: 20-year follow-up of five randomized trials. *Lancet* **376** (9754), 1741–50.

Rubin GP, Hungin AP, Kelly PJ, and Ling J (2000) Inflammatory bowel disease: epidemiology and management in an English general practice population. *Alimentary Pharmacology & Therapeutics* **14** (12), 1553–9.

Ruidavets J-B, Ducimetière P, Evans A, Montaye M, *et al.* (2010) Patterns of alcohol consumption and ischaemic heart disease in culturally divergent countries: the Prospective Epidemiological Study of Myocardial Infarction (PRIME). *BMJ (Clinical Research Ed)* **341**, c6077.

Shah SS, Bhatia SJ, and Mistry FP (2001) Epidemiology of dyspepsia in the general population in Mumbai. *Indian Journal of Gastroenterology* **20** (3), 103–6.

Shaib Y and El-Serag HB (2004) The prevalence and risk factors of functional dyspepsia in a multiethnic population in the United States. *The American Journal of Gastroenterology* **99** (11), 2210–16.

Smith L and Foxcroft DR (2009) *Drinking in the UK: An exploration of trends*. York: Joseph Rowntree Foundation.

Stanghellini V (1999) Three-month prevalence rates of gastrointestinal symptoms and the influence of demographic factors: results from the Domestic/International Gastroenterology Surveillance Study (DIGEST). *Scandinavian Journal of Gastroenterology, Suppl.* **231**, 20–8.

Talley NJ (2005) American Gastroenterological Association medical position statement: evaluation of dyspepsia. *Gastroenterology* **129** (5), 1753–5.

Towler BP, Irwig L, Glasziou P, Weller D, *et al.* (2000) Screening for colorectal cancer using the faecal occult blood test, hemoccult. *Cochrane Database of Systematic Reviews* [Online] **2**, CD001216.

Tuyns AJ and Pequignot G (1984) Greater risk of ascitic cirrhosis in females in relation to alcohol consumption. *International Journal of Epidemiology* **13** (1), 53–7.

Vial M, Grande L, and Pera M (2010) Epidemiology of adenocarcinoma of the esophagus, gastric cardia, and upper gastric third. *Recent Results in Cancer Research* **182**, 1–17.

Weingarten MA, Zalmanovici A and Yaphe J (2008) Dietary calcium supplementation for preventing colorectal cancer and adenomatous polyps. *Cochrane Database of Systematic Reviews* [Online] **1**, CD003548.

WHO (2011a) European Health for All Database (HFA-DB). http://www.euro.who.int/en/what-we-do/data-and-evidence/databases/european-health-for-all-database-hfa-db2; [Accessed 28 November 2011].

WHO (2011b) *Global status report on alcohol and health.* Geneva: World Health Organization.

Table 11.2 Model answer

Study type	Advantages	Disadvantages
Case-control	Rapid, inexpensive	Cannot determine whether *H. pylori* infection preceded, or is the consequence of, gastric cancer
Cohort study	Can determine temporal sequence of infection and gastric cancer	Expensive, very time-consuming.
		Long latent period between infection (normally in childhood) and development of gastric cancer (disease predominantly of the elderly)
Case-control study within a cohort (nested case-control)	Rapid, inexpensive, can determine temporal sequence of infection and gastric cancer	
Experimental study, for example, RCT of eradication therapy	Could provide a definite answer?	Time-consuming, expensive, very long follow-up period required, possibly decades. Preventing contamination of the control arm would be difficult. The disease process may be initiated at a very early stage with the result that prevention of infection rather than eradication is required to effect a reduction in gastric cancer occurrence

12 Renal diseases

DAMIAN FOGARTY AND PETER MAXWELL

CHAPTER CONTENTS

The epidemiology of kidney failure, both acute and chronic, is reviewed. Kidney failure represents a significant public health issue given the hardship of living with advanced chronic kidney disease and the costs of managing end-stage renal disease by dialysis and/or transplantation. Acute kidney injury is associated with prolonged hospitalization and greatly increased mortality compared to persons without kidney disease. An understanding of the epidemiology of kidney failure is vital to the planning of renal services. The scope for primary and secondary prevention of kidney disease will be reviewed.

Introduction

The kidneys' network of glomerular capillary vessels receive about 25 per cent of the resting cardiac output. Around one million glomeruli in each kidney filter fluid across large surface areas of capillary basement membrane. Kidney function is normally defined by the glomerular filtration rate (GFR) which, in healthy individuals, is in the range of 90–140 mL/min. Up to 180 litres of glomerular filtrate, containing water, electrolytes, and simple unbound chemical compounds, enters the renal tubules each day. Tubular reabsorption of water and solutes occurs before the urine is finally voided. The kidney has excretory, regulatory, endocrine, and metabolic functions and these normal physiological processes are disrupted in patients with acute kidney failure (usually termed *acute kidney injury*) or chronic kidney failure (usually designated as *chronic kidney disease* (CKD) by clinicians). The kidneys are vulnerable to so called pre-renal injury from defects in renal perfusion (hypotension, renal artery atherosclerosis). Pathological damage to nephrons (glomeruli and tubules) can occur from ischaemia, diabetes, high blood pressure, sepsis, autoimmune inflammation, and certain toxins (including prescribed drugs). Finally, adequate drainage of the renal tracts and bladder is essential since obstruction of either the ureters or bladder outlet can also cause kidney failure. The main causes of CKD are diabetes, hypertension, and atherosclerotic renal vascular disease. Usually people with kidney failure only develop symptoms when they have lost a substantial amount of renal function. Potentially life-threatening kidney failure is present when the GFR is less than 10 mL/per min (~ 10 per cent of normal), and patients will usually need some form of renal replacement therapy in order to survive. Acute kidney injury (AKI) and chronic kidney disease (CKD) are epidemiologically distinct with some degree of overlap, and acute renal failure can progress to chronic disease. All forms of kidney failure are defined by a reduced GFR, which is immediately apparent by oliguria or anuria in the case of AKI but in CKD the fall in GFR is typically insidious and asymptomatic until it is less than 30 per cent of normal. Serum creatinine levels, which reflect the ability of the kidney to excrete metabolized muscle protein, tend to be used to make the provisional diagnosis. However, due to the non-linear (exponential) relationship between serum creatinine and GFR, an elevated serum creatinine is a relatively late marker for loss of renal function. Serum creatinine only rises above the reference range when ~ 50 per cent of kidney function has been lost. Formula-based estimated GFR (eGFR) measurements, using serum creatinine values, are now established in routine clinical practice and have been modified and incorporated into clinical practice guidelines (Levey *et al.* 2009). The typical eGFR formula requires simple input data such as the age, gender, ethnicity, in addition to serum creatinine. Until the introduction of eGFR, a high proportion of patients who eventually needed renal replacement therapy (RRT) were referred at a late stage of kidney failure. To some extent this was because routine kidney function tests failed to alert clinicians to the severity of the kidney failure (Kee *et al.* 2005). Such late referral often meant poor RRT planning for both the patient and the health service. Furthermore, patients referred at a later stage had poorer outcomes (more hospitalizations and higher mortality) than those whose kidney failure was diagnosed at least 6 to 12 months before dialysis (Stack 2003).

The definitions of both AKI and CKD have been revised in the last 10 years. The lack of a single highly specific and sensitive marker means that effective definitions for kidney diseases often rely on multiple parameters. The spectrum of published AKI definitions is striking with over 30 reported in the literature, ranging from relatively modest increases in serum creatinine concentration to the most severe forms such as AKI requiring dialysis (Mehta and Chertow 2003). Additionally, it has become apparent that the clinical overlap between AKI and CKD is much wider than previously appreciated. Patients can be left with significant CKD following a single episode of AKI and multiple AKI insults may contribute to incremental progression of CKD in some individuals (Coca *et al.* 2009).

12.1 Acute kidney disease

Acute kidney injury (AKI), formerly called Acute renal failure, occurs when there is a decline in GFR that occurs rapidly within a period of hours to a few weeks. AKI in general is seen in hospitalized patients undergoing medical and surgical interventions although it can start *de novo* in the community. The incidence of AKI is set to increase in an ageing population. Until recently no single definition of AKI was used consistently in epidemiological studies making it difficult to compare AKI reported in publications and over time. In 2004 a consensus group described a new classification to improve comparability in AKI studies (Bellomo *et al.* 2004). It is important to recognize that the reported incidence and outcomes of AKI depend substantially on how the condition is defined.

AKI is traditionally explained in terms of pre-renal, renal, or post-renal risk factors. In pre-renal AKI there is a decreased perfusion of the normal kidneys as occurs in hypotensive states. The kidneys respond to the reduced perfusion in various physiological ways such as activating the renin–angiotensin–aldosterone system (which results in enhanced renal sodium and water reabsorption), in an effort to restore perfusion to the kidneys. If the blood pressure improves and renal perfusion increases then the GFR will rise and AKI will usually rapidly resolve. Post-renal or obstructive AKI occurs when there is impaired drainage from the renal tracts or obstruction at the level of the bladder outlet. The aetiology of obstructive AKI is age and gender related. Post-renal AKI is commonly caused by obstruction to the bladder outlet due to prostatic enlargement in older men or pelvic cancer in women. It is easily diagnosed by an ultrasound scan of the renal tracts and bladder.

AKI may also occur secondarily to prolonged pre-renal insults, often as a complication of trauma, sepsis, or surgery. Persistent hypotension results in hypoxic injury to kidney cells and subsequent renal tubular cell necrosis. Acute tubular necrosis and pre-renal AKI account for about three-quarters of all the AKI identified in hospital. AKI may more rarely occur due to primary renal diseases such as proliferative glomerulonephritis or secondary to a systemic disorder such as small vessel vasculitis or multiple myeloma. Sometimes the injury is predominantly to the tubules and interstitial structures following an allergic reaction to drugs, e.g. proton pump inhibitors or antibiotics. It is increasingly appreciated that AKI often occurs in patients with pre-existing CKD—so-called acute-on-chronic kidney disease (AoCKD). This is best thought of as an acute deterioration in renal function occurring in an individual with limited renal reserve (Hsu *et al.* 2009).

AKI is often reversible if promptly recognized, investigated, and managed appropriately. AKI is reported to complicate up to five per cent of all hospital admissions. In a study of over five million hospital admissions in the USA the AKI rate was 14.6 cases per 1000 discharges in 1992 and increased to 36.4 cases per 1000 discharges in 2001 (Xue *et al.* 2006) though case identification was incomplete. Applying laboratory definitions of AKI (an acute rise in serum creatinine), much higher incidences of AKI have been observed. In 2003, in a well-defined Scottish region, the incidences of AKI and AoCKD were 1811 and 336 per million population (pmp), respectively, each year. The median age for AKI was 76 years and for AoCKD was 80.5 years. Sepsis was a precipitating factor in half of these patients (Ali *et al.* 2007). The same authors repeated this study a few years later and found that the AKI incidence had risen to 2147 pmp per year (Ali *et al.* 2011). A higher proportion of patients with AKI were now referred to specialists and treatment with RRT was almost four times more common.

Increasing age, pre-existing CKD, other co-morbid diseases, certain procedures (e.g. radiology with contrast agents), and drugs (particularly hypotensive, diuretic agents and NSAIDs) are the common risk factors for AKI. It is likely that future AKI incidence rates will rise in high and in middle income countries with ageing of these populations and with their dependence on medical therapies and interventions that form part of the AKI risk profile.

12.2 Chronic kidney disease

Chronic kidney disease (CKD) is a collective term covering a number of primary disease processes that result in structural and/or functional kidney abnormalities

persisting for at least three months (Levey *et al.* 2005). Abnormal urinalysis with proteinuria and/or haematuria, abnormal kidney structure and/or histology, with or without a decreased glomerular filtration rate (GFR < 60 mL/min/1.73m²) are the defining presentations. CKD typically causes a decline in GFR over months or years although with effective treatment this progression is not always inevitable. CKD is subdivided into five stages according to the measured GFR (Table 12.1) reflecting the observation that CKD progresses slowly through these stages before a minority reach end-stage renal disease (ESRD). This is represented in Fig. 12.1.

The CKD staging system has two important implications: firstly, it suggests that if CKD is detected at an early stage, intervention may prevent or slow progression to more advanced stages (Foley 2010); and, secondly, it reflects the observation that as GFR declines the risk for the patient and associated complications change. Thus staging allows for structuring therapy and prioritizing interventions for the management of CKD (Fogarty and Taal 2011).

The diagnosis of CKD stage 1 or stage 2 is based on the presence of either albuminuria (micro- or macroalbuminuria), haematuria, or structural kidney disease. Patients with CKD stage 1 and 2 do not have specific renal failure symptoms, or complications such as renal anaemia or metabolic renal bone disease. The emphasis at these early stages should be on identifying any specific renal diseases, appropriate referral to a nephrologist and reduction of cardiovascular risk. Population surveys from the USA estimate the prevalence of CKD stage 1 at 5.7 per cent and stage 2 at 5.4 per cent of the total US population (Anon 2007).

Cardiovascular mortality increases substantially below a GFR of 45 mL/min/1.73m² (Quinn *et al.* 2011). The aims of management within CKD stage 3 are to identify specific renal diseases, correct reversible causes of renal dysfunction, prevent or slow the progression of CKD, reduce cardiovascular risk, and to provide treatment of CKD complications of CKD.

Patients with CKD stage 4 have much higher cumulative risks for cardiovascular death or progression to ESRD than those with earlier CKD. Almost 65 per cent of patients with CKD stage 4 will have either a renal or

Table 12.1 Internationally agreed staging system for chronic kidney disease (CKD) with associated complications and clinical strategy

CKD stage	Description	Glomerular filtration rate (mL/min/1.73m²)[1]	Complications and risks	Clinical strategy
1	Mild kidney damage not yet detectable by change in renal function	≥ 90 (but evidence of structural problems, e.g. cysts or scars or evidence of damage with albuminuria or haematuria)	Asymptomatic. Hypertension[2] in ~ 30%	Diagnostic tests to detect treatable disease. Blood pressure and vascular risk assessment and lowering
2	Mild/moderate ↓ in kidney function	60–89	Asymptomatic. Hypertension[2] in ~ 50%	As above and estimating and retarding progression
3a	Moderate ↓ in kidney function	45–59	Asymptomatic. Hypertension in ~ 70% [2,3]	As above and screening for complications
3b	Moderate–severe ↓ in kidney function	30–44	Hypertension in ~ 85% Anaemia in up to 20% [2,3]	
4	Severe ↓ in kidney function	15–29	Anaemia more common and evolving mineral bone disorder[2,3]	As above and preparing for renal replacement therapy
5	Established kidney failure	≤ 15	As above and evolving uraemia[2,3]	
Acute kidney injury (AKI)	Onset in days or weeks Due to rapid changes in renal function assessment of baseline glomerular filtration rate (GFR) on its own cannot establish a diagnosis. It is important to see changes in GFR along with urine output.		Mortality of hospitalized patients with AKI needing dialysis is > 50%	Critical care setting and renal replacement therapy usually needed

Notes

[1] 1.73m² is the standardized body surface area

[2] Hypertension and anaemia rates from the UK Neoerica Study (Stevens *et al.* 2007)

[3] Prevalence of CKD and co-morbid illness in elderly patients in the United States: results from the Kidney Early Evaluation Program (KEEP) (Stevens *et al.* 2010).

a cardiovascular event over the ensuing five years. As the GFR falls below 20 mL/min/1.73m² the focus moves to treating the advanced CKD complications and planning for RRT (Abboud and Henrich 2010).

Many community-based surveys in the USA, UK and elsewhere have highlighted that the prevalence of CKD is much higher than previously appreciated and appears to be increasing especially in countries with rising prevalence of diabetes and hypertension (Table 12.2).

In a study based on primary care data across over 300 general practices in Italy, ICD-9-codes for CKD were reported in 2.5 per cent of the cohort compared to an age adjusted eGFR based CKD diagnosis of 9.3

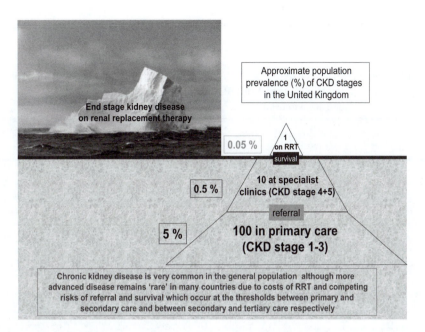

Figure 12.1 A schematic representation on the relative prevalence of patients with stages of chronic kidney disease (CKD) using the analogy of the iceberg. For every one patient on renal replacement therapy (RRT) with dialysis or a kidney transplant there are 10 more patients with advanced CKD attending specialists and 100 patients with earlier forms of CKD in the community. This is a simplification as the prevalence of RRT patients in the UK is 1 in 1000 and in the US is almost 2 in 1000 of the population. The competing risks that influence whether a patient may move to the next level of care is highlighted by the thresholds where *referral* and *survival* influence the numbers and also type of patients who are studied in either a specialist clinic or dialysis/transplant population.

per cent (Minutolo *et al*. 2008). The infrequent use of CKD diagnostic codes suggests that awareness of CKD in primary care is still relatively low. This is relevant to studies of CKD where the patients may be ascertained based on some other factor (such as diabetes or symptoms) rather than the biochemical definition of CKD by eGFR measurement. Interestingly, among patients with decreased kidney function (by GFR), primary care practitioners correctly diagnosed CKD (with ICD codes) in only 15.2 per cent of such patients. Furthermore specific diagnoses of CKD, such as diabetic nephropathy and hypertensive nephropathy, were rarely reported (0.1 per cent and 0.5 per cent, respectively) despite a high prevalence of diabetes (11.1 per cent) and hypertension (34.1 per cent) in the group of patients with eGFR < 60 mL/min/1.73 m². Since this study in 2003 there has been a global initiative to educate primary care practitioners on the appropriate interpretation of serum creatinine and the utility of estimated GFR in

the early detection of CKD patients. In the UK there is evidence that this approach is reaping benefits with CKD patients referred earlier to renal services (with higher GFRs at time of referral) and a lower proportion of patients starting dialysis in an unplanned fashion (Gilg *et al*. 2011). The only 'disadvantage' of this earlier recognition is that many more elderly patients with non-progressive CKD are being assessed at hospital clinics. In Canada there is now evidence that the reporting of estimated GFR has substantially increased referral to specialists and should in time improve the outlook for these patients (Hemmelgarn *et al*. 2010).

12.3 End-stage renal disease

Not all patients with CKD stage 4 will progress to CKD stage 5 and end-stage renal disease (ESRD). Many have stable but impaired kidney function and will die

Table 12.2 Prevalence and incidence of chronic kidney disease (CKD) in UK, US, and other international groups. Note the increase in prevalence over short periods of time due to newer and broader definitions.

Prevalence rate (%)	Definition of CKD (creatinine μmol/L; eGFR and albuminuria)	Population studied and location	Author, year
3%	Creatinine >141 in men	US population sample (NHANES III, 1988–94)	(Coresh et al. 2001)[1]
	Creatinine >124 in women		
11%	CKD stages 1–4 i.e. eGFR >15 mL/min/1.73m^2	US population sample (NHANES III, 1988–94)	(Coresh et al. 2003)
9.3%	CKD stages 3–5	Italy. Primary care: 451,548 individuals in the entire practice population, only 77,630 (17.2%) underwent serum creatinine testing	(Minutolo et al. 2008)
7.3%	CKD stages 3–5	UK Primary Care Trust 185,434 aged > 15 years	(Richards et al. 2008)
6.8%	CKD stages 3–5	Spain	(de Francisco et al. 2007)
13.1%	CKD stages 1–4 i.e. eGFR >15 mL/min/1.73m^2	US (NHANES III, 1999–2004)	(Coresh et al. 2007)
Incidence rates per year			
1,701 per million population	> or = 150 μmol/L for 6 months	UK laboratory data	(Drey et al. 2003)
2,435 pmp	≥ 180 μmol/L in men and ≥ 135 μmol/L in women	UK laboratory data	(John et al. 2004)

[1] Definition in this era used an elevated creatinine alone.

from other competing causes, especially cardiovascular disease and cancer. This potential for a **survival bias** is also important in comparing any study where the inclusion criteria include the 'acceptance' on to a form of onerous dialysis treatment. In many low- and middle-income countries very few patients will be recorded with ESRD (Fig. 12.2) and an estimated 80 per cent of patients on RRT live in North America, Europe, and Japan (Weening 2004). A high prevalence but low awareness of CKD in Taiwan is suggested to account for its high rate of ESRD and highlights that education on CKD prevention is critical for both physicians and the public (Hsu et al. 2006).

ESRD is an irreversible loss of renal function and is fatal unless treated by renal replacement therapy (RRT), either from dialysis or transplantation. Usually ESRD is associated with an absolute reduction in GFR below 10 mL/min/1.73m^2 and an elevated serum creatinine (above 500 μmol/L in men and 300 μmol/L in women). Registries which collate information on incidence and prevalence of ESRD define a new patient as one who is accepted for treatment and dialysed or transplanted for more than 90 days (three months). This definition would exclude an individual with newly diagnosed ESRD who died within three months and, therefore, leads to an underestimate of the true incidence

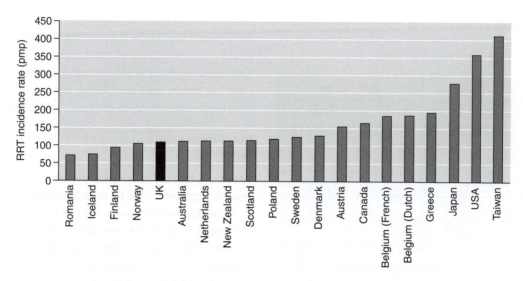

Figure 12.2 Crude renal replacement therapy (RRT) incidence rates for 2004 to 2008 combined for several countries with complete coverage of their populations. The UK incidence rate is similar to many other Northern European countries and Australasia, but remains lower than Belgium, Greece, US, Japan and Taiwan.
Reproduced from Gilg J *et al., Nephron Clin Pract* 2011; 199(Suppl.2):c1-c25, with permission from S Karger AG.

of ESRD, which is also compounded by exclusion of patients who have not been accepted for RRT.

Aetiology

Table 12.3 shows the underlying causes of renal failure in the UK and in the USA and a comparison of disease specific incidence rates. These striking variations in incidence rates reflect many differences between the two nations including ethnic mix and acceptance rates for RRT.

In North America and most European countries, diabetic nephropathy has emerged as the most common cause of ESRD. A majority of patients with diabetic nephropathy have type 2 diabetes although the lifetime risk of ESRD is higher in patients with Type 1 diabetes.

A significant proportion of patients with ESRD present late with advanced renal failure, hypertension, and small kidneys on ultrasound scan. The precise aetiology of their renal disease is often undetermined although individual clinicians may attribute this to hypertensive nephrosclerosis or glomerulonephritis (not biopsy proven). Variation in clinical diagnostic practice and certainty will account for some of the apparent differences in clinical diagnoses when national ESRD registries are compared.

Dialysis services in the USA have a longer history of development and were federally funded from the early 1970s onwards. The UK, with a more restricted NHS structure, was slower to develop RRT services and initially patients were only accepted for dialysis treatment if they were deemed fit enough for a subsequent renal transplant. This resulted in inequity of access to RRT, amounting to a major injustice through the 1980s and even early 1990s (Feest *et al.* 2005). Since then a large increase in funding for renal services has allowed more liberal acceptance criteria for chronic dialysis. The growth in UK RRT population is shown by modality in Fig. 12.3.

Trends

The incidence of ESRD is rising worldwide reflecting both a true increase in incidence of CKD and an increased acceptance of patients with ESRD for RRT. Worldwide incidence is rising at eight per cent per annum in comparison to population growth of 1.3 per cent (Dirks *et al.* 2006). There are many reasons why the rates of ESRD may increase and these are listed in Table 12.4.

Historically, the largest increases occurred when funding for the expensive treatments of dialysis and kidney transplantation was provided (Feest *et al.* 1990).

Table 12.3 Primary renal diagnosis for patients starting renal replacement therapy (RRT) in 2009. Rates are quoted as rates per million population (pmp)

Diagnosis	National rate	
	UK[1] 109 pmp	USA[2] 348 pmp[3]
Diabetes	24.4	154.1
Hypertension[4]	12.6	101.0
Glomerulonephritis	11.1	23.8
Polycystic kidneys[5]	6.4	8.3
Pyelonephritis[6]	7.1	4.9
Other	15.0	46.2
Unknown/missing	30.7	16.9

[1] UK Renal Registry Thirteenth Annual Report (2011).
[2] United States Renal Data System (2011).
[3] Differences in absolute rates of end-stage renal disease (ESRD) diagnoses between UK and USA populations reflect multiple factors including diagnostic coding practices in each country, age structure of the ESRD population, and, most importantly, the ethnic mix and acceptance rates for RRT. So, for instance, the 2009 incident rate for African-American patients initiating on haemodialysis at 928 pmp is 3.7 times greater than the rate of 251 among white patients in the US.
[4] This includes renal vascular disease in the UK figures.
[5] Note the similar rates for this genetic disease between the UK and the USA. Polycystic kidney disease is much less amenable to treatment that substantially reduces progression.
[6] In the US this group have a code termed 'other urological'.

More recently the increase in incidence reflects demographic factors such as an ageing population and in some countries an increased need due to the effects of higher prevalence rates of advanced kidney disease due especially to type 2 diabetes. The health care systems in these countries may also influence RRT. In an elegant study it was noted that although the CKD prevalence in Norway was similar to that in the USA the ESRD prevalence was much lower in Norway compared to the USA (Hallan et al. 2006). This suggests that Norwegian patients with CKD were much less likely to progress to ESRD compared to Americans with CKD and may reflect differences in effectiveness of CKD management in the different countries (Fig. 12.4).

Ensuring equitable access to kidney services has been a key theme for any developed nation and its health system. Historically there was ample evidence that patients of lower socio-economic status were at higher risk of renal failure than the better off in black and in white populations in the US (Klag et al. 1997). It has been assumed that this reflects higher rates of underlying risk factors such as diabetes, hypertension, and smoking that are also socio-economically distributed.

....

Question 1

Assuming that the causes and prevalence of CKD remain constant for the foreseeable future, but that the survival of patients with CKD and end-stage renal disease improves, what will happen to the numbers of patients needing dialysis as we move forward 10 and 20 years? Use Figs. 12.1–12.4 to explore this.

....

Epidemiology

The marked geographic variation in acceptance rates for ESRD between countries and within regions cannot be entirely explained by differences in population, age structure, ethnicity, or co-morbidity. Variation in the provision of RRT reflects clinical, societal, and economic factors. Previously in the UK, older patients with ESRD were not accepted for RRT but age is no longer recognized as a bar to treatment and it is ethically unacceptable to deny life-sustaining treatment to older people. Indeed, the perceived quality of life of older dialysis patients is reported to be comparable to others of the same age (Lamping et al. 2000). Variations also exist within regions of the UK with England having lower acceptance rates than Wales, Northern Ireland, or Scotland despite having a higher proportion of ethnic minorities (Gilg et al. 2011). People of Asian and Afro-Caribbean descent have higher rates of CKD: African-Americans have four times higher RRT acceptance rates compared to whites which has been attributed to much higher prevalence rates of hypertension (USRDS 2011). In the UK, prevalence rates have risen from under 400 prevalence pmp in 1993 to 794 pmp in 2009 and continue to increase at a rate of 3.5 per cent per annum (Steenkamp et al. 2011). Furthermore, the relative proportions of ESRD patients treated by dialysis versus transplantation

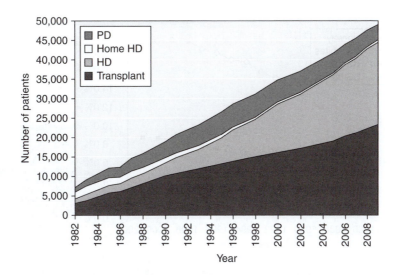

Figure 12.3 Growth in prevalent patients by treatment modality at the end of each year 1982–2009. Recent growth is 3.3 per cent per annum across the UK. Prevalence has almost doubled from 1993 to 2009.

Reproduced from the UK Renal Registry. **www.renalreg.com**. PD: Peritoneal dialysis; HD: Haemodialysis.

Table 12.4 Factors that associate with an increase in renal replacement therapy rates

Factors	Class of effect
Economically developed nation (can afford 'expensive' treatments such as dialysis/transplantation)	Macro-health care system related
Increased acceptance among patients Increased acceptance among doctors offering this complex/onerous treatment	Macro-behaviour related
Ageing population Higher proportion of Asian patients Higher proportion of black patients	Demography of population
↑ Diabetes in population ↑ Hypertension in population ↑ Vascular disease in population	Increased risk factors for development
Reduced deaths from vascular disease Reduced deaths from cancer	Reduced competing risks

are changing. Whilst renal transplantation provides the most cost-effective form of RRT, it is difficult to substantially increase the overall rate of transplantation although some countries, notably Spain, have achieved this with a multifaceted approach (Matesanz *et al.* 1994). Nevertheless, demand for kidney

transplantation has, and will continue, to outstrip supply of donor organs. Although living kidney donors are increasingly being used, the number of deceased donor kidney procedures has fallen over the last 15 years (NHS Blood and Transplant 2012). In addition, many ESRD patients accepted for RRT are not suitable

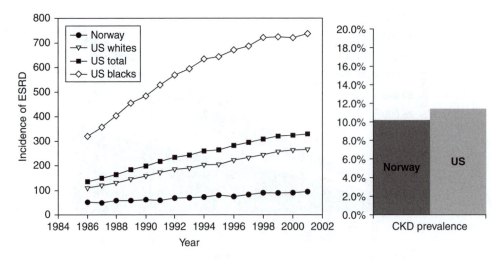

Figure 12.4 Left panel: annual incidence of end-stage renal disease (ESRD) (per million inhabitants) in Norway and the United States from 1986–2002. Note the almost threefold difference of ESRD rates between Norway and US white population. Right panel: prevalence of chronic kidney disease (CKD), the forerunner to ESRD in both countries. Total CKD prevalence in Norway was 10.2 per cent. Reported US CKD prevalence was 11.0 per cent in 1988 to 1994 and 11.7 per cent in 1999 to 2000 and averaged here as 11.4 per cent.

Reproduced from Hallan SI *et al.*, 'International comparison of the relationship of chronic kidney disease and prevalence of ESRD risk.' *Journal of the American Society of Nephrology*, 2006, with permission from the American Society of Nephrology.

for transplantation in view of their multiple medical problems and advanced age. It is currently unusual for renal transplantation to be performed in persons over 70 years of age and since the median age of new dialysis patients across many countries is ~ 65 years of age it is evident that renal transplantation will not be the usual form of RRT for most patients. The majority of ESRD patients will be treated by maintenance chronic dialysis that is often provided as hospital-based haemodialysis; lower cost options such as peritoneal dialysis are also used (Lindholm and Davies 2011) but may be less suitable for some elderly patients with very poor renal function or limited social support.

Survival

The annual mortality for a dialysis population approaches 15–20 per cent which is much higher than for many cancers. This high mortality is usually attributed to the excess cardiovascular risk in patients with CKD. Clustering of 'classic' cardiovascular risk factors such as older age, male gender, hypertension, diabetes, and smoking accounts for some, but not all, of the increased risk. Survival on dialysis is also reduced by advanced age, late referral for dialysis, the type of renal disease,

and the quality of the dialysis delivered. Primary renal diseases such as glomerulonephritis or polycystic kidney disease have a better prognosis than renal failure secondary to diabetic nephropathy or atherosclerotic renal vascular disease even when matched for age at RRT commencement. This demonstrates that comparisons between individual renal units or between countries are difficult to interpret without adjusting for case-mix—the burden of other co-morbid medical problems in addition to the renal failure. Some studies may report all those on dialysis yet these may include young adults with congenital kidney diseases and older persons with diabetes or myeloma as a cause of their renal failure. Such heterogeneity needs to be accounted for in studies using appropriate statistical applications (see Chapter 6, section 6.4).

....

Question 2

Why is the age of patients starting on dialysis in London much younger (approximate median age 55 years old) than the age of those on dialysis in rural Scotland and Northern Ireland (approximate median age 65)?

....

12.4 Prevention of end-stage renal disease

Diabetes is the leading cause of ESRD; in the USA up to 50 per cent of cases are directly attributed to diabetes and up to 40 per cent of cases worldwide (Atkins 2005). Fuelled by the rapid rise in non-communicable disease, overweight and obesity in middle-income, and increasingly in low-income countries, the prevalence of diabetes has risen three- to fivefold in countries such as India, China, Indonesia, and Thailand in the past 25 years (Yoon *et al.* 2006). Fig. 12.5 shows the number of new cases of ESRD attributed to diabetes between 1980 and 2004 in Australia. The manyfold increase in the numbers of patients is almost entirely due to the rise in the numbers of type 2 diabetics. Similar findings have been reported from Japan (Yamagata *et al.* 2008).

The heavy burden and healthcare costs associated with ESRD are likely to be beyond the means of the majority of middle- and low-income countries and cost-effective solutions are urgently required to prevent an epidemic of diabetes associated nephropathy and ESRD. In high-income countries such as the USA the most cost-effective solution was to treat all diabetic patients with ACE-inhibitors at a 1999 cost of US$320 per annum which compares favourably with the very large future costs of transplantation or dialysis (Golan *et al.* 1999). Similar calculations for low- and middle-income

countries suggest a cost of US$1100 for each QALY saved (Dirks *et al.* 2006). This compares to US$11,000 per QALY saved for a transplant, US$71,000 for home dialysis, and US$114,000 for hospital dialysis (costs for the year 2000). Control of the obesity epidemic is both feasible and possible given the necessary political will, and is discussed in further detail in Chapter 9.

Patients with ESRD receiving RRT are at high risk of developing cardiovascular disease, although the mechanism underlying this is uncertain. A recent trial of lipid-lowering in CKD and ESRD patients suggested a significant reduction in risk of a CVD event in CKD patients but not in those with ESRD (Baigent *et al.* 2011).

Web addresses

United Kingdom Renal Registry (2010)
www.renalreg.com
United Kingdom National Health Service Blood and Transplant (2011)
http://www.uktransplant.org.uk/ukt/
United States Renal Data System (2011)
http://www.usrds.org/atlas.aspx

References

Abboud H and Henrich WL (2010) Clinical practice. Stage IV chronic kidney disease. *The New England Journal of Medicine* **362** (1), 56–65.

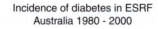
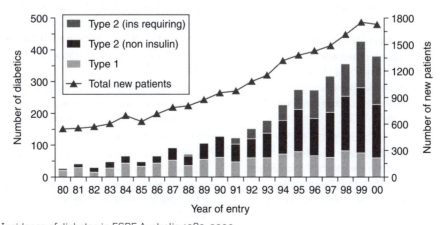

Figure 12.5 Incidence of diabetes in ESRF Australia 1980–2000.

Reproduced with permission from Atkins, R.C. (2005) The epidemiology of chronic kidney disease. *Kidney International*, Supplement. (94), S14–18.

Ali T, Khan I, Simpson W, Prescott G, *et al.* (2007) Incidence and outcomes in acute kidney injury: a comprehensive population-based study. *Journal of the American Society of Nephrology: JASN* **18** (4), 1292–8.

Ali T, Tachibana A, Khan I, Townend J, *et al.* (2011) The changing pattern of referral in acute kidney injury. *QJM: Monthly Journal of the Association of Physicians* **104** (6), 497–503.

Anon (2007) Prevalence of chronic kidney disease and associated risk factors—United States, 1999–2004. *Morbidity and Mortality Weekly Report* **56** (8), 161–5.

Atkins RC (2005) The epidemiology of chronic kidney disease. *Kidney International. Supplement* (**94**), S14–18.

Baigent C, Landray MJ, Reith C, Emberson J, *et al.* (2011) The effects of lowering LDL cholesterol with simvastatin plus ezetimibe in patients with chronic kidney disease (Study of Heart and Renal Protection): a randomized placebo-controlled trial. *Lancet* **377** (9784), 2181–92.

Bellomo R, Ronco C, Kellum JA, Mehta RL, *et al.* (2004) Acute renal failure—definition, outcome measures, animal models, fluid therapy and information technology needs: the Second International Consensus Conference of the Acute Dialysis Quality Initiative (ADQI) Group. *Critical Care* **8** (4), R204–212.

Coca SG, Yusuf B, Shlipak MG, Garg AX, *et al.* (2009) Long-term risk of mortality and other adverse outcomes after acute kidney injury: a systematic review and meta-analysis. *American Journal of Kidney Diseases* **53** (6), 961–73.

Collins AJ, Foley RN, Herzog C, Chavers B, *et al.* (2011) US Renal Data System 2010 Annual Data Report. *American Journal of Kidney Diseases* **57** (1 Suppl 1), A8, e1–526.

Coresh J, Wei GL, McQuillan G, Brancati FL, *et al.* (2001) Prevalence of high blood pressure and elevated serum creatinine level in the United States: findings from the third National Health and Nutrition Examination Survey (1988–1994). *Archives of Internal Medicine* **161** (9), 1207–16.

Coresh J, Astor BC, Greene T, Eknoyan G, *et al.* (2003) Prevalence of chronic kidney disease and decreased kidney function in the adult US population: Third National Health and Nutrition Examination Survey. *American Journal of Kidney Diseases* **41** (1), 1–12.

Coresh J, Astor BC, Greene T, Eknoyan G, *et al.* (2007) Prevalence of chronic kidney disease in the United States. *JAMA* **298** (17), 2038–47.

de Francisco ALM, De la Cruz JJ, Cases A, de la Figuera M, *et al.* (2007) Prevalence of kidney insufficiency in primary care population in Spain: EROCAP study. *Nefrología* **27** (3), 300–12.

Dirks J, Remuzzi G, Horton S, Schieppati A, *et al.* (2006) Diseases of the Kidney and the Urinary System. In: Jamison DT, Breman JG, Measham AR, Alleyne G, *et al.* (eds) *Disease Control Priorities in Developing Countries*, 2nd edn, pp. 695–706. Washington, DC: World Bank/ Oxford University Press.

Drey N, Roderick P, Mullee M, and Rogerson M (2003) A population-based study of the incidence and outcomes of diagnosed chronic kidney disease. *American Journal of Kidney Diseases* **42** (4), 677–84.

Feest TG, Mistry CD, Grimes DS, and Mallick NP (1990) Incidence of advanced chronic renal failure and the need for end stage renal replacement treatment. *BMJ (Clinical Research Ed)* **301** (6757), 897–900.

Feest TG, Rajamahesh J, Byrne C, Ahmad A, *et al.* (2005) Trends in adult renal replacement therapy in the UK: 1982–2002. *QJM: Monthly Journal of the Association of Physicians* **98** (1), 21–8.

Fogarty DG and Taal MW (2011) A stepped care approach to the management of chronic kidney disease. In: Taal MW, Chertow GM, Marsden PA, Skorecki A, *et al.* (eds) *Brenner and Rector's: The Kidney*, 9th edn; pp. 2205–39. Philadelphia: Elsevier.

Foley RN (2010) Temporal trends in the burden of chronic kidney disease in the United States. *Current Opinion in Nephrology and Hypertension* **19** (3), 273–7.

Gilg J, Castledine C, Fogarty D, and Feest T (2011) UK Renal Registry 13th Annual Report (December 2010): Chapter 1: UK RRT incidence in 2009: national and centre-specific analyses. *Nephron. Clinical Practice* **119** Suppl. 2c1–25.

Golan L, Birkmeyer JD, and Welch HG (1999) The cost-effectiveness of treating all patients with type 2 diabetes with angiotensin-converting enzyme inhibitors. *Annals of Internal Medicine* **131** (9), 660–7.

Hallan SI, Coresh J, Astor BC, Asberg A, *et al.* (2006) International comparison of the relationship of chronic kidney disease prevalence and ESRD risk. *Journal of the American Society of Nephrology: JASN* **17** (8), 2275–84.

Hemmelgarn BR, Zhang J, Manns BJ, James MT, *et al.* (2010) Nephrology visits and health care resource use before and after reporting estimated glomerular filtration rate. *JAMA* **303** (12), 1151–8.

Hsu C-C, Hwang S-J, Wen C-P, Chang H-Y, *et al.* (2006) High prevalence and low awareness of CKD in Taiwan: a study on the relationship between serum creatinine and awareness from a nationally representative survey. *American Journal of Kidney Diseases* **48** (5), 727–38.

Hsu C, Chertow GM, McCulloch CE, Fan D, *et al.* (2009) Non-recovery of kidney function and death after acute on chronic renal failure. *Clinical Journal of the American Society of Nephrology: CJASN* **4** (5), 891–8.

John R, Webb M, Young A, and Stevens E (2004) Unreferred chronic kidney disease: a longitudinal study. *American Journal of Kidney Diseases* **43** (5), 825–35.

Kee F, Reaney EA, Maxwell AP, Fogarty DG, *et al.* (2005) Late referral for assessment of renal failure. *Journal of Epidemiology and Community Health* **59** (5), 386–8.

Klag MJ, Whelton PK, Randall BL, Neaton JD, *et al.* (1997) End-stage renal disease in African-American and white men. 16-year MRFIT findings. *JAMA* **277** (16), 1293–8.

Lamping DL, Constantinovici N, Roderick P, Normand C, *et al.* (2000) Clinical outcomes, quality of life, and costs in the North Thames Dialysis Study of elderly people on dialysis: a prospective cohort study. *Lancet* **356** (9241), 1543–50.

Levey AS, Eckardt K-U, Tsukamoto Y, Levin A, *et al.* (2005) Definition and classification of chronic kidney disease: a position statement from Kidney Disease: Improving Global Outcomes (KDIGO). *Kidney International* **67** (6), 2089–100.

Levey AS, Stevens LA, Schmid CH, Zhang YL, *et al.* (2009) A new equation to estimate glomerular filtration rate. *Annals of Internal Medicine* **150** (9), 604–12.

Lindholm B and Davies S (2011) End-stage renal disease in 2010: Timing of dialysis initiation and choice of dialysis modality. *Nature Reviews. Nephrology* **7** (2), 66–8.

Matesanz R, Miranda B, and Felipe C (1994) Organ procurement in Spain: impact of transplant coordination. *Clinical Transplantation* **8** (3 Pt. 1), 281–6.

Mehta RL and Chertow GM (2003) Acute renal failure definitions and classification: time for change? *Journal of the American Society of Nephrology: JASN* **14** (8), 2178–87.

Minutolo R, De Nicola L, Mazzaglia G, Postorino M, *et al.* (2008) Detection and awareness of moderate to advanced CKD by primary care practitioners: a cross-sectional study from Italy. *American Journal of Kidney Diseases* **52** (3), 444–53.

Quinn MP, Cardwell CR, Kee F, Maxwell AP, *et al.* (2011) The finding of reduced estimated glomerular filtration rate is associated with increased mortality in a large UK population. *Nephrology, Dialysis, Transplantation* **26** (3), 875–80.

Richards N, Harris K, Whitfield M, O'Donoghue D, *et al.* (2008) The impact of population-based identification of chronic kidney disease using estimated glomerular filtration rate (eGFR) reporting. *Nephrology, Dialysis, Transplantation* **23** (2), 556–61.

Stack AG (2003) Impact of timing of nephrology referral and pre-ESRD care on mortality risk among new ESRD patients in the United States. *American Journal of Kidney Diseases* **41** (2), 310–18.

Steenkamp R, Castledine C, Feest T, and Fogarty D (2011) UK Renal Registry 13th Annual Report (December 2010): Chapter 2: UK RRT prevalence in 2009: national and centre-specific analyses. *Nephron. Clinical Practice* **119** Suppl. 2c27–52.

Stevens LA, Li S, Wang C, Huang C, *et al.* (2010) Prevalence of CKD and comorbid illness in elderly patients in the United States: results from the Kidney Early Evaluation Program (KEEP). *American Journal of Kidney Diseases* **55** (3 Suppl 2), S23–33.

Stevens PE, O'Donoghue DJ, de Lusignan S, Van Vlymen J, *et al.* (2007) Chronic kidney disease management in the United Kingdom: NEOERICA project results. *Kidney International* **72** (1), 92–9.

Stewart JH, McCredie MRE, and Williams SM (2006) Geographic, ethnic, age-related and temporal variation in the incidence of end-stage renal disease in Europe, Canada and the Asia-Pacific region, 1998–2002. *Nephrology, Dialysis, Transplantation* **21** (8), 2178–83.

Udayaraj U, Ben-Shlomo Y, Roderick P, and Casula A (2010) Social deprivation, ethnicity, and access to the deceased donor kidney transplant waiting list in England and Wales. *Transplantation* **90** (3), 279–85.

USRDS, 30/04/2011, 2011-last update, *U S Renal Data System, USRDS 2010 Annual Data Report: Atlas of Chronic Kidney Disease and End-Stage Renal Disease in the United States, National Institutes of Health, National Institute of Diabetes and Digestive and Kidney Diseases, Bethesda, MD, 2010. Chapter 2 Incidence and Prevalence*. http://www.usrds.org/2010/pdf/v2_02.pdf [Accessed: 30 April 2011].

Weening JJ (2004) Advancing nephrology around the globe: an invitation to contribute. *Journal of the American Society of Nephrology: JASN* **15** (10), 2761–2.

Xue JL, Daniels F, Star RA, Kimmel PL, *et al.* (2006) Incidence and mortality of acute renal failure in Medicare beneficiaries, 1992 to 2001. *Journal of the American Society of Nephrology: JASN* **17** (4), 1135–42.

Yamagata K, Iseki K, Nitta K, Imai H, *et al.* (2008) Chronic kidney disease perspectives in Japan and the importance of urinalysis screening. *Clinical and Experimental Nephrology* **12** (1), 1–8.

Yoon K-H, Lee J-H, Kim J-W, Cho JH, *et al.* (2006) Epidemic obesity and type 2 diabetes in Asia. *Lancet* **368** (9548), 1681–8.

Model answers

Question 1

There will be a substantial increase in the number of patients requiring dialysis due to growth in the number of prevalence cases.

Question 2

Much higher rates of ethnic minorities in London with ~ 20 per cent of some areas being non-white. The average difference in age between white and non-white patients starting dialysis is almost eight years. In addition, there are more deprived areas in inner cities and previous data reveals that this is also associated with younger age of onset of end-stage renal failure (Stewart *et al.* 2006; Udayaraj *et al.* 2010).

13 Neurological diseases

STANLEY HAWKINS, JAMES MORROW, AND JACKIE PARKES

CHAPTER CONTENTS

This chapter deals with the major diseases considered to have a neurological basis in ICD-10 including Parkinson's disease, multiple sclerosis, epilepsy, and cerebral palsy. Dementia and Alzheimer's disease (Chapter 14) and vascular causes of neurological deficit (Chapter 7) are reviewed elsewhere.

Introduction

Neurological diseases are associated with damage to a particular region of the brain or nervous system. This group of diseases can be particularly difficult to diagnose. This poses problems, not only for the clinician, but also for epidemiologists. Difficulty in accurately diagnosing neurological disease hampers **case ascertainment**, thus reducing the robustness of incidence and prevalence data, precluding reliable assessment of secular trends, and reducing confidence in aetiological findings. Estimates of disease occurrence have been made for the wealthier countries, where patients and their families have full access to neurological services, the best estimates coming from large prospective studies. Available data are summarized in Table 13.1. In developing countries the problem is even more acute, because even death certification of neurological diseases is unreliable, and these diseases are therefore very under-researched outside industrial nations.

At least six per cent of the population have a neurological disorder in their lifetime, and the prevalence of the disorders discussed in this chapter together exceed the lifetime prevalence rate for completed stroke (Table 13.1). Both cerebral palsy and multiple sclerosis contribute more strongly towards **disability-adjusted life-years (DALYs)** because of their earlier ages of onset. Epilepsy is the commonest neurological disorder but, unlike other significant neurological disease, may remit completely in some patients. We look first at Parkinson's disease, the commonest of the movement disorders.

13.1 Parkinson's disease

In his 1817 monograph *The Shaking Palsy*, James Parkinson described the major features of the illness that now bears his name from his observation of patients in London. The pathology of Parkinson's disease begins on one side of the brain, principally in the basal ganglia, producing clinical manifestations in the contralateral limbs. The pathological hallmark of the condition is the loss of pigmented dopaminergic neurons in the substantia nigra with associated eosinophilic, cytoplasmic inclusions called Lewy bodies in the surviving neurons. The deficiency of dopamine in the brain, first described by Hornykiewicz in

Table 13.1 Epidemiological indicators for neurological diseases

Disease	Incidence rate (age and sex adjusted per 100,000 per year)	Lifetime prevalence per 1000
Parkinson's disease	19	2
Multiple sclerosis	7	2
Epilepsy	46	4
Cerebral palsy	3	3
Stroke	205	9

Reproduced from MacDonald BK, Cockerell OC, Sander JW, and Shorvon SD (2000) 'The Incidence and Lifetime Prevalence of Neurological Disorders in a Prospective Community-Based Study in the UK'. *Brain* **123** (4), 665–76, with permission from Oxford University Press.

1959, led to the therapeutic use of levodopa (L-dopa) and dopamine agonists that act directly on dopamine receptors within the brain, which today are the mainstays of the treatment of Parkinson's disease. Indeed, it is considered that if a patient has a response to L-dopa he or she is more likely to have classical (idiopathic) Parkinson's disease, the commonest form of the disease.

Parkinson's disease is the next most important neurological disease associated with ageing after dementia (see Chapter 14) and, in common with this condition, is set to increase worldwide as populations begin to age.

Diagnosis and clinical course

Parkinson's disease is the clinical syndrome of involuntary asymmetrical tremor (a rhythmic oscillation of one or more body parts) associated with poverty and slowness of movement (bradykinesia), cogwheel rigidity, and postural gait changes. Despite almost two centuries of research into this disease, the diagnosis is still based on clinical examination. Parkinsonism or 'secondary Parkinsonism' relates to a syndrome of many conditions similar to Parkinson's disease except that these conditions have an identifiable cause, such as neuroleptic drugs or carbon monoxide exposure; usually they have a more severe disease course, which may be manifested as early gait disorder. Falls tend to occur within the first year; urinary incontinence,

orthostatic hypotension, dysarthia, or dementia are likely to follow within the first four years (Samii *et al.* 2004). In a community-based series, idiopathic Parkinson's disease accounted for 75–80 per cent of all Parkinsonian syndromes with a prevalence of about 360 per 100,000 (Tanner and Ben-Shlomo 1999). Several other degenerative brain diseases can produce manifestations of atypical Parkinsonism, including multiple system atrophy, progressive supranuclear palsy, corticobasal degeneration, and dementia with Lewy bodies.

As there is no diagnostic test, with autopsy remaining the best reference for diagnosis, it is important to determine the accuracy of clinical diagnosis (Rao *et al.* 2003). It has been shown that even practising neurologists cannot always distinguish between different forms of Parkinsonism. One hundred cases accumulated in the Parkinson's Brain Bank in London showed that only 75 per cent of Parkinsonian syndromes conformed pathologically to a diagnosis of idiopathic Parkinson's disease. The remaining cases had alternative pathologies, so cases confidently diagnosed by competent consultant neurologists were found to have atypical pathology. However, using more modern methods, the accuracy was recently reported to be 90 per cent (Hughes *et al.* 2002).

Inevitably, there is thus strong motivation to find biomarkers that reflect pathological change and response to treatment. Clinical, imaging, biochemical and genetic factors are being actively sought; probably

Box 13.1 Characteristics of the ideal biomarker that is designed to reflect a change in pathological or clinical trait X

- Close (first-degree) association with X without relying on intermediate variables, thereby minimizing the risk of dissociation.
- It must sensitively reflect even small changes in X.
- Treatment has no direct effect on the biomarker; it only changes with a true change in X.
- The biomarker changes linearly (either negatively or positively) in response to a change in X.
- Measurements are reproducible at a different time or in a different centre.

- The biomarker should ideally capture all changes in X so that no information is lost.
- The optimal clinical biomarker should be cheap, non-invasive, and quick to measure by untrained staff.
- Appropriately thorough validation of the listed criteria (depends on the use of the biomarker and implications of error).

Michell AW, Lewis SJG, Foltynie T, and Barker RA. (2004). 'Biomarkers and Parkinson's Disease'. *Brain* **127**, 1693–705.

a combination of several biomarkers will be needed, the likelihood being that none will fulfil all the criteria listed in Box 13.1 (Michell *et al.* 2004).

Descriptive epidemiology

Parkinson's disease is a disease of ageing. Incidence is very low before age 50 years (less than 10 per 100,000 population), and is usually associated with a hereditary form of Parkinsonism after which there is a gradual increase in incidence rising steeply after the age of 60 years, and increasing to at least 200 per 100,000 at age 80 years (Tanner and Ben Shlomo 1999). Prevalence is somewhat higher. In the USA, crude prevalence of Parkinson's disease for all ages is approximately 150 per 100,000, ranging from 30 per 100 000 in those younger than 50 years to 800 per 100,000 in 75- to 80-year-olds. It has generally been reported that mortality is higher in Parkinsonian patients than in the general population and this appears to be mainly due to the increased risk of dementia, which is two to six times higher in Parkinson disease patients (de Lau and Breteler 2006). Twentyfold worldwide variation in risk of Parkinson's disease has been reported, but whether this indicates genetic or environmental factors is not clear. Men have approximately twice the incidence and prevalence of Parkinson's disease as women. In a Finnish study, there was no difference in relative risk in men compared with women in 1971 but 20 years later men had an almost twofold greater risk, suggesting a possible environmental causative factor to which men may be more exposed or are more susceptible than women.

Aetiology

The 1917–18 influenza pandemic probably caused *encephalitis lethargica*—characterized by high fever, headache, double vision, delayed physical, and mental response, and lethargy—which led to a severe form of Parkinsonism; more recent studies have failed to link infectious agents with Parkinsonism. In the 1980s a proportion of narcotics abusers on the west coast of the USA developed a severe L-dopa responsive form of Parkinson's disease after contaminated injections with a mitochondrial protoxin. Subsequent studies then indicated that certain pesticides like paraquat and rotenone, which had similar activity, can reproduce the pathology of Parkinson's disease in animals, and a recent meta-analysis in human studies suggested an odds ratio of 1.9 (95% CI 1.5–2.5) for pesticide exposure in Parkinsonian disease (Priyadarshi *et al.* 2000). A recent study in California in agricultural workers found that combined exposure to three agents (ziram, maneb, and paraquat) increased risk of Parkinson's disease threefold (Wang *et al.* 2011).

People who have smoked cigarettes are less likely to develop Parkinson's disease. The inverse dose–response association with smoking—heavier smokers having lower risk than lighter smokers—has been a consistent aetiological finding in both retrospective and prospective studies (Fratiglioni and Wang 2000). Earlier case-control studies suggested a lower risk in people who have high dietary intake of vitamin C and/ or antioxidants. More recent prospective cohort studies have been inconclusive (de Lau and Breteler 2006).

Question 1

What explanations could there be for the negative association between smoking and risk of Parkinson's disease?

Genetic factors

Recently, pedigrees of dominantly inherited 'Parkinson's disease' were reported, which were identified to be idiopathic Parkinson's. The genes associated with these pedigrees are called 'Park' genes and at least twelve have been described (de Lau and Breteler 2006). The product of these genes, α-synuclein, is a major protein component of Lewy bodies. It is hypothesized that the pathogenesis of Parkinson's disease involves the abnormal folding, aggregation, and deposition of α-synuclein as key steps in mediating neuronal dysfunction and degeneration, and that certain mutations may predispose to this.

As the population ages, Parkinson's disease is set to become more common. The challenge of making a valid diagnosis is probably largely responsible for the paucity of population-based studies providing accurate data about incidence, prevalence, and mortality. If adequate biomarkers can be uncovered, diagnostic reliability will improve leading to better studies which, with developing genetic insights, will allow wider scope for treatment and prevention of this important disorder.

13.2 Multiple sclerosis

Multiple sclerosis is the commonest disabling neurological disease in young Caucasian adults, and is second only to trauma as the leading cause of acquired neurological disability. Worldwide there are around 2.5 million affected individuals. Annual health expenditure on this disease in the UK is approximately £1.2 billion including indirect costs such as loss of earnings, child care, and similar expenditure.

This is a chronic inflammatory disease of the central nervous system, characterized by large multiple focal areas of *demyelination*, and is so called because multiple areas of sclerosis (hardening) are observed at autopsy. The first evidence of pathology is a breakdown of the blood–brain barrier, which allows activated lymphocytes to leak into the brain, leading to inflammation and loss of myelin surrounding the axons of neurons (Compston and Coles 2008). These lesions, or plaques, vary in age and are distributed throughout the central nervous system from the cerebrum through the length of the spinal cord, corresponding to the scattering of clinical symptoms in time and space. They were first noted in 1865 by the French neurologist Charcot. There is limited capacity for remyelination and, as the disease progresses over time, repeated episodes of inflammation and demyelination lead to loss of nerve cells and fibres, frequently culminating in severe disability. Although the pathological basis for these changes is unknown, the pattern is similar to that in autoimmune disorders.

Disease description and clinical course

The clinical course is characterized by episodes of variable activity called relapses, separated by remissions or periods of quiescence. Symptoms vary both between and within individuals, reflecting the functional anatomy of impaired axonal conduction at affected sites, and include limb weakness, disturbed vision, sensory loss or imbalance, bladder and bowel incontinence, pain, and fatigue; cognitive disturbance is observed in up to 65 per cent of patients. The course is heterogeneous but two major subtypes are generally recognized: *relapsing-remitting*, seen in around 85 per cent of cases and *primary progressive* in the remainder. In the former there are usually phases of relapse with recovery, with gradually poorer recovery and accumulating residual deficit, culminating in *secondary progressive* disease in which, after about 15–20 years, there is increasing disability without any clear clinical relapses. For a proportion of relapsing–remitting patients the disease runs a *benign* course with full recovery between episodes and no significant disability up to 15 years after disease onset, although, even here, sufficient follow-up usually reveals disabling disease. About five per cent of patients have very rapid progression of disability, and this is labelled *acute* or the *Marburg variant*.

Diagnosis

Because no single clinical feature or test is sufficient for the diagnosis of multiple sclerosis, diagnostic criteria have included a combination of clinical and paraclinical studies. Revised diagnostic criteria incorporating evidence from magnetic resonance imaging classify individuals into three categories: (i) multiple sclerosis, for which a minimum of two attacks affecting more than one anatomical site are required; (ii) possible multiple sclerosis; and (iii) not multiple sclerosis (McDonald *et al.* 2001; Polman *et al.* 2011).

Descriptive epidemiology

Accurately estimating the prevalence and incidence is not straightforward. Incidence and prevalence figures have largely been derived from cross-sectional surveys, yielding incidence rates of around one to ten per 100,000 person-years and prevalences of 120–200 per 100,000. It appears that the prevalence is increasing worldwide (Benito-Leon 2011), probably in part due to increasing incidence, earlier diagnosis, and improved survival due to better management. Several studies have shown that multiple sclerosis is associated with an elevated risk of death. In a large study of patients from the Danish multiple sclerosis registry, the median survival time from onset was ten years shorter for multiple sclerosis patients than for the age-matched general population, representing a threefold increase in the risk of death. More than half died from the disease itself, but excess mortality was also observed for several other diseases, and from accidents and suicide (Brønnum-Hansen *et al.* 2004).

....

Question 2

Why is the prevalence of multiple sclerosis up to 500 times higher than disease incidence?
....

Greater precision in measuring disease burden can be gained from prospective studies. In the Danish registry, operating since 1948, nearly all Danish residents in whom the disease was diagnosed by a neurologist have been registered, and the diagnosis has been reviewed and classified, according to standardized diagnostic criteria, with overall diagnostic accuracy and completeness estimated at 94 per cent and 90 per cent, respectively. A UK study using capture-recapture techniques (see Chapter 2) demonstrated that the north-south gradient in the prevalence of multiple sclerosis was not an artefactual finding (Forbes and Swingler 1999). A recent study from Portugal suggested that prevalence figures may be overestimated if crude prevalence figures are used unadjusted for age and delay in diagnosis (de Sá *et al.* 2012).

Aetiology and risk factors

The cause of multiple sclerosis is unknown but it is clear that both environmental and genetic factors are involved. Significant geographical and ethnic differences in occurrence are observed. Among Eskimos, the Aboriginals of Australia, and the Bantu people of Southern Africa the disease is virtually unknown; and in Indians, Chinese, and Japanese the distribution of lesions is different to that in people of European ancestry. These findings cannot be explained on the basis of population genetics alone. Outside Europe, prevalence rates among white people are half those documented for many parts of northern Europe. It has been suggested that adult immigrants retain the risk factor of their country of origin, whereas their children tend towards the risk factor of their host country. The hypothesis that an environmental factor acquired in childhood conveys a risk of developing multiple sclerosis in later life is supported by two *migrant* studies: firstly, there is a low, second-generation risk in emigrants from high-risk countries such as the UK to South Africa; and secondly, that immigrants to the UK from areas of low risk (for example, West Indies) have a low prevalence, but their British-born children have the same high prevalence as British Caucasians. Migrant studies and their methodological limitations have been reviewed in detail elsewhere (Gale and Martyn 1995).

Recently sunlight and sunlight exposure have been studied in detail. There have been several interesting observations: the prevalence of multiple sclerosis in French agricultural workers is associated with the change of sunlight exposure from north to south of France, relapses are more common in spring than autumn in the northern and southern hemispheres, and the risk of developing the disease is greater in infants born in the spring. The hypothesis is that since vitamin D is synthesized in the skin as a consequence of exposure to ultraviolet light, vitamin D deficiency can predispose to this disorder and possibly modulate its clinical course. But there are a number of issues unexplained by epidemiological studies conducted to date (Ascherio *et al.* 2010) and interventional studies using vitamin D supplementation are being planned in Canada and in Europe.

The *clusters* of the disease observed in several isolated populations, most notably the Faroe Islands, are considered by some to point to evidence for a transmissible agent, as the epidemic occurred after the occupation by British troops between 1941 and 1944. It has been hypothesized that exposure to ubiquitous infectious agents may trigger the immune system to react against the brain; possible candidates include: *Chlamydia pneumoniae*, human herpes virus 6, measles, herpes simplex, HSV-6, and Epstein–Barr virus (EBV). A recent review reported that multiple sclerosis was more than 10 times greater in EBV-positive individuals than in those who were EBV-negative (Ascherio and Munger 2010), although 90 per cent of the world's population is infected with EBV (Pohl 2009). Noninfectious agents may also be implicated in disease risk or modulation, but evidence for a role for smoking or low antioxidant levels is weak or conflicting.

Increased disease risk is seen within families; risk is highest in identical monozygotic (MZ) twins (20–35 per cent), then dizygotic (DZ) twins and other siblings (2–5 per cent), then parents, and finally first cousins, whereas the frequency in adoptees is similar to that in the general population. If multiple sclerosis showed simple Mendelian inheritance, the risk in MZ twins would be close to unity, but as this is not so it indicates that multiple sclerosis is a complex trait in which susceptibility is determined by several genes acting independently (*epistatically*). In common with most other complex traits, no major susceptibility gene has been identified, but regions of interest have been provisionally identified. Multiple sclerosis affects twice as many women as it does men, mimicking the ratio seen in other putative autoimmune diseases. The lifetime risk for a young woman in Northern Ireland or Scotland of developing the disease is about one in 130 (Gray *et al.* 2008). Susceptibility seems to be conferred by genes within the major histocompatibility complex, although recent studies indicate that other loci are also involved and a possible role for cell-mediated immune mechanisms (Sawcer *et al.* 2011). The relative rarity of multiple sclerosis, and the complexities and heterogeneity of the disorder, suggest that large studies and pooled data from several investigations will be required to properly elucidate its genetic nature. Along with these, advances in technology are likely to make genetic studies more fruitful. Nevertheless, multiple sclerosis presents major obstacles for both patient and researcher, and there is much to understand before preventive and therapeutic modalities can be designed.

Therapy

There have been considerable recent advances in the treatment of multiple sclerosis. In particular, interferon-beta has been demonstrated in several independent, multicentre clinical trials to lower unequivocally the biological activity of relapsing-remitting and secondary progressive disease, and of clinically isolated syndromes. The results of these trials have been consistent, demonstrating a reduction in both disease activity and cumulative disability, using a combination of clinical MRI outcome measures and, more recently, measures of brain atrophy (Miller 2004). On balance, convincing evidence is provided to support the notion that there is a clinically relevant dose–response in the use of interferon-beta to treat patients with relapsing/remitting disease, although this remains an active area of current research. Natalizumab, a humanized monoclonal antibody against activated lymphocyte trafficking through the brain is recommended for very active relapsing-remitting disease, and new therapies are under development.

....

Question 3

You have resources to set up a register for multiple sclerosis. What factors are important to maximize the potential of the register?

....

13.3 Epilepsy

The term *epilepsy* encompasses several syndromes whose cardinal feature is a predisposition to recurrent unprovoked seizures. Although epilepsy is the most common serious neurological condition, affecting 40 million people worldwide, its epidemiology remains poorly understood. Various factors contribute to this deficiency; differences in inclusion criteria can elevate (for example, inclusion of febrile seizures) or deflate (exclusion of non-active epilepsies) prevalence figures, cases ascertained using hospital records may underestimate true community levels, while coding errors also lead to inaccuracies.

Definition and classification of epilepsy

An epileptic *seizure* is an intermittent, stereotyped disturbance of behaviour, emotion, motor function, or sensation accompanied by an abnormal cortical neuronal discharge, which may lead to altered consciousness. Anyone can have a seizure if the circumstances are appropriate, and triggers such as hormonal changes, stress, or fever may provoke onset. Those with a low seizure threshold are more at risk of developing epilepsy. An isolated seizure does not necessarily warrant the diagnosis of epilepsy, which is specifically defined as a disorder in which the individual has a tendency to experience spontaneous and *recurrent* seizures. For most epidemiological studies, two unprovoked seizures on separate occasions are necessary to define the disease (Hauser *et al*. 1998). For many patients, epilepsy is relatively short-lived, over two-thirds entering early remission, after which relapse is uncommon.

Essential for epidemiological investigation, accurate *classification* of seizures is also required to ensure appropriate management (Panayiotopoulos 2005). Unfortunately, this is not straightforward. The most widely used classification, developed by the International League Against Epilepsy, and recently revised, takes account of the clinical manifestations of a seizure, which depend on where in the brain the discharge originates and spreads. The two main types are: (primary) *generalized* in which both cerebral hemispheres are affected simultaneously, usually resulting in loss of consciousness and motor or sensory symptoms, and *partial* (or focal) affecting only part of the brain, sometimes without impaired consciousness. *Secondary generalized* seizures are partial seizures that spread to become generalized. Electroencephalograph (EEG) recordings may assist the clinical classification as different seizure types are usually accompanied by characteristic EEG changes. However, *inter-ictal* EEGs (between attacks) tend to be of limited value.

It is recognized that, even in tertiary epilepsy centres, it may not be possible to clinically classify up to 20 per cent of epilepsy or seizure types (Seino 2006).

....

Question 4

(a) Accurate case definition is an essential part of epidemiology, but diagnosing seizure may not be straightforward. What other conditions may be confused with seizure?

(b) Apart from drug toxicity what other *personal* issues would arise from being (mis)diagnosed with epilepsy?

....

Descriptive epidemiology

A meta-analysis of incidence studies of epilepsy reported an overall incidence rate (omitting febrile and single convulsions) of around five per 100,000 per year (Kotsopoulos *et al*. 2002). In the 1958 UK national child development study cohort, based on over 17,000 children born in March 1958, the cumulative incidence of confirmed epilepsy was 8.4 per 1000 by the age of 23 years, with an active prevalence of 6.3 per 1000. Lifetime prevalence has been estimated at two to five per cent, far in excess of the active prevalence of 6–10 cases per 1000, confirming the self-limiting nature of most seizures. Of the approximately 160,000 people in the UK with active epilepsy, around 25,000 have more than one major seizure per month, and over double this number have a similar rate of minor attacks. Up to 20,000 have advanced disease with attendant handicaps that may necessitate institutional care. Risk at birth is about one per cent until the age of 20 years, rising to three per cent by the age of 75 years (cumulative incidence). Summary descriptive data by age are shown in Fig. 13.1.

Individuals with epilepsy are known to have greater risk of death than the general population, particularly among the young and in the first five to ten years after diagnosis. The UK National General Practice Study of Epilepsy, a prospective, population-based study of people with newly diagnosed epilepsy, estimated that life expectancy can be reduced by up to two years for people with a diagnosis of idiopathic/cryptogenic epilepsy, and the reduction can be up to ten years in people with symptomatic epilepsy. Reductions in life expectancy are highest at the time of diagnosis and diminish with time (Gaitatzis and Sander 2004). After 1950, epilepsy mortality declined steeply in people younger than age 20 years. For young and middle-aged adults, the rate of decline was lower, whereas in people aged 65 years and over, mortality initially declined but rose again from 1974 onwards. There was general evidence of a fall in epilepsy mortality with each successive birth cohort after 1905, in parallel with improvements in antenatal care and perinatal mortality (O'Callaghan *et al.* 2000).

Aetiology and risk factors

Onset of epilepsy is age-related, with many seizures occurring in infancy and childhood, but the incidence is also high in later life (see Fig. 13.1); there is also

an upward secular trend in epilepsy among individuals aged 60 years and above, probably because of an ageing population with longer life expectancy and increased risk of diseases such as stroke. A 34 per cent increase in the proportion of incidence cases in those aged 65 years or more between 1985 and 1994 has been described in the Rochester, Minnesota, population.

Environmental factors

In many cases of epilepsy no specific cause can be found (idiopathic or cryptogenic epilepsy), but this number is decreasing in favour of the symptomatic epilepsies with the use of high-resolution MRI which may demonstrate structural cortical lesions previously undetected by a computed tomography brain scan or even first-generation MRI scanners (Panayiotopoulos 2005).

A national UK study found the following aetiologies: cerebrovascular disease (15 per cent), cerebral tumours (six per cent), alcohol (six per cent), trauma (two per cent), developmental (eight per cent); any other causes, including specific epilepsy syndromes, were rare. However, age of diagnosis was very important in determining cause, with epilepsy in children largely due to developmental conditions, infections, and, to a lesser extent, trauma. In young adults, trauma was the major risk, whereas in middle age, trauma and tumour accounted for the bulk of disease, with cerebrovascular aetiology becoming steadily more important with advancing age. In this latter group, degenerative conditions also led to epilepsy.

Febrile convulsions in infancy, particularly complex febrile convulsions, are associated with subsequent risk of epilepsy in cohort studies, and a recent community-based study reported a twofold increase in risk of epilepsy in the most socio-economically deprived fifth of the population in a UK region (Heaney *et al.* 2002). These latter findings suggest associations with birth defects, trauma, infection, and poor nutrition, which are known to be more common in non-affluent populations.

Brain injury accounts for approximately 13 per cent of epilepsy of presumed cause; the severity of the injury is directly related to the subsequent incidence of epilepsy, and the period of risk appears extend to up to 20

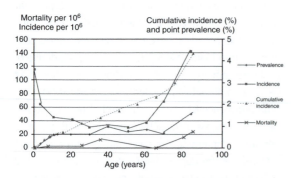

Figure 13.1 Epidemiological indicators for epilepsy by age in population-based studies in Rochester, Minnesota. Adapted from Annegers, J. F. (2004). 'Epilepsy', in L. M. Nelson. C. M. Tanner, S. K. Van Den Eeden, and V. M. McGuire, (eds.), *Neuroepidemiology. From Principles to Practice*, with permission from Mayo Clinic Proceedings.

years after the insult (Annegers *et al.* 1998). A shorter period of risk follows bacterial meningitis of up to five years, with a fivefold increase in risk. Viral encephalitis carries a tenfold increase in risk and the period of risk is again 15 or more years. Taken together, all brain infections are believed to account for up to five per cent of epilepsy cases. Cerebrovascular disease is the major cause of seizures in the elderly, but there are few valid data on the magnitude of the effect or its duration. Seizures occurring for the first time in late life, without a predisposing cause, may indicate increased risk of stroke (Cleary *et al.* 2004). Brain tumours account for around 12 per cent of acquired epilepsy, with risk being greatest in 25–64-year-olds. Almost one-third of individuals with newly diagnosed brain tumours develop seizures. Developmental and degenerative diseases also increase the risk of epilepsy.

Genetic factors

Although seizure disorders aggregate in families, there are very few Mendelian seizure disorders. On the other hand, mutations in over 70 genes now define biological pathways leading to epilepsy, and the list of genes will certainly expand (Noebels 2003). Better understanding of the molecular and cellular circumstances that predispose to seizure could have implications for prevention and development of more effective anticonvulsive treatments, possibly including gene therapies. An unresolved puzzle is why risk is higher in children whose mother has epilepsy rather than the father. At least 12 forms of epilepsy have been demonstrated to possess some genetic basis. For example, LaFora disease (progressive myoclonic, type 2), an autosomal recessive disorder and a particularly aggressive epilepsy, is characterized by the presence of glycogen-like Lafor bodies in the brain.

Treatment and prevention

Although a novel (medical or surgical) treatment option for epilepsy was marketed almost every year during the past decade, many patients still experience uncontrolled seizures or have adverse effects (Nguyen and Spencer 2003). Treatment effectiveness can be monitored by seizure diaries, and quality of life scales have also been designed for people with epilepsy.

Epilepsy raises additional problems in women of childbearing years; female hormones can influence seizure control and drug treatments can affect hormonal contraception, fertility, and the developing embryo. Previous studies have shown an increased risk of major congenital malformations (neural tube defects in particular) from prenatal exposure to sodium valproate and carbamazepine. As folate has been shown to protect against neural tube defects in the general population extrapolations have been made to the epilepsy population and folate supplementation is now recommended for all female patients with epilepsy contemplating pregnancy of childbearing age who are taking these drugs. However, recent studies have cast doubt on the additional protective value of this supplementation in this population (Morrow *et al.* 2009) and suggested that the defects may be due alternate mechanisms. Teratogenic effects of current and newer drugs and possible effects on cognitive and behavioural development of the offspring are increasingly being explored. A UK and Ireland register of women who take epilepsy drugs during pregnancy has been established. This register has shown differences in teratogenic risk associated with individual antiepileptic drugs taken throughout pregnancy, with the highest risks associated with sodium valproate (Morrow *et al.* 2006). Similar initiatives have been established in the USA and Europe. More recently there has been concern not only of drug links to structural defects but also to neurocognitive and neurodevelopmental delay (Meador *et al.* 2009).

In the UK and in the USA there has been a decline in mortality from epilepsy (O'Callaghan *et al.* 2000), but maternal mortality rates in women with epilepsy remain unchanged. This is possibly because of increased maternal awareness of the teratogenic potential of the antiepileptic drugs leading to non-compliance but may also be due to changing clearance rates during pregnancy in those drugs deemed 'safer' to the fetus (Cantwell *et al.* 2011).

Epilepsy can perhaps be best viewed as a heterogeneous disorder with different aetiologies in the young and in the elderly and consequently requiring differing strategies towards prevention.

······························
Question 5

Table 13.2 shows mortality data from community-based studies of epilepsy. Why do you think there is such disparity in the risks of death?
······························

13.4 Cerebral palsy

Introduction

Cerebral palsy is a disorder of voluntary movement and posture caused by damage to the developing brain affecting 2–2.5 per 1000 of the population in the developed and developing world (Odding et al. 2006). It is the commonest cause of motor impairment in childhood and is often associated with other impairments affecting intellect, vision, hearing, communication, behaviour, and can include seizure disorders. As might be expected, those with the more severe and complex forms of cerebral palsy are at higher risk of early mortality, although developments in medical care, for example, artificial feeding, antibiotics, and respiratory management, have increased life expectancy. Consequently, an estimated 85 per cent or more of people

with cerebral palsy survive to age 20 years, and this has implications for health and social services provision as well as medico-legal settlements (Hemming et al. 2006).

Definition

The term *cerebral palsy* is considered an umbrella term for a collection of disorders affecting voluntary movement and posture resulting in loss of motor function. Cerebral palsy is generally caused by lesion/s or malformation/s in the developing brain occurring some time during pregnancy, delivery, or in the neonatal period and is sometimes referred to as 'early impairment' or 'congenital' cerebral palsy. With developments in MRI it is estimated that most cases (80 per cent) have observable neuropathology, the most common being white matter lesions (about 50 per cent), followed by grey matter and deep cortical lesions (20 per cent), with brain malformations comprising less than 10 per cent (Bax et al. 2006). While the brain-based problem is non-progressive, the clinical presentation of cerebral palsy can change over time as a result of growth and maturation, sometimes leading to improved function, but at other times giving rise to complications such as

Table 13.2 Community-based studies of all-cause mortality in epilepsy

Study setting	Methods	Follow-up	Age	SMR* (95% CI)
Rochester Minnesota, USA	Retrospective incidence cohort	34 years	All	2.1 (1.9–2.5)
UK	Prospective incidence cohort	14 years	All	2.1 (1.8–2.4)
Iceland	Retrospective incidence cohort	30 years	All	1.6 (1.2–2.2)
Sweden	Prospective incidence cohort	11 years	All?	2.5 (1.6–3.8)
France	Prospective incidence cohort	1 year	All	9.4 (8–11)
Switzerland	Retrospective incidence cohort	10 years	All	7.0 (6.2–8.4)
Wales	Retrospective incidence cohort	6 years	All	2.1 (1.7–2.6)
Canada	Retrospective incidence cohort	15 years	Children 1 month–6 years	8.8 (4.1–13.4)

*SMR: standard mortality ratio.
Adapted from Gaitatzis A and Sander JW (2004) 'The Mortality of Epilepsy Revisited'. *Epileptic Disorders* **6**, 3–13.

muscle contractures, bony deformities, and deteriorating abilities. Cerebral palsy can also occur after the neonatal period in early childhood and has been referred to as 'late impairment' or 'post-neonatal' cerebral palsy. This subgroup accounts for an estimated 7–14 per cent of all cases and, from an aetiological perspective, represents a distinct group with childhood infections, trauma, surgical complications, and non-accidental injury as the main causes.

Clinical presentation

There are three main cerebral palsy subtypes. In the context of 'early impairment cerebral palsy', spastic subtypes are the commonest affecting about 80–85 per cent of cases, and present with velocity-related increased muscle tone in one or more limbs—called bilateral spastic cerebral palsy where both sides of the body are affected; and unilateral cerebral palsy where only side of the body is affected. Spastic cerebral palsy is associated with damage to the motor cortex and internal capsule of the brain. Dyskinetic cerebral palsy (fewer than 10 per cent of early impairment cases) presents with slow, writhing, and involuntary movements, with fluctuating tone and total body involvement due to damage in the basal ganglia. Ataxic cerebral palsy (fewer than five per cent of early impairment cases) presents as short and jerky movements with low tone, and is associated with damage to the cerebellum. It is also possible to have 'mixed' subtypes (for example spastic-dyskinetic or spastic-ataxic), where there is increased tone, usually in the legs, accompanied by slow and writhing, or short and jerky, movements as a result of damage to the pyramidal and extrapyramidal structures of the brain.

Aetiology

The following discussion is confined to early impairment cerebral palsy. The precise causes of cerebral palsy are unknown and the opportunities for primary prevention remain limited (Nelson 2003). This is because the timing of adverse events during fetal and infant development is difficult to assign, and is also associated with many possible biological factors (MacLennan et al. 1999). However, it is important to distinguish between those born at term (37+ weeks), which constitute approximately half of all cases of cerebral palsy affecting one per 1000 live births, those born preterm (less than 37 weeks), and very prematurely (less than 32 weeks). These scenarios represent different causal pathways in cerebral palsy (Stanley et al. 2000). For example, more than 75 per cent of cerebral palsy in term infants is believed to be of prenatal origin and related more to cerebral malformations, intrauterine infection, or placental insufficiency, whereas fewer than 10 per cent are related to possible intrapartum events, of which suboptimal care is only one possibility (Krägeloh-Mann and Cans 2009). Evidence to support prenatal aetiology includes an excess of congenital malformations and growth restriction among infants with cerebral palsy born at term when compared with the unaffected population. Most cerebral palsy in preterm babies (75–90 per cent) is believed to be of perinatal origin. Evidence to support this includes abnormal brain scans taken in the first week of life in infants who subsequently develop cerebral palsy.

The preterm brain is prone to damage of the white matter caused by bleeding and ischaemia due to inadequate regulation of cerebral blood flow. These complications can span the antenatal, intrapartum, and post-natal periods, but in preterm babies most complications are thought to occur post-natally (Stanley et al. 2000). The periventricular region of the brain is particularly vulnerable to fluctuations in perfusion during weeks 26–36 of development (Hagberg et al. 1993). This contrasts with the brain of babies born at term, where regulation of the cardiovascular system is well established, but the brain's oxygen requirements are greater. At term, several areas of the brain are particularly sensitive to the effects of asphyxia and oxygen deprivation; these include the cortical and subcortical areas, the basal ganglia, and thalamus.

Risk factors

It is well established that birthweight and gestational age are strongly and inversely associated with the risk for cerebral palsy. Although gestational age is the single, strongest determinant of cerebral palsy

(Stanley *et al.* 2000), birthweight-specific rates are most often cited in epidemiological studies. Birthweight is used as a proxy for gestational age (or maturity) as it is easier to measure and more readily available. Fig. 13.2 shows the relation between birthweight and cerebral palsy. These data are from the geographically defined case register, the Northern Ireland Cerebral Palsy Register, and comprise 893 early impairment cases born during 1981–97 when there was a total of 412,256 live births, giving an overall prevalence of 2.2 (95 % CI 2.0–2.3) per 1000 live births (Parkes *et al.* 2005).

....

Question 6

The risk of cerebral palsy increases with decreasing birthweight. Why then in Fig. 13.2 is the rate of cerebral palsy among those born 1000–1499 g greater than those born less than 1000 g?
....

Birthweight and gestation have independent effects on the risk of cerebral palsy and represent the scenarios of being born too small and/or too soon. The relative risk of cerebral palsy among babies born very prematurely (less than 32 weeks) is up to 100 times greater than risk in those born at term (37+ weeks). The risk of cerebral palsy among babies born very small (less than 1500 g) is about 70 times greater

than that in those of normal birthweight (2500 g+). These higher risks are particularly evident if the rate of cerebral palsy is expressed per neonatal survivors and not live births. This is because mortality is highest among the smallest and most premature infants (up to 50 per cent for the most extreme groups). Rates based on neonatal survivors tend to be higher than rates based on live births as the population 'at risk' has been depleted. However, the attributable risk of very premature and small babies developing cerebral palsy is small, as these births constitute only about one per cent of all live births in developed countries.

The risk of cerebral palsy also increases when the weight for gestational age is well above the norm (large for gestational age) or below the norm (small for gestational age) (Jarvis *et al.* 2003). The risk increases tenfold in the case of babies who are small for gestational age, although this increase mainly affects those born at term (37+ weeks) or moderately preterm (32–37 weeks) but not the premature (less than 32 weeks). Antibiotic treatment for spontaneous preterm labour appears to be associated with increased risk of cerebral palsy (Marlow *et al.* 2012).

Another important risk factor for cerebral palsy is multiple birth, mainly related to the higher rate of premature birth among this group. Twins (who represent around two per cent of all births) constitute about 10 per cent of all cerebral palsy cases, and the rate of cerebral palsy among this group is sevenfold that for singletons (Williams *et al.* 1996). The origin of cerebral palsy in multiple births stems from poor uterine growth, complications of preterm delivery, congenital malformations, placental complications, and, in monozygotic multiple pregnancies, from problems related to shared blood supply and, if monochorionic, to cord entanglement. It has been postulated that the death of a monozygotic co-fetus may be a significant cause of spastic cerebral palsy (Pharoah and Cooke 1997). This is associated with the increased risk of sharing a vascular supply and developing twin-to-twin transfusion syndrome, which has a poor outcome. The early detection and recording of multiple pregnancies and their outcome (including early losses) is important, and could provide important clues about the causal mechanisms.

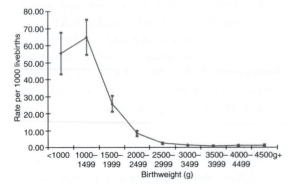

Figure 13.2 Birthweight-specific prevalence of cerebral palsy per 1000 livebirths for the birth period 1983–97 in Northern Ireland (excludes 1988).

Trends in prevalence

It is difficult to be definitive about trends in cerebral palsy between 1950 and 1970 because reports conflict. The Surveillance of Cerebral Palsy in Europe project (SCPE) (Anon 2002) reported an increase in the overall rate of cerebral palsy during the 1970s, which stabilized during the late 1980s. The apparent, but relatively small, increase during this time has been attributed to an increase in the survival of low and very low birthweight babies. Secular trends in the prevalence of cerebral palsy can only really be understood when rates are stratified by birthweight or gestational age. Most case registers of cerebral palsy have reported statistically significant increases in the rates of cerebral palsy among the very low birthweight group (less than 1500 g) in the 1980s, but before 1985 in particular. It is unclear to what extent these increases represent improved survival of already compromised babies or the improved survival of babies at higher risk of developing cerebral palsy because of their prematurity, or elements of both.

More recently, the SCPE group reported stable rates of cerebral palsy for normal birthweight infants in Europe up to 1998. This was also associated with a significant decline in bilateral spastic cerebral palsy (typically a more severe subtype) and a significant increase in unilateral spastic cerebral palsy (typically less severe) among this birthweight group (Sellier et al. 2010). Since 1990 there has been a decline in the cerebral palsy rate among infants born of moderate and very low birthweight, with a similar reduction in the frequency of bilateral spastic cerebral palsy among babies weighing 1000–1499 g (Platt et al. 2007). While these findings suggest a more optimistic clinical picture, the overall prevalence of cerebral palsy and in normal birthweight infants has remained remarkably stable over the last 30 years, despite significant decreases in perinatal and neonatal mortality in the developed world (Cans et al. 2008). It is possible that the increase in the proportion of multiple births during the 1980s and 1990s as result of reproductive technologies may have contributed at least in part to this stability (Cans et al. 2008). A registry study in Australia found no improvement in survival of children born between 1970 and 2004 (Reid et al. 2012).

Establishing reliable prevalence rates of cerebral palsy

Surveillance of cerebral palsy cannot be based on a simple case count as the condition varies by type, severity, aetiology, and pathology and is difficult to define and classify in a standardized way. The ability to group together similarly defined cases of cerebral palsy and clinical subtypes is essential to reliably monitor

Box 13.2 Methodological issues when comparing cerebral palsy prevalence rates between populations

Case definition	• Conforms with international definition (SCPE 2000*) • Inclusion/exclusion criteria stated • Differentiation of congenital and post-natal cases
Case ascertainment	• Geographically defined register with multiple sources of ascertainment • Professional and voluntary sectors should be checked for cases
Denominator data	• Match to case register geographic area • Basic data required are live-births, infant and child mortality, and population at risk
Incidence and prevalence	• Prevalence is the preferred measure as cases may only be detected at five years of age or more • Based on neonatal survivors
Age at ascertainment	• Incomplete registration may result if cases ascertained before five years of age
Deaths, immigration, and emigration	• Flagging of cases using NHS central register may be useful to follow removals within the UK

*Surveillance of Cerebral Palsy in Europe project (Anon 2000).

geographic and temporal trends, undertake aetiological research, and plan services. Several important methodological issues are worthy of note in the interpretation or compilation of statistics on cerebral palsy (see Box 13.2).

Routine child-health information systems have been found to be incomplete and are an unreliable source of information on children with cerebral palsy, partly because they tend to adopt a simple case-count approach. In contrast, successful case registers of cerebral palsy tend to use predetermined inclusion criteria, multiple, and overlapping sources of ascertainment, a standardized approach to classification, and active surveillance of a geographic population over time (Cans *et al.* 2008). In particular, follow-up of infants up to at least five years of age is important to establish eligibility for inclusion, and monitoring the population for emigration, migration, and death also assists accuracy.

CONCLUSIONS

Cerebral palsy is likely to affect 2–2.5 per 1000 of the population for the foreseeable future. Continued surveillance of cerebral palsy over time is required to monitor the effect of improved survival of very small and premature infants, the severity of the condition, and the effect of new technologies such as assisted reproduction. International collaboration on conditions such as cerebral palsy offers an important way forward.

Web addresses

European Collaboration on Cerebral Palsy
http://www-rheop.ujf-grenoble.fr/scpe2/site_scpe/index.php.

Further reading

Nelson LM, Tanner CM, Van Den Eeeden SK, and McGuire VM (eds) (2004) *Neuroepidemiology*. New York: Oxford University Press.

Stanley F, Blair E, and Alberman E. (2000) *Cerebral Palsies: Epidemiology and Causal Pathways. Clinics in Developmental Medicine*. London: MacKeith Press.

References

Annegers JF (2004) Epilepsy. In: Nelson LM, Tanner CM, Van Den Eeden SK, and McGuire, VM (eds) *Neuroepidemiology. From Principles to Practice*. Oxford: Oxford University Press.

Annegers JF, Hauser WA, Coan SP, and Rocca WA (1998) A population-based study of seizures after traumatic brain injuries. *The New England Journal of Medicine* **338** (1), 20–4.

Anon (2000) Surveillance of cerebral palsy in Europe: a collaboration of cerebral palsy surveys and registers. *Surveillance of Cerebral Palsy in Europe (SCPE)* **42** (12), 816–24.

Anon (2002) Prevalence and characteristics of children with cerebral palsy in Europe. *Developmental Medicine and Child Neurology* **44** (9), 633–40.

Ascherio A and Munger KL (2010) Epstein–Barr virus infection and multiple sclerosis: a review. *Journal of Neuroimmune Pharmacology* **5** (3), 271–7.

Ascherio A, Munger KL, and Simon KC (2010) Vitamin D and multiple sclerosis. *Lancet Neurology* **9** (6), 599–612.

Bax M, Tydeman C, and Flodmark O (2006) Clinical and MRI correlates of cerebral palsy: the European Cerebral Palsy Study. *JAMA* **296** (13), 1602–8.

Benito-León J (2011) Multiple sclerosis: is prevalence rising and if so why? *Neuroepidemiology* **37** (3–4), 236–7.

Brønnum-Hansen H, Koch-Henriksen N, and Stenager E (2004) Trends in survival and cause of death in Danish patients with multiple sclerosis. *Brain: A Journal of Neurology* **127** (Pt. 4), 844–50.

Cans C, De-la-Cruz J, and Mermet M (2008) Epidemiology of cerebral palsy. *Paediatrics and Child Health* **18** (9), 393–8.

Cantwell R, Clutton-Brock T, Cooper G, Dawson A, *et al.* (2011) Saving Mothers' Lives: Reviewing maternal deaths to make motherhood safer: 2006–2008. The Eighth Report of the Confidential Enquiries into Maternal Deaths in the United Kingdom. *BJOG: An International Journal of Obstetrics and Gynaecology* **118** Suppl. 11–203.

Cleary P, Shorvon S, and Tallis R (2004) Late-onset seizures as a predictor of subsequent stroke. *Lancet* **363** (9416), 1184–6.

Compston A and Coles A (2008) Multiple sclerosis. *Lancet* **372** (9648), 1502–17.

de Lau LML and Breteler MMB (2006) Epidemiology of Parkinson's disease. *Lancet Neurology* **5** (6), 525–35.

de Sá J, Alcalde-Cabero E, Almazán-Isla J, Sempere A, *et al.* (2012) Capture-recapture as a potentially useful procedure for assessing prevalence of multiple sclerosis: methodologic exercise using portuguese data. *Neuroepidemiology* **38** (4), 209–16.

Forbes RB and Swingler RJ (1999) Estimating the prevalence of multiple sclerosis in the United Kingdom by using capture-recapture methodology. *American Journal of Epidemiology* **149** (11), 1016–24.

Fratiglioni L and Wang HX (2000) Smoking and Parkinson's and Alzheimer's disease: review of the epidemiological studies. *Behavioural Brain Research* **113** (1-2), 117–20.

Gaitatzis A and Sander JW (2004) The mortality of epilepsy revisited. *Epileptic Disorders: International Epilepsy Journal with Videotape* **6** (1), 3–13.

Gale CR and Martyn CN (1995) Migrant studies in multiple sclerosis. *Progress in Neurobiology* **47** (4–5), 425–48.

Gray OM, McDonnell GV, and Hawkins SA (2008) Factors in the rising prevalence of multiple sclerosis in the north-east of Ireland. *Multiple Sclerosis* **14** (7), 880–6.

Hagberg B, Hagberg G, and Olow I (1993) The changing panorama of cerebral palsy in Sweden. VI. Prevalence and origin during the birth year period 1983–1986. *Acta Paediatrica* **82** (4), 387–93.

Hauser WA, Rich SS, Lee JR, Annegers JF, *et al.* (1998) Risk of recurrent seizures after two unprovoked seizures. *The New England Journal of Medicine* **338** (7), 429–34.

Heaney DC, MacDonald BK, Everitt A, Stevenson S, *et al.* (2002) Socioeconomic variation in incidence of epilepsy: prospective community based study in south east England. *BMJ (Clinical Research Ed)* **325** (7371), 1013–16.

Hemming K, Hutton JL, and Pharoah POD (2006) Long-term survival for a cohort of adults with cerebral palsy. *Developmental Medicine and Child Neurology* **48** (2), 90–5.

Hughes AJ, Daniel SE, Ben-Shlomo Y, and Lees AJ (2002) The accuracy of diagnosis of Parkinsonian syndromes in a specialist movement disorder service. *Brain: A Journal of Neurology* **125** (Pt. 4), 861–70.

Jarvis S, Glinianaia SV, Torrioli M-G, Platt M-J, *et al.* (2003) Cerebral palsy and intrauterine growth in single births: European collaborative study. *Lancet* **362** (9390), 1106–111.

Kotsopoulos IAW, van Merode T, Kessels FGH, de Krom MCTFM, *et al.* (2002) Systematic review and meta-analysis of incidence studies of epilepsy and unprovoked seizures. *Epilepsia* **43** (11), 1402–9.

Krägeloh-Mann I and Cans C (2009) Cerebral palsy update. *Brain and Development* **31** (7), 537–44.

MacDonald BK, Cockerell OC, Sander JW, and Shorvon SD (2000) The incidence and lifetime prevalence of neurological disorders in a prospective community-based study in the UK. *Brain: A Journal of Neurology* **123** (Pt. 4) 665–76.

McDonald WI, Compston A, Edan G, Goodkin D, *et al.* (2001) Recommended diagnostic criteria for multiple sclerosis: guidelines from the International Panel on the diagnosis of multiple sclerosis. *Annals of Neurology* **50** (1), 121–7.

McDonnell GV and Hawkins SA (1998) An epidemiologic study of multiple sclerosis in Northern Ireland. *Neurology* **50**, 423–8.

MacLennan A (1999) A template for defining a causal relation between acute intrapartum events and cerebral palsy: international consensus statement. *BMJ (Clinical Research Ed)* **319** (7216), 1054–9.

Marlow N, Pike K, Bower E, Brocklehurst P, *et al.* (2012) Characteristics of children with cerebral palsy in the ORACLE children study. *Developmental Medicine and Child Neurology* **54** (7), 640–6.

Meador KJ, Baker GA, Browning N, Clayton-Smith J, *et al.* (2009) Cognitive function at 3 years of age after fetal exposure to antiepileptic drugs. *The New England Journal of Medicine* **360** (16), 1597–1605.

Michell AW, Lewis SJG, Foltynie T, and Barker RA (2004) Biomarkers and Parkinson's disease. *Brain: A Journal of Neurology* **127** (Pt. 8), 1693–1705.

Miller DH (2004) Biomarkers and surrogate outcomes in neurodegenerative disease: lessons from multiple sclerosis. *NeuroRx: The Journal of the American Society for Experimental NeuroTherapeutics* **1** (2), 284–94.

Morrow J, Russell A, Guthrie E, Parsons L, *et al.* (2006) Malformation risks of antiepileptic drugs in pregnancy: a prospective study from the UK Epilepsy and Pregnancy Register. *Journal of Neurology, Neurosurgery, and Psychiatry* **77** (2), 193–8.

Morrow JI, Hunt SJ, Russell AJ, Smithson WH, *et al.* (2009) Folic acid use and major congenital malformations in offspring of women with epilepsy: a prospective study from the UK Epilepsy and Pregnancy Register. *Journal of Neurology, Neurosurgery, and Psychiatry* **80** (5), 506–11.

Nelson KB (2003) Can we prevent cerebral palsy? *The New England Journal of Medicine* **349** (18), 1765–9.

Nguyen DK and Spencer SS (2003) Recent advances in the treatment of epilepsy. *Archives of Neurology* **60** (7), 929–35.

Noebels JL (2003) The biology of epilepsy genes. *Annual Review of Neuroscience* **26**, 599–625.

O'Callaghan FJ, Osmond C, and Martyn CN (2000) Trends in epilepsy mortality in England and Wales and the United States, 1950–1994. *American Journal of Epidemiology* **151** (2), 182–9.

Odding E, Roebroeck ME, and Stam HJ (2006) The epidemiology of cerebral palsy: incidence, impairments and risk factors. *Disability and Rehabilitation* **28** (4), 183–91.

Panayiotopoulos CP (2005) Clinical aspects of the diagnosis of epileptic seizures and epileptic syndromes. In: *The Epilepsies*, pp. 1–19. Oxfordshire: Blandon Medical Publishing.

Parkes J, Dolk H and Hill N (2005) *Children and Young People with Cerebral Palsy in Northern Ireland (birth years 1977 –1997): A Comprehensive Report from the Northern Ireland Cerebral Palsy Register*. Belfast: Queen's University Belfast.

Pharoah PO and Cooke RW (1997) A hypothesis for the aetiology of spastic cerebral palsy—the vanishing twin. *Developmental Medicine and Child Neurology* **39** (5), 292–6.

Platt MJ, Cans C, Johnson A, Surman G, *et al.* (2007) Trends in cerebral palsy among infants of very low birthweight (< 1500 g) or born prematurely (< 32 weeks) in 16 European centres: a database study. *Lancet* **369** (9555), 43–50.

Pohl D (2009) Epstein–Barr virus and multiple sclerosis. *Journal of the Neurological Sciences* **286** (1–2), 62–4.

Polman CH, Reingold SC, Banwell B, Clanet M, *et al.* (2011) Diagnostic criteria for multiple sclerosis: 2010 revisions to the 'McDonald Criteria'. *Annals of Neurology* **69** (2), 292–302.

Priyadarshi A, Khuder SA, Schaub EA, and Shrivastava S (2000) A meta-analysis of Parkinson's disease and exposure to pesticides. *Neurotoxicology* **21** (4), 435–40.

Rao G, Fisch L, Srinivasan S, D'Amico F, *et al.* (2003) Does this patient have Parkinson disease? *JAMA: The Journal of the American Medical Association* **289** (3), 347–53.

Reid SM, Carlin JB, and Reddihough DS (2012) Survival of individuals with cerebral palsy born in Victoria, Australia, between 1970 and 2004. *Developmental Medicine and Child Neurology* **54** (4), 353–60.

Samii A, Nutt JG, and Ransom BR (2004) Parkinson's disease. *Lancet* **363** (9423), 1783–93.

Sawcer S, Hellenthal G, Pirinen M, Spencer CCA, *et al.* (2011) Genetic risk and a primary role for cell-mediated immune mechanisms in multiple sclerosis. *Nature* **476** (7359), 214–19.

Seino M (2006) Classification criteria of epileptic seizures and syndromes. *Epilepsy Research* **70** Suppl. 1S27–33.

Sellier E, Surman G, Himmelmann K, Andersen G, *et al.* (2010) Trends in prevalence of cerebral palsy in children born with a birthweight of 2,500 g or over in Europe from 1980 to 1998. *European Journal of Epidemiology* **25** (9), 635–42.

Stanley F, Blair E, and Alberman E (2000) *Cerebral Palsies: Epidemiology and Causal Pathways. Clinics in Developmental Medicine*. London: MacKeith Press.

Tanner CM and Ben-Shlomo Y (1999) Epidemiology of Parkinson's disease. In: Stern GM (ed) *Parkinson's Disease: Advances in Neurology*, **80**, pp. 153–9. Philadelphia: Lippincott, Williams & Wilkins.

Wang A, Costello S, Cockburn M, Zhang X, *et al.* (2011) Parkinson's disease risk from ambient exposure to pesticides. *European Journal of Epidemiology* **26** (7), 547–55.

Williams K, Hennessy E, and Alberman E (1996) Cerebral palsy: effects of twinning, birthweight, and gestational age. *Archives of Disease in Childhood. Fetal and Neonatal Edition* **75** (3), F178–82.

Model answers

Question 1

- The association may be due to chance: but over 40 studies, some prospective, have reported the same finding.

- Reverse causality is also ruled out because in prospective studies individuals without disease would have been non-smokers long before disease onset; prospective studies also overcome the problem of recall bias which can occur in case-control studies.

- The association may be real, and animal studies suggest that nicotine protects against experimental Parkinsonism.

- Alternatively, it has been suggested that decreased smoking in Parkinson's disease is a sign of the conservative personality that has been noted in patients before their diagnosis.

Question 2

Incidence is rare, but as multiple sclerosis often occurs in young people and has no cure and a relatively low excess mortality, patients generally survive for a long time after diagnosis, thus making the number of people with the disease much higher than the number of new cases.

Question 3

- Accurate demographic data to determine denominator: for example, census.
- Sources of data: in-patient and outpatient clinics, individual physicians, especially neurologists, health insurance organizations, multiple sclerosis societies, and support organizations.
- Diagnostic criteria to validate diagnosis.
- Success depends on the probability that an individual with multiple sclerosis is diagnosed and that this individual is identified by the search, which is determined in part by the completeness of the provider lists.

Question 4

(a) Syncope, pseudo-seizures, transient ischaemic attack, breath-holding episodes, and narcolepsy, etc.

(b) A diagnosis of epilepsy may preclude certain types of employment and, unless treatment renders the patient seizure-free continuously for a minimum period of 12 months, a driving licence cannot be issued.

Question 5

Because the population at risk appears to be similar for all cohorts it is likely that differences in the case-definition of epilepsy in the various studies account for the discrepancies in the mortality rates.

Question 6

It is likely that the prenatal mortality rate is higher in fetuses under 1000 g in weight. Additionally these deaths are likely to occur as miscarriages (before 24 weeks) rather than as stillbirths (after 24 weeks).

14 Mental disorders

MICHAEL DONNELLY, SINEAD MCGILLOWAY,
TONY O'NEILL, AND JOHN YARNELL

CHAPTER CONTENTS

Four major disorders of mental health are discussed in this chapter, focusing on the problem of disease definition and their descriptive epidemiology. These include: disorders of the mind (psychoses), mood (depression and anxiety), memory (dementia), and cognition (learning disability). Suicide, which is frequently associated with mental disorder, is also discussed (although it is classified by the International Classification of Disease (ICD) with 'accidents, poisoning and violence' based on the external cause (mode) of death or injury. Related disorders including epilepsy and alcohol and substance abuse are considered in Chapters 13 and 20 respectively.

Introduction

Mental health problems can profoundly affect the quality of life of individuals and their families. They are common throughout the world and have important impacts on society and also on the physical health of individuals (Kessler *et al.* 2009). Furthermore, neuro-psychiatric diseases, as a whole, account for about 28 per cent of the global burden of disease (Prince *et al.* 2007) (see Fig. 14.1) and this burden may be greater in high-income (32 per cent) versus low-income countries (26 per cent). This chapter considers four major disorders; these may be defined as: '*clinically significant conditions characterized by alterations in thinking, mood (emotions), or behaviour associated with personal distress and/or impaired functioning*' (WHO 2001).

People who experience a psychotic illness such as *schizophrenia* tend to lose their grasp or understanding of reality. More common illnesses such as *anxiety* and *depression* tend to be less severe. These illnesses frequently overlap and people with schizophrenia may also have a very high rate of depression and anxiety disorders (Achim *et al.* 2011). There are many types of mental illness, as well as conditions relating to developmental or behavioural irregularities (collectively termed *learning disabilities*); in addition to drug misuse, eating problems, sexual difficulties, and personality disorder.

A major problem in the study of mental disorders is lack of clarity about classification (Kraemer *et al.* 2004). Depression, anxiety, and personality problems tend to be understood best within a dimensional framework in which these traits are present as part of a continuum on a quantitative scale. However, the main classification systems, ICD and the *Diagnostic and Statistical Manual of Mental Disorders* (DSM) (American Psychiatric Association), use a categorical

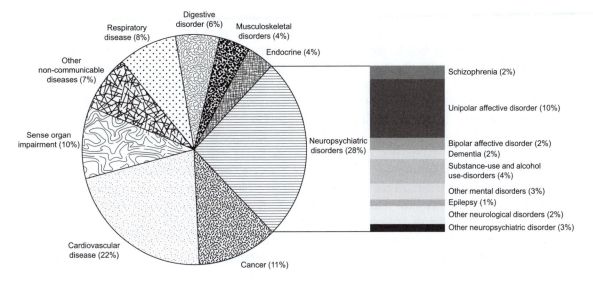

Figure 14.1 Global burden of neuropsychiatric diseases.
Reproduced from Prince M, Patel V, Saxena S, Maj M, *et al.* (2007) 'No health without mental health'. Lancet **370** (9590), 859–77, with permission from Elsevier.

or disease-based clinical approach, although the original intention for the DSM was that it should be based on dimensional criteria (Kraemer *et al.* 2004). While the categorical approach has clinical value, it often obscures the reality of the underlying quantitative trait. For example, moving the definition of schizophrenia from a narrow to a broad category, points to a different set of causes (Weiser *et al.* 2005). There is also a problem of co-morbidity; using a categorical system may lead to a patient receiving several diagnoses but they may be understood more easily at an individual level as a single process within a clear aetiological framework (Aragona 2009). Thus, there may be a 'disconnect' between useful measures from clinical and epidemiological perspectives.

It is often difficult to determine accurate incidence and prevalence rates in the population. For example, factors such as illness thresholds tend to influence observed epidemiological rates. Prevalence estimates based on clinical, treated populations often underestimate 'true' population prevalence whilst epidemiological studies based on population surveys using questionnaires or rating scales are often based on a cut-off point or threshold value denoting 'disease'. The illness threshold or cut-off point used, will clearly influence the reported prevalence. Beginning in the 1990s, WHO adopted standardized mental health questionnaires to measure the prevalence and incidence of mental disorders in all countries and found a point prevalence of 10 per cent across the globe and a lifetime prevalence of 25 to 30 per cent (Demyttenaere *et al.* 2004). However, it is important to note that an individual with mental illness must be understood within their particular cultural and social context. For this reason, ICD-10 includes a number of categories which are specific to particular cultures, e.g., *amok, dhat, susto, and koro* which are discussed elsewhere (Patel *et al.* 2012).

Any understanding of mental illness must embrace a developmental approach as nearly all mental disorders have their onset in early to late adolescence (Cicchetti and Toth 2009; Cohen *et al.* 2003); there are many possible trajectories and relatively few studies have incorporated longitudinal designs. Cross-sectional studies provide insights about associations between mental illness and risk factors but, often, these are confounded and it is not possible to discern causal direction. For example, what is the relationship between family environment and genetic factors? Most mental disorders have a substantial heritable component, but a recent review concluded that psychiatric disorders such as bipolar disorder, schizophrenia, and Alzheimer's disease were no more likely to be heritable than were behavioural disorders, such as anorexia nervosa or addiction (Bienvenu *et al.* 2011). Summary estimates for heritability from this review were as follows: bipolar disorder (85 per cent), schizophrenia (81 per cent), Alzheimer's disease (75 per cent), cocaine use disorder (72 per cent), anorexia nervosa (60 per cent), alcohol dependence (56 per cent), sedative use disorder (51 per cent), cannabis use disorder (48 per cent), panic disorder (43 per cent), stimulant use disorder (40 per cent), major depressive disorder (37 per cent), and generalized anxiety disorder (28 per cent).

In many countries, there have been dramatic changes from the 19th-century moral view of mental disorders to a more enlightened contemporary view (Fabrega 1991). Thus, many find the term 'illness' pejorative and prefer to emphasize 'mental health' in a positive sense. However, despite advances in mental health care, stigma remains a serious problem for people with a mental illness and it is a major obstacle to help-seeking (Callard *et al.* 2012). Mental disorders also have a wide range of different symptoms and also tend to vary in terms of their impact. Furthermore, the economic burden in terms of direct health care costs and loss of productivity is considerable and, in Europe, brain disorders were estimated to result in an annual cost of almost €800 billion in 2010. The costs of individual mental and physical brain disorders are shown in Fig. 14.2.

Although the economic costs associated with mental disorders are high, a large proportion of cases which could benefit from treatment go unrecognized or untreated. A global survey by a WHO Mental Health consortium found that the 'treatment gap' for untreated

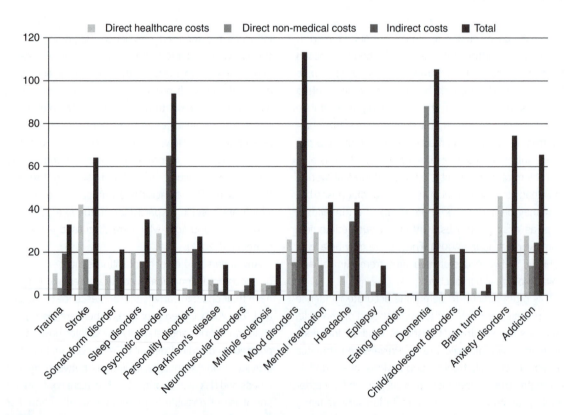

Figure 14.2 Direct, indirect, and total costs estimated for brain disorders in Europe in 2010 (€billions).
Reproduced from Olesen J *et al*, The economic cost of brain disorders in Europe, *European Journal of Neurology*, 2011, with permission from John Wiley and Sons.

Box 14.1 Prevalence estimates for major mental disorders in the general population

Type of disorder	Prevalence (%)
Any mental disorder	28–29
Schizophrenia	0.7–1.0
Unipolar depression	1.9–3.2
All forms of depression	9.6–20.4
Anxiety (generalized)	3–5
Dementia	5–8 (> 65 years) 20–34.5 (> 85 years)
Learning disability	0.3–0.4 (severe) 2.5–3.0 (mild)

Data from: Kessler *et al.* (1994), WHO (2001), Launer *et al.* (1999), and Fryers (2002).

serious mental illness reached up to 50 per cent in high-income countries and 85 per cent in low- and middle-income countries (Demyttenaere *et al.* 2004).

The remainder of this chapter focuses on the epidemiology of the major disorders including: schizophrenia; depression and anxiety; dementia; and learning disability. The estimated point prevalence of each is shown in Box 14.1. Suicide and parasuicide are more appropriately described using mortality and incidence data; these are discussed in the concluding section of the chapter.

14.1 Schizophrenia

Definition

Although psychosis and mental deterioration have been described from antiquity, schizophrenia was first described by the German psychiatrist Kraepelin in the late 19th century. Kraepelin adopted a strictly descriptive approach and his separation of schizophrenia from bipolar disorder (see 'Depression and anxiety' section) has been influential ever since. However, the Swiss psychiatrist Bleuler was the first to use the term

schizophrenia from the Greek words *schizein*, meaning *to split* and *phren*, meaning *mind* to describe the condition. The term is perhaps unfortunate as it suggests that the condition is literally a 'split mind' and that the person has multiple personalities. In reality, most individuals with schizophrenia live rewarding lives and have intact personalities. However, the illness in acute episodes can be characterized by marked and sometimes bizarre disturbances in cognitive, emotional, and social functioning, all of which may profoundly affect the quality of life of patients and their families (Wilkinson *et al.* 2000).

Schizophrenia is the most heterogeneous of all the mental disorders, with a clinical picture that may vary widely from one individual to the next; the ICD-10 classification of mental disorders describes nine different sub-types, including paranoid schizophrenia and simple schizophrenia. However, during the course of an illness a person may have several of these diagnoses and, perhaps, the illness may be understood better by adopting a longitudinal, developmental perspective. The illness may be continuous or episodic in nature and may also show high inter-individual variability. There are many groups of symptoms and these groups may reflect different neurobiological substrates. The symptom groups are described as positive, negative, disorganized, and cognitive. Catatonic symptoms are very rare now and are probably of limited diagnostic significance (van der Heijden *et al.* 2005). It is unclear why the clinical picture has changed over the years. Clinical diagnosis can be challenging and subjective, as described in classic experiments using actors in mental hospitals in the USA in the 1970s (Rosenhan 1973).

Key symptoms are usually classified into positive and negative symptoms which can co-exist. Positive symptoms usually accompany an acute episode, and include delusions (false unrealistic beliefs) and hallucinations (sensory experiences without a stimulus such as hearing voices). Negative symptoms reflect an absence or a reduction in normal behaviour and refer mainly to flat affect (impaired or absent emotional expression and responsiveness), apathy, and severe social impairment. Disorganized symptoms include incoherent thinking and chaotic social relationships, which may present great difficulty for a person in terms of reintegrating into family and community living.

Cognitive problems may also be present and can have an enormous impact on a person's day-to-day living although they are often under-recognized. These include: difficulties with executive functioning, planning, working memory, attention, problem solving, verbal reasoning, inhibition, mental flexibility, multitasking, and initiation and monitoring of actions. Increasingly, schizophrenia is seen as part of a neuro-developmental spectrum that includes autism (Owen *et al.* 2011). The disorder may affect many aspects of patients' lives, placing them at increased risk of developing problems such as homelessness, depression, substance abuse, and suicide. Substance abuse, in particular, has been estimated to occur in more than one-third of people with schizophrenia in the UK, whereas estimates from the USA suggest a figure closer to half. The treatment of such co-morbidity may present considerable difficulties for addiction and mental health services, particularly where the health care facilities are configured separately or operate within different ideological frameworks. Furthermore, there is, as yet, little evidence to inform appropriate service development in this area (Weaver *et al.* 1999).

Epidemiology

The lifetime prevalence of schizophrenia is approximately one per cent. The idea that the incidence of schizophrenia is similar in all countries has been challenged and some authors (McGrath *et al.* 2004) have suggested that there is a fivefold range in estimates (7.7 and 43.0 cases per 100,000 population). Onset typically occurs in late adolescence or early adulthood; men are twice as likely to develop schizophrenia as women, and also tend to have poorer long-term outcomes. It has been estimated that approximately 13 per cent of people with mental disorders who present to their general practitioner have schizophrenia, but many of these patients may avoid contact with primary and secondary services for many years owing to the nature of the illness and the continuing perceived stigma.

Multiple factors appear to be involved in the aetiology of schizophrenia. Convincing evidence has accumulated from family, twin, and adoption studies to illustrate the significant contribution of genetic factors, while environmental influences (for example, obstetric complications) have also been implicated (Thomas *et al.* 2001). The risk of developing schizophrenia increases dramatically if a sibling or parent has schizophrenia (around nine and 12 times higher, respectively, than the general population). Advances in molecular genetics have led to an increased understanding of the complex genetic architecture that underlies schizophrenia. The complexity is not surprising given the likely heterogeneity and multiple factors. The genes have been described as: 'small, often non-specific and embedded in causal pathways of stunning complexity' (Kendler 2005). The most recent genome-wide association scan (Ripke *et al.* 2011) in schizophrenia, comprised a consortium that included most of the case-control samples in the developed world. A two-stage design was used with a total sample of 51,695 individuals. The research programme reported seven genome-wide significant findings. The variation in these genes produces a very small increase in risk but they appear to be compatible with the neurodevelopmental nature of schizophrenia. The study also confirmed that schizophrenia is a classical polygenetic disorder. A previous paper (Purcell *et al.* 2009) produced a 'polygene' score made up of common variation at hundreds and perhaps thousands of loci. This paper also suggested that there was a substantial overlap with the genetic risk for schizophrenia and bipolar disorder. Copy number variants (CNVs) are structural variants in genomic structure, either deletions or replications and they contribute to normal variability as well as to disease risk. There has been increased interest in their contribution to the overall genetic risk for schizophrenia. A recent review (Bassett *et al.* 2010) suggested that three deletions cited at 22q11.2, 1q21.1, and 15q13.3 contribute to two per cent of the overall incidence of schizophrenia. The review also suggests that other relatively rare CNVs may be detected with increased sophistication in detection. The three most common CNVs are connected with epilepsy, autism, and mental retardation. However, people with these deletions can present with schizophrenia alone. This suggests that the expression of these deletions may be influenced by epigenetic factors such as imprinting (see also Chapter 19). In common with other major psychiatric disorders epigenetic mechanisms are believed to account for much of the 'missing heritability' of these disorders where currently-associated genetic polymorphisms account for only a minute fraction of the overall heritability (Rutten and Mill 2009).

Epidemiological studies have identified several other socio-economic and cultural factors that may interact with genetic influences, including parental age at conception, membership of (non-white) ethnic minorities, nutritional deficiencies, and a history of taking drugs such as lysergic acid diethylamide (LSD), and heavy use of cannabis (see Chapter 20). A comprehensive review of studies that looked at the relationship between psychotic symptoms and cannabis, produced evidence to suggest that cannabis showed an increased risk of psychosis independent of confounding and transient psychotic intoxication effects. The increased risk was modest but showed a dose–response effect. The authors estimated that the use of cannabis increased the risks of a psychotic outcome by 1.4 times and, given a figure of 40 per cent for this exposure in the UK, cannabis use would account for about 14 per cent (95% CI 7–19%) of new cases (Moore et al. 2007). Social difficulties and deterioration at an individual level rather than at a socio-economic level, and beginning at school age, have been associated with the development of psychoses in a major cohort study in Sweden (Zammit et al. 2010). There is also a highly replicated association with the urban environment (Kelly et al. 2010) and, in the UK, in a meta-analysis of studies conducted between 1950 and 2009, Caribbean, African, and Asian minority groups had severalfold higher relative risks than the background population (Kirkbride et al. 2012).

Treatment and prevention

The strong genetic predisposition to schizophrenia makes attempts at primary prevention difficult, particularly as the genetic risk is likely to be complex. However, the *stress-vulnerability model* provides a useful framework within which psychosocial and environmental factors may mediate this genetic vulnerability and ultimately prevent the full-blown expression of the illness. According to this model, the development and natural history of schizophrenia depend on a delicate balance between vulnerability and stress on the one hand (to which people with schizophrenia are particularly sensitive), and the individual's strengths and environmental supports on the other. Within this framework, it is desirable to reduce, as far as possible, any environmental stressors in the lives of those who are most at risk, or in the early stages of the illness to prevent the development of, or reduce, symptoms. It is also important that patients effectively manage any stress that they do encounter in their lives through the development of appropriate coping skills and/or participation in meaningful daytime activities. Evidence from randomized controlled trials (RCTs) suggests that cognitive behavioural therapy could have an important role in reducing the levels of psychotic symptoms (Lincoln et al. 2012).

A large body of research has found an association between 'expressed emotion' among family members and relapses (but not onset) in patients who have been diagnosed with schizophrenia. Thus, the type and amount of social and emotional stress (for example, hostility or emotional over-involvement) to which people with schizophrenia are exposed within the family milieu may often influence their path of recovery. However, research focusing on attempts to detect at-risk individuals so as to implement early interventions, is in its infancy. Consequently, pharmacological treatment and maintenance regimens remain the mainstay of secondary prevention with psychosocial interventions (designed to improve social and daily living skills) and/or rehabilitation such as specialist day care or training and supported (sheltered) employment schemes (McGilloway and Donnelly 2000).

The described interventions are important, not only in promoting recovery, but also in helping to prevent the typically high rates of suicide among people with schizophrenia. Approximately five per cent die prematurely in this way (Mueser and McGurk 2004), while the lifetime occurrence of attempted suicide (parasuicide) in this group has been estimated to range from 18 per cent to 55 per cent. The risk of both is significantly increased by the presence of depressive symptoms and/or substance abuse. The fatality rate of suicide attempts has also been reported to be greater in people with schizophrenia when compared with those with other psychotic illnesses. Furthermore, the risk of suicide is compounded by the tendency for people with schizophrenia failing to present to their general practitioner, or to avoid contact with them after discharge from psychiatric hospitals. However, in high-income countries, the development in recent years of more accessible and less stigmatized community-based psychiatric clinics has gone some way towards addressing this issue.

14.2 Depression and anxiety

Definitions

Depression is one of the most prevalent and costly of all the mental disorders and a leading (and growing) cause of disability worldwide, affecting as many as one in four people over their lifetime. It is important to distinguish between depression as a symptom and depressive disorder. The latter is broadly categorized within ICD-10 into depressive episode and recurrent depressive disorder. Depressive disorder is characterized by a prevailing feeling of sadness and varying degrees of emotional and social withdrawal, often involving a loss of (or impaired) self-esteem, sleep, concentration, appetite, and/or libido. Symptoms may vary from mild to severe and are usually of an episodic and recurrent nature, although approximately 20 per cent of sufferers have chronic depression without remission (Thornicroft and Sartorius 1993). Chronic depression with or without remission and characterized by depressed mood is termed *unipolar disorder*. This is already a leading cause of global disability and is predicted, by 2030, to become the leading cause of disability in high income countries, and the second most common cause globally (Saraceno *et al.* 2009). Depressive symptoms may also be seen in *bipolar affective disorder*. This describes a condition characterized by episodes of

mania (that is, euphoria, irritability, and distractibility) and depression. People with depression have a high rate of co-morbid chronic physical conditions such as stroke or heart disease, diabetes mellitus, or Alzheimer's disease. Elderly people with depression are also more at risk of developing Alzheimer's disease and of being admitted to nursing-home care than their non-depressed counterparts. Unfortunately, many depressive disorders in the elderly population go undetected and untreated because they tend to be viewed as part of the ageing process and may not be reported by older people. Additionally, the presence of depression in all age groups can lead to a myriad of attendant physical symptoms such as chronic pain, headaches, and digestive disorders (*somatoform disorders*). It is also the mental disorder that is most frequently linked to suicide (see section 14.5). It has been estimated that one in six of all patients with clinical depression take their own life (Gunnell and Frankel 1994), but this figure excludes the potentially large 'at risk' group of people who do not seek or receive treatment. Paradoxically, the risk of suicide increases when treatment is started as most relevant medications cause motor symptoms which can increase anxiety levels.

Depression co-exists commonly with anxiety, an overwhelming, uncontrollable, and irrational apprehension and/or fear experienced during normal day-to-day activities. Clinical anxiety may cluster with other mental disorders and is much more intensive, debilitating, and longer-lasting than periods of anxiety that may be experienced as part and parcel of everyday life. According to ICD-10, anxiety refers to a family of disorders, some of which may also co-occur and which may share common diagnostic criteria and aetiologies. Major categories include *phobic anxiety disorders* and other anxiety disorders including *generalized anxiety disorder*, which is one of the most common (and often untreated) forms of anxiety. The sufferer may be described as a 'chronic worrier' who is persistently and uncontrollably anxious about everyday matters and events irrespective of their perceived importance. Reactions to severe stress such as *post-traumatic stress disorder (PTSD)* are also classed with anxiety disorders.

Epidemiology

Both depression and anxiety (or at least certain forms of anxiety such as generalized anxiety disorder) are almost twice as common in women as in men and may occur at any point in the lifespan. However, there is increasing evidence to suggest that these disorders are becoming more prevalent among teenagers and adolescents, many of whom rarely seek help. The most recent estimates from the Global Burden of Disease project show a lifetime prevalence for unipolar depressive episodes of 3.2 per cent for women compared with 1.9 per cent for men (WHO 2001). However, when all forms of depression (stand-alone or co-morbid) are taken into account, these figures rise dramatically to 20.4 per cent for women and 9.6 per cent for men (WHO 2001). The corresponding prevalence rates in any 12-month period are 9.5 per cent and 5.8 per cent, respectively. Similarly, the lifetime prevalence for generalized anxiety disorder in the general population has been reported to be as high as five per cent (Wittchen et al. 1994). The World Mental Health Survey Initiative (Kessler 2009) conducted epidemiological studies of anxiety, depression, and substance disorders in 20 countries in five WHO world regions and found, for example, 12-month prevalence rates for the combined group of non-psychotic mental disorders ranging from six per cent in Nigeria to 27 per cent in the USA. A UK survey of 10,000 adults in private households (OPCS 1995) found that one in seven had a psychiatric disorder, the most common of which included anxiety-depressive disorder (seven per cent) and generalized anxiety disorder (three per cent). The higher prevalence of both depression and anxiety among women appears to be due to a complex interplay of biological, socio-cultural, and psychological/behavioural factors. Twin studies suggest that there is a modest genetic component to depression and anxiety and that the genetic risk is entirely shared. This implies that environmental factors determine the type of symptoms that someone has, given their genetic background (Kendler et al. 1992).

Many people may develop neurotic illnesses such as depression and anxiety without ever being treated or receiving a formal diagnosis. However, the prevalence rates for (diagnosed) depression and anxiety, as well as age at onset and the course of the illness, vary widely across populations. Several social and economic factors have been identified as important in explaining this variation, the most important of which would appear to be poverty and deprivation. Fig. 14.3 indicates that the prevalence of depression is higher in low-income groups in both high- and low-income countries.

The relation between poverty and mental health is not straightforward and involves many potentially mediating factors. A Swedish follow-up study of first

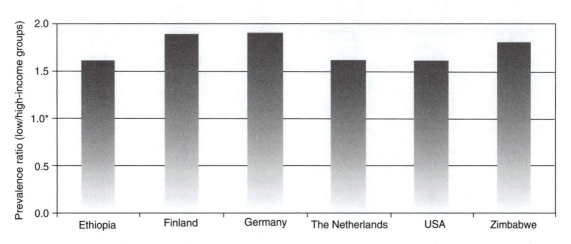

Figure 14.3 Prevalence ratio of depression in low- versus high-income groups (selected countries).

Reproduced wth permission from World Health Report 2001. Available at: **www.who.int**.

*1.0 = no difference between groups.

psychiatric admissions during 1997–1999 showed that the incidence of depression (and psychoses) increased significantly with rising levels of urbanization, after controlling for age and gender (Sundquist *et al.* 2004). Level of urbanization was assessed by dividing the study population (4.4 million) into five equal groups according to the population density of area of residence. The authors found that those living in more densely populated areas had a 12–20 per cent greater risk of developing depression than those in more sparsely populated regions (Table 14.1). Depression was defined using several diagnostic codes within the ICD-9 and ICD-10 classification systems as well as additional specialized classification systems for mental disorder.

Table 14.1 Population and age-adjusted incidence rates for depression in a general population aged 25–64 years in Sweden[1]

Variable	Female rate (95% CI)	Male rate (95% CI)
Urbanization		
Q1 (lowest)	84 (82–86)	67 (65–69)
Q2	87 (85–89)	66 (64–68)
Q3	90 (88–92)	66 (64–68)
Q4	107 (104–109)	71 (69–73)
Q5 (highest)	122 (120–125)	87 (85–90)
Marital status		
Living alone	135 (133–138)	103 (100–105)
Married/ co-habiting	79 (76–81)	53 (51–54)
Education		
Low	129 (126–132)	88 (86–90)
Middle	93 (91–95)	68 (66–70)
High	82 (80–84)	58 (56–59)

[1] Incidence rate per 100,000 person-years.

Sundquist K, Frank G, and Sundquist J (2004). 'Urbanisation and Incidence of Psychosis and Depression'. *British Journal of Psychiatry* **184**, 293–8.

The relation between poverty and mental disorders such as depression and anxiety is multi-dimensional and may encompass other socio-environmental risk factors, such as political instability and conflict. Natural disasters and major epidemics may also play an important role. For example, a diagnosis of human immuno-deficiency virus/acquired immunodeficiency syndrome (HIV/AIDS) often gives rise to extreme stigma and discrimination and, in turn, to high levels of depression and/or anxiety among sufferers and their families. Major life events such as bereavement or marital breakdown, and the extent of social support, are additional risk factors for developing depression and anxiety.

Question 1

Previous studies of possible urban–rural differences in mental health are inconsistent. Why do you think this might be?

Treatment and prevention

Most depressive and anxiety disorders tend to be self-limiting but can, nonetheless, be extremely debilitating and distressing. There is little evidence for the effectiveness of approaches to primary prevention per se (WHO 2001), but a range of interventions has been shown to be effective, not only for reducing symptoms of depression and anxiety, but also in screening, educating, and supporting at-risk groups such as mothers with post-natal depression (Cooper and Murray 1998). However, these kinds of initiatives are relatively uncommon, especially within primary care where most of these disorders are first recognized and treated. Thus, antidepressant and anxiolytic (anti-anxiety) medication remain the most commonly used forms of treatment designed to reduce or alleviate symptoms in the short term, to prevent a relapse and, ultimately (and more challengingly), to promote a full recovery. However, these do not work for everyone and there is evidence to suggest that they are more effective for the treatment of moderate and severe depression than for milder forms of the illness (National Institute for Health and Clinical Excellence (NICE) 2004). Some people may also experience adverse side effects such as physical addiction, especially if medicated for a prolonged period. Furthermore, evidence on the apparent links between newer antidepressant medication, such as selective serotonin re-uptake inhibitors and an increased risk of suicide, has led to a ban on their use in children (under 18 years of age) (Gunnell and Ashby 2004). However, increased prescribing of these drugs has coincided with an overall drop in the suicide rate in many countries, although the evidence is weak owing to the difficulty in disentangling the effects of medication from the many other factors that may influence suicide rates. Clearly, further research in this area is required to determine the long-term safety of antidepressant prescribing.

Increasingly, the value of psychological therapies in the treatment and management of both depression and anxiety; cognitive behavioural therapy (CBT), interpersonal psychotherapy (IPT), and various forms of counselling are all used as forms of treatment, often with medication. Cognitive behavioural therapy is primarily aimed at changing negative and maladaptive thought patterns. Interpersonal psychotherapy, on the other hand, helps patients to improve their interpersonal and social skills and to derive greater benefit from their social interactions. Both of these forms of therapy have been found to be effective, to a greater or lesser degree, in alleviating the symptoms of depression. The evidence for their effectiveness is derived mainly from several controlled studies, one of the largest and most widely cited of which was conducted by the National Institute for Mental Health in the USA (Elkin *et al.* 1985). The findings indicated that, although pharmacological therapy led to a more rapid improvement during the 16-week treatment period, all three forms of treatment including CBT and IPT achieved significant and equivalent degrees of success when compared with the placebo group. Many other studies have since been conducted (e.g. Ward *et al.* 2000) which suggest that some time-limited therapies such as CBT and non-directive counselling can be as effective as medication, but only for mild to moderate depression. A controlled, cluster-based trial in a low-income country (rural Uganda) suggested that CBT may provide a low cost, safer, alternative to pharmacological treatment for depression (Bolton *et al.* 2003).

14.3 Dementia

Definition

Dementia is a syndrome characterized by a progressive decline in cognitive and functional abilities. Clinicians would usually require that the symptoms and signs persist for six months before a provisional diagnosis is made. Onset is usually gradual and the main symptoms include: a loss of recent memory; a decreased ability to perform activities of daily living; impaired judgement; disorientation; changes in personality; a deterioration in language skills; and behavioural disturbance. Affective changes such as depression are also common. It is important to evaluate the nature and degree of co-morbidity among older people when assessing their mental health status. In particular, it is necessary that epidemiological and clinical assessments take account of the possibility of misclassifying depression as dementia (so-called pseudo-dementia).

Epidemiology

Dementia may result from a range of different diseases, although there is considerable uncertainty about their aetiology. Most cases are caused by neurodegenerative disease (e.g. Alzheimer's disease, dementia with Lewy bodies, frontotemporal dementia) and/or cerebrovascular disease (e.g. vascular dementia). Other causes include the effects of alcohol, trauma (e.g. subdural haematoma, dementia pugilistica), infection (e.g. HIV, neurosyphilis), prion disease (e.g. Creutzfeldt–Jakob disease (CJD)), and metabolic and nutritional deficiencies. There is some variation between studies in estimates of different types of dementia. Alzheimer's disease appears to be the most common dementia accounting for up to two-thirds of cases. Alzheimer first described the characteristic pathology of the brain plaques and neurofibrillary tangles in his patient who died in 1906 after a five-year progressive loss of cognitive ability. Today, early-onset Alzheimer's disease occurring before the age of 65 years is distinguished from the much commoner late-onset disease occurring mainly in the mid-70s onwards. The second most common type of dementia is vascular dementia (accounting for an estimated 20 per cent), characterized by small vessel disease and areas of brain infarction (multi-infarct dementia). Approximately, 10 per cent of cases have Lewy bodies in the brain at autopsy, which may be associated clinically with dementia with Lewy bodies, or Parkinson's disease dementia. The remaining 10 per cent of cases is made up of less common causes listed earlier. People with Down's syndrome carry a high lifetime risk of dementia, with a tendency to develop Alzheimer's disease in late middle-age.

A key task in psychiatric epidemiology is to identify and describe disorders such as dementia. Thus, a number of scales and interview schedules have been developed to assess the presence of dementia and other disorders. Typically, a brief screening measure such as the Mini-Mental State Exam (MMSE) is used initially, followed by a more detailed clinical assessment. The MMSE is an interviewer-administered scale and individuals who score below a certain cut-point are designated a 'case', indicating that they have significant cognitive impairment. There is some uncertainty about which cut-point should be used to define a 'case'—a common methodological problem in epidemiology for most risk factors based on continuous distributions, whether measured by questionnaire or using a physiological measured variable. Different cut-points will lead to variations in estimates of prevalence and incidence. However, in general, research suggests that the widely used MMSE appears to be a valid test for detecting dementia. For example, a cut-point of 21/22 on the MMSE had a sensitivity of 96 per cent and a specificity of 80 per cent for a diagnosis of dementia in community epidemiological studies (see Chapter 5). Some studies suggest that higher cut-points may be required with graduates or other similar professional and literate populations. There is growing interest in the use of biomarkers, especially neuroimaging to identify and quantify pathology relevant to dementia. Recent guidelines on the diagnosis of Alzheimer's disease and mild cognitive impairment for clinical and research use have been issued by the Alzheimer's Association and the National Institute on Aging (USA) (Jack et al. 2011).

Both the incidence and prevalence of dementia increase exponentially with age (Lobo et al. 2000). Overall, approximately one in 20 people over 65 years and one in three people over 85 years old have dementia, whilst around only one in 1000 people under 65 years develops the illness. Globally, in 2005, it was estimated that 24.4 million people lived with dementia, rising to 81.1 million in 2040, a doubling every 20 years in line with the ageing of the world populations (Ferri et al. 2005). Overall prevalence rates for dementia appear to be higher in women particularly since life expectancy is several years longer.

Population studies using MMSE screening assessments characteristically reveal a higher prevalence rate than clinically-based epidemiological studies (Anstey et al. 2010). Incidence studies are less common, but a prospective study in China found that the incidence of dementia was higher than that found in several Western studies (Chen et al. 2011). This study also found that the incidence rate for dementia was 2.5 times greater in women, and significantly (statistically) higher in smokers, those with angina, those with certain psychosocial characteristics, and in those with only a primary education. Living with one or more close relatives appeared to be a protective factor. Similar findings have been found in prospective studies in Europe and North America and most studies report associations between cardiovascular risk factors and both Alzheimer's disease and vascular dementia.

Heritability estimates vary between 58–79% for Alzheimer's disease (Jones et al. 2010), but early and late onset disease should be distinguished. In early onset disease, three genes have been identified as having an effect on risk; the amyloid precursor protein and two presenilin genes. These are Mendelian autosomal dominant disorders, responsible for up to 10 per cent of early-onset Alzheimer's disease. Apolipoprotein E is the main susceptibility locus for late onset disease and, in the many populations studied, has a population attributable risk of 10 per cent. Possession of the $\epsilon 4$ allele confers an increased risk, but many individuals with this allele survive into old age without developing dementia. The allele $\epsilon 2$ appears to reduce the

Table 14.2 Odds of developing incident dementia by 10 years by Apo E genotype

Genotype	Overall genotype frequency (%)	OR*	95% CI
ε2/ε2	7	0.5	0.0–5.7
ε2/ε3	14	0.6	0.3–1.1
ε2/ε4	3	0.6	0.2–2.3
ε3/ε3	62	1.0	
ε3/ε4	19	2.3	1.5–3.6
ε4/ε4	2	5.0	1.9–13.0

*OR adjusted for age, sex, education, and social class.
Reproduced from Keage HAD, et al, 'APOE and ACE polymorphisms and dementia risk in the older population over prolonged follow-up: 10 years of incidence in the MRC CFA study', *Age and Ageing* **39**, 1 2010, with permission from Oxford University Press.

risk of dementia. Some typical risks, shown as odds ratios, taken from a major British study of incident cases of dementia at 10 years of follow-up, are shown in Table 14.2.

Recent genome-wide association studies (GWAS) have identified at least two further loci of genome-wide significance (Seshadri *et al.* 2010) but their contribution to overall risk is small. Several of these new genes, along with ApoE, are involved with lipid metabolism in the brain (Jones *et al.* 2010) and an improved understanding of their biological pathways should lead to the possibility of preventive interventions.

....
 Question 2

Why do you think that there have been fewer published incidence studies of dementia than studies of the prevalence of dementia?
....

Treatment and prevention

Currently, there are no fully effective treatments for dementia, though in recent years a variety of approaches have been developed. NICE has recommended the use of several cholinesterase-inhibiting drugs for mild to moderate Alzheimer's disease (see

NICE guidelines March 2011). Current treatment options do not offer a 'cure' for dementia, but instead delay or control symptoms. Consequently, an assessment of **quality of life** may be a more meaningful outcome measure with which to assess the effectiveness of the interventions and available services for dementia. A recent systematic review of 127 observational studies, 22 RCTs, and 16 systematic reviews reported that smoking habits, ApoE ε4 genotype, and some medical conditions were consistently related to the risk of dementia. Several observational studies also suggested that Mediterranean diet, vegetable consumption, and dietary ω-3 fatty acids were associated with a reduced risk (Plassman *et al.* 2010). Evidence for possible preventive benefits from lifestyle changes were limited, although one RCT with high-quality evidence reported a small, sustained benefit from cognitive training (Willis *et al.* 2006) and a small RCT of physical activity found that it sustained cognitive function (Lautenschlager *et al.* 2008). Treatment of hypertension has been shown to reduce cognitive decline and active management of other vascular risk factors seems prudent, despite absence of evidence of benefit. The most recent Cochrane review of the use of statins reported negative outcomes in two large RCTs with 20,000+ and 5800 subjects respectively, but follow-up was limited to five years (McGuinness *et al.* 2009). One observational study reported that dementia developed in midlife smokers who possessed an ε4 genotype, but not in others (Rusanen *et al.* 2010). Randomized controlled trials are needed to assess single and multiple risk factor reduction strategies on dementia incidence and several such trials are ongoing, in France, Finland, and the USA. There is an urgent need for good quality evidence and viable preventive interventions for this growing public and personal health problem.

14.4 Learning disability

Definition

Various terms such as 'learning disability' (used in 47 WHO countries, e.g. UK), 'intellectual disability' (used in 83 WHO countries, e.g. USA), or 'mental retardation' (the term used in the WHO ICD-10 and in 111 WHO countries) refer to people with intellectual impairment and impaired functioning or adaptive behaviour. Learning disability is a permanent condition that tends to be present from birth and has a lasting effect on development. Intellectual impairment is usually defined as an IQ score lower than 50 for individuals with severe disability and between 50 and 70 for those with the milder form (see Fryers (2002) for discussion of key issues including the problems associated with definition). In addition, up to 40 per cent of people with this disorder also have a mental illness, and there is a high level of physical ill health. For example, people with learning disability tend to have higher levels of epilepsy, sensory impairments, osteoporosis, musculoskeletal problems, dysphagia, and nutritional problems when compared with the general population.

There is a lack of consensus about the most appropriate way to define and describe people with this disorder. The inadequacy of using any single definition is evident from epidemiological studies, which tend to report significant levels of variation and complexity in impairments and disabilities among people with the disorder. While these terms may be stigmatizing to varying degrees, it is important to try to arrive at an accurate definition for the purposes of planning, organizing, and delivering appropriate and necessary services. Epidemiology can provide a framework within which to conduct a needs assessment of the population with learning disabilities and to plan the provision of health and social services (Rees *et al.* 2004).

Epidemiology

Fryers (2002), in his overview of the difficulties surrounding the definition, categorization, and epidemiology of learning disability, noted that incidence and prevalence are variable owing to its heterogeneous nature, the many different types, the wide array of aetiological factors, and the dynamic processes of inception, mortality, and migration. These points should be borne in mind when reading epidemiological studies of the disorder.

A recent systematic review and meta-analysis of the prevalence of intellectual disability across 52 countries found a rate of 10.4 per 1000 population (Maulik *et al.* 2011). However, prevalence rates varied according to variables such as income group of country (from 16.4 per 1000 in low-income countries, 15.9 per 1000 in middle income countries to 9.2 per 1000 in high-income countries), age group (18.3 per 1000 child/adolescent population; 4.9 per 1000 adult population), and study design (9.7 per 1000 for cross-sectional studies; 13.2 for cohort studies). The much lower prevalence rates in high income countries may be due to effective screening services and better antenatal care and maternal and child health care provision. The meta-analysis is instructive regarding the kind of factors that need to be considered when reading and interpreting epidemiological data. For example, methodological issues such as different methods of assessing or diagnosing learning disability may produce different prevalence estimates: studies in the review that used a psychometric measure reported an overall estimate of 14.3 per 1000 population whereas studies that used the ICD or DSM system reported 8.7 per 1000. In broad terms, reviews of prevalence studies of people with learning disability known to service providers have found three to four people with severe disability and between 25 and 30 people with less severe disability in every 1000 of the general population. Studies that have screened whole populations of people with severe disorder have found six per 1000 of the population. Prevalence rates vary according to gender, age, ethnic background, and socio-economic circumstances. Lesser disability is more common among people from families with low incomes and adverse or unstable backgrounds (Fryers 2002).

Learning disability comprises a very heterogeneous group of syndromes and conditions with different aetiologies (see Box 14.2). Down's syndrome represents the largest single cause. A social model of disability tends to view the disorder in terms of developmental delay that is due to differences in learning opportunities and receipt of appropriate interventions rather than to biological causes per se (Chappell *et al.* 2001). Screening for Down's syndrome is discussed in Chapter 5, and congenital anomalies are described in Chapter 16.

Box 14.2 Aetiology of learning disabilities

Genetic exposures

Dominant genes causing gross disease of the brain

Tuberose sclerosis, neurofibromatosis

Recessive genes causing metabolic disorders affecting

Amino acids (for example, phenylketonuria, homocystinuria), urea cycle (citrullinuria, aminosuccinicaciduria), lipids (Tay–Sachs, Gaucher's, and Niemann–Pick diseases), carbohydrate (galactosaemia), mucopolysaccharidoses (Hurler's syndrome)

Chromosome abnormalities

Down's syndrome, Klinefelter syndrome, Turner syndrome

X-linked disorders

Fragile X syndrome, Lesch–Nyhan syndrome

Cranial malformations

Hydrocephalus, microcephalus

Polygenic factors influencing the normal distribution of intelligence

Non-specific learning disability

Antenatal exposures

Infections (rubella, cytomegalovirus, syphilis, toxoplasmosis), intoxications (lead, certain drugs, alcohol), physical damage (injury, radiation, hypoxia), endocrine disorders (hypothyroidism, hypoparathyroidism), fetal malnutrition (including iodine deficiency, a common cause in developing countries, see Chapter 9)

Perinatal exposures

Birth asphyxia, kernicterus, intraventricular haemorrhage

Post-natal exposures

Injury (accidental, child abuse), infections (encephalitis, meningitis), lead intoxication.

Reproduced from Gelder *et al.*, *Oxford Textbook of Psychiatry*, 1994, with permission from Oxford University Press.

Severe disability is associated with genetic or biological factors such as Down's syndrome and Fragile X syndrome. Causes may also be classified according to the time (ante-, peri-, or post-natal) of damage to the development of the central nervous system. Antenatal factors such as rubella or toxins (e.g. fetal alcohol syndrome) contribute 50–70 per cent of cases. Perinatal damage such as asphyxia during birth accounts for 10–20 per cent of cases whereas post-natal damage (5–10 per cent) may be due to factors such as meningitis, encephalitis, and accidental or deliberate injury. Severe learning disability in four out of five children is caused by genetic and biological factors compared with between one and two out of five with less severe disability. The aetiology of the latter is more likely to involve a combination of genetic and environmental factors.

There is considerable developmental variation among people with the same genetic condition; also, social factors have a bearing on development and on the severity of the impact of a biological impairment. For example, early intervention strategies may be successful in ameliorating the effects of Down's syndrome (Cunningham 1996), although few controlled studies have been conducted. The personality, family

background, and social environment of each individual with the disorder, as well as the nature and degree of their disability, will determine the kind of life that they will experience. The majority (around 80 per cent) are classified as 'mild' and most tend to be able to live in their respective communities without needing support or supervision, in contrast to people with 'severe' disability who require formal services and support from health and social services and other agencies (and the committed support of families). Children with mild disease may not be identified or detected formally until they attend school whereas people with severe disability tend to be known from birth. Indeed, Fryers (2002) makes the important point that mild learning disability is socially determined to a large degree.

Treatment and prevention

Disability that is due to causes such as hypothyroidism, phenylketonuria, rubella infection, and kernicterus can be successfully prevented using public health measures such as rubella immunization and neonatal screening; disability from other causes such as chromosome defects, rare single-gene disorders, drug exposures, exposure to lead, and head injury can be reduced by methods such as the use of educational programmes, genetic counselling, prenatal and neonatal diagnosis, and other prevention strategies (see Table 14.3 for a list of relevant services for prevention). In particular, there is an urgent need to develop, provide, and improve appropriate genetic screening and maternal and child health care in low- to middle-income countries given current epidemiological data pointing to much higher prevalence rates and the increasing population of children and adolescents in countries such as Bangladesh, Pakistan, India, and Nigeria. While the diagnosis or detection of the disorder and the identification of genetic conditions are very important tasks, the prognosis or the quality of life of individuals may be influenced significantly by the availability of opportunities in areas such as specific interventions, education, vocational training and employment, and support to live 'ordinary lives' (Gates 2002). Similar to mental disorders such as schizophrenia and depression, learning disability is associated with stigma and discrimination and special efforts are required to educate the general population.

14.5 Suicide and parasuicide

Definition

Suicide refers to acute self-inflicted death which, in the UK, can only be labelled as such after a coroner's investigation, and frequently an open or accidental verdict is made which falls short of suicide. This practice varies considerably between different countries owing to legal, cultural, and religious factors, thereby making comparisons of suicide rates difficult. The same is true for attempted suicide (parasuicide), although comparisons over time can be made within countries. The term 'parasuicide' was coined to describe deliberate self-harm inflicted with no intent to die. In practice, 'intent' can be difficult to evaluate and the distinction between attempted suicide and parasuicide is frequently blurred in epidemiological studies. In most countries, attempted suicides are referred to the psychiatric services for assessment and possible intervention, and most studies suggest

Table 14.3 Services for the prevention of learning disabilities

Preconceptual services
Immunization of adolescent girls against rubella
Genetic counselling
General advice on diet, avoidance of tobacco and alcohol consumption, and avoidance of drug abuse and HIV
Pre-natal
Identification of 'at risk' pregnancies
Monitoring alpha-fetoprotein (AFP) levels, etc., provision of amniocentesis
Blood tests
Diagnostic ultrasound services
Advice and counselling on termination of pregnancy
Perinatal/neonatal
High quality obstetric and neonatal care
Neonatal screening and treatment of specific conditions
Surgical intervention to prevent or reduce impairments
Injection of anti-D immunoglobulin to prevent antibody formation in mothers at risk of future rhesus incompatibility
Phenylketonuria (PKU) screening
Post-natal
Immunization
Control of infection and complications in children already suffering a specific impairment
General support to families at risk

Source: Felce D, Taylor D, and Wright K (1994). 'Learning Disabilities', in A Stevens and J Raffery (eds) *Health Care Needs Assessment: The Epidemiologically Based Needs Assessment Reviews*, 1st edn. Oxford: Radcliffe Medical Press.

that attempted suicide/parasuicide is a highly heterogeneous condition with considerable variation in the level of intent and the possibility of repeated attempts.

Epidemiology

Suicide is one of the three leading causes of death among 15- to 34-year-olds in the developed world. However, in many countries, even in Europe, the incidence is severalfold higher in the elderly, particularly in men (see Fig. 14.4). 'Global' mortality rates from suicide have been estimated to be as high as 16 per 100,000 whereas the rate of attempted suicide may be up to 20 times more common again (WHO 2001). Suicide rates worldwide vary considerably and, as noted above, are notoriously difficult to estimate, compare, and interpret. It has been estimated that almost 90 per cent of the 800,000 people who commit suicide come from low- and middle-income countries; more than 50 per cent are between 15 and 44 years old (Prince *et al.* 2007). Rates in low- and middle-income countries are almost double those in high-income countries and usually rates are two to eight times higher in men than in women (Hawton *et al.* 2012). Exceptionally, higher rates of suicide are reported in younger women in China and in India, particularly in rural areas (Pitman *et al.* 2012). However, international data show considerable variability in the age groups at greatest risk, as illustrated in Fig. 14.4. This may be due to social and cultural pressures, but a need for further research is indicated.

Parasuicide, in contrast, is much more common, particularly among females, and the highest rates are found in young adults. Repeated episodes are common, but parasuicide is also a major risk factor for completed suicide with 30–47 per cent of such cases having had an episode of parasuicide (Welch 2001). A recent national British survey indicated that suicidal thoughts are more common in women than men, possibly because of different patterns of help-seeking

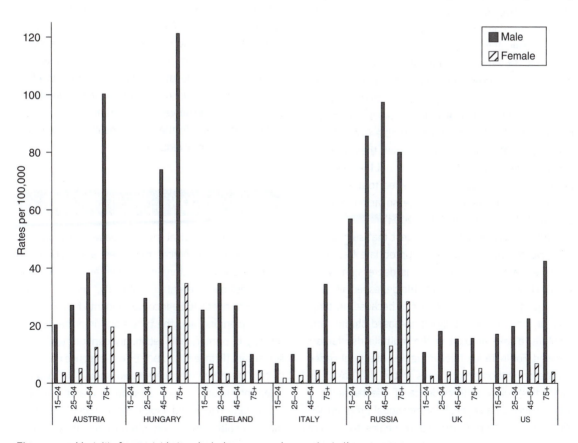

Figure 14.4 Mortality from suicide in selected age groups by country in the year 2000.
Data obtained from the WHO (2001).

behaviour and/or the use of more lethal methods by men (Gunnell *et al.* 2004). However, Gunnell *et al.* indicate that fewer than one in 200 of those who develop such thoughts actually go on to die by suicide. Nonetheless, these gender-related differences may be important for identifying at-risk individuals and developing appropriate measures for suicide prevention.

Potential for prevention

Several important risk factors for suicide, in addition to depression and schizophrenia, have been identified. These include: alcohol/substance abuse; previous and/or family history of suicide; childhood abuse; deliberate self-harm; and chronic physical illness (Torpy *et al.* 2005). Arguably, the heterogeneous nature and methods of suicide coupled with its multifactorial aetiology hinder attempts to develop adequate and systematic preventive measures. However, the strong links between suicidal behaviour and mental ill health suggest that the effective, timely, and appropriate identification and treatment of mental disorders, including depression, represent an important element of any suicide prevention programme. Evidence from the UK suggests that more than a fifth of suicides among people with mental illness are preventable (Department of Health 2001). As mentioned earlier, there remains considerable debate as to whether or not the increased prescribing of antidepressants has led to a reduction in suicidal behaviour. The evidence, so far, remains circumstantial (Gunnell and Ashby 2004).

There is good evidence to suggest that suicide can be prevented by the early and appropriate treatment of some mental disorders such as depression (WHO 2001). However, prevention of suicide, especially among young people, is controversial because, in large part, of the paucity of population-based studies and a failure to take account of the multiple risk factors involved. For instance, a recent review of school-based suicide prevention programmes in the US (based on 13 studies) found little evidence of effectiveness, or of replication of any effects of individual programmes (Miller *et al.* 2009). Dedicated strategies to prevent suicide aimed at developing and promoting effective clinical practice have also been implemented. These include, primarily, training and education programmes for general practitioners and other health professionals designed to improve the recognition, assessment, and treatment of individuals presenting a risk of suicide. For example, a Swedish study by Rutz *et al.* (1992) reported a decline in suicide rates after the implementation of a training programme for general practitioners. A RCT indicated that post-crisis contact between mental health professionals and individuals at risk for suicide (and who refuse ongoing treatment) was effective in reducing suicide rates during the two-year period after discharge from hospital (Motto and Bostrom 2001).

Public awareness and education programmes have been designed to overcome the stigma commonly associated with suicide and mental illness in general, but few appear to have been evaluated. In a review of suicide prevention measures, reducing the means of suicide appeared to offer some empirical evidence of benefit, particularly if the mode of suicide is common in the population (Mann *et al.* 2005). The role of the media, both positive and negative, in publicizing modes of suicide is discussed elsewhere (Yip *et al.* 2012). Systematic evidence for the effectiveness of any single suicide prevention programme still appears to be lacking and further public health research and actions are urgently required.

CONCLUSION

Future epidemiological studies, based on biological and socio-psychological measures are required to improve our understanding of mental disorders and their possible prevention. Globally, mental health awareness needs to be incorporated into health policy, service planning and the provision, organization and delivery of primary and secondary general health and social care (Prince *et al.* 2007). Cost-effective packages of care have been evaluated and should be incorporated into health service development and planning, particularly in low- and middle-income countries where mental health services are often rudimentary or non-existent (Saraceno *et al.* 2009).

Further reading

Tsuang MT, Tohen M, and Jones P (eds) (2011) *Textbook in Psychiatric Epidemiology*, 3rd edn. New York: Wiley.

World Mental Health Initiative: Global Perspectives from the WHO World Mental Health Surveys. Available at: www.hcp.med.harvard.edu/wmh/

References

Achim AM, Maziade M, Raymond E, Olivier D, *et al.* (2011) How prevalent are anxiety disorders in schizophrenia? A meta-analysis and critical review on a significant association. *Schizophrenia Bulletin* **37** (4), 811–21.

Anstey KJ, Burns RA, Birrell CL, Steel D, *et al.* (2010) Estimates of probable dementia prevalence from population-based surveys compared with dementia prevalence estimates based on meta-analyses. *BMC Neurology* **10**, 62.

Aragona M (2009) The role of comorbidity in the crisis of the current psychiatric classification system. *Philosophy, Psychiatry, & Psychology* **16** (1), 1–11.

Bassett AS, Scherer SW, and Brzustowicz LM (2010) Copy number variations in schizophrenia: critical review and new perspectives on concepts of genetics and disease. *The American Journal of Psychiatry* **167** (8), 899–914.

Bienvenu OJ, Davydow DS, and Kendler KS (2011) Psychiatric 'diseases' versus behavioral disorders and degree of genetic influence. *Psychological Medicine* **41** (1), 33–40.

Bolton P, Bass J, Neugebauer R, Verdeli H, *et al.* (2003) Group interpersonal psychotherapy for depression in rural Uganda: a randomized controlled trial. *JAMA* **289** (23), 3117–24.

Callard F, Sartorius N, Arboleda-Flórez J, Bartlett P, *et al.* (eds) (2012) *Mental Illness, Discrimination and the Law.* Chichester: John Wiley & Sons.

Chappell AL, Goodley D, and Lawton R (2001) Making connections: the relevance of the social model of disability for people with learning difficulties. *British Journal of Learning Disabilities* **29**, 45–50.

Chen R, Hu Z, Wei L, Ma Y, Liu Z, *et al.* (2011) Incident dementia in a defined older Chinese population. *PLoS ONE* **6** (9): e24817.

Cicchetti D and Toth SL (2009) The past achievements and future promises of developmental psychopathology: the coming of age of a discipline. *Journal of Child Psychology and Psychiatry, and Allied Disciplines* **50** (1–2), 16–25.

Cohen P, Kasen S, Chen H, Hartmark C, *et al.* (2003) Variations in patterns of developmental transitions in the emerging adulthood period. *Developmental Psychology* **39** (4), 657–69.

Cooper PJ and Murray L (1998) Postnatal depression. *BMJ (Clinical Research Ed)* **316** (7148), 1884–6.

Cunningham C (1996) *Understanding Down syndrome.* Cambridge: Brookline Books.

Demyttenaere K, Bruffaerts R, Posada-Villa J, Gasquet I, *et al.* (2004) Prevalence, severity, and unmet need for treatment of mental disorders in the World Health Organization World Mental Health Surveys. *JAMA* **291** (21), 2581–90.

Department of Health (2001) *Safety First: Five Year Report of the National Confidential Inquiry into Suicide and Homicide by People with Mental Illness.* London: Department of Health.

Elkin I, Parloff MB, Hadley SW, and Autry JH (1985) NIMH Treatment of Depression Collaborative Research Program. Background and research plan. *Archives of General Psychiatry* **42** (3), 305–16.

Fabrega H (1991) The culture and history of psychiatric stigma in early modern and modern Western societies: A review of recent literature. *Comprehensive Psychiatry* **32** (2), 97–119.

Felce D, Taylor D, and Wright K (1994) Learning Disabilities. In: Stevens A and Raffery J (eds). *Health Care Needs Assessment: The Epidemiologically Based Needs Assessment Reviews,* 1st edn. Oxford: Radcliffe Medical Press.

Ferri CP, Prince M, Brayne C, Brodaty H, *et al.* (2005) Global prevalence of dementia: a Delphi consensus study. *Lancet* **366** (9503), 2112–17.

Fryers T (2002) Mental retardation: public health approaches to intellectual impairment and its consequences. In: Detels R, McEwen J, Beaglehole R, and Tanaka H (eds) *Oxford Textbook of Public Health: Volume 3.* Oxford: Oxford University Press.

Gates B (2002) *Learning Disabilities: Towards Inclusion.* London: Churchill Livingstone.

Gelder M, Gath D, and Mayou R (eds) (1994) *Concise Oxford Textbook of Psychiatry.* Oxford: Oxford University Press.

Gunnell D and Ashby D (2004) Antidepressants and suicide: what is the balance of benefit and harm. *BMJ (Clinical Research Ed)* **329** (7456), 34–8.

Gunnell D, Harbord R, Singleton N, Jenkins R, *et al.* (2004) Factors influencing the development and amelioration of suicidal thoughts in the general population. Cohort study. *The British Journal of Psychiatry: The Journal of Mental Science* **185**, 385–93.

Gunnell D and Frankel S (1994) Prevention of suicide: aspirations and evidence. *BMJ (Clinical Research Ed)* **308** (6938), 1227–33.

Hawton K, Saunders KEA, and O'Connor RC (2012) Self-harm and suicide in adolescents. *Lancet* **379** (9834), 2373–82.

Jack CR, Albert MS, Knopman DS, McKhann GM, *et al.* (2011) Introduction to the recommendations from the National Institute on Aging—Alzheimer's Association workgroups on diagnostic guidelines for Alzheimer's disease. *Alzheimer's and Dementia* **7** (3), 257–62.

Jones L, Harold D, and Williams J (2010) Genetic evidence for the involvement of lipid metabolism in Alzheimer's disease. *Biochimica Et Biophysica Acta* **1801** (8), 754–61.

Keage HAD, Matthews FE, Yip A, Gao L, *et al.* (2010) APOE and ACE polymorphisms and dementia risk in the older population over prolonged follow-up: 10 years of incidence in the MRC CFA Study. *Age and Ageing* **39** (1), 104–11.

Kelly BD, O'Callaghan E, Waddington JL, Feeney L, *et al.* (2010) Schizophrenia and the city: A review of literature and prospective study of psychosis and urbanicity in Ireland. *Schizophrenia Research* **116** (1), 75–89.

Kendler KS, Neale MC, Kessler RC, Heath AC, *et al.* (1992) A population-based twin study of major depression in women. The impact of varying definitions of illness. *Archives of General Psychiatry* **49** (4), 257–66.

Kendler KS (2005) 'A gene for . . .': the nature of gene action in psychiatric disorders. *The American Journal of Psychiatry* **162** (7), 1243–52.

Kessler RC, McGonagle KA, Zhao S, Nelson CB, *et al.* (1994) Lifetime and 12-month prevalence of DSM-III-R psychiatric disorders in the United States. Results from the National Comorbidity Survey. *Archives of General Psychiatry* **51** (1), 8–19.

Kessler RC, Aguilar-Gaxiola S, Alonso J, Chatterji S, *et al.* (2009) The global burden of mental disorders: an update from the WHO World Mental Health (WMH) surveys. *Epidemiologia E Psichiatria Sociale* **18** (1), 23–33.

Kirkbride JB, Errazuriz A, Croudace TJ, Morgan C, *et al.* (2012) Incidence of schizophrenia and other psychoses in England, 1950–2009: a systematic review and meta-analyses. *PloS One* **7** (3), e31660.

Kraemer HC, Noda A, and O'Hara R (2004) Categorical versus dimensional approaches to diagnosis: methodological challenges. *Journal of Psychiatric Research* **38** (1), 17–25.

Launer LJ, Andersen K, Dewey ME, Letenneur L, *et al.* (1999) Rates and risk factors for dementia and Alzheimer's disease: results from EURODEM pooled analyses. EURODEM Incidence Research Group and Work Groups. European Studies of Dementia. *Neurology* **52** (1), 78–84.

Lautenschlager NT, Cox KL, Flicker L, Foster JK, *et al.* (2008) Effect of physical activity on cognitive function in older adults at risk for Alzheimer disease: a randomized trial. *JAMA* **300** (9), 1027–37.

Lincoln TM, Ziegler M, Mehl S, Kesting M-L, *et al.* (2012) Moving from efficacy to effectiveness in cognitive behavioral therapy for psychosis: a randomized clinical practice trial. *Journal of Consulting and Clinical Psychology* **80** (4), 674–86.

Lobo A, Launer LJ, Fratiglioni L, Andersen K, *et al.* (2000) Prevalence of dementia and major subtypes in Europe: A collaborative study of population-based cohorts. Neurologic Diseases in the Elderly Research Group. *Neurology* **54** (11 Suppl. 5), S4–9.

McGilloway S and Donnelly M (2000) Work, rehabilitation and mental health. *Journal of Mental Health* **9**, 199–210.

McGrath J, Saha S, Welham J, El Saadi O, *et al.* (2004) A systematic review of the incidence of schizophrenia: the distribution of rates and the influence of sex, urbanicity, migrant status and methodology. *BMC Medicine* **213**.

McGuinness B, Craig D, Bullock R, and Passmore P (2009) Statins for the prevention of dementia. *Cochrane Database of Systematic Reviews* **2**, CD003160.

Mann JJ, Apter A, Bertolote J, Beautrais A, *et al.* (2005) Suicide prevention strategies: a systematic review. *JAMA* **294** (16), 2064–74.

Maulik PK, Mascarenhas MN, Mathers CD, Dua T, *et al.* (2011) Prevalence of intellectual disability:

a meta-analysis of population-based studies. *Research in Developmental Disabilities* **32** (2), 419–36.

Miller DN, Eckert TL, and Mazza JJ (2009) Suicide prevention programs in the schools: A review and public health perspective. *School Psychology Review* **38** (2), 168–88.

Moore THM, Zammit S, Lingford-Hughes A, Barnes TRE, *et al.* (2007) Cannabis use and risk of psychotic or affective mental health outcomes: a systematic review. *Lancet* **370** (9584), 319–28.

Motto JA and Bostrom AG (2001) A randomized controlled trial of postcrisis suicide prevention. *Psychiatric Services (Washington, D.C.)* **52** (6), 828–33.

Mueser KT and McGurk SR (2004) Schizophrenia. *Lancet* **363** (9426), 2063–72.

National Institute for Health and Clinical Excellence (2004) *Management of Depression in Primary and Secondary Care* (Clinical Guideline 23). London: NICE.

NICE (2011) *Alzheimer's disease-donepezil, galantamine, rivastigmine and memantine*. NICE. Available from: http://www.nice.org.uk/guidance/index.jsp?action=byID&o=13419

Olesen J, Gustavsson A, Svensson M, Wittchen H-U, *et al.* (2012) The economic cost of brain disorders in Europe. *European Journal of Neurology* **19** (1), 155–62.

OPCS (1995) *OPCS surveys of Psychiatric Morbidity in Britain. Bulletin 1: The prevalence of psychiatric morbidity among adults living in private households: Report 1.* London: HMSO.

Owen MJ, O'Donovan MC, Thapar A, and Craddock N (2011) Neurodevelopmental hypothesis of schizophrenia. *The British Journal of Psychiatry: The Journal of Mental Science* **198** (3), 173–5.

Patel V, Flisher AJ, and Cohen A (2012) Global mental health. In: Merson MH, Black RE, and Mills AJ (eds) *Global Health: Diseases, Programs, Systems, and Policies,* 3rd edn, pp. 445–80. Burlington, MA: Jones and Bartlett Learning.

Pitman A, Krysinska K, Osborn D, and King M (2012) Suicide in young men. *Lancet* **379** (9834), 2383–92.

Plassman BL, Williams JW, Jr, Burke JR, Holsinger T, *et al.* (2010) Systematic review: factors associated with risk for and possible prevention of cognitive decline in later life. *Annals of Internal Medicine* **153** (3), 182–93.

Prince M, Patel V, Saxena S, Maj M, *et al.* (2007) No health without mental health. *Lancet* **370** (9590), 859–77.

Purcell SM, Wray NR, Stone JL, Visscher PM, *et al.* (2009) Common polygenic variation contributes to risk of schizophrenia and bipolar disorder. *Nature* **460** (7256), 748–52.

Rees S, Cullen C, Kavenagh S, and Lelliott H (2004). Learning disabilities. In: Stevens A, Raffery R, and Mant J (eds) *Health Care Needs Assessment: The epidemiologically based needs assessment reviews,* 2nd edn. Oxford: Radcliffe Medical Press.

Ripke S, Sanders AR, Kendler KS, Levinson DF, *et al.* (2011) Genome-wide association study identifies five new schizophrenia loci. *Nature Genetics* **43** (10), 969–76.

Rosenhan DL (1973) On being sane in insane places. *Science (New York, N.Y.)* **179** (4070), 250–8.

Rusanen M, Rovio S, Ngandu T, Nissinen A, *et al.* (2010) Midlife smoking, apolipoprotein E and risk of dementia and Alzheimer's disease: a population-based cardiovascular risk factors, aging and dementia study. *Dementia and Geriatric Cognitive Disorders* **30** (3), 277–84.

Rutten BPF and Mill J (2009) Epigenetic mediation of environmental influences in major psychotic disorders. *Schizophrenia Bulletin* **35** (6), 1045–56.

Rutz W, von Knorring L, and Wålinder J (1992) Long-term effects of an educational program for general practitioners given by the Swedish Committee for the Prevention and Treatment of Depression. *Acta Psychiatrica Scandinavica* **85** (1), 83–8.

Saraceno B, Freeman M, and Funk M (2009) Public mental health. In: Detels, R, Beaglehole R, Lansang MA, and Gulliford M (eds) *Oxford Textbook of Public Health, Volume 3,* 5th edn; pp. 1081–100. Oxford: Oxford University Press.

Seshadri S, Fitzpatrick AL, Ikram MA, DeStefano AL, *et al.* (2010) Genome-wide analysis of genetic loci associated with Alzheimer disease. *JAMA* **303** (18), 1832–40.

Sundquist K, Frank G, and Sundquist J (2004) Urbanisation and incidence of psychosis and depression: follow-up study of 4.4 million women and men in Sweden. *The British Journal of Psychiatry: The Journal of Mental Science* **184**, 293–8.

Thomas HV, Dalman C, David AS, Gentz J, *et al.* (2001) Obstetric complications and risk of schizophrenia. Effect of gender, age at diagnosis and maternal history of psychosis. *The British Journal of Psychiatry: The Journal of Mental Science* **179**, 409–14.

Thornicroft G and Sartorius N (1993) The course and outcome of depression in different cultures: 10-year follow-up of the WHO Collaborative Study on the Assessment of Depressive Disorders. *Psychological Medicine* **23** (4), 1023–32.

Torpy JM, Lynm C, and Glass RM (2005) JAMA patient page. Suicide. *JAMA* **293** (20), 2558.

van der Heijden FMMA, Tuinier S, Arts NJM, Hoogendoorn MLC, *et al.* (2005) Catatonia: disappeared or under-diagnosed? *Psychopathology* **38** (1), 3–8.

Ward E, King M, Lloyd M, Bower P, *et al.* (2000) Randomised controlled trial of non-directive counselling, cognitive-behaviour therapy, and usual general practitioner care for patients with depression. I: clinical effectiveness. *BMJ (Clinical Research Ed)* **321** (7273), 1383–8.

Weaver T, Renton A, Stimson G, and Tyrer P (1999) Severe mental illness and substance misuse. *BMJ (Clinical Research Ed)* **318** (7177), 137–8.

Weiser M, van Os J, and Davidson M (2005) Time for a shift in focus in schizophrenia: from narrow phenotypes to broad endophenotypes. *The British Journal of Psychiatry: The Journal of Mental Science* **187**, 203–5.

Welch SS (2001) A review of the literature on the epidemiology of parasuicide in the general population. *Psychiatric Services (Washington, D.C.)* **52** (3), 368–75.

Wilkinson G, Hesdon B, Wild D, Cookson R, *et al.* (2000) Self-report quality of life measure for people with schizophrenia: the SQLS. *The British Journal of Psychiatry: The Journal of Mental Science* **177**, 42–6.

Willis SL, Tennstedt SL, Marsiske M, Ball K., *et al.* (2006) Long-term effects of cognitive training on everyday functional outcomes in older adults. *JAMA* **296** (23), 2805–14.

Wittchen HU, Zhao S, Kessler RC, and Eaton WW (1994) DSM-III-R generalized anxiety disorder in the National Comorbidity Survey. *Archives of General Psychiatry* **51** (5), 355–64.

World Health Organization (2001) World Health Report. *Mental Health: New Understanding, New Hope*. Geneva: World Health Organization.

Yip PSF, Caine E, Yousuf S, Chang S-S, *et al.* (2012) Means restriction for suicide prevention. *Lancet* **379** (9834), 2393–9.

Zammit S, Lewis G, Rasbash J, Dalman C, *et al.* (2010) Individuals, schools, and neighborhood: a multilevel longitudinal study of variation in incidence of psychotic disorders. *Archives of General Psychiatry* **67** (9), 914–22.

Model answers

Question 1

Firstly, the relation between the two is complex owing to the potential range of other influential factors (for example, socio-economic status, gender, and ethnicity) that most studies are unable to account for in their entirety. For example, social networks are generally better developed in rural than in urban areas and these may act as a 'buffer' against the more adverse living circumstances and daily life stress typically encountered in cities. This may, in turn, result in fewer psychiatric admissions from rural areas. Methodologically, however, it is difficult to obtain a measure of social support within large-scale studies other than perhaps marital status, which is too simplistic and differs by gender. Despite the potentially greater likelihood of supportive relationships, rural living may also be typified by factors that may, in the long term, precipitate mental ill health, such as limited access to appropriate support services. A second methodological difficulty relates to how urbanization is measured. In the study by Sundquist *et al.* (2004), it was calculated (correctly) as population density, but other studies have used self-report estimates, or the number of addresses per unit area, neither of which is a sufficiently precise or unbiased measure of the actual number of people in any area (Sundquist *et al.* 2004). Thirdly, the number of psychiatric beds may differ across urban and rural areas and may, therefore, bias the results (although this was not found in the Sundquist study), as would perhaps the effects of selective urban-rural migration.

Question 2

Incidence studies tend to be more difficult and costly because they involve identifying and selecting a large cohort of people who do not have dementia at the outset of a study and then following-up these study participants and assessing them over a significant period.

15 Musculoskeletal diseases

MADELINE ROONEY

CHAPTER CONTENTS

This chapter reviews the epidemiology of four of the most common musculoskeletal disorders: rheumatoid arthritis, osteoarthritis, osteoporosis, and backache.

Introduction

Musculoskeletal disorders are extremely common and include more than 150 different diseases and syndromes. The most common worldwide are rheumatoid arthritis, osteoarthritis, osteoporosis, spinal disorders (backache), and limb trauma. These disorders have a major impact on society owing to their frequency, chronicity, and resultant disability. At any one time (point prevalence) approximately five per cent of adults in Western populations will have a musculoskeletal disability, with a higher prevalence in women and the elderly. Furthermore, the prevalence of these disabilities is set to increase markedly in coming decades as the world's population continues to age. Musculoskeletal conditions are the second most common reason for consulting a doctor in most countries, are the commonest cause of long-term sickness absence in developed countries, and are one of the most common reasons for claiming disability benefit. Patients suffering from these disorders experience greatly reduced quality of life (QoL), especially in physical functioning (Fig. 15.1), and the associated pain and physical disability also affect the social functioning and mental health of patients.

In Fig. 15.1 standardized QoL scales were used in different patient groups in a total of 15,000 patients. Physical and mental functioning were compared for various disorders. Healthy individuals (data not shown) tended to have higher scores on both scales. In general, the results suggest that many diseases have an impact of similar magnitude on the physical and mental QoL, although it should be recognized that these assessments are based on the subjective assessments of patients and may also reflect, in part, coping behaviors.

15.1 Rheumatoid arthritis

Definition

Rheumatoid arthritis (RA) is a chronic, multisystem, autoimmune disorder of unknown cause, the major characteristic of which is chronic symmetrical erosive synovitis, usually involving the peripheral joints. There are no unique clinical or laboratory features that define the disease, and RA is defined according to the joint American and European guidelines (Aletaha *et al.* 2010; Box 15.1).

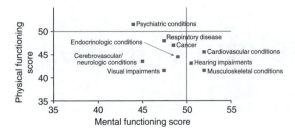

Figure 15.1 The position of disease clusters with respect to physical and mental functioning.

Reproduced form Sprangers MA, de Regt EB, and Andries F (2000) 'Which Chronic Conditions are Associated with Better or Poorer Quality of Life?' *Journal of Clinical Epidemiology* **53**, 895–907, with permission from Elsevier.

Note: Mean scores have been set at 50 to facilitate comparison of the two aspects of functioning.

Non-articular manifestations of RA include subcutaneous nodules, vasculitis, pericarditis, pulmonary nodules, intestinal fibrosis, neuritis, and episcleritis or scleritis.

Incidence and prevalence

Rheumatoid arthritis occurs throughout the world and affects all races. Most studies of the occurrence of RA have examined prevalence rather than incidence of the disease and estimates of point prevalence in developed countries vary between 0.5 and one per cent (500–1000 per 100,000 population). Throughout the world, RA is more common in women than men with a female : male ratio of disease prevalence of approximately 2.5 : 1, although there is variation between populations. In the UK, the annual incidence is 36 per 100,000 in women and 14 per 100,000 in men (Symmons *et al.* 1994). The age and sex distribution of incidence of RA is shown in Fig. 15.2. Incidence increases with increasing age but appears to fall in elderly women. The disease occurs at an earlier age in women than in men: peak age of incidence is around 55–64 years of age in women and 10 years later in men.

Time trends and geographic distribution

Evidence from skeletal remains indicates that RA occurred in native North American populations for several thousand years but was unknown in Europe before the 15th century, when it may have been imported by early explorers of the 'New World' (Rothschild *et al.* 2004). The incidence of RA in Europe appears to have increased rapidly during the 19th and early 20th centuries, possibly related to industrialization, but has fallen in westernized populations over the past 50 years. There is substantial geographic variation in the prevalence of RA. It is rare in rural Africa, and in urban and rural settings in China,

Box 15.1 Current criteria for the diagnosis of rheumatoid arthritis

- Involvement of one large joint gives 0 points
- Involvement of 2–10 large joints gives 1 point
- Involvement of 1–3 small joints (with or without involvement of large joints) gives 2 points
- Involvement of 4–10 small joints (with or without involvement of large joints) gives 3 points
- Involvement of more than 10 joints (with involvement of at least one small joint) gives 5 points
- Serological parameters—including the 'rheumatoid factor' as well as 'ACPA'—ACPA stands for *anti-citrullinated protein antibody*:
- Negative RF *and* negative ACPA gives 0 points
- Low-positive RF *or* low-positive ACPA gives 2 points

- High-positive RF *or* high-positive ACPA gives 3 points
- Acute phase reactants: one point for elevated erythrocyte sedimentation rate ESR, or elevated CRP value (C-reactive protein)
- Duration of arthritis: one point for symptoms lasting six weeks or longer

Values range from 0–10, values of six or greater indicate definite **rheumatoid arthritis**.

Reproduced from Aletaha D *et al.* '2010 rheumatoid arthritis classification criteria: an American College of Rheumatology/European League Against Rheumatism collaborative initiative'. *Annals of the Rheumatic Diseases* **69** (9), 2010, with permission from BMJ Publishing Ltd.

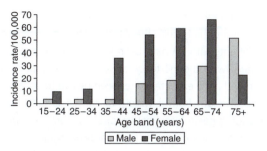

Figure 15.2 Age- and sex-specific incidence of rheumatoid arthritis.
Reproduced from Symmons DP, Barrett EM, Bankhead CR, Scott, DG, and Silman AJ (1994). 'The Incidence of Rheumatoid Arthritis in the United Kingdom: Results from the Norfolk Arthritis Register'. *British Journal of Rheumatology* **33** (8), 735–9, with permission from Oxford University Press.

Indonesia, and the Philippines (around 0.4 per cent), whereas the prevalence in India is similar to that in the West (approximately 0.75 per cent). The highest prevalence has traditionally been seen in Pima Indians in North America, although there have been declines in the prevalence in this group in the past few decades. In the UK the prevalence of RA appears to have fallen over the last 40 years in women, but not in men (Symmons *et al.* 2002). Similar trends have been observed in other western countries. One plausible hypothesis is the introduction of the contraceptive pill, known to have a protective effect. The geographic distribution and time trends underline the contribution of environmental and lifestyle factors to the development of this disease.

Aetiology and risk factors

The aetiology of RA is unknown but probably results from an interaction between exposure to environmental agents and genetic susceptibility. Family studies indicate a genetic predisposition; 10 per cent of patients have a first-degree relative with the disease and monozygotic twins are four times more likely to be concordant for disease than dizygotic twins. Approximately 70 per cent of patients with RA express the class II major histocompatibility complex (MHC) gene product HLA-DRB1, compared with 28 per cent of control subjects; this association has been seen in many

populations but is strongest in Caucasians. These alleles encode amino acid sequences at prominent positions on the antigen binding site; this resulted in the 'shared epitope' (SE) hypothesis and an elegant link between genetics and the environment (Gregerson *et al.* 1987), though this hypothesis remains unproven. Furthermore, the under representation of this allele in non-hospital based studies suggests that HLA DRB1 is a severity gene rather than a susceptibility gene. Other genetic factors involving mediators of inflammation, novel non-inherited maternal alleles, and autoimmunity are also under investigation.

Hormonal factors are thought to be important in the development of RA. Women have a higher incidence than men, onset during pregnancy is rare, and pregnancy is associated with remission of disease, while exacerbations may occur post-delivery. However, a meta-analysis of studies examining the association between oral contraceptive use and development of RA has failed to demonstrate that oral contraceptives protect against RA (Pladevall-Vila *et al.* 1996), though there is some evidence that contraceptive use results in milder RA and that patients have a better long-term outcome (Spector and Hochberg 1990).

One of the most important developments in the last five years has been the association between RA and anti-cyclic citrullinated protein antibodies (anti-CCP). Anti-CCP antibodies are a better predictor of disease severity and long-term joint damage (OR 4.0) than the presence of rheumatoid factor (RF) (Avouac *et al.* 2006). The association between anti-CCP and severe disease has been confirmed in several studies. Its prognostic importance is shown by its inclusion in the 2010 American College Criteria for RA (Aletaha *et al.* 2010). Furthermore, anti-CCP (and RF) positivity determines the first choice of biological therapy to be used in the treatment of RA.

Smokers of both sexes have an increased risk of developing RF and anti-CCP positive, but not RF and anti-CCP negative, RA. The increased risk occurs after a long duration, but moderate intensity, of smoking and may remain for several years after smoking cessation. Obesity has been strongly associated as a risk factor in anti-CCP negative RA but not in anti-CCP positive RA. Alcohol consumption is protective in RF and anti-CCP positive disease (Pederson *et al.* 2006; Klareskog *et al.* 2006).

The role of diet in the epidemiology of RA has been infrequently investigated. Fish oils have a beneficial effect on the symptoms of established RA, but it is not known whether they reduce the risk of developing the disease. There is emerging evidence that high intake of fruit and vegetables and antioxidants may be protective against RA (Cerhan *et al.* 2003). A recent systematic review of the literature by was unable to identify any dietary intervention that significantly affected outcome, probably due to sample size and study design (Smedslund *et al.* 2010).

Many patients attribute their RA to either physical or psychological trauma but there is no robust evidence to support this notion, and, although recent infection has been implicated in triggering RA, no specific organism has been identified. Although environmental exposures are undoubtedly important in the development of RA, the evidence is insufficient to identify possible preventive measures.

Natural history

The course of RA varies considerably between patients; some experience only a brief mild oligo-articular arthritis with minimal joint damage, whereas others develop a chronic destructive arthritis with marked functional impairment and disability. Within a decade of diagnosis between 50 and 60 per cent of patients are too disabled to remain economically active. Several factors appear to be associated with the development of disabling disease. Patients who are RF-positive and/ or anti-CCP positive are more likely to develop erosive disease than those who are RF and anti CCP-negative. Later onset of the disease is associated with more rapid progression and women have a worse functional outcome than men, although sex does not appear to influence radiological progression. There is some evidence that use of oral contraceptives or hormone replacement therapy may have a positive long-term effect on the outcome of RA among women. Socio-economic disadvantage is also associated with a worse clinical course (and earlier mortality) in RA patients, which does not appear to result from systematic differences

in treatment but probably from differences in individual susceptibility and other lifestyle factors.

Patients with RA have been shown to have approximately twice the mortality rate of the general population and a life expectancy reduced by five to 10 years. Risk of death from a variety of causes is increased, including gastrointestinal, respiratory, cardiovascular, and infectious diseases, with cardiovascular disease contributing up to 40 per cent of the observed excess mortality.

In recent years the association between chronic inflammation and cardiovascular damage in RA has been established. Maradit-Kremers *et al.* (2005) noted that RA patients experienced more acute myocardial infarctions (OR 3.2, 95% CI 1.2–8.7) and more silent infarctions (OR 5.9, 95% CI 1.3–26.6) than a control group. Research suggests that the presence of RA in conjunction with other risk factors such as smoking and hyperlipidaemia further increases the risk of heart disease in these patients.

The treatment of RA has been revolutionized over the last ten years with the advent of biological therapies (Curtis and Singh 2011). These drugs targeted at specific components of the inflammatory cascade have had a significant impact on controlling disease with few short-term side effects. However, since many of these, such as anti-TNF, are directed against highly conserved molecules (which are probably important for survival), there are concerns regarding long-term side effects. Thus clinicians need to be vigilant and all patients in the UK are placed on a long-term data base so that side effects can be closely monitored. The National Institute for Health and Clinical Excellence (NICE) (UK) has developed guidelines for their use in RA and other inflammatory musculoskeletal disorders. Costs are high and treatment is long-term. In 2007 the estimated worldwide cost of biological therapy was €7 billion. With the advent of new agents, this cost will only increase. A recent systematic review on the use and timing of biological intervention in RA provides an excellent summary of our current knowledge of these agents (Nam *et al.* 2010). There is little doubt however that the early introduction of aggressive therapy significantly improves outcome (Goekoop-Ruiterman *et al.* 2005).

Quality of life

Management of RA is aimed at relieving symptoms, modifying the disease process, and minimizing disability associated with the disease; the overall goal is to maximize the patient's QoL. As the course of RA can extend over many years, with periods of remission and relapse, and because early and continuous treatment with toxic drugs has now become standard management, the measurement of health-related QoL in this patient group has assumed increasing importance. There is an increasing consensus that the evaluation of health and health care should comprise an assessment of (1) health status and (2) QoL, as well as (3), the usual physiopathological measures relating to the presence, nature, and severity of a disease. According to Gill and Feinstein (1994), these three dimensions provide doctors with a comprehensive outcome assessment, a better understanding of the complex relationship between physiological and psychosocial health, and a measure of the effect of illness and chronic disease on a patient's life. Because of the long-term nature of the disease, clinical outcomes such as mortality, survival, and relapse rates are less appropriate and less informative for RA and other chronic conditions in which the main goal of treatment and care is to improve, or at least maintain, QoL. In addition, clinical outcomes tend to be assessed by doctors, whereas health status and QoL tend to be self-assessed, thereby providing a patient perspective of the consequences of a disease. Health status measures such as the Short-Form 36 health survey questionnaire (Ware and Sherbourne 1992) provide important information (usually in a self-report format) about aspects of the quality of a patient's health, for example pain, functioning, and mood. Health status may be assessed by a health care professional or a family carer as well as by a patient, whereas each individual patient assesses QoL. Thus, QoL measures provide an opportunity and means of eliciting and recording the unique perspective of each patient on their condition and how it affects their daily life. Measures tend to be questionnaire based and it is important that a relevant, condition-specific measure is applied to the appropriate patient group which is sufficiently sensitive to assess each patient's status and

which can also detect any changes in QoL over time. Many compendiums of QoL scales such as EuroQol, arthritis impact measurement scales, and other outcome measures are readily available (see, for example, Bowling 1995). Health-related quality of life studies in RA reveal *significant differences* in pain, functional disability, fatigue, and mental problems compared to control populations. Factors such as socio-economic and educational status significantly influence outcome.

....

Question 1

What is the most important reason for the use of QoL scales for the clinician specializing in musculoskeletal disease?

Question 2

For which other diseases may QoL scales be especially relevant?

....

Juvenile idiopathic arthritis

Whilst less common than adult RA, next to childhood asthma, juvenile idiopathic arthritis (JIA) is one of the commonest chronic group of diseases of childhood. Juvenile idiopathic arthritis is comprised of seven subgroups according to the International League of Associations for Rheumatology (ILAR) criteria. In the vast majority of cases JIA is not adult RA beginning in childhood. The genetics of JIA are different to that observed in adult RA, though, in keeping with adult disease, the aetiology is thought to be a combination of environmental and genetic factors. The concordance in monozygotic twins was reported to be 25 per cent in eight twin pairs in Finland (Thompson and Donn 2002).

Oligo-articular JIA, in which less than four joints are involved, accounts for some 60 per cent of all cases. Joint erosions are less common in JIA possibly because of the different mechanisms involved but are more likely due to the superior powers of repair in children. However, a consequence of arthritis occurring in a growing joint is the development of growth abnormalities. Some 15 per cent of children with JIA develop an asymptomatic anterior uveitis, which if undetected and/or untreated can lead to functional blindness. The epidemiology of JIA (where robust figures exist) is fairly similar worldwide with reported prevalence rates varying from 0.07–4 per 100,000 population, probably reflecting changes in diagnostic criteria over time and the mode of acquisition of data (Manners and Bower 2002).

Natural history

Juvenile idiopathic arthritis is a potentially destructive disease. Predictors of a poor outcome include: young age at onset, persistently raised inflammatory markers, systemic subtype of disease, and those children with true RA commencing in late childhood.

Prior to the use of aggressive therapies, studies in the 1970s have observed an overall mortality of just under 9 per cent, primarily due to infection and amyloidosis. Chronic disability was common, with a significant minority requiring wheelchairs and special education provision. With early intervention and current aggressive treatments including methotrexate and biological agents (Lovell *et al.* 2008) it is now rare to see a child with severe mobility problems and mortality is now estimated at 0.5–1 per cent, primarily among children with the systemic subtype of JIA (Petty 1999).

15.2 Osteoarthritis: definition and natural history

Osteoarthritis (OA), until relatively recently, was considered to be part of normal ageing, which is reflected in terms such as 'degenerative' or 'wear and tear'. Currently, despite some controversy, OA is defined as a disease characterized by focal areas of loss of articular cartilage within synovial joints, which are associated with hypertrophy of bone (osteophytes and subchondral bone sclerosis) and thickening of the capsule. The disease is defined as primary, where no cause can be identified for premature joint failure, and secondary, where conditions such as inflammatory joint disease (see RA, section 15.1), injury, or neurological and metabolic conditions impair the joint, predisposing it to failure. Clinically, the condition is characterized by joint pain, tenderness, limitation of movement, crepitus, occasional effusion, and, as reflected in the name, inflammation. It can occur in any joint but is most common in the hip, knee, and the joints of the hand, foot, and spine. Inclusion in the disease definition of changes made visible by X-ray cannot distinguish between symptomatic and relatively asymptomatic OA. However, in an attempt to reduce overestimation of disease burden, epidemiological studies use definitions that combine X-ray findings and joint pain.

Most people with OA have relatively mild symptoms, but for an appreciable minority, the condition is more aggressive. In this group, fraying and fibrillation of cartilage results in development of synovitis, ultimately the loss of articular cartilage and bone-on-bone contact within the joint results in increasing pain and disability. Narrowing of joint spaces apparent on X-rays of knees appears to be a strong predictor of future progression, and is also a significant predictor of total joint arthroplasty (Wolfe and Lane 2002).

Incidence and prevalence

Osteoarthritis was estimated to be the eighth leading non-fatal burden of disease in the world in 1990, accounting for 2.8 per cent of total years of living with disability. In general, it is more prevalent in Europe and the USA than in other parts of the world.

Few data are available on the incidence of OA because of the difficulty of defining it and in determining its onset. A study from Australia which sought to calculate the incidence indicated that the disease is more common among women in all age groups (2.95 per 1000 population versus 1.71 per 1000 in men). For women, the highest incidence is among those in the 65–74 year age group, reaching 13.5 per 1000 population per year, whereas for men, the highest incidence occurs among those aged over 75 years (nine per 1000 population per year). More recent radiological longitudinal surveys in the UK suggest that the incidence may be much higher, with 20–30 women per 1000 aged 50–60 years developing new radiological knee, hip, or spinal OA each year (Hassett *et al.* 2003).

Prevalence is also problematic to measure accurately. Worldwide estimates are that 9.6 per cent of men and 18.0 per cent of women aged 60 years and above have symptomatic disease. Most attempts to estimate the prevalence are based on radiographic surveys of populations and indicate that prevalence increases indefinitely with age; changes are uncommon in persons under the age of 40 years but are seen in more than 50 per cent of people over the age of 65 years, and almost universally after 85 years. Men are affected more often than women among those aged less than 45 years, whereas in the over 55-year-old age group it is women who experience more disease. Radiographic studies of North American and European populations aged over 45 years show higher rates for OA of the knee: 14 per cent for men and 23 per cent for women.

Symptomatic, radiographically confirmed OA of the knee has been found among three per cent of women aged 45–65 years. Hip OA is slightly less common, with a radiographic prevalence of 1.9 per cent among men and 2.3 per cent among women aged 45 years or more in one Swedish survey (Danielsson and Lindberg 1997).

Time trends

Not surprisingly, because of the difficulty of defining and measuring the disease, there are few data on trends in the incidence of OA, and whether incidence is changing is not clear. Two Nordic studies used proxy measures to assess trends. The first, from Norway, reported that the incidence of OA-specific disability pensions increased over the 30 years from 1968 to 1997 while the second, an Icelandic study, found an increase in the rate of new hip replacements from 1982 to 1996. However, it has been suggested that this reflects improved access to surgery rather than an upward trend in incidence. In the USA, pharmacological treatment for OA decreased from 49 per cent of visits (1989–91) to 46 per cent (1992–94) to 40 per cent (1995–98), which supports this view. As the incidence and prevalence of the disease rise with increasing age, extended life expectancy will result in greater numbers of people with the condition. The burden will be the greatest in low income countries, where life expectancy is increasing and access to arthroplasty and joint replacement is poor.

Risk factors

The main risk factors are age, a positive family history, female sex, obesity, and joint trauma. Modifiable factors, including obesity, injury, quadriceps strength, malalignment of the joint, and occupational activities, contribute to the onset and progression of joint disability.

Obesity is a risk factor for the development of OA of the hand, knee, and hip and for progression in the knee and hip. It was generally believed that the obesity was secondary to inactivity brought about by the painful joints. However, well-designed epidemiological studies now show that the risk begins as early as the third decade of life. For every two units increase in body mass index (BMI) (equivalent to about 5 kg), the risk of OA of the knee is increased by 36 per cent. Conversely, for every 5 kg decrease in body weight during the preceding 10 years, the risk of OA of the knee declines by more than 50 per cent. People classified as obese (BMI > 30 kg/m^2) have a 20-fold risk of developing bilateral OA of the knee (Hart *et al.* 1999).

Trauma and certain physically demanding activities or occupations are also risk factors for the development of OA of the knee and hip. Farming presents the greatest relative risk: 4.5 for those who work in farming for 1–9 years and 9.3 for those who farm for more than 10 years. The strongest association with occupational activity has been shown with OA of the knee in men. It is estimated that up to 30 per cent of OA in this joint is attributable to occupational activity that involves repeated knee bending, kneeling, squatting, or climbing. These activities increase the risk two- to fourfold and, if combined with heavy lifting of more than 25 kg on a regular basis, increase risk fivefold. Strong interactions are shown between occupational knee bending and obesity (risk increased 10–15 times), and between age and injury to the knee. Klussmann *et al.* (2010) have recently demonstrated an association between knee bending and loading in women.

Family history of OA is a well-documented risk factor, with the occurrence of Heberden's nodes having autosomal dominant inheritance. Despite this strong association, no single gene defect has been identified. Studies of twins now suggest that the heritability component of osteoarthritis may be as high as 60–65 per cent for hip and hand osteoarthritis, and around 40–50 per cent for knee osteoarthritis. Whilst no single gene has been identified as pivotal, a number of genes primarily associated with collagen and cartilage matrix have been associated with the disease.

All races can be affected by OA, but some Asians have a much lower prevalence in the hip and hand, but a higher prevalence in the knee. More disease is seen in the knee in Chinese women when compared with North American women, and is independent of weight and anatomical alignment of the lower limbs. Why this might be so is suggested in a study that investigated the association between squatting and risk of OA, a common daily posture in China (Zhang *et al.* 2004).

Treatment issues

Although pharmacotherapy has a major role in treatment of OA, hip and knee joint replacements are also of great importance as they are among the most cost-effective interventions available. Ninety per cent of total hip replacements and over 95 per cent of total knee replacements are performed for OA. The difficulties in measuring incidence and prevalence of OA complicate the assessment of **population need** for total joint replacement surgery. Many aspects need to be considered, not only incidence and prevalence, but also disease progression, and patients' preferences for surgery, and doctors' propensity for recommending it. Such factors were considered in studies of the need for total hip and knee surgery in England. The authors estimated that, whereas hip replacement rates were closely in line with need, a doubling of the current rate of knee replacement surgery would be required just to meet existing need (Jüni *et al.* 2003). This **unmet need** was not just the result of health care services' inability to keep up with demand, but also of patients and doctors not considering, or offering, knee replacement as a treatment option. However the outcome following total knee replacement appears to be less favourable than that for hip.

15.3 Osteoporosis

Osteoporosis is a condition of decreased bone mass. This results in increased bone fragility and thus an increase risk of fracture though loss of bone mass is not the only contributor to fracture; brittleness is another. Thus children with low bone mass are much less likely to fracture following trauma, probably because of the flexibility of young bones. The clinical diagnosis of osteoporosis is defined according to the WHO criteria (see 'Evaluation of bone mineral density measurements' section) according to bone mineral density (BMD), with osteoporosis defined as a BMD which predicts a twofold increased risk of fracture. This diagnosis is of particular importance in the elderly who are at risk of falling, often causing fracture of the neck of the femur at the hip joint, or Colles' fracture of head of the radius at the wrist. In a systematic review of the literature, hip fracture resulted in a fatal outcome at one year from eight to 36 per cent (Abrahamsen *et al.* 2009).

In healthy young adults, bone strength far exceeds the loads that are normally applied to bone during activities of daily living. Thus there is a large 'safety factor' in this age group. However, with increased age there is a reduction in bone mass and impairment of bone architecture. This coupled with increasing brittleness with age results in decreased strength.

Evaluation of bone mineral density measurements

Several technologies now exist which measure BMD, including single and dual energy absorptiometry, dual-energy X-ray absorptiometry (DEXA), and quantitative computed tomography. However the most widely used and validated today is DEXA. These technologies vary in their accuracy, which can be compared to a 'gold standard' where BMD is measured in animals, and animal bone is then evaluated chemically (WHO 1994). Accuracy may also depend on the precise skeletal site being assessed and the amount of fat tissue interposed between the instrument and the bone. However, when evaluating the usefulness of different screening techniques it is also important to consider the population variance in BMD. The distribution of BMD in young adults is shown in Fig. 15.3.

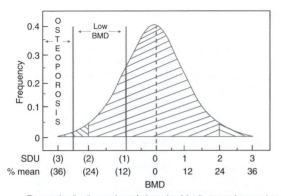

The curve describes the normal range for bone mineral density expressed as percentage positive or negative deviation from the mean, or in units of standard deviation (SDU).

Figure 15.3 Distribution of bone mineral density (BMD) in a young, normal population and definition of osteoporosis. Adapted from World Health Organization (1994). *Assessment of Fracture Risk and Application to Screening for Postmenopausal Osteoporosis.* WHO Technical Report Series No. 843, with permission from the World Health Organization.

Bone mineral density is calculated in g/cm². The BMD of the patient is compared with the young adult reference mean BMD and expressed as a standard deviation (SD) score or 'T' score. Osteoporosis is defined as a BMD T score more than 2.5 SD below the young adult reference mean. It should be noted that the WHO definition of osteoporosis with T scores refers only to postmenopausal women and men over 50 years and must not be used to evaluate the risk of fracture in the young adult population. Furthermore, the evaluation of a patient with suspected osteoporosis must involve a thorough clinical history, physical examination, and BMD measurement. Table 15.1 illustrates some of the more important modifiable and non-modifiable risk factors for osteoporosis.

There has been much debate about the value of BMD measurement as a screening tool. The National Screening Committee (2012) has not been able to recommend this based on current methods and evidence. Combinations of risk factors increase the risks of sustaining a fracture (Table 15.2), but most people with these risk factors will not experience an adverse outcome. Thus, among the key reasons for the decision of the National Screening Committee, is the relatively poor ability of the test to predict which *individuals* will sustain a fracture. It is crucial, when any diagnostic or screening test is being evaluated, to consider its place in a clinical pathway designed to improve patient outcomes. No test should be ordered unless the result will be likely to affect the outcome for the patient. Screening of all women is not recommended, but selected high-risk women are routinely screened in North America (Anon 2001). Arguments have been made for (Dequeker and

Table 15.1 Risk factors for osteoporosis

Not modifiable	Possibly modifiable
Personal history of adult fracture	Low bone mineral density
History of fracture in first-degree relative	Current cigarette use Low body weight (< 127 pounds or 57 kg)
Caucasian and Asian race	Oestrogen deficiency including menopause onset at younger than 45 years
Advanced age	Alcoholism
Female sex	Lifelong low calcium intake
Glucocorticoid use	Recurrent falls
Dementia	Inadequate physical activity
Poor health/frailty	Discontinuation or non-compliance of anti-resorptive therapy

Table 15.2 Population relative risk of fracture by number of risk factors

| | Women aged 50–60 years | | Annual absolute fracture risk for women aged: | |
Risk factors	Prevalence of factor (%)	Relative risk if have factor versus average risk	50–54 years (%)	55–59 years (%)
No risk factors	58.3	0.5	0.7	0.8
One risk factor	32.8	1.2	1.5	1.9
Two risk factors	7.6	2.7	3.5	4.3
Three risk factors	1.4	5.9	7.6	9.4
After bone densitometry				
One risk factor, BMD > mean	14.3	0.6	0.8	1.0
One risk factor, BMD in second quarter	8.5	1.1	1.5	1.8
Two risk factors, BMD > mean	2.9	1.4	1.7	2.8
One risk factor, BMD in lowest quarter	10.1	2.0	2.5	3.2
Two risk factors, BMD in second lowest quarter	2.0	2.4	3.0	3.8
Three risk factors, BMD above mean	0.4	2.8	3.6	4.5
Two risk factors, BMD in lowest quarter	2.6	4.0	5.2	6.5
Three risk factors, BMD in second lowest quarter	0.1	4.8	6.2	7.6
Three risk factors, BMD in lowest quarter	0.9	7.8	10.1	12.5

The non-spine fracture incidence for Caucasian British women aged 52 years is 1.3 per cent, and for women aged 57 years is 1.6 per cent. BMD, bone mineral density.

Modified from Torgerson DJ, Igesisias CP, Reid DM (2001). 'The Economics of Fracture Prevention', in DH Barlow, RM Francis, and A Miles (eds), *The Effective Management of Osteoporosis*. London: Aesculapius Medical Press, 111–21.

Luyton 2001) and against (Wilkin and Devendra 2001) the use of bone densitometry as a screening tool. An evaluation of four different selection criteria in a cohort of 2365 postmenopausal women from Canada showed that an alternative set of decision rules was superior to that recommended in national guidelines to predict risk of hip fracture (Cadarette *et al.* 2001).

Prevention of hip fractures

Sustaining a fracture, particularly a hip fracture in old age, is not a trivial affliction. The Scottish Inter-collegiate Guidelines Network (SIGN) guidelines have identified four factors that significantly increase the risk of a hip fracture and should be addressed:

previous low-impact fracture, family history of fracture, smoking, and low BMD. Any strategy to prevent or treat osteoporosis therefore must incorporate a programme not only to improve BMD but also to prevent falls. Intensive multifactorial preventive strategies that include exercise, reduction in medications, and environmental modifications can reduce falls by 30 per cent (Carter *et al.* 2001). At a minimum, the risk factors for falls to predict hip fracture should be recorded and acted upon for all frail elderly, whether in hospital or community. Some of these risks are illustrated in Table 15.3 and many are amenable to simple interventions.

However, the condition needs to be tackled on multiple fronts, with, for example, advice on diet (and calcium supplementation where necessary). Effective treatment (with bone strengthening agents such as bisphosphonates or bone forming agents such as teraparatide) are the cornerstone of treatment for established disease. An important lesson

Table 15.3 Host risk factors for falls among the elderly for which the evidence is strong or moderate

Demographic characteristics
Older age
Female sex
Functional level
Limitations in activities of daily living and instrumental activities of daily living
Cane/walker use
History of falls
Gait, balance, strength
Slow walking speed
Postural sway
Low lower-extremity strength
Low upper-extremity strength
Impaired reflexes

Sensory
Poor vision
Lower-extremity sensory perception
Chronic illnesses
Parkinson's disease
Other neuromuscular disease
Stroke
Urinary incontinence
Arthritis
Acute illness
Medications, alcohol
Several medications used
Hypnotics
Sedatives
Antidepressants
Antiparkinsonism drugs
Mental status
Cognitive impairment
Depression

Reproduced from Kelsey JL and Sowes MF (2004). 'Musculoskeletal Diseases', in R Detels, J McEwen, R Beaglehole, and H Tanaka (eds.), *Oxford Textbook of Public Health* (4th edn). Oxford: Oxford University Press. (Modified from Grisso *et al.* (1991)).

to be drawn from the debates about the measurement of BMD must be that the outcome of any intervention (whether diagnostic or therapeutic) must be seen against a broad canvas. Low BMD is of itself asymptomatic, it is its consequence, fracture, that is the problem. Thus, the benefit of a **systems approach** lies in seeing our actions and intervention to combat the consequences of osteoporosis in their place, as part of a system or environment that can either enhance or erode our health (see Fig. 15.4).

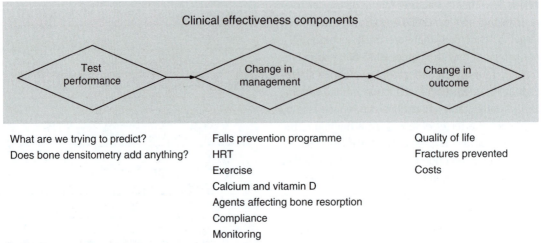

Figure 15.4 A systems approach to the evaluation of bone densitometry.

15.4 Backache

More than two-thirds of adults in Western countries will at some time suffer from low back pain (LBP) (Deyo and Weinstein 2001) but, fortunately, although LBP consists of a variety of entities with somewhat different aetiologies, most episodes are self-limiting. Nevertheless, the condition is a leading cause of sickness absence and retirement due to ill health. The epidemiology and management of the condition were well reviewed in the 1990s by the Clinical Standards Advisory Group (1994) and by the Royal College of General Practitioners (1996), and the guidance from these is still valid. Data from an official survey in the UK revealed a prevalence of LBP of 37 per cent. Maniadakis and Gray (2000) calculated that this equated to a loss of 116 million working days and a conservative estimated loss of revenue of over £3–10 billion. They estimated that the annual total direct and indirect cost of LBP was between £6–12 billion.

Epidemiology

Any strategy to reduce morbidity has to start with an appreciation of the epidemiology and risk factors. In a review of studies, the population annual prevalence was reported to lie between 15 and 45 per cent and the point prevalence averaged 30 per cent. In surveys of the general population, LBP is found equally in men and women and is most common in the elderly (Andersson 1999). Up to 60 per cent of people with LBP will also have neck pain, and LBP is frequently associated with other complaints. There is conflicting evidence for a relation between LBP prevalence and social class, and this may be largely related to occupation. It seems clear that back pain is more common in people in heavy manual occupations who undertake heavy lifting, and it has been reported to be more common among smokers. On both counts, the health service itself needs to target its training programmes towards especially vulnerable staff such as nurses. A recent review of trials of primary prevention in the workplace concluded that there was little evidence to support the use of education in lifting techniques or for lumbar supports but there was some evidence to recommend an exercise programme (van Poppel *et al.* 2004).

Psychological factors are often quoted as being important to the aetiology of LBP, but it is difficult to distinguish those that preceded acute symptoms from those that followed. Nevertheless, such factors have to be borne in mind when decisions about patient management are being made in primary care. In a longitudinal study in the UK, it was noted that

90 per cent of patients were no longer consulting their general practitioner three months after the initial consultation, but, on interview, most had continued symptoms and disability 12 months later (Croft *et al.* 1998).

Clinical management

The most important underlying principle to guide management of LBP in primary care is early and effective *triage*. Box 15.2 summarizes the main points for triage and initial management.

Most cases can and should be managed without recourse to secondary care, which should be reserved for those who have failed to settle within six to eight weeks. Consensus evidence suggests that there should be a gradual increase in physical activity with no initial bed rest (Royal College of General Practitioners 1996). The types of hospital service most likely to prove effective are those that offer multi-disciplinary assessment from the outset, including psychosocial and vocational advice, and input from rehabilitation and pain management specialists. In certain defined cases, manipulative treatment or surgery can be beneficial. In a systematic review of the literature on the management of LBP, Liddle *et al.* (2004) found no specific management superior (possibly due to the differences in trial design), but concluded that self-help and active management were superior to passive approaches. A recent systematic review of the cost-effectiveness of general practice care concluded that adding advice, education and exercise, or exercise and behavioural counselling, to usual general practice was more cost-effective than GP care alone (Lin *et al.* 2011). A systematic review and meta-analysis of the efficacy, cost-effectiveness, and safety of complementary medicine for LBP (also for neck pain) included data from 147 RCTs concluded that complementary therapies including spinal manipulation were more effective than no treatment or usual care at short-term follow-up (Furlan *et al.* 2012).

Box 15.2 Diagnostic triage for back pain

Diagnostic triage is the differential diagnosis between:

1. Simple backache (non-specific low back pain)
2. Nerve root pain
3. Possible serious spinal pathology

1 Simple backache: specialist referral not required

- Presentation 20–55 years
- Lumbrosacral, buttock, and thighs
- 'Mechanical' pain
- Patient well

2 Nerve root pain: specialist referral not generally required within first 4 weeks, provided resolving

- Unilateral leg pain worse than low back pain
- Radiates to foot or toes
- Numbness and parathesia in same distribution

*Straight leg raising (test)

- SLR* reproduces leg pain
- Localized neurological signs

3 Red flags for possible serious spinal pathology: prompt referral (less than 4 weeks)

- Presentation under 20 years or onset over 55 years
- Non-mechanical pain
- Thoracic pain
- Past history: carcinoma, steroids, HIV
- Unwell, weight loss
- Widespread neurology
- Structural deformity

Cauda equina syndrome: immediate referral

- Sphincter disturbance
- Gait disturbance
- Saddle anaesthesia

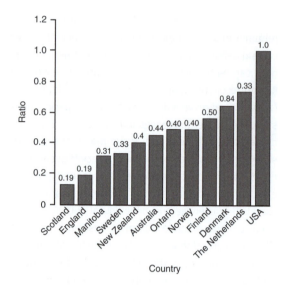

Figure 15.5 Rates of surgery for back pain in 11 countries and Canadian provinces as a proportion of those in the USA. Reproduced from Andersson BJ (1999). 'Epidemiological features of chronic low back pain', *Lancet* **354**, 581–5, with permission from Elsevier.

....

Question 3

How would you interpret the data shown in Fig. 15.5?

Question 4

What additional data would be helpful?
....

Further epidemiological studies and RCTs will be required for all musculoskeletal disorders because of their uncertain aetiologies, and a likely increase in the prevalence of these disorders in an ageing population. Whilst no single method of treatment is superior, current advice would be that any appropriate active intervention is better than none. In addition, QoL outcome measurements for these disorders will require further development.

Web addresses

Guidelines for BMD measurements (SIGN)
www.sign.ac.uk

Further reading

Kelsey JL and Hannan MT (2009) Musculoskeletal diseases. In: Detels R, Beaglehole R, Lansang MA, and Gulliford M (eds), *Oxford Textbook of Public Health*, 5th edn, pp. 1117–31. Oxford: Oxford University Press.

References

Abrahamsen B, van Staa T, Ariely R, Olson M, *et al.* (2009) Excess mortality following hip fracture: a systematic epidemiological review. *Osteoporosis International* **20** (10), 1633–50.

Aletaha D, Neogi T, Silman AJ, Funovits J, *et al.* (2010) 2010 rheumatoid arthritis classification criteria: an American College of Rheumatology/European League Against Rheumatism collaborative initiative. *Annals of the Rheumatic Diseases* **69** (9), 1580–8.

Andersson GB (1999) Epidemiological features of chronic low-back pain. *Lancet* **354** (9178), 581–5.

Anon (2001) Osteoporosis prevention, diagnosis, and therapy. *JAMA* **285** (6), 785–95.

Avouac J, Gossec L, and Dougados M (2006) Diagnostic and predictive value of anti-cyclic citrullinated protein antibodies in rheumatoid arthritis: a systematic literature review. *Annals of the Rheumatic Diseases* **65** (7), 845–51.

Bowling A (1995) *Measuring Disease. A Review of Quality of Life Measurement Scales.* Milton Keynes: Open University Press.

Cadarette SM, Jaglal SB, Murray TM, McIsaac WJ, *et al.* (2001) Evaluation of decision rules for referring women for bone densitometry by dual-energy x-ray absorptiometry. *JAMA* **286** (1), 57–63.

Carter ND, Kannus P, and Khan KM (2001) Exercise in the prevention of falls in older people: a systematic literature review examining the rationale and the evidence. *Sports Medicine (Auckland, N.Z.)* **31** (6), 427–38.

Cerhan JR, Saag KG, Merlino LA, Mikuls TR, *et al.* (2003) Antioxidant micronutrients and risk of rheumatoid arthritis in a cohort of older women. *American Journal of Epidemiology* **157** (4), 345–54.

Cherkin DC, Deyo RA, Loeser JD, Bush T, *et al.* (1994) An international comparison of back surgery rates. *Spine* **19** (11), 1201–6.

Clinical Standards Advisory Group (1994) *Epidemiology Review: The Epidemiology and Cost of Back Pain.* London: HMSO.

Croft PR, Macfarlane GJ, Papageorgiou AC, Thomas E, et al. (1998) Outcome of low back pain in general practice: a prospective study. *BMJ (Clinical Research Ed)* **316** (7141), 1356–9.

Curtis JR and Singh JA (2011) Use of biologics in rheumatoid arthritis: current and emerging paradigms of care. *Clinical Therapeutics* **33** (6), 679–707.

Danielsson L and Lindberg H (1997) Prevalence of coxarthrosis in an urban population during four decades. *Clinical Orthopaedics and Related Research* **342**, 106–10.

Dequeker J and Luyten FP (2001) Bone densitometry is not a good predictor of hip fracture. *BMJ (Clinical Research Ed)* **323** (7316), 797–9.

Deyo RA and Weinstein JN (2001) Low back pain. *The New England Journal of Medicine* **344** (5), 363–70.

Furlan AD, Yazdi F, Tsertsvadze A, Gross A, et al. (2012) A systematic review and meta-analysis of efficacy, cost-effectiveness, and safety of selected complementary and alternative medicine for neck and low-back pain. *Evidence-Based Complementary and Alternative Medicine: eCAM* 2012: 953139. Epub 2011 24 November.

Gill TM and Feinstein AR (1994) A critical appraisal of the quality of quality-of-life measurements. *JAMA* **272** (8), 619–26.

Goekoop-Ruiterman YPM, de Vries-Bouwstra JK, Allaart CF, van Zeben D, et al. (2005) Clinical and radiographic outcomes of four different treatment strategies in patients with early rheumatoid arthritis (the BeSt study): a randomized, controlled trial. *Arthritis and Rheumatism* **52** (11), 3381–90.

Gregersen PK, Silver J, and Winchester RJ (1987) The shared epitope hypothesis. An approach to understanding the molecular genetics of susceptibility to rheumatoid arthritis. *Arthritis and Rheumatism* **30** (11), 1205–13.

Grisso JA, Kelsey JL, Strom BL, Chiu GY, et al. (1991) Risk factors for falls as a cause of hip fracture in women. The Northeast Hip Fracture Study Group. *The New England Journal of Medicine* **324** (19), 1326–31.

Hart DJ, Doyle DV, and Spector TD (1999) Incidence and risk factors for radiographic knee osteoarthritis in middle-aged women: the Chingford Study. *Arthritis and Rheumatism* **42** (1), 17–24.

Hassett G, Hart DJ, Manek NJ, Doyle DV, et al. (2003) Risk factors for progression of lumbar spine disc degeneration: the Chingford Study. *Arthritis and Rheumatism* **48** (11), 3112–17.

Jüni P, Dieppe P, Donovan J, Peters T, et al. (2003) Population requirement for primary knee replacement surgery: a cross-sectional study. *Rheumatology (Oxford, England)* **42** (4), 516–21.

Kelsey JL and Sowes MF (2004) Musculoskeletal Diseases. In: Detels R, McEwen J, Beaglehole R, and Tanaka H (eds) *Oxford Textbook of Public Health*, 4th edn, pp. 1117–31. Oxford: Oxford University Press.

Klareskog L, Padyukov L, Lorentzen J, and Alfredsson L (2006) Mechanisms of disease: Genetic susceptibility and environmental triggers in the development of rheumatoid arthritis. *Nature Clinical Practice. Rheumatology* **2** (8), 425–33.

Klussmann A, Gebhardt H, Nübling M, Liebers F, et al. (2010) Individual and occupational risk factors for knee osteoarthritis: results of a case-control study in Germany. *Arthritis Research & Therapy* **12** (3), R88.

Liddle SD, Baxter GD, and Gracey JH (2004) Exercise and chronic low back pain: what works? *Pain* **107** (1–2), 176–90.

Lin C-WC, Haas M, Maher CG, Machado LAC, et al. (2011) Cost-effectiveness of general practice care for low back pain: a systematic review. *European Spine Journal* **20** (7), 1012–23.

Lovell DJ, Reiff A, Ilowite NT, Wallace CA, et al. (2008) Safety and efficacy of up to eight years of continuous etanercept therapy in patients with juvenile rheumatoid arthritis. *Arthritis and Rheumatism* **58** (5), 1496–1504.

Maniadakis N and Gray A (2000) The economic burden of back pain in the UK. *Pain* **84** (1), 95–103.

Manners PJ and Bower C (2002) Worldwide prevalence of juvenile arthritis why does it vary so much? *The Journal of Rheumatology* **29** (7), 1520–30.

Maradit-Kremers H, Crowson CS, Nicola PJ, Ballman KV, et al. (2005) Increased unrecognized coronary heart disease and sudden deaths in rheumatoid arthritis: a population-based cohort study. *Arthritis and Rheumatism* **52** (2), 402–11.

Nam JL, Winthrop KL, van Vollenhoven RF, Pavelka K, et al. (2010) Current evidence for the management of rheumatoid arthritis with biological disease-modifying antirheumatic drugs: a systematic literature review informing the EULAR recommendations for the management of RA. *Annals of the Rheumatic Diseases* **69** (6), 976–86.

National Screening Committee (2012) Screening for Osteoporosis in Postmenopausal Women: a draft report for the UK National Screening Committee. Available at: http://www.screening.nhs.uk/osteoporosis

Pedersen M, Jacobsen S, Klarlund M, Pedersen BV, et al. (2006) Environmental risk factors differ between rheumatoid arthritis with and without auto-antibodies against cyclic citrullinated peptides. Arthritis Research & Therapy 8 (4), R133.

Petty RE (1999) Prognosis in children with rheumatic diseases: justification for consideration of new therapies. Rheumatology (Oxford, England) 38 (8), 739–42.

Pladevall-Vila M, Delclos GL, Varas C, Guyer H, et al. (1996) Controversy of oral contraceptives and risk of rheumatoid arthritis: meta-analysis of conflicting studies and review of conflicting meta-analyses with special emphasis on analysis of heterogeneity. American Journal of Epidemiology 144 (1), 1–14.

Rothschild BM, Coppa A, and Petrone PP (2004) 'Like a virgin': Absence of rheumatoid arthritis and treponematosis, good sanitation and only rare gout in Italy prior to the 15th century. Reumatismo 56 (1), 61–6.

Royal College of General Practitioners (1996) Clinical Guidelines for the Management of Acute Low Back Pain. London: RCGP.

Smedslund G, Byfuglien MG, Olsen SU and Hagen KB (2010) Effectiveness and safety of dietary interventions for rheumatoid arthritis: a systematic review of randomized controlled trials. Journal of the American Dietetic Association 110 (5), 727–35.

Spector TD and Hochberg MC (1990) The protective effect of the oral contraceptive pill on rheumatoid arthritis: an overview of the analytic epidemiological studies using meta-analysis. Journal of Clinical Epidemiology 43 (11), 1221–30.

Sprangers MA, de Regt EB, and Andries F (2000) Which chronic conditions are associated with better or poorer quality of life? Journal of Clinical Epidemiology 53, 895–907.

Symmons DP, Barrett EM, Bankhead CR, Scott DG, et al. (1994) The incidence of rheumatoid arthritis in the United Kingdom: results from the Norfolk Arthritis Register. British Journal of Rheumatology 33 (8), 735–9.

Symmons D, Turner G, Webb R, Asten P, et al. (2002) The prevalence of rheumatoid arthritis in the United Kingdom: new estimates for a new century. Rheumatology (Oxford, England) 41 (7), 793–800.

Thomson W and Donn R (2002) Juvenile idiopathic arthritis genetics - what's new? What's next? Arthritis research 4 (5), 302–6.

Torgerson DJ, Iglesias CP, and Reid DM (2001) The economics of fracture prevention. In: Barlow DH, Francis RM, and Miles A (eds). The Effective Management of Osteoporosis, pp. 111–21. London: Aesculapius Medical Press.

van Poppel MNM, Hooftman WE, and Koes BW (2004) An update of a systematic review of controlled clinical trials on the primary prevention of back pain at the workplace. Occupational Medicine (Oxford, England) 54 (5), 345–52.

Ware JE Jr and Sherbourne CD (1992) The MOS 36-item short-form health survey (SF-36). I. Conceptual framework and item selection. Medical Care 30 (6), 473–83.

Wilkin TJ and Devendra D (2001) Bone densitometry is not a good predictor of hip fracture. BMJ (Clinical Research Ed) 323 (7316), 795–7.

Wolfe F and Lane NE (2002) The longterm outcome of osteoarthritis: rates and predictors of joint space narrowing in symptomatic patients with knee osteoarthritis. The Journal of Rheumatology 29 (1), 139–46.

World Health Organization (1994) Assessment of fracture risk and application to screening for postmenopausal osteoporosis. WHO Technical Report Series No. 843. Geneva: World Health Organization.

Zhang Y, Hunter DJ, Nevitt MC, Xu L, et al. (2004) Association of squatting with increased prevalence of radiographic tibiofemoral knee osteoarthritis: the Beijing Osteoarthritis Study. Arthritis and Rheumatism 50 (4), 1187–92.

Model answers

Question 1

Musculoskeletal disease does not cause death in the short-term; however, pain and disability can severely restrict movement and the ability to perform activities of daily living. This will have an effect on QoL, so QoL scales are an important means of assessing remission, progression of disease, and response to treatment.

Question 2

Similarly, other diseases that may be long term and debilitating include mental disorders, certain cancers, chronic cardiovascular diseases such as angina and stroke, and chronic lung and kidney disease.

Question 3

There is a more than a tenfold difference between rates for surgical intervention for back pain between the UK and USA. In part this may reflect a conservative attitude towards intervention on the part of the UK surgeons (and also those in Manitoba), but it may also reflect the availability of the service. It would be helpful to know where the optimal intervention rates lie in relation to the current evidence-base for surgical intervention (see also Cherkin *et al.* 1994).

Question 4

From the perspective of audit it would be helpful to have an estimate of the complication rate of surgery.

16 Maternal and child health

HEATHER REID, JOHN YARNELL, AND HELEN DOLK

CHAPTER CONTENTS

This chapter introduces the topics of fertility (its influence on population structure and trends worldwide) and infertility. Global trends in maternal and child mortality are reviewed and major causes of death and opportunities for their prevention in neonates, infants, and children are discussed. Surveillance and screening for congenital anomalies conclude this chapter.

Introduction

The delivery of a healthy baby who survives to adulthood is not only a potentially desirable outcome for any mother it is one of the most valuable assets a community can enjoy. In 2008 almost nine million children below the age of five years and more than a quarter of a million women died from complications of pregnancy, childbearing, or unsafe abortion (Black *et al.* 2010). The vast majority of these deaths occurred in low- and middle-income countries where poverty is widespread, effective public health programmes and clinical care services are often poor or absent, and malnutrition, both overt and at subclinical, micronutrient level, affects many women of childbearing age and their infants. The health of both are jeopardized by impaired immunity resulting from poor nutrition, and the suboptimal physical and mental development which ensue. The reproductive performance of women, their survival and fertility, and the survival of the infants and children they bear are widely accepted as summary markers of the general health status of a population. Measurement of these markers provide some insights into the range and quality of health care services for women and their infants, and also enable the monitoring of the impact of changing health care practices. These are key indicators of progress in achieving the Millennium Development Goals, which are discussed in Chapter 22. As we saw in Chapter 1, even simple hygienic measures, poorly understood at the time of Semmelweis, greatly improved the chance of survival of mothers and infants in 19th-century Vienna by reducing the risk of puerperal fever (Chapter 1). Maternal and child health are fundamental to the population science of demography and are important determinants of life expectancy, as discussed in Chapter 2. They can also improve our understanding of the health effects of changes in other sectors such as agriculture, education, and fiscal policy (see also Chapter 1, Fig. 1.1 and Chapter 22). The key indicators to be considered here relate to the patterns of fertility, maternal, perinatal, and infant mortality, and congenital malformation in the population.

16.1 Fertility and infertility

The capacity to control or improve fertility is the out-come of a range of interrelated factors shaped by educational, socio-economic, cultural and educational circumstances; contraceptive practice and effective-ness, marriage and cohabitation trends, sexual mores and practice, female expectations and aspirations, availability of abortion, all influence the pattern of reproduction. Taking the example of England and Wales from 1830 to 2000 there was an overall fall from about 140 live births per 1000 women of fertile age (taken as 15–44 years) to 50 live births per 1000 (see Fig. 16.1). This pattern reflects the net effect of many fac-tors including political stability and economic growth (rising trend), war and economic depression (declining trend), and widespread availability of contraception (declining trend).

As discussed in Chapters 1 and 2 following industri-alization and economic growth in the late 19th and the first half of the 20th centuries, many leading countries in Europe and North America progressed through the stages of the demographic and health transition with declining birth and death rates and improving life expectancies. At the beginning of the 21st century the demographic transition is almost complete in most of these countries with low death rates and low, or very low, birth rates; population growth may be stabilized, declining, or boosted by new immigration. In many of these countries there has been a marked reduction in childbearing among younger women and reproduc-tive rates have risen among older women suggesting a postponement of childbearing to the 30s or 40s (Botting et al. 2001). In the past 25 years the propor-tion of births in England and Wales in women aged 30 years or above has doubled, and the proportion to mothers aged 35 years or more has trebled in the past 10 years.

The demographic transition has begun in many parts of the world and there has been a global decline in the **total fertility rate** (the average number of live births per woman of reproductive age) from 5.0 in 1950 to 2.5 in 2011 when the world populations were 2.5 billion and 7.0 billion, respectively (Bloom 2011). In Asia and in Latin America the rates were about six in 1950 and have fallen to levels similar to those in Europe and North America in 2011 (between 1.6 and 2.2). In Africa the rates were slightly higher at 6.6 and have fallen to 4.4. Fertility rates are the major determi-nant of population growth, although migration is also important for some countries. Population projections for the world regions are shown in Fig. 16.2a. Projected fertility trends are shown in Fig. 16.2b.

Population structure Declining fertility in most high income countries and improved survival of both the very young and the elderly has led to alteration in the demo-graphic profile of such countries. Fig. 16.3a shows the proportion of the total population in each age stratum by sex in Europe in 2010. This pattern shows similar pro-portions for all age groups except for the most elderly. In contrast, the World population (Fig. 16.3b) shows a burgeoning younger population as death rates decline globally but birth rates decline to a lesser degree.

India's population structure (Fig. 16.3c) shows the pyramidal structure typical of countries passing through the stages of the demographic transition while Fig. 16.3d shows the pattern for sub-Saharan Africa which is at the earliest stage of transition. Finally, Fig. 16.3e shows the population structure for China which has been shaped by the one-child policy and periods of rapid cultural change.

Mortality or morbidity rates, which compare different countries, clearly require adjustment for differing pop-ulation age structures. The World Health Organization adopted a new World Reference Standard in 2001 con-structed for the period 2000–2025 which removed the effects of historical events such as wars and famine.

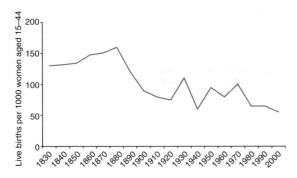

Figure 16.1 General fertility rate, England and Wales, 1830–2000.

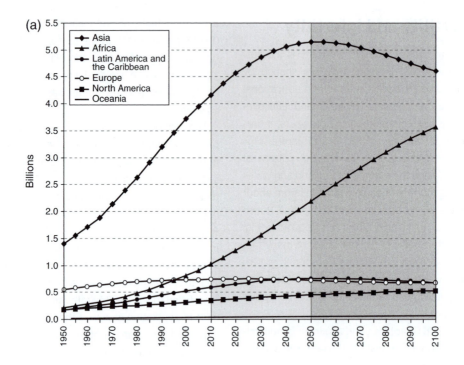

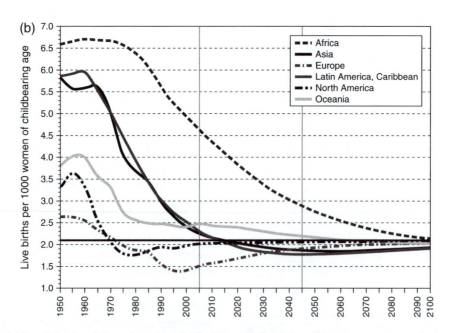

Figure 16.2 (a) Population trends in world regions. (b) Fertility rates (total) in world regions.
Reproduced from World Population Prospects, 2010 Revision, with permission from the United Nations.

(a) **World 2010**   **6,908,689,000** population

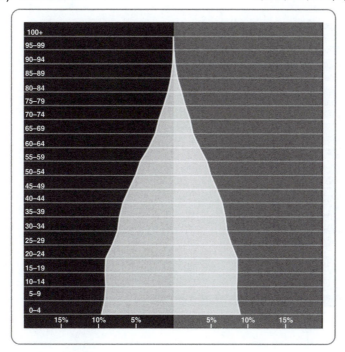

(b) **Europe 2010**   **732,760,000** population

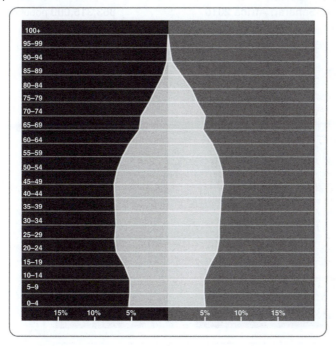

Figure 16.3 (a–e) Population pyramids in world, subregions, and selected countries in 2010.

Reproduced with permission from **http://www.populationpyramid.net**

(c) **India 2010**   **1,214,465,000** population

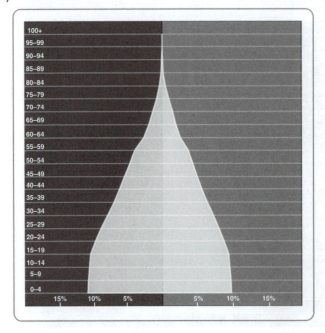

(d) **Sub-Saharan Africa 2010**   **863,315,000** population

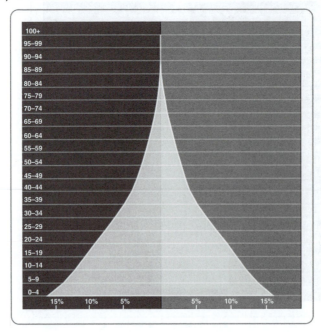

Figure 16.3 (*continued*)

(e) **China 2010**   **1,354,148,000** population

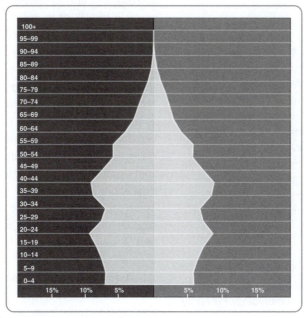

Figure 16.3 (*continued*)

Age-adjusted rates based on the new standard are not comparable to the former world standard rates. Age-standardized rates based on a European Standard population are also used as well as individual regional or country standards.

Apart from the social and cultural factors influencing fertility two 'medical' interventions have had an important role. These are developments in assisted reproduction techniques, which are common in high-income and in some middle-income countries, and the legalization and liberalization of abortion which has occurred worldwide, but to a very variable extent depending on the prevailing cultural norms in each country.

Assisted reproduction Human fertility is low compared with most other species, and the chance of pregnancy per menstrual cycle in the most fertile couples is about 33 per cent. Within a year of regular intercourse 90 per cent of fertile couples should become pregnant, but a delay of more than one year is usually the accepted criterion to define sub-fertility and initiate investigations. A woman's fertility declines with age, and one effect of choosing to defer childbirth to later years has been to increase referrals for infertility investigations and treatment. In an Australian study 17 per cent of women aged 28 to 33 years reported infertility; 72 per cent of these sought treatment but only 50 per cent received hormone treatment or *in vitro* fertilization (IVF) (Herbert *et al.* 2009). Many assisted conception technologies exist with a bewildering array of acronyms—but all with the aim of bringing sperm and egg together to promote fertilization, achieve pregnancy, and to see that result in a healthy baby. The three main types of assisted conception are:

1. Intrauterine insemination (IUI)—prepared sperm are pipetted in the uterus at a time when ovulation is likely or assisted.

2. *In vitro* fertilization (IVF)—fertilization is aided by mixing sperm and eggs in the laboratory.

3. Intracytoplasmic sperm injection (ICSI)—a single sperm is injected directly into the egg cytoplasm to achieve fertilization.

In the UK guidelines rule that all patients considering an assisted pregnancy must be informed of the live birth rate per treatment cycle started, sometimes called the 'take-home baby' rate for the centre providing the

Box 16.1 About the Human Fertilisation and Embryology Authority.

The Human Fertilisation and Embryology Authority (HFEA) was set up in August 1991 by the Human Fertilisation and Embryology Act 1990. The first statutory body of its type in the world, the HFEA's creation reflected public and professional interest in the potential future of human embryo research and infertility treatments, and a widespread desire for statutory regulation of all related procedures.

The HFEA's principal tasks are to license and monitor clinics that carry out *in vitro* fertilization, donor insemination, and human embryo research. The HFEA also regulates the storage of gametes (sperm and ova) and embryos.

service; and all clinical pregnancies and their outcome from these various techniques must be reported to the UK Human Fertilisation and Embryology Authority (HFEA), see Box 16.1.

The live birth rates from the different techniques vary but are around 20 per cent per treatment cycle started. The cause of the infertility, ages of partners, sperm quality, and duration of infertility all affect the outcome but maternal age is a major determinant of success, whatever the method. Only one per cent of live births in the UK are from assisted conceptions, but an increasing proportion of multiple births stem from these procedures. In women under 40 years of age, the HFEA has proposed that a maximum of two eggs are used per treatment cycle (three or more can be used in women over 40 years of age). A recent review and meta-analysis of studies of complications associated with IVF/ICSI singleton pregnancies (multiple pregnancies are established to be at higher risk of adverse pregnancy outcomes) found a higher risk of ante-partum haemorrhage (OR 2.5, 95% CI 2.3–2.7), congenital anomalies (1.8, 95% CI 1.3–2.1), and several other adverse events (Pandey *et al.* 2012).

16.2 Abortion

Spontaneous abortion or miscarriage is a common outcome of pregnancy with an international average of approximately 15 per cent (Vogel and Motulsky 2002); if occurring very early in pregnancy it may be unrecognized but, for epidemiological and legal purposes in the UK, it is defined as the expulsion of a fetus or dead-born infant occurring before 24 weeks of pregnancy. Spontaneous abortion is associated with a higher than average prevalence of congenital anomaly, often due to chromosomal abnormalities. The issue of viability is controversial and definitions of 20 to 22 weeks are common worldwide. Following the introduction of the Abortion Act of 1967 in England, Wales, and Scotland sepsis deaths and complications from illegal abortions fell sharply while the incidence of legal abortion rose gradually from five to 18 per 1000 women aged 15–44 years and access to contraceptive services has increased (Rowlands 2007). About 30 per cent of these procedures are induced medically before 12 weeks of pregnancy.

In 2008 there were an estimated 43.8 million induced abortions worldwide with rates of 28 per 1000 women aged 15–44 years, down from 35 per 100 women in 1995 (Sedgh *et al.* 2012). Almost half (49 per cent) were classified as unsafe by WHO when conducted by untrained or lay persons or in environments below the minimum medical standards (Grimes *et al.* 2006). The proportion of unsafe abortions was 100 per cent in Central and South America and 97 per cent in Africa as a whole but was about 60 per cent in South and West Asia and in South Africa. In Eastern Europe the proportion was five per cent compared to less than 0.5 per cent in the rest of Europe and in North America. Unsafe abortion is estimated to cause 13 per cent of maternal deaths worldwide and leave five million women with permanent disabilities each year (WHO 2010). Some 84 countries from more than 190 worldwide were deemed to have liberal abortion policies and induced abortion rates tended to be lower in these countries (Sedgh *et al.* 2012).

The widespread availability of effective contraception and of safe termination of unwanted pregnancies have had a strong influence on maternal reproductive behaviour and outcome. Religious, cultural, and economic factors limit the availability or acceptability of some services in many countries but the benefits of integrated programmes for sexual and reproductive health in low- and middle-income countries (see

Box 16.2 Packages of care for low- and middle-income countries.

> 1) Family planning
> 2) Safe abortion care
> 3) Pregnancy care
> 4) Childbirth care
> 5) Postpartum care of the mother
> 6) Care of the newborn
> 7) Care during infancy and childhood
>
> Reproduced from WHO (2010). Packages of Interventions for Family Planning, Safe Abortion care, Maternal, Newborn and Child Health. WHO, Geneva. Available at: **http://whqlibdoc.who. int/hq/2010/WHO_FCH_10.06_eng.pdf**, with permission from WHO.

Box 16.2) considerably outweigh the costs associated with their introduction (Singh *et al.* 2006). Integrated packages for use in low- and middle-income countries have been proposed by WHO (WHO 2010).

....

Question 1

Summarize the methods of birth control, their relative effectiveness, advantages, and disadvantages.

....

16.3 Maternal mortality

In the 19th century it was recognized that pregnancy and childbirth were often hazardous times for both mother and baby. At the time of Semmelweis in the mid-19th century maternal mortality was as high as 10 per cent. Simple hygienic measure introduced by Semmelweis reduced this to 1 per cent. In the UK at the end of the 19th century five women died in every 1000 pregnancies. Effective treatment of common, serious complications of pregnancy was extremely limited, regular antenatal supervision was unusual, and the specialty of obstetrics was undeveloped. Obstetrics represents a classical example of the practice of prevention by surveillance during pregnancy and appropriate early intervention. In the UK and other industrialized countries progress was slow until the 1940s when a number

of key scientific and social developments occurred which have reduced the maternal mortality to 0.14 per 1000 'maternities' (total pregnancies; miscarriages, stillbirths, and livebirths). Here, we can use a more precise denominator since the data for miscarriages, stillbirths, and livebirths are available, although miscarriages may be estimated. In low- and middle-income countries only data for livebirths are commonly available. Measures to prevent or treat the sepsis, haemorrhage, and toxaemia, which had hitherto threatened the lives of many women, were of major importance but, so too were the establishment of routine antenatal care, and a wide range of schemes related to education and social welfare. Together these improved not just the nature, availability, and organization of maternity care but also the health of the women who required it. In the UK a confidential enquiry into maternal deaths was introduced in 1952 which focused attention on collecting comprehensive, valid information on all the deaths. This helped to distinguish direct and indirect deaths which are shown in Box 16.3.

In low- and middle-income countries up to 80 per cent of maternal deaths are due to direct causes; haemorrhage (25 per cent), sepsis (15 per cent), and eclampsia (12 per cent) are the commonest causes (Rahman and Menken 2012), although worldwide 13 per cent of maternal deaths are attributable to unsafe abortion and 17 per cent are associated with HIV/AIDS (Hogan *et al.* 2010). In high-income countries indirect deaths are responsible for more than 50 per cent of maternal deaths from causes such as cardiovascular disease. Worldwide it was estimated that there were 342,900 maternal deaths in 2008 compared to more than half a million deaths in 1980. Using the indicator maternal mortality ratio (MMR) (the number of maternal deaths per 100,000 livebirths) the global figure fell from 422 in 1980 to 320 in 1990 and to 251 in 2008. Maternal mortality ratios remain very high in some countries, e.g. Afghanistan 1575, Central African Republic 1570, and remain high in many countries in sub-Saharan Africa. Over 50 per cent of all maternal deaths occurred in six large countries India, Nigeria, Pakistan, Afghanistan, Ethiopia, and the Democratic Republic of Congo (Hogan *et al.* 2010). Table 16.1 shows the maternal mortality by world region in 1990 and in 2010.

Box 16.3 Direct and indirect causes of maternal deaths.

Direct	From obstetric complications of the pregnant state (pregnancy, labour, and puerperium) from interventions, omissions, incorrect treatment, or from a chain of event resulting from any of these.
Indirect	From previous existing disease or disease that developed during pregnancy and which was not due to direct obstetric causes, but which was aggravated by the physiologic effects of pregnancy.
Late	Between 42 days and one year after termination of pregnancy, miscarriage, or delivery that are due to direct or indirect maternal causes.
Coincidental	Deaths from unrelated causes that happen to occur in pregnancy or the puerperium.

Reproduced from Weindling AM 'The confidential enquiry into maternal and child health (CEMACH)'. *Archives of Disease in Childhood* **88** (12), 2003, with permission from BMJ Publishing Group Ltd.

In contrast many middle-income countries have experienced improved MMRs such as China (MMR 40), Sri Lanka (MMR 30), and Malaysia (MMR 42). In high-income countries rates are below 10 in countries in Western Europe and in some countries in Central Europe. In North America the 2008 MMRs are reported to be 17 in the USA and seven in Canada. Possible reasons for the increase in MMR in the USA are discussed elsewhere (Bingham *et al.* 2011). Many high-income countries, in addition to low- and middle-income countries, show strong socio-economic gradients in maternal mortality.

Progress towards achieving the Millennium Goal of reducing maternal mortality by 75 per cent by 2015 has been variable; they have been achieved or on track in many countries, but unlikely to be achieved in others including many countries in sub-Saharan Africa that have not experienced significant economic growth or development and have also been severely affected by HIV/AIDS. However, the global initiative to increase access to anti-retroviral drugs and implementation of low cost initiatives could accelerate progress towards achieving significant reductions in the heavy burden of maternal mortality in these countries. Examples of successful programmes and of low-cost interventions are discussed in detail elsewhere (Coeytaux *et al.* 2011; WHO 2010; Liang *et al.* 2012).

16.4 Infant and child mortality

At the beginning of the 20th century infant mortality (deaths in the first year of life) in Britain was about 140 per 1000 livebirths. Effective preventive or therapeutic measures to combat infection were not available, malnourishment was widespread, and the particular requirements of the premature infant were not understood. However, as with maternal mortality, the second half of the 20th century saw the mortality rate in infants begin to fall steeply, from 30 in 1950 to 18 in 1970, and to 6 per 1000 livebirths in 2006 (Norman *et al.* 2008). As noted in Chapter 1 the majority of the decline in infant mortality occurred long before the introduction of immunization against childhood infections.

At the beginning of the 21st century infant mortality in sub-Saharan Africa is about 80 per 1000 livebirths but deaths under five years of age approach 140 per 1000 livebirths (Skolnik 2012). Child deaths are lower in other world regions and 70 per cent of the child deaths occur in the first year of life. Epidemiological indicators used to examine infant and child health are shown in Box 16.4.

In high-income countries over 50 per cent of infants who die now do so in the first week of life, the majority on the first day. The longer a baby lives the greater its chances of continuing to survive. It was recognized that these very early post-natal deaths were often part of a continuum of threats to the fetus, and, whether a particular infant died shortly before or after birth, was often largely a matter of chance. The index perinatal mortality encompasses stillbirths and deaths in the first week of life and tends to be measured in high income countries

Table 16.1 Maternal mortality in WHO regions 1990 to 2010

Region	MMR					% change in MMR between 1990 and 2010	Average annual % change in MMR between 1990 and 2010
	1990	1995	2000	2005	2010		
Africa	820	800	720	600	480	−42	−2.7
Americas	100	91	80	68	63	−40	−2.5
Eastern Mediterranean	430	410	360	300	250	−42	−2.6
Europe	44	37	29	22	20	−54	−3.8
South-East Asia	590	460	370	270	200	−66	−5.2
Western Pacific	140	100	77	60	49	−66	−5.2
World	400	360	320	260	210	−47	−3.1

Trends in estimates of maternal mortality ratio (MMR, maternal deaths per 100,000 live births) by 5-year periods, 1990–2010, by WHO region

Reproduced with permission from *Trends in maternal mortality: 1990 to 2010*. WHO, UNICEF, UNFPA and The World Bank estimates. Available from: **http://www.who.int/reproductivehealth/publications/monitoring/9789241503631/en/index.html**.

Box 16.4 Epidemiological indicators in infant and child health.

- Child mortality under five years per 1000 livebirths
- Infant mortality per 1000 livebirths (deaths in the first year of life)
- Post-neonatal mortality per 1000 livebirths (deaths between 28 days and the end of the first year)
- Neonatal mortality rate per 100 livebirths (deaths in the first 28 days)
- Perinatal mortality rate per 1000 total births (livebirths and stillbirths) (deaths in the first seven days of life)

with available data. Neonatal mortality includes deaths in the first four week (28 days) of life and generally has a different pattern of causes than that later in childhood. Infant mortality was formerly used as the standard index in high income countries. Child mortality (deaths under five years) tends to be used as the most robust index for global and regional comparisons. Some of the technical difficulties in obtaining accurate estimates of child deaths under the age of five years are discussed in more detail elsewhere (Black *et al.* 2010).

Stillbirths and deaths that occur in the first week of life (early neonatal deaths) often have many common causes and determinants which could be attributed to obstetric events and are termed perinatal deaths. A stillbirth refers to a baby that is born with no signs of life. This can occur either before labour (antepartum) or during labour (intrapartum). Stillbirths may occur because of pregnancy complications or maternal disease, although the reason for a large number of stillbirths is undetermined. Measuring the true rate of stillbirth is often challenging as in some societies the child is not recognized or named until the newborn has survived the initial period. Causes of neonatal deaths and stillbirths tend to be similar and are often related to the events during pregnancy, delivery, and the neonatal period. Some of the main causes of neonatal death include congenital malformation, extreme prematurity, obstetric complications before or during delivery. Causes are assigned based on the likely timing of the damage that may have caused the death, i.e. before labour (e.g. congenital anomalies, infection, immaturity), during or shortly after (e.g. asphyxia or trauma), or post-neonatal (e.g. sudden infant death, infection, or other external factors). Recent

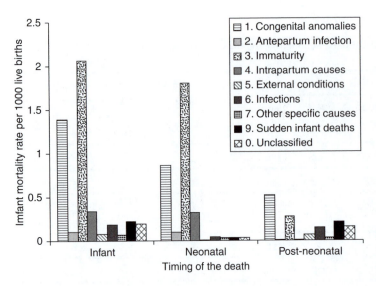

Figure 16.4 Causes of death during infancy, and in neonatal and post-neonatal periods in England and Wales in 2007.

data for infant, neonatal, and post-neonatal mortality (deaths between 28 days and one year) for England and Wales are shown in Fig. 16.4.

In the normally formed infant, birth weight is the major determinant of survival. The immature infant, born too small, accounts for almost 50 per cent of neonatal mortality and over 10 per cent of post-neonatal mortality. Low birth weight may be the result of failure to grow appropriately *in utero* or of delivery at an early gestational age. For infants who thrive appropriately, but are born early, a clinical reason for the premature onset of labour is not clear in about 50 per cent of cases; but characteristics associated with preterm birth include multiple pregnancy, smoking, history of previous preterm birth, and non-white ethnic origin in UK data (Critchley *et al.* 2004). In turn infant mortality is also associated with multiple births, maternal age, marital status, socio-economic position, and mother's country of birth. The reasons for failure of an infant to grow appropriately *in utero* may be congenital or environmental, fetal or maternal, in origin. The sex of the infant, maternal parity and size, smoking, ethnicity, maternal disease, and nutrition are contributory factors. Developments in neonatal intensive care have contributed enormously to improved survival of the premature newborn. Infants born at 27/28 weeks of gestation now have survival rates of almost 90 per cent (Critchley *et al.* 2004). To what extent this increased survival seen in recent years equates with subsequent well-being awaits the results of longer term follow-up. Studies in the 1980s of infants born before 29 weeks found approximately one-third to be profoundly disabled; more recently a figure of 10 per cent has been reported (Tin *et al.* 1997). The level of disability increases with lowering of gestational age at birth. The clinical, psychological, social, economic, and ethical aspects of extending care to infants of increasingly low gestational age should be reviewed and subjected to public debate.

Large numbers of children die soon after birth: many of them in the first four weeks of life, and most of those during the first week. About 41 per cent of deaths worldwide occur within the first month of life. Neonatal rather than perinatal mortality is often used as a global indicator due to challenges in measuring accurately number of stillbirths. As child mortality decreases, neonatal deaths now account for a higher proportion of all child deaths. Almost all regions have seen a slower rate of decline in neonatal deaths. Of the 7.7 million deaths reported in 2010 in children under the age of five years, 3.1 million were in the neonatal period (Rajaratnam *et al.* 2010). Globally, neonatal mortality has declined 28 per cent between 1990 and 2010 from 32 to 23 deaths per 1000 livebirths. The fastest reduction in neonatal mortality was in North Africa, Eastern Asia, Latin America, and the Caribbean.

Child mortality under five years is now the most common global indicator used and is a key indicator of

Under-five mortality rate, by Millennium Development Goal region,
1990 and 2010 (deaths per 1000 live births)

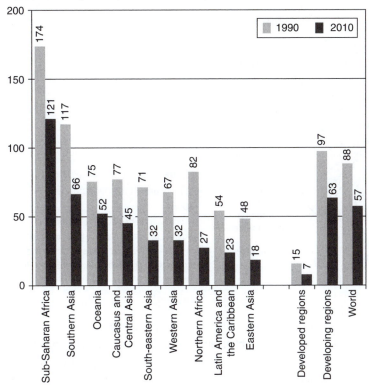

Figure 16.5 Child mortality rate under five years in WHO regions in 1990 and 2010.
Reproduced from *Levels and Trends in Child Mortality*, 2011, with permission from Unicef.

the health of a nation. It is associated with a variety of factors such as maternal health, quality and access to healthcare, and public health practices, and reducing the child mortality rates worldwide is a major goal of the Millennium Declaration (Chapter 22) (Lozano *et al.* 2011) Data developed and used by a UN inter-agency group are shown in Fig. 16.5 for world regions.

Out of the nine regions classed as developing, child mortality has declined by more than 50 per cent in 20 years in five of them, with the highest reductions in North Africa (67 per cent) and Eastern Asia (63 per cent). In sub-Saharan Africa and in Oceania, the decline has been only 30 per cent and child mortality, as with maternal mortality, remains very high in sub-Saharan Africa. Maternal and child mortality are closely correlated although the death of the mother is far less likely than the death of her child. In sub-Saharan Africa one in eight children die before the age of five (129 deaths per 1000 livebirths), nearly twice the average in low- and

middle-income regions overall and around 18 times the average in developed regions. Southern Asia has the second highest rate; 69 deaths per 1000 livebirths or about one child in 14.

Some 50 per cent of the world's deaths under five years of age in 2010 occurred in five large countries; India, Nigeria, Democratic Republic of the Congo, Pakistan, and China, a similar distribution to that for maternal mortality. In China child mortality decreased by 70 per cent and neonatal causes became more common (Rudan *et al.* 2010). Across the globe child mortality tends to be higher in rural areas and there is a strong gradient with socio-economic position and with the level of the mother's education. Infectious diseases caused 68 per cent of child deaths with the largest percentages due to pneumonia (18 per cent), diarrhoea (15 per cent), and malaria (eight per cent). More than 90 per cent of the deaths due to malaria and to HIV/ AIDS occurred in the African Region. In neonates

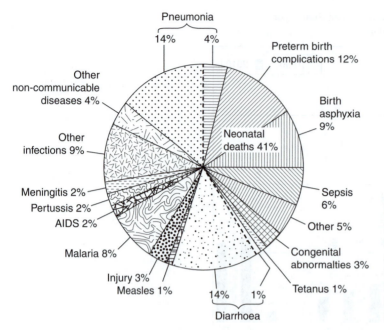

Figure 16.6 Global causes of death in infancy and in the neonatal period in 2008.

Reproduced from Black A *et al*, 'Global, regional, and national causes of child mortality in 2008: a systematic analysis', *Lancet* **375**, (9730) 1969–1987, 2010, with permission from Elsevier.

(40 per cent of these deaths) the most important causes worldwide were preterm birth complications (12 per cent), birth asphyxia (nine per cent), sepsis (six per cent), and pneumonia (four per cent). The major causes of death in children under five years and in neonates are shown in Fig. 16.6, but their distribution varies across the world regions.

Many low cost-effective interventions have been shown to reduce child mortality. Ninety per cent of child deaths occurred in 42 countries in 2000 and it has been estimated that six million child deaths could prevented annually at an annual global cost of US$5.1 billion (Bryce *et al.* 2005). Tables 16.2a and 16.2b show the running costs of effective preventive measures and treatments, respectively.

16.5 Sudden unexpected death in infancy

A number of terms have been used, often interchangeably, to refer to a sudden unexpected death in infancy. Most commonly referred to in lay terms as 'cot death', the term sudden infant death syndrome (SIDS) was first used in the late 1960s and is defined

as: 'the sudden death of an infant under one year of age, which remains unexplained after a thorough case investigation, including performance of a complete autopsy, examination of the death scene, and review of the clinical history.' (Hunt and Hauck 2006). It is by definition a diagnosis of exclusion; therefore variations in the degree of care or detail with which the post-mortem is conducted, in the interpretation of findings by different pathologists, or in the range of other investigations undertaken, will have considerable influence on the published figures. Comparisons of SIDS rates should be made with caution unless the evidence for this final diagnosis is clear. Sudden infant death syndrome was first introduced as a cause of death internationally in the ninth revision of the International Classification of Disease in 1975 and engendered a number of epidemiological observational studies, both case-control and cohort, and some community and national trials which promoted the policy of placing infants in the supine sleeping position from the early 1990s. Secular trends in deaths from SIDS and accidental suffocation/strangulation in Canada are shown in Fig. 16.7a. Fig. 16.7b shows that the decline in mortality from SIDS has occurred in many high income countries,

Table 16.2a Estimated annual costs of providing preventive interventions for child survival at coverage levels in the year 2000 and with universal coverage

	Running costs for 2000 coverage levels	Additional running costs to provide universal coverage
Breastfeeding	102	414
Insecticide-treated materials	1	77
Complementry feeding	46	158
Zinc	0	301
Delivery with skilled attendant	502	653
Newborn temperature management	19	79
Haemophilus influenzae type b (Hib) vaccine	66	1051
Water and sanitation	1889	753
Antenatal steroids	61	420
Vitamin A	129	271
Tetanus toxoid	71	161
Nevirapine and replacement feeding	1	82
Antibiotics for premature rupture of membranes	44	52
Measles vaccine	39	30
Antimalarial intermittent preventive treatment in pregnancy	0	26
Cost of additional Expanded Programme on Immunization vaccines	245	165
Total	3215	4693
Data are million US $		

Reproduced from Bryce J *et al*, 'Can the world afford to save the lives of 6 million children each year?', *Lancet* **365** (9478), 2193–2200, with permission from Elsevier.

although it is reported to a variable extent in different countries.

Despite the decline in the incidence of SIDS in high-income countries it remains a leading cause of infant mortality, particularly in the post-neonatal period. Sudden infant death syndrome occurs more commonly in infants under six months of age and recent meta-analyses of bed sharing have confirmed this as a strong risk factor. In an analysis of 11 studies the overall OR for bed sharing was 2.9 (95% CI 2.0–4.2), which increased to 6.3 (95% CI 3.9–10.0) with smoking mothers, and was 10.4 (95% CI 4.4–24.2) for infants less than 12 weeks of age (Vennemann *et al.* 2012). In contrast breastfeeding appears to be protective and a meta-analysis of 18 studies reported the fully adjusted OR to be 0.6 (95% CI 0.4–0.7) for infants who had received breast milk for any duration (Hauck *et al.* 2011).

There is a strong association with deprivation and poverty in many studies, documented in a large study

Table 16.2b Estimated annual costs of providing treatments for child survival at coverage levels in the year 2000 and with universal coverage

	Running costs for 2000 coverage levels without expanded prevention savings	Running costs for 2000 coverage levels (after savings from expanded prevention)	Additional running costs to provide universal coverage
Oral rehydration therapy	29	14 (15)	124
Antibiotics for neonatal sepsis	101	22 (79)	17
Antibiotics for pneumonia	290	151 (139)	332
Antimalarials	200	38 (162)	46
Zinc	0	0 (0)	150
Newborn resuscitation	19	19 (0)	35
Antibiotics for dysentery	284	134 (150)	333
Vitamin A*	52	0 (52)	0
Total	975	378 (597)	1037

Data are million US$. *With universal measles vaccine coverage there would be no need for treatment with vitamin A.

Reproduced from Bryce J *et al*, 'Can the world afford to save the lives of 6 million children each year?', *Lancet* **365** (9478), 2193–2200, with permission from Elsevier.

of all singleton births in Scotland during the period 1985 to 2008 (Wood *et al.* 2012). Soft bedding has been reported as a risk factor in some studies and more deaths occur in boys than in girls. Ethnic and cultural factors are also relevant and, in the USA, SIDS is reported more frequently in infants of African Americans, Native Americans, and Alaska Natives. In a New Zealand review of autopsy cases 83 per cent of SIDS occurred in the infants of Maori or Pacific Islander mothers (Hutchinson *et al.* 2011). Risk factors both environmental and possible genetic factors have been reviewed in detail elsewhere (Hunt and Hauck 2006; Moon 2007). Environmental risk factors are shown in Table 16.3.

In a study in 20 regions of Europe of 745 cases of sudden infant deaths and 2411 controls, 48 per cent of cases were attributable to sleeping on the side or prone. Mothers who smoked formed 27 per cent of cases (10 per cent controls) but the relative risk of smoking almost trebled from 5.6 to 14.8 if the mother shared the bed with the infant (Carpenter *et al.* 2004).

Recommendations in the UK for the prevention of sudden infant death for parents and professionals are shown in Box 16.5.

....

Question 2

Why may residual confounding be a particular problem in observational studies of SIDS?
....

16.6 Congenital anomalies

How frequent are congenital anomalies? Two to four per cent of babies are diagnosed with one or more major malformations or chromosomal anomalies, with serious medical, functional or cosmetic consequences. The exact prevalence found in any survey of births depends crucially on the rather arbitrary division between 'major and 'minor' anomalies as 'minor' anomalies are much more common. The reported

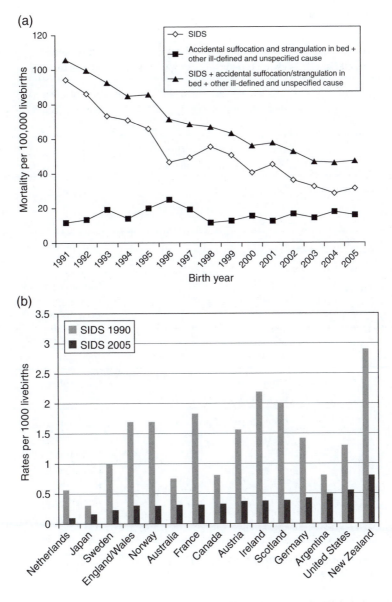

Figure 16.7 (a) Trends in SIDS in Canada 1991–2005 (b) SIDS mortality rates in selected countries in 1990 and 2005.
(a) Reproduced from Gilbert *et al.* (2012) 'Paediatric and Perinatal Epidemiology'. **26** (2), 124–130. (b) Reproduced from Hauck RF, Tanabe KO, 2008, 'International trends in sudden infant death syndrome: stabilization of rates requires further action', *Pediatrics* **122**(3), 660–6 and Hauck RF and Tanabe, 2010, 'International trends in sudden infant death syndrome and other unexpected deaths in infancy', *Current Paediatric Reviews* **95** (101), 1–24, with permission from the National SIDS/SUID Resource Centre, Georgetown University.

prevalence also depends on ascertainment methods of the survey. Population-based congenital anomaly registries accessing multiple sources of clinical information and at least covering diagnoses made in the first year of life provide the most reliable prevalence estimates. A network of such registries exists in Europe (EUROCAT) providing particularly extensive and readily available data. Population-based and hospital-based registries worldwide contribute to the International Clearinghouse for Birth Defects Surveillance and Research. Web addresses are appended to this chapter.

Table 16.3 Putative risk factors for sudden infant death syndrome

Maternal characteristics	Birth characteristics	Pregnancy characteristics	Family characteristics	Post-natal characteristics	Time of death and position at death
Lower socio-economic status	First born	Younger age of mother at first pregnancy	Larger family size	Use of prone sleeping position	Age 1–6 months
Teenage mother	Multiple birth	Late attendance at antenatal clinic	School age sibling(s)	Use of side sleeping position	Winter
Unmarried mother	Low birthweight	Non-attendance at antenatal classes		Infection Maternal and paternal smoking	Weekends
Younger school-leaving age	Male infant	Higher parity		Bed sharing	Between midnight and 6am
Less formal education		Short inter-pregnancy interval		Not room sharing with adult(s) Prone position	
Depression		Short gestation		Not breastfeeding Non-use of pacifier	
Illegal drug use		Intrauterine growth retardation		Overheating	Covers over face/head
Race/ethnicity		Maternal smoking		Overwrapping/overdressing Non-attendance for post-natal health check Admission to a special baby care unit	

Reproduced from Sullivan F and Barlow S, 'Review of risk factors for Sudden Infant Death Syndrome', *Paediatric and Perinatal Epidemiology*, 2001, with permission from John Wiley and Sons.

Question 3

What does 'population-based' mean and why is it important for a registry to be population-based? [see Chapter 2]

Since congenital anomalies, particularly chromosomal anomalies, are selectively lost as spontaneous abortions (see 'Abortion' section), the term **prevalence** (rather than **incidence**) was adopted to recognize the fact that we only count cases among those who survive the early fetal period. For *prevalence at birth* the numerator is the number of babies born, both liveborn and stillborn, with congenital anomalies, while the denominator is the total number of live- and stillbirths in a given population. It should be remembered that differences in birth prevalence between populations, or between groups with different environmental exposures, may reflect differences in survival of affected fetuses during pregnancy rather than differences in incidence. *Live-birth prevalence*, which is more readily measured where

Box 16.5 Key health messages for new parents

Back to sleep

Babies should be put down to sleep lying on their backs, unless there is a substantial medical reason not to do so. Sleeping on the back is preferable to sleeping on the side, and sleeping on the front should be avoided.

Feet to foot; head uncovered

Babies should sleep in such a way that their head does not become covered during sleep. This is most easily achieved by putting a baby to sleep with his or her feet close to or touching the foot of the cot. Blankets are preferred to duvets, and should be tucked in so that the baby's head is exposed and uncovered without a hat.

Not too hot

Although it is important to prevent a baby becoming cold, becoming too hot is also a danger. Room heating is not required at night except when the weather is very cold. Babies' bedrooms should be at a temperature overnight which is comfortable for a lightly clothed adult (usually 16–20°C).

Smoke-free zone

Cigarette smoking in pregnancy and around babies increases the risk of cot death. Although giving up would be the best option, a baby will be partly protected if his or her sleeping place is regarded as a smoke-free zone, whether the baby is asleep there or not.

Prompt medical advice

The risk of cot death may be reduced by seeking prompt medical advice for babies who become unwell, particularly those with a raised temperature, breathing difficulties, and who are less responsive than usual. A proportion may have acute infections amenable to treatment.

Bed sharing for comfort, not sleep

While it is likely to be beneficial for parents to take their baby into bed with them to feed or comfort, it is preferable to place the baby back into a cot to sleep. This is especially important if the parents smoke or have consumed alcohol.

Reproduced from Weindling AM 'The confidential enquiry into maternal and child health (CEMACH)'. *Archives of Disease in Childhood* **88** (12), 2003, with permission from BMJ Publishing Group Ltd.

registration of stillbirths is incomplete, counts cases among livebirths only.

In the last few decades in Europe, prenatal diagnosis of congenital anomalies has become common. Prenatal diagnosis can prepare both family and health care professionals for birth, and improve early treatment. In case of severe congenital anomalies, it can also give the mother the option to terminate the pregnancy (Dommergues *et al.* 2010), but this is not legal in many countries worldwide (for example, it is not legal in Ireland and Malta in Europe, nor in many countries of South America and Africa). In order to compare prevalence rates between populations in relation to possible underlying environmental causes without confounding by differences in prenatal diagnosis and termination of pregnancy, it is now common to calculate a 'total' or 'adjusted' **prevalence rate** including terminations of pregnancy for fetal anomaly (TOPFA)

in the numerator. The vast majority of these terminations would have been live- or stillborn if the congenital anomaly had not been prenatally diagnosed. It is very important that health information systems should include TOPFA so that trends in total prevalence of congenital anomalies can be assessed. Increasing termination rates for congenital anomaly are leading to slight decreases in perinatal mortality rates.

Table 16.4 shows the total prevalence and livebirth prevalence of selected subgroups of congenital anomaly in Europe, as well as the proportion of TOPFA among all cases.

Congenital heart disease is responsible for a third of all major congenital anomalies. The prevalence is reported to be higher in Asia than in Europe (van der Linde *et al.* 2011). Surgical intervention has improved survival in infants with congenital heart disease and, in high income countries, adults who have received

Table 16.4 Total and livebirth prevalence (per 10,000 births) and proportion of terminations of pregnancy for fetal anomaly (TOPFA) for selected congenital anomalies in Europe 2005–2009*

Congenital anomaly subgroup**	Total prevalence	Livebirth prevalence	Proportion of TOPFA among all cases (%)
Non-chromosomal anomalies			
Central nervous system	23.0	9.8	53.1
Neural tube defects	10.2	2.0	76.0
Congenital heart defects	59.5	53.9	7.7
Severe congenital heart defects	17.6	14.1	17.0
Orofacial clefts	14.2	12.9	7.9
Limb defects	34.1	30.2	9.2
Urinary system	30.3	25.9	12.7
Musculoskeletal	8.4	5.5	30.7
Chromosomal anomalies	40.2	15.1	59.1
Down's syndrome	22.3	9.2	56.6

Source: EUROCAT network of population-based registries (**http://www.eurocat-network.eu/accessprevalencedata/prevalencetables**, accessed 12/12/11).
*Based on data from the following EUROCAT registries: Styria (Austria), Hainaut (Belgium), Zagreb (Croatia), Odense (Denmark), Isle de la Reunion (France), Paris (France), Mainz (Germany), SE Ireland, Emilia Romagna (Italy), Tuscany (Italy), Malta, N Netherlands (NL), S Portugal, Basque Country (Spain), Vaud (Switzerland), Ukraine, East Midlands & South Yorkshire (UK), Northern England (UK), Thames Valley (UK), Wales (UK), Wessex (UK).
**Note that a case with more than one type of anomaly can be counted in more than one anomaly subgroup, but only once in each subgroup.

cardiac surgery in infancy for cardiac anomalies represent an important group of cardiac patients at greater risk themselves of cardiac complications of pregnancy.

Neural tube defects, including spina bifida and anencephaly, represent about five per cent of congenital anomalies in Europe, and 10 per cent of perinatal deaths due to congenital anomaly according to EUROCAT data. In low income countries, 29 per cent of neonatal deaths reported to be due to a congenital anomaly, were in infants with a neural tube defect (NTD) (Blencowe *et al.* 2010). Very high prevalence rates have been reported from urban and rural areas of India (Cherian *et al.* 2005).

What causes congenital anomalies? Approximately 15 per cent of cases of congenital anomaly recorded by European registries have a chromosomal anomaly (Table 16.3). It has been estimated that seven to eight

per cent of cases have a single gene defect with autosomal dominant, autosomal recessive or X-linked inheritance (Mueller and Young 2001), although some of these are diagnosed in later childhood. EUROCAT records a prevalence of six per 10,000 for genetic syndromes diagnosed prenatally or in the first year of life. A number of malformations, including neural tube defects, certain cardiac defects, hypospadias, cleft lip and cleft palate, renal agenesis, congenital dislocation of the hip, and talipes are attributed to multifactorial aetiologies (Mueller and Young 2001), where the pattern of recurrence within families suggests that many genetic factors are involved, interacting with environmental exposures. Few cases, less than 10 per cent, can be attributed to a single environmental exposure with known teratogenic effects such as antiepileptic drugs (see Chapter 13), maternal rubella infection, or high alcohol exposure (Table 16.5). Even in many of these

Table 16.5 Risk factors for congenital anomalies

Risk factor	Comment
Older maternal age	Chromosomal anomalies; little or no effect for non-chromosomal
Young maternal age (< 20)	Fivefold excess of gastroschisis, not a strong risk factor for other anomalies
Low socio-economic status	Higher risk of non-chromosomal anomalies
Epilepsy	Two- to threefold risk associated with certain anticonvulsant drugs
Diabetes	Teratogenic if good level of glycaemic control not achieved
Obesity	Obesity is a risk factor for many types of congenital anomaly; evidence for overweight is less clear (Stothard *et al.* 2009)
Rubella, cytomegalavious, toxoplasmosis	Maternal rubella infection was one of the earliest known risk factors for congenital anomalies
Fever/hyperthermia	Well-established cause of NTDs and probably other congenital anomalies
Thalidomide	Caused many thousands of babies to be born with limb and other defects in the late 1950s, when prescribed for nausea in pregnancy, until withdrawal in 1961
Isotretinoin	A vitamin A derivative acne treatment which is highly teratogenic causing central nervous system, cardiac and ear defects, hence strictly controlled prescriptions with Pregnancy Prevention Programme
Smoking	Not as strongly associated with congenital anomaly risk as with many other disease outcomes
Low folic acid status	Can be remedied by periconceptional folic acid supplementation or food fortification. Women must take supplements starting before conception for this to be an effective preventive measure
High vitamin A intake	Threshold dose unclear
Alcohol	Threshold dose unclear; microcephaly, heart defects, dysmorphic facial features, learning disabilities
Assisted reproductive therapy	A range of congenital anomalies including imprinting disorders
Radiation	Central nervous system malformations, mainly microcephaly

apparently environmental cases, genetic factors may play a role in determining susceptibility to the exposure, since not all exposed fetuses (even at a relevant dose and time of pregnancy) are affected.

An environmental cause can have preconceptional mutagenic action (i.e. changing genes, maternal or paternal) or postconceptional teratogenic action. Post-conceptional action is generally during the first trimester of pregnancy when most organogenesis occurs,

although relevant exposures may have occurred earlier if their effects are indirect (e.g. effects on endocrine function) or if a chemical has a long biological half-life in the body (e.g. PCBs). The development of the brain remains subject to adverse influences well into the second trimester and beyond. The fact that most organogenesis occurs very early in pregnancy, often before pregnancy is confirmed, is extremely important for prevention, as it means that primary prevention of congenital anomalies involves preconceptional care, not waiting until the woman attends for antenatal care. Folic acid for the prevention of NTDs provides a classic example of this.

A *teratogen* is a chemical or an agent which can cause a malformation in animals or in humans. However, whether an agent acts as a teratogen in a human pregnancy is crucially dependent on dose. Animal experiments show that a vast array of chemicals, if given in high enough doses early in pregnancy, will cause fetal malformation. The agent will be considered teratogenic if it leads to fetal malformation at doses *without* significant maternal toxicity. For practical purposes, each agent can be considered to have a 'threshold dose' above which it starts to cause fetal malformation, and below which the developing fetus is unaffected or is able to self-regulate or repair damage. For the protection of humans, it is important to determine whether the highest exposures experienced in the population are anywhere near the estimated 'threshold range' (taking into account also the likely variation of individual thresholds depending on other genetic and environmental factors). The thalidomide tragedy first brought the world's notice to the potential for drugs to affect the developing fetus; since then testing regimens have been instituted to improve drug safety for pregnant women. These testing regimens are far from perfect, requiring extrapolation from animal evidence to humans. Pregnant women are excluded from clinical trials, so post-marketing drug surveillance or pharmacovigilance aims to detect any increase in malformations associated with maternal drug intake. Pregnancy is often a contraindication to drug prescription, whether based on evidence of teratogenic effect, or lack of relevant evidence. A busy medical practitioner should consider the possibility of pregnancy before prescribing any drug not established as non-teratogenic.

··

Question 4

The epidemiological approach (for example, a case-control study) can be contrasted to case reports or case series where one or more cases are described in the literature where the mother took a certain drug and had a child with a birth defect. Why is the interpretation of case reports limited?

··

When dealing with 'cause', we do not simply have a horizontal array of different biological, chemical, or physical agents, but also vertical causal pathways and networks which determine exposure to these proximate agents. For example, maternal rubella infection and rubella vaccination policy are at different levels in the causal network leading to congenital rubella syndrome (characterized by eye defects, heart defects, and deafness); folic acid intake, both dietary and supplemental, social class and economic prosperity are all parts of the causal network for neural tube defects. Non-conformity to best clinical practice is part of the causal network leading to malformations caused by maternal epilepsy and diabetes (Table 16.5). Preventive strategies use knowledge at more than one level in these causal networks.

Folic acid and neural tube defects Periconceptional folic acid is now well established as preventing neural tube defects (NTDs) and possibly a range of other congenital anomalies including congenital heart disease. During the 1970s and 1980s, the main evidence for a protective effect was from case-control and non-randomized intervention studies. Many of these studies were carried out in the UK and Ireland, where, at that time, the total prevalence of NTDs was three to four times higher than in other European countries, although the difference is now very small (Busby *et al.* 2005).

··

Question 5

One of the criticisms of case-control studies is the possibility of 'maternal recall bias'. How do you think this might apply to case-control studies of maternal nutrition in pregnancy?

··

In 1991, the results of a randomized trial were published which confirmed the evidence from previous studies that periconceptional folic acid supplementation could prevent NTDs (Anon 1991). The trial concerned NTD 'recurrence' rather than 'occurrence', i.e. women entered into the trial already had a child with a NTD and therefore were at higher risk of having another NTD pregnancy than other women. There was other evidence, however, that the results of this recurrence trial would also be applicable to women without a previously affected child. Underlying biological mechanisms have been further elucidated; homozygotes for variants of the gene for the MTHFR enzyme which impair folate metabolism are at greater risk of NTDs (Brody *et al.* 2002).

Unfortunately, epidemiological studies show that disappointing progress has been made translating research into practice. Most pregnant women either do not take supplements at all, or do not start before conception (trial results show beneficial effects if supplementation starts preconceptionally). As a result the prevalence of NTDs has not fallen dramatically in Europe (EUROCAT 2009). There is evidence that socio-economic differences in access to health promotion messages and in pregnancy planning may be increasing inequalities in the prevalence of NTD-affected pregnancies (De Walle *et al.* 1998). Women may assume that 'healthy eating' leads to sufficient folic acid intake, but this has been shown to be very unlikely (Cuskelly *et al.* 1996). More than 50 countries of the world, including the USA, Canada, and several countries in South America, but not yet European countries, have therefore introduced fortification of staple foods with folic acid as the most effective preventive strategy (Crider *et al.* 2011; De Wals *et al.* 2007). Research has suggested a role for folic acid in protecting against cardiovascular disease and Alzheimer's disease, which would be an additional strong argument for fortification.

Environmental pollution and congenital anomalies While there is much interest in the potential role of environmental pollutants in causing congenital anomalies (outside of environmental disaster situations), it has been difficult to establish a strong evidence base. Since congenital anomalies are rare outcomes (even rarer when considering specific types of congenital anomaly), large populations need to be studied. Exposure can occur via air, food, water, or soil in various settings: personal, domestic, occupational, recreational, community. Exposure may be cumulative via a number of different exposure pathways. Little is known about the effect of chemical mixtures in the environment. Environmental

contaminants for which there is a growing evidence base include pesticide exposures (occupational, domestic, and drift from agricultural land) (Shirangi *et al.* 2011), solvents (particularly occupationally exposed groups such as in leather work or hairdressing), air pollutants (Vrijheid *et al.* 2011), by-products of drinking water chlorination (Niewenhuijsen *et al.* 2009), and unspecified releases from landfill sites (Vrijheid 2000). Hypospadias is a congenital anomaly characterized by abnormal position of the penile meatus and is one of a range of reproductive abnormalities (including also reduced fertility) that have been linked to endocrine-disrupting chemical exposures (Toppari *et al.* 1996). A huge variety of chemicals have endocrine-disrupting properties, including dioxins, organochlorine pesticides, phthalates (plasticizers found in a range of products including personal care products and packaging), some flame retardants, and some heavy metals.

··

Question 6

A particular problem for epidemiological studies is difficulty in estimating individual exposure to environmental contaminants leading to considerable *exposure misclassification*. What would you imagine to be sources of exposure misclassification when studying the risks associated with drinking water contaminants? What would you expect misclassification of exposure to do to the estimates of risk obtained by the study?

··

Reports in the media of a 'cluster' of birth defects, often associated with suspected local contamination of air or water, are relatively frequent. A random distribution of cases in space and time is not a regular distribution, and there will be patches of a denser concentration of cases. A community may become aware of an aggregation of cases in their area, and seek the nearest reason such as a waste site or power line. The problem has been likened to the 'Texan sharpshooter' who draws his gun and fires at the barn door, and only afterwards goes and draws the target in the middle of the densest cluster of bullet holes. Investigating clusters to distinguish 'random' clusters from clusters where there is a single cause is a difficult task for public health practitioners. Most of the well documented instances in the literature where a cluster was observed which was subsequently established as due to environmental contaminants have been related to food exposures with high relative risk (Dolk and Vrijheid 2003), including the Minnamata incident in Japan where fish and shellfish were contaminated with methylmercury, PCB contamination of cooking oil in Taiwan and Japan, and pesticide over-use at a fish farm in Hungary.

Man-made environmental disasters are characterized by very high levels of exposure to chemicals or to radiation, and congenital anomalies are one of the potential effects of short-term high exposure. It is often difficult to document congenital anomalies in the aftermath of a disaster, especially when the population has been wholly or partially evacuated. Exposure may be long-lasting in the area (e.g. after the Chernobyl nuclear disaster) but also bring great socio-economic hardships which in themselves affect the risk of congenital anomaly. There may be a high degree of mistrust between the community and those held responsible for the disaster which affects information gathering and transparency. Intensive study of Hiroshima survivors has established a link between exposure to radiation in the 8–15th week of pregnancy and microcephaly and mental retardation. Research on the population exposed to dioxins in an industrial accident in Seveso, Italy, in 1984 did not find an increase in congenital anomalies.

....

Question 7

Do some literature research of scientific and grey literature on a man-made environmental disaster that has happened in or near your country. Find out what is known about how many pregnant women were exposed, the nature of the exposure, the number of children born with birth defects among the exposed, the types of birth defects documented, and any sources of bias which may affect the interpretation of the known information.

....

Web addresses

Confidential Enquiry into Maternal and Child Health (CEMACH 2005)
www.cemach.org.uk

Department of Health (2005) SIDS: Advice for parents
www.dh.gov.uk/publications

EUROCAT (2004) Database of population registries
www.eurocat.ulster.ac.uk/pubdata/tabl; www.hfea.gov.uk

Office of National Statistics
www.statistics.gov.uk

PatientPlus (contraception)
www.patient.co.uk/.

US Census Bureau (2005) International database: summary statistics
www.census/gov/ipc/idbsum.html

EUROCAT (European Surveillance of Congenital Anomalies)
www.eurocat-network.eu

International Clearinghouse for Birth Defects Surveillance and Research
www.icbdsr.org

References

Anon (1991) Prevention of neural tube defects: results of the Medical Research Council Vitamin Study. *MRC Vitamin Study Research Group Lancet* **338** (8760), 131–7.

Bingham D, Strauss N, and Coeytaux F (2011) Maternal mortality in the United States: a human rights failure. *Contraception* **83** (3), 189–93.

Black RE, Cousens S, Johnson HL, Lawn JE, *et al.* (2010) Global, regional, and national causes of child mortality in 2008: a systematic analysis. *Lancet* **375** (9730), 1969–87.

Blencowe H, Cousens S, Modell B, and Lawn J (2010) Folic acid to reduce neonatal mortality from neural tube disorders. *International Journal of Epidemiology* **39** Suppl. 1 i110–21.

Botting B on behalf of the Editorial Board (2001) *Trends in Reproductive Epidemiology and Women's Health*. Confidential Enquiry into Maternal Deaths in the United Kingdom. 5th Report. London: Royal College of Obstetricians and Gynaecologists.

Brody LC, Conley M, Cox C, Kirke PN, *et al.* (2002) A polymorphism, R653Q, in the trifunctional enzyme methylenetetrahydrofolate dehydrogenase/methenyl-tetrahydrofolatecyclohydrolase/formyltetrahydrofolate-synthetase is a maternal genetic risk factor for neural tube defects: report of the Birth Defects Research Group. *American Journal of Human Genetics* **71** (5), 1207–15.

Bryce J, Black RE, Walker N, Bhutta ZA, *et al.* (2005) Can the world afford to save the lives of 6 million children each year? *Lancet* **365** (9478), 2193–200.

Busby A, Abramsky L, Dolk H, Armstrong B, *et al.* (2005) Preventing neural tube defects in Europe: a missed opportunity. *Reproductive Toxicology (Elmsford, NY)* **20** (3), 393–402.

Carpenter RG, Irgens LM, Blair PS, England PD, *et al.* (2004) Sudden unexplained infant death in 20 regions in Europe: case control study. *Lancet* **363** (9404), 185–91.

Cherian A, Seena S, Bullock RK, and Antony AC (2005) Incidence of neural tube defects in the least-developed area of India: a population-based study. *Lancet* **366** (9489), 930–1.

Coeytaux F, Bingham D, and Langer A (2011) Reducing maternal mortality: a global imperative. *Contraception* **83** (2), 95–8.

Crider KS, Bailey LB, and Berry RJ (2011) Folic acid food fortification—its history, effect, concerns, and future directions. *Nutrients* **3** (3), 370–84.

Critchley H, Bennett P, and Thornton S (2004) *Preterm Birth*. London: RCOG Press.

Cuskelly GJ, McNulty H, and Scott JM (1996) Effect of increasing dietary folate on red-cell folate: implications for prevention of neural tube defects. *Lancet* **347** (9002), 657–9.

De Walle HE, van der Pal KM, de Jong-van den Berg LT, Schouten J, *et al.* (1998) Periconceptional folic acid in The Netherlands in 1995. Socioeconomic differences. *Journal of Epidemiology and Community Health* **52** (12), 826–7.

De Wals P, Tairou F, Van Allen MI, Uh S-H, *et al.* (2007) Reduction in neural-tube defects after folic acid fortification in Canada. *The New England Journal of Medicine* **357** (2), 135–42.

Dolk H and Vrijheid M (2003) The impact of environmental pollution on congenital anomalies. *British Medical Bulletin* **68**, 25–45.

Dommergues M, Mandelbrot L, Mahieu-Caputo D, Boudjema N, *et al.* (2010) Termination of pregnancy following prenatal diagnosis in France: how severe are the fetal anomalies? *Prenatal Diagnosis* **30** (6), 531–9.

EUROCAT (2009) Special Report: Prevention of Neural Tube Defects by Periconceptional Folic Acid Supplementation in Europe, EUROCAT Central Registry, University of Ulster. Available at: **www.eurocat-network.eu**.

Gilbert NL, Fell DB, Joseph KS, Liu S, *et al.* (2012) Temporal trends in sudden infant death syndrome in Canada from 1991 to 2005: contribution of changes in cause of death assignment practices and in maternal and infant characteristics. *Paediatric and Perinatal Epidemiology* **26** (2), 124–30.

Grimes DA, Benson J, Singh S, Romero M, *et al.* (2006) Unsafe abortion: the preventable pandemic. *Lancet* **368** (9550), 1908–19.

Hauck FR, Thompson JMD, Tanabe KO, Moon RY, *et al.* (2011) Breastfeeding and reduced risk of sudden infant death syndrome: a meta-analysis. *Pediatrics* **128** (1), 103–10.

Herbert DL, Lucke JC, and Dobson AJ (2009) Infertility, medical advice and treatment with fertility hormones and/or in vitro fertilisation: a population perspective from the Australian Longitudinal Study on Women's Health. *Australian and New Zealand Journal of Public Health* **33** (4), 358–64.

Hogan MC, Foreman KJ, Naghavi M, Ahn SY, *et al.* (2010) Maternal mortality for 181 countries, 1980–2008: a systematic analysis of progress towards Millennium Development Goal 5. *Lancet* **375** (9726), 1609–23.

Hunt CE and Hauck FR (2006) Sudden infant death syndrome. *CMAJ: Canadian Medical Association Journal.* **174** (13), 1861–9.

Hutchison BL, Rea C, Stewart AW, Koelmeyer TD, *et al.* (2011) Sudden unexpected infant death in Auckland: a retrospective case review. *Acta Paediatrica (Oslo, Norway: 1992)* **100** (8), 1108–12.

Liang J, Li X, Dai L, Zeng W, *et al.* (2012) The changes in maternal mortality in 1000 counties in mid-Western china by a government-initiated intervention. *PloS One* **7** (5), e37458.

Lozano R, Wang H, Foreman KJ, Rajaratnam JK, *et al.* (2011) Progress towards Millennium Development Goals 4 and 5 on maternal and child mortality: an updated systematic analysis. *Lancet* **378** (9797), 1139–65.

Moon RY (2011) SIDS and other sleep-related infant deaths: expansion of recommendations for a safe infant sleeping environment. *Pediatrics* **128** (5), e1341–67.

Mueller RF and Young ID (2001) *Emery's Elements of Medical Genetics*, 11th edn. Edinburgh: Churchill Livingstone, Harcourt Publishers Ltd.

Nieuwenhuijsen MJ, Martinez D, Grellier J, Bennett J, *et al.* (2009) Chlorination disinfection by-products in drinking water and congenital anomalies: review and meta-analyses. *Environmental Health Perspectives* **117** (10), 1486–93.

Norman P, Gregory I, Dorling D, and Baker A (2008) Geographical trends in infant mortality: England and Wales, 1970–2006. *Health statistics quarterly / Office for National Statistics* (40), 18–29.

Pandey S, Shetty A, Hamilton M, Bhattacharya S, *et al.* (2012) Obstetric and perinatal outcomes in singleton pregnancies resulting from IVF/ICSI: a systematic review and meta-analysis. *Human Reproduction Update* **18** (5), 485–503.

Rahman MO and Menken J Reproductive health. In: Merson MH, Black RE, & Mills AJ (eds) (2012) *Global Health: Diseases, Programs, Systems, and Policies*, 3rd edn, pp. 115–76. Burlington: Thomas and Bartlett Learning.

Rajaratnam JK, Marcus JR, Flaxman AD, Wang H, *et al.* (2010) Neonatal, postneonatal, childhood, and under-5 mortality for 187 countries, 1970–2010: a systematic analysis of progress towards Millennium Development Goal 4. *Lancet* **375** (9730), 1988–2008.

Rowlands S (2007) Contraception and abortion. *JRSM* **100** (10), 465–8.

Rudan I, Chan KY, Zhang JSF, Theodoratou E, *et al.* (2010) Causes of deaths in children younger than 5 years in China in 2008. *Lancet* **375** (9720), 1083–9.

Sedgh G, Singh S, Shah IH, Ahman E, *et al.* (2012) Induced abortion: incidence and trends worldwide from 1995 to 2008. *Lancet* **379** (9816), 625–32.

Shirangi A, Nieuwenhuijsen M, Vienneau D, and Holman CDJ (2011) Living near agricultural pesticide applications and the risk of adverse reproductive outcomes: a review of the literature. *Paediatric and Perinatal Epidemiology* **25** (2), 172–91.

Singh S (2006) Hospital admissions resulting from unsafe abortion: estimates from 13 developing countries. *Lancet* **368** (9550), 1887–92.

Skolnik R (2012) *Global Health 101*, 2nd edn. Burlington MA: Jones & Bartlett Learning.

Stothard KJ, Tennant PWG, Bell R, and Rankin J (2009) Maternal overweight and obesity and the risk of congenital anomalies: a systematic review and meta-analysis. *JAMA* **301** (6), 636–50.

Sullivan FM and Barlow SM (2001) Review of risk factors for sudden infant death syndrome. *Paediatric and Perinatal Epidemiology* **15** (2), 144–200.

Tin W, Wariyar U, and Hey E (1997) Changing prognosis for babies of less than 28 weeks' gestation in the north of England between 1983 and 1994. Northern Neonatal Network. *BMJ (Clinical Research Ed)* **314** (7074), 107–11.

Toppari J, Larsen JC, Christiansen P, Giwercman A, *et al.* (1996) Male reproductive health and environmental xenoestrogens. *Environmental Health Perspectives* **104** Suppl. 4, 741–803.

UNICEF (2011) *Levels and Trends in Child Mortality: Report 2011.* Available at: www.childinfo.org/publications

van der Linde D, Konings EEM, Slager MA, Witsenburg M, *et al.* (2011) Birth prevalence of congenital heart disease worldwide: a systematic review and meta-analysis. *Journal of the American College of Cardiology* **58** (21), 2241–7.

Vennemann MM, Hense H-W, Bajanowski T, Blair PS, *et al.* (2012) Bed sharing and the risk of sudden infant death syndrome: can we resolve the debate? *The Journal of Pediatrics* **160** (1), 44–8.e2.

Vogel F and Motulsky AG (2002) Human and medical genetics. In: Detels R, McEwen J, Beaglehole R, and Tanaka H (eds) *Oxford Textbook of Public Health*, pp. 131–48. Oxford: Oxford University Press.

Vrijheid M (2000) Health effects of residence near hazardous waste landfill sites: a review of epidemiologic literature. *Environmental Health Perspectives* **108** Suppl. 1101–12.

Vrijheid M, Martinez D, Manzanares S, Dadvand P, *et al.* (2011) Ambient air pollution and risk of congenital anomalies: a systematic review and meta-analysis. *Environmental Health Perspectives* **119** (5), 598–606.

Weindling AM (2003) The confidential enquiry into maternal and child health (CEMACH). *Archives of Disease in Childhood* **88** (12), 1034–7.

WHO (2010) *Packages of Interventions for Family Planning, Safe Abortion care, Maternal, Newborn and Child Health.* Geneva: WHO. Available at: http://whqlibdoc. who.int/hq/2010/WHO_FCH_10.06_eng.pdf

Wood AM, Pasupathy D, Pell JP, Fleming M, *et al.* (2012) Trends in socioeconomic inequalities in risk of sudden infant mortality, other causes of infant mortality, and stillbirth in Scotland: population based study. *BMJ (Clinical Research Ed)* **344**, e1552.

Model answers

Question 1

Legally available methods of birth control appear to be culturally determined in the majority of countries, but culture would include social, religious, and economic aspects of each society. What appears inescapable is that birth control is popular with women as it permits control over the size of family achieved, or indeed, in well developed countries in which gender equality is socially and legally the norm, whether any children are desirable. Methods of birth control are discussed in detail elsewhere (see PatientPlus (contraception) in Web addresses section).

Question 2

Residual confounding occurs when factors which have not been considered in the analysis may contribute to the results. Socio-economic factors are strongly (but not exclusively) associated with SIDS but are also linked to a large number of behavioural and environmental factors which may not have been considered in the analysis.

Question 3

Population-based means referring to a geographically defined population. It is used in contrast to 'hospital-based' referring to births or patients of one or more hospitals. Hospital-based studies can be biased due to selective referral of high-risk pregnancies or affected children to tertiary centres and therefore give artificially high prevalence rates.

Question 4

In a series of case reports, it is often impossible to tell whether the drug exposure and congenital anomaly are associated by chance or whether it is truly unusual, as there is no measure of the frequency of the drug exposure in the population, or the frequency of the congenital anomaly in the population. The first case report may elicit similar case reports, and their similarity may be due to reporting bias rather than any specificity of association between the drug and the congenital anomaly.

Question 5

Mothers taking part in retrospective case-control studies who have experienced a poor pregnancy outcome may be particularly likely to link coincidental events in pregnancy with their poor outcome. For studies of maternal nutrition mothers may be more likely to remember what they perceive as poor nutritional practices.

Question 6

Variability in amounts of tap water drunk and variability in levels of contaminants in tap water both predispose to the possibility of exposure misclassification. Exposure misclassification would be most likely to reduce the size of the estimates of risk obtained in a study.

17 Neoplasms

LESLEY ANDERSON, LIAM MURRAY, AND JOHN YARNELL

CHAPTER CONTENTS

This chapter briefly reviews the pathology of cancer and how information on cancer incidence is collected (cancer registration). The epidemiology of selected cancers is reviewed. These include: skin cancers, the hormone-related cancers (breast, prostate, ovary), cancers of the oesophagus, stomach and liver, and haematopoietic cancers. Finally genetic, lifestyle, environmental, occupational, and dietary risk factors, and the prospects for cancer prevention, are discussed. Respiratory and colorectal cancers are discussed in Chapters 8 and 11, respectively.

Introduction

What is cancer?

Cancer is the result of a breakdown in the normal growth of body cells. It is ultimately a disease of the genetic material that regulates cell growth, is very common in human populations, and can be induced also in laboratory animals. Based on data from the USA in 2006/8 it was estimated that American men had a lifetime risk of developing an invasive cancer of 45 per cent (risk of dying 23 per cent); for women the risks were 38 per cent and 20 per cent respectively (American Cancer Society 2012). Almost every type of cell in the human body is capable of malignant change and over 200 forms of cancer have been described. There is ongoing debate about the exact mechanisms by which this transformation occurs, but it is agreed that cancer is the result of cumulative, acquired (somatic) mutations in genes that regulate cell growth, the expression of other genes, and cell death.

Only 5–10 per cent of cancers are caused by inherited mutations which have passed from the parental germ cells and are present in all cells. Three kinds of cancer genes contribute to the successful malignant transformation of a pre-cancerous cell: *tumour suppressor genes* restrict the ability of cells to divide, and have an important regulatory role in the normal cell. Mutations that permanently disable these genes, or reduce their capacity to regulate cell division, contribute to malignant change; *proto-oncogenes* also have roles in growth regulation but mutations which lead to the development of *oncogenes* characteristically enhance the usual function of the gene; *microRNA genes* which regulate gene expression. Currently these mechanisms are relevant to the development of new therapeutic agents (Croce 2008) rather than for cancer epidemiology. Some general properties of malignant cells are shown in Box 17.1.

It has been estimated that for most normal cells sufficient mutations to promote malignant change

Box 17.1 Properties of cancer cells

- They continue dividing in situations in which normal cells would wait for a chemical signal, for example in response to injury.
- They do not respond to signals to stop dividing.
- Normally damaged cells self-destruct (a process termed apoptosis), but this does not happen in cancer cells despite significant DNA damage.
- Cancer cells have the ability to promote the growth of blood vessels (angiogenesis) to provide nutrients for tumour growth.
- Cancer cells, unlike normal cells, are not limited in the number of times they can divide.
- Cancer cells invade nearby tissue and then metastasize to distant parts of the body.

would not occur naturally during the current normal lifespan of a human being, but many agents present in the environment are known to promote this by causing mutations in relevant genes. These agents include many chemicals, viruses, reproductive hormones, and ionizing radiation, among others. Industrial carcinogens, including those found in food and drink, are classified according to their known or suspected toxicity in humans or other animals. Common carcinogenic agents are discussed further in section 17.5.

17.1 Cancer registration

Epidemiological information on cancer in various countries is available from mortality data; but these records do not count people cured from their cancer or in long-term remission, or those who die of other causes, and may not give an accurate idea of cancer burden. For example, epithelial skin cancers, which are the commonest cancers in most countries, tend not to be invasive and can be readily treated. Thus the high incidence rates for these cancers are not reflected at all in mortality data. Cancer registration, the systematic recording of details on cancer cases, provides an

estimate of incidence and often provides additional information such as histological and clinical data which allow the separation of primary and secondary tumours. Histological grading is very important from the perspective of prognosis for many types of cancer and different cell types at the same site may have different risk factors (see 'Oesophagus' section for oesophageal cancers). Secondary tumours occur by metastatic spread in the lymphatic or blood systems. The most common secondary sites are liver, bone, lung, and brain. Such information is used for 'staging' of tumours at diagnosis and during treatment.

Two types of cancer registry are common: (1) hospital-based, which are selective in nature and of limited representativeness; and (2) community-based, which record all cancer cases arising in a defined population. The latter are an invaluable part of any rational programme of cancer control. They assist in planning services and in evaluating treatment and prevention for the population concerned. They provide a data resource for aetiological studies, and are used for monitoring cancer risk in occupational groups and other cohorts of individuals exposed to various carcinogens.

All relevant epidemiological disease measures can be made from cancer registries which can provide reliable population-based data with follow-up (see Chapter 2). These include **incidence (rate), cumulative incidence, prevalence, mortality, case-fatality, survival** (five-year survival rates are the standard measure used by registries globally), **life-years lost**, and **disability-adjusted life-years (DALYs)**. The last two measures require population-based life tables, usually available only for large geographical regions and countries.

The World Health Organization established the International Agency for Research on Cancer (IARC) in 1965 to promote international collaboration in cancer research. One of its key functions has been to collate, help validate, and publish data from cancer registries across the globe in a series of volumes *Cancer in Five Continents (CI5)*. Incidence and mortality data for the world and the estimated number of deaths and incident cases for the WHO world regions are shown in Fig. 17.1a,b and in Fig. 17.2a–f, respectively.

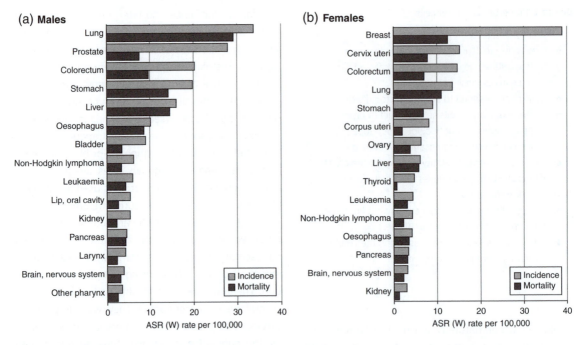

Figure 17.1 (a,b) Incidence of the most common cancers worldwide in 2008.

Reproduced with permission from Ferlay J, Shin HR, Bray F, Forman D, Mathers C, and Parkin DM. *GLOBOCAN 2008, Cancer Incidence and Mortality Worldwide: IARC CancerBase No 10* [Internet]. Lyon, France: International Agency for Research on Cancer; 2010. Available from: **http://globocan.iarc.fr**

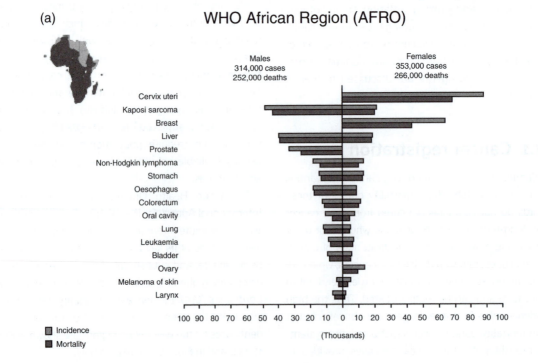

Figure 17.2 (a–f) Incidence and mortality of cancers by WHO World Regions.

Reproduced with permission from IARC (2008) World cancer report 2008. Available at: **http://www.iarc.fr/en/publications/pdfs-online/wcr/2008/**

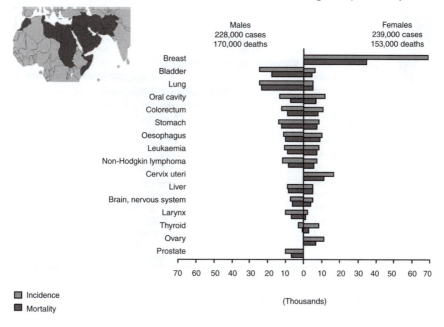

(b) WHO Eastern Mediterranean Region (EMRO)

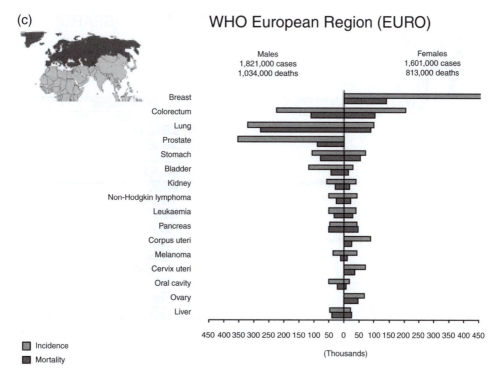

(c) WHO European Region (EURO)

Figure 17.2 *(continued)*

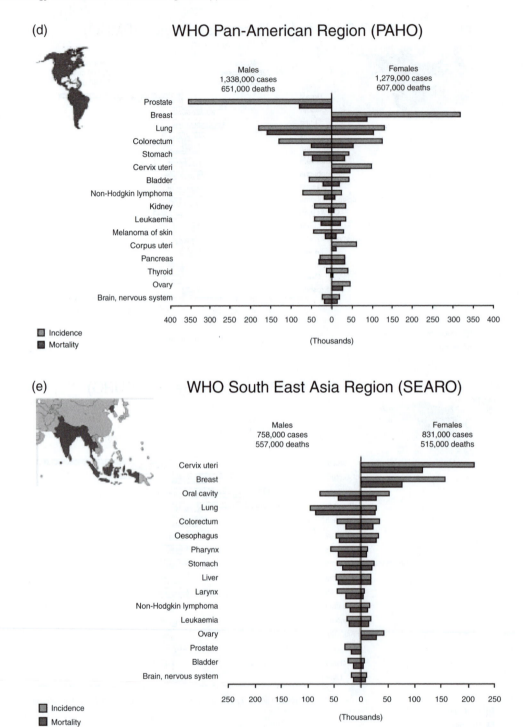

Figure 17.2 (*continued*)

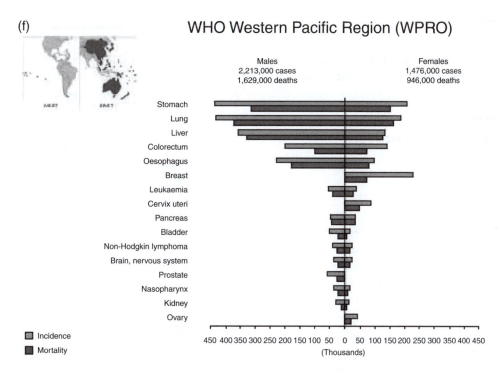

(f)

WHO Western Pacific Region (WPRO)

Males
2,213,000 cases
1,629,000 deaths

Females
1,476,000 cases
946,000 deaths

Stomach
Lung
Liver
Colorectum
Oesophagus
Breast
Leukaemia
Cervix uteri
Pancreas
Bladder
Non-Hodgkin lymphoma
Brain, nervous system
Prostate
Nasopharynx
Kidney
Ovary

■ Incidence
■ Mortality

450 400 350 300 250 200 150 100 50 0 50 100 150 200 250 300 350 400 450
(Thousands)

Figure 17.2 *(continued)*

17.2 Common cancers

Cancer is a major cause of morbidity and mortality worldwide and in high-income countries is second only to all cardiovascular diseases as the leading cause of death. Worldwide the number of cases of cancer has doubled in the past 30 years and, in 2008, at least 12 million people developed a potentially invasive cancer, more than seven million died from the disease, and about 25 million were living with the disease (IARC 2008a,b). By 2030 these figures are expected to increase 2.5 to 3-fold.

In Fig. 17.1a,b global incidence and mortality data are shown for the 15 commonest cancers worldwide. For women breast and cervical cancer rank one and two in terms of incidence, and for men lung, prostate, and bladder cancer rank one, two, and seven, respectively, although bladder cancer does not appear in the top 15 cancers for women. The gap between mortality and incidence provides an overall measure of the case-fatality of the cancers at specific sites but clinical and

histological factors are of major importance in determining individual case-fatality.

Fig. 17.2a–f show the distribution of cancer deaths in the world regions, which may be underestimated in regions with partial or inadequate cancer registration. Nevertheless the pattern of cancer deaths is likely to reflect the overall distribution for the relevant region and it is striking that these differ markedly. For example, stomach cancer predominates in the Western Pacific region, which includes China and Japan, and stomach cancer is more important than colorectal cancer in the Eastern Mediterranean region, which includes Afghanistan and Pakistan. Bladder cancer is ranked first or first equal in men in this last region. Cervical cancer predominates in Africa and in South East Asia (a region which includes India and Bangladesh) and liver cancer is important in the Western Pacific and in Africa. South East Asia features uniquely oral cancers high in the rankings and Africa likewise registers Kaposi's sarcoma (see Chapter 18).

Question 1

How would you investigate the causes of the distributions of cancers shown in the world regions?

a) **In general terms?**

b) **For as many specific cancers as possible?**

In summary the five major sites worldwide are breast, prostate, lung, colorectal, and cervix (IARC 2008a) Non-melanoma skin cancer, which is easily treated, usually by surgery, accounts for 25 per cent of cancer cases but has a very small proportion of deaths and is not usually included in routine cancer statistics. Cancers at several sites are related to hormones that affect local tissue as part of normal physiological functioning. Not all cancers at these sites are hormone-dependent for their growth but, for those that are, this provides a valuable opportunity for therapy. Sites that have such cancers include the breast, prostate, endometrium, and ovary.

Cancer trends

Crude mortality rates suggest that cancer incidence has increased during the 20th century. Increased life expectancy with an ageing population is a major factor contributing to the increase. Age-standardization (see Chapter 16) is important when comparing different time periods or countries with different population structures, and allows us to detect differences in mortality or incidence that are not due to changes in the age structure of the population. Other reasons for the upward trend in cancer incidence include: improved diagnosis, control of competing causes such as infections and heart disease, and the effect of changing lifestyle and exposure to risk factors. Strong, established risk factors include *tobacco, alcohol, radiation* from medical procedures and from the environment, increased exposure to *ultraviolet radiation* for melanoma, *human papilloma virus* subtypes for cervical cancer, *hepatitis B and C* for primary liver cancer, *human herpes virus 8* infection (often additionally with

HIV) for Kaposi's sarcoma worldwide, and *HIV infection* and lymphomas. *Obesity* is an emerging risk factor that is linked to endometrial, breast, colon, and possibly renal and prostate cancers. Invasive cancers characteristically possess long *incubation periods* from acute or chronic exposures to risk factors. For example, lung cancer can result from exposure to tobacco smoke during a 40-year period or more and can appear after cessation of smoking. Thus lung cancer mortality in women is predicted to rise, particularly in high-income countries, in line with trends in cigarette smoking in these counties during the past three decades.

Cancer rates may also increase substantially for a limited period during the **prevalence round** if a new screening test is introduced when more cancers will be detected at an earlier stage (see Chapter 5).

Skin cancers

Skin cancers are most common in white populations across the globe, with rates severalfold higher in white people than in races with all other shades of skin pigmentation. Most skin cancers appear to be caused by excessive exposure to the sun. Within countries rates vary with latitude, which support this view, but tar and arsenic are also established risk factors. *Basal cell cancer (rodent ulcer)* is the most common type of skin cancer, accounting for 50 per cent of cases. It grows slowly, mainly affecting people over 60 years of age, usually appearing on the face or ears. It rarely metastasizes but can cause local damage and so warrants treatment. A quarter of skin cancers are squamous cell tumours, which may spread but can be treated successfully by surgery. *Melanoma* of the skin accounts for only two per cent of male and three per cent of female cancers, and accounts for about one per cent of cancer deaths despite the fact that five-year survival in Europe approaches 90 per cent in many high-income countries. The median age at diagnosis, 57 years, is relatively young for cancer. Rates have increased over recent decades, probably because of increased exposure to ultraviolet radiation, both of duration and pattern. Prevention by taking care in the sun, avoiding sunbed use, and early detection are key public health strategies. In Australia, stabilization of the incidence rates for melanoma in white Australians attests to the success of a national public health campaign to reduce exposure to solar radiation.

Breast cancer

Breast cancer is the most common cancer in women but about one per cent of cases occur in men. In 2009, 22 European Member States were running or establishing breast cancer screening programmes. In most European and other developed countries, screening by mammography is offered to all women in their 50s and 60s and detects tumours earlier than they would present clinically. Recent evidence has shown that screening women of younger and older ages is also adequately efficient in early detection. Breast cancer, like most cancers, increases with age and over 50 per cent of cases are diagnosed over the age of 60 years. Other risk factors include a family history of breast or ovarian cancer which is reported in up to 27 per cent of breast cancer cases, although only 5.7 per cent of all postmenopausal breast cancers are inherited (Barnes *et al.* 2011). Family history carries a two to threefold increase in risk as does a history of benign breast disease (fibroadenoma and fibrocystic disease). Mutations of *BRCA1/BRCA2* account for approximately four per cent of all breast cancers and carry a lifetime risk of more than 50 per cent. Early menarche, late menopause, nulliparity, first birth after age 30 years, and lack of breastfeeding of offspring, are all weak risk factors, as is exposure to oestrogen through hormone replacement therapy of more than five years' duration (RR up to 1.6). Other risk factors are a previous history of breast cancer and exposure to ionizing radiation. Alcohol consumption is an established risk factor with a 40 per cent increase in risk at higher levels of consumption (five or more drinks per day) (and an 80 per cent increase in risk for colorectal cancer at this level of consumption). Obesity is associated with a doubling of risk (100 per cent) in postmenopausal women, which may be mediated by hyperinsulinaemia (Gunter *et al.* 2009). Exercise of four or five hours per week has been associated with a reduced risk. Breast cancer is more common in affluent populations, which may reflect lower levels of parity and delayed age at

first pregnancy. The outlook in breast cancer is good, with average survival relative to the general population almost 80 per cent at five years (see Table 17.1). Most breast tumours are sensitive to the effects of oestrogen (oestrogen-receptor positive) and respond to oestrogen antagonists such as tamoxifen.

Trends in breast cancer: period and cohort effects

Age adjustment will take account of changes in the age structure of the population over time but changes in trends may be also due to **period** and **cohort effects**. A period effect influences disease rates in all ages at a single point in time. A good example occurred in America when, in 1974, Betty Ford, the wife of the President, was diagnosed with breast cancer. This resulted in more openness about breast cancer and an increase in breast cancer rates in all age groups. This may reflect over-diagnosis at that point of time and under-diagnosis in other periods. An initial increase in breast cancer incidence may also be predicted on the introduction of population-wide screening programmes (see Chapter 5). A cohort effect relates to specific birth cohorts. For example, women born in 1900 to 1930 in the USA had higher rates of non-parity than women born from 1930 to 1945. Non-parity (nulliparity) is an independent risk factor for breast cancer, and the effect may be amplified by the absence of the protective effect on breast cancer of breastfeeding. We can predict a future cohort effect with current levels of non-parity, late age at first pregnancy and low breastfeeding levels, leading to increased levels of breast cancer in the current cohort of women, particularly in high income countries.

Prostate cancer

This is the third most common cancer in males. It accounts for one in seven cancers diagnosed in men. Age is a risk factor and over half the cases are over 74 years at diagnosis. The average age at diagnosis is falling due to the use of prostate-specific antigen (PSA) testing in younger men, which has resulted in an increase in the detection of this cancer (see Chapter 5). The rates of prostate cancer vary widely internationally

Table 17.1 European cancer survival: patients diagnosed 1995–1999 and followed up to end of 2002

	Lung*	Breast	Colon	Stomach	Prostate	All
			Age-standardized 5-year relative survival			
Denmark	7.9	77.5	49.3	14.4	47.7	–
Finland	9.7	83.5	59.1	27.6	79.6	55.7
Iceland	15.0	88.0	56.9	26.5	79.3	56.6
Norway	10.9	82.4	57.0	21.9	74.5	53.6
Sweden	13.0	84.6	57.7	22.1	77.5	58.3
Ireland	9.8	73.8	52.2	18.0	71.3	45.5
England	8.4	77.3	49.9	16.1	69.7	46.2
Northern Ireland	10.2	77.6	53.4	17.2	60.8	44.6
Scotland	8.0	74.9	51.6	15.7	67.5	43.0
Wales	9.0	76.9	50.8	15.9	68.7	48.4
Austria	14.4	80.0	58.7	30.3	86.7	56.1
Belgium	16.5	77.3	56.4	31.5	83.3	54.2
France	12.9	83.1	58.0	26.0	78.3	52.4
Germany	13.2	78.3	57.9	27.5	81.6	52.3
Netherlands	13.4	81.3	56.8	18.1	78.9	51.0
Switzerland	13.9	82.0	59.1	27.2	82.3	55.0
Italy	12.8	82.7	58.7	31.7	79.1	51.8
Malta	8.7	76.1	49.7	18.9	71.2	48.6
Portugal	12.8	77.2	51.9	28.1	82.3	52.2
Slovenia	8.8	71.9	45.8	20.7	58.2	41.5
Spain	10.7	80.3	54.9	27.8	75.4	49.3
Czech Republic	8.2	69.2	46.9	18.0	54.4	42.5
Poland	9.2	73.7	38.7	14.4	60.5	38.6
Europe	**12.0**	**79.4**	**54.5**	**24.5**	**76.4**	**50.3**

*Includes bronchus and trachea.
Reproduced from Sant M *et al*, 'EUROCARE-4. Survival or cancer patients diagnosed in 1995–1999', *European Journal of Cancer* **45** (6), 931–91, 2009, with permission from Elsevier.

with the highest rates in the USA and Canada, and the lowest in Korea and Japan. High rates are found in black populations and the lowest in Japanese, but both Japanese Americans and black Americans have higher rates than men in their native countries. Some of this variation may be due to access to PSA testing as there is less variation in deaths from prostate cancer, but this is unlikely to fully explain the excess in black rather than white Americans. The variation may also reflect an environmental aetiology possibly related to diet and behavioural factors. Carriers of *BRCA1* and *BRCA2* mutations have a four to fivefold increase in risk and a family history of prostate cancer confers a two- to threefold increase (Boffetta and La Vecchia 2009).

Prostate cancer may also be hormone-dependent as the prostate gland is dependent on androgens for its growth and function. Bilateral orchidectomy and chemical forms of anti-androgenic treatments are used to treat prostate cancer and can produce significant remission in many cases, although five-year survival is slightly lower than that for breast cancer (Table 17.1).

Endometrial and ovarian cancer

Endometrial cancer is also hormone related and is the sixth most common cancer in women worldwide, with 66 per cent of cases occurring in high-resource countries. The major risk factor is obesity which carries an attributable risk of 50 per cent (Reeves *et al.* 2007), and nulliparity, infertility, and late menopause are associated with a doubling of risk as is the case for unopposed oestrogen therapy (Boffeta and La Vecchia 2009). Combined oral contraceptives appear to reduce the risk by up to 50 per cent. With the developing global epidemic of obesity in low- and middle-income countries endometrial cancer incidence is predicted to increase substantially in the next decades.

Ovarian cancer is the seventh most common cancer in females worldwide and the third most common gynaecological cancer after cervical and uterine cancer. It often presents late as symptoms are vague. It is more common with increasing age and with affluence. A woman's ovulatory history plays an important role in the risk of developing the disease. As in the case of breast cancer, nulliparity is a risk factor. There is a decreasing risk with each pregnancy whereas oral contraception and premature menopause each have a protective effect. Epidemiological studies of risk factors for ovarian cancer tend to be case-control rather than cohort studies, because there are few established cohorts of women of sufficient size and length of follow-up to give an adequate number of ovarian cancer cases. About 10 per cent of ovarian cancers are due to genetic factors associated with a faulty copy of the *BRCA1 or BRCA2* gene.

Cervix uteri

Cervical cancer is the second most common cancer in women worldwide and causes about a quarter of million deaths annually, 85 per cent of these in low- and middle-income countries (Tay 2012). The highest incidence is in WHO's South East Asia region which includes India, Bangladesh, and Thailand where it is the leading cancer (Fig. 17.2e).

Epidemiological studies have long shown associations between sexual activity and the development of this cancer, but in recent decades international studies showed that certain human papillomaviruses (HPV) were necessary (but not sufficient) causes. Human papillomavirus occurs in almost all cases of this cancer but in only 5–40 per cent of controls (Clifford *et al.* 2005). Human papillomavirus infection tends to persist only in cases, and typically cellular transformation of the cervix may take 10–15 years or more. The widespread use of vaccines in young girls containing HPV-16 and HPV-18, which account for 70 per cent of cases worldwide, is likely to have a significant impact on the prevalence of disease in future generations.

Stomach

This is the fourth most common cancer worldwide, and is the leading cancer in the Far East (Japan and China) (see Fig. 17.2f). In most countries incidence has fallen sharply during the latter part of the 20th century, and dietary and other changes in salt intake, increase in refrigeration, reduction in nitrates, and increase in antioxidant foods have been linked with this decline. The disease is twice as common in men as in women, and it is more common in the poor. Alcohol and tobacco may contribute to its development (Perez-Perez *et al.* 2004), but the worldwide prevalence and trends in *Helicobacter pylori* can explain 50 per cent of the global burden of the disease (Parkin 2006). Precursor conditions for gastric cancer such as atrophic gastritis are strongly associated with chronic *H. pylori* infection and the epidemiology of this widespread infection, which is more common in low- and middle-income countries, and becoming less common in high-income countries, is discussed further in Chapters 11 and 18.

Oesophagus

These cancers are regionally distributed across the globe (the highest prevalence is in the Western Pacific region, Fig. 17.2f) and are derived from two different cellular origins: squamous cell cancers represent 90 per cent or more of these cancers worldwide while adenocarcinoma cancers occur in high-income countries (up to 80 per cent). Squamous cell tumours tend to occur in the upper two-thirds of the oesophagus and adenocarcinomas in the lower third.

Tobacco smoking and alcohol consumption are strong risk factors for squamous cell cancers and obesity and tobacco are risk factors for adenocarcinoma. It is believed that gastrointestinal reflux related to obesity may be the mechanism of this association. A recent large cohort study found that increasing body mass index was linked to the risk of developing oesophageal or gastric cardia (at the junction of the oesophagus and stomach) cancer (Merry *et al.* 2007).

The incidence of squamous cell cancers are stable or in decline in the world regions while adenocarcinoma has shown a marked increase in high-income countries, possibly partially explained by trends in overweight and obesity, although the role of misclassification has also been investigated (Pohl and Welch 2005).

Liver

Primary liver cancer is a major cause of mortality in the Far East, in China, and in other countries of the Western Pacific (Fig. 17.2f) and it is closely linked with early childhood infection with hepatitis B and C viruses. It is estimated that 54 per cent of cases worldwide are linked with hepatitis B virus and 31 per cent with hepatitis C. Food contaminated with aflatoxins from *Aspergillus* fungi has been also associated with primary liver cancer, and alcohol, through its role in the development of cirrhosis, and tobacco, are also important factors, particularly in regions with a low prevalence of hepatitis B infection (Boffetta and La Vecchia 2009).

Mother-to-child transmission is common in high-prevalence areas for hepatitis B and WHO initiatives in these regions include vaccination during the perinatal period which has become well established in the past decade. Hepatitis C is not preventable by vaccination at present, but detection and medical treatment of carriers may represent one strategy towards prevention.

17.3 Haematological malignancies

Haematological cancers are the most common cancers in childhood and collectively account for approximately six to eight per cent of all cancers diagnosed annually. They arise in haemopoietic tissue associated with blood, bone marrow, and lymphoid tissue, including the spleen. They comprise a broad range of diseases, with significant variation in their presentation, natural history, treatment, and prognosis. The main groupings are *acute and chronic leukaemias, Hodgkin's and non-Hodgkin's lymphoma, myeloma*, and other *lymphoproliferative* malignancies. Leukaemias are confined to blood cells but lymphomas are usually solid tumours at sites of lymphocyte proliferation, with some overlap with lymphocytic leukaemias.

The diagnosis and classification of haematological malignancies has evolved in parallel with developments in laboratory techniques ranging from microscopy through cytochemical staining and antibody detection to DNA analysis. The ability to define subgroups is increasingly important as treatment is tailored, not only to specific types of leukaemia and lymphoma, but also on the basis of their prognostic group. The latest WHO classification uses cellular origin (B, T and natural killer cells) as its basis. Such changes in nomenclature pose problems both for registration systems

Table 17.2   Haematological cancers: worldwide incidence and mortality rates and risk factors

	Age-standardized incidence rate per 100,000[*]	Age-standardized mortality rate per 100,000[*]	Risk factors (strength of relationship)[**]
Leukaemias	5.0	3.6	Ionizing radiation++ Smoking+, some occupational carcinogens+ (e.g. benzene)
Lymphoma			
Hodgkins	1.0	0.4	Epstein–Barr virus+
Non-Hodgkins	5.1	2.7	Viral infections of lymphocytes++

Sources: *IARC (2008a)
**Doll and Peto (2003).
+, weak: ++, moderate: +++, strong.
Reproduced from *Oxford Textbook of Medicine 4e* edited by David A Warrell, Timothy M Cox and John D Firth (2003) Ch. 'Epidemiology of Cancer' by R Doll and R Peto pp. 193–218, with permission of Oxford University Press.

and for epidemiologists interested in examining trends in the incidence of these diseases over time. In an attempt to produce more meaningful epidemiological data for this group of disorders, several specialist registries have been established (Cartwright *et al.* 1999). New techniques and strategies may be required to advance our understanding of the causes of childhood leukaemias (Wiemels 2012). Incidence and mortality rates standardized to the world population of haematological cancers are shown in Table 17.2.

Acute myeloid leukaemia

This is a leukaemia of the myeloid cells of the bone marrow and may occur *de novo* or following the development of a pre-leukaemic condition. The reported incidence varies widely throughout the world; the European incidence rate is estimated as 3.6 per 100,000 population. It is rare in children and young adults, but the incidence rises with increasing age. Below age 65 years, *de novo* acute myeloid leukaemia (AML) predominates. There is a slight male preponderance of cases and an apparent slow decline in numbers of cases over time, possibly because of a rise in cases presenting in the pre-leukaemic phase. Aetiological factors that have been suggested include smoking, and exposure to ionizing radiation, benzene, and chloramphenicol.

Acute lymphoblastic leukaemia

Acute lymphoblastic leukaemia (ALL) is a leukaemia of lymphoid precursor cells of either B- or T-cell origin and there are several subtypes. It is the commonest cancer of childhood and has a characteristic peak of incidence among two- to seven-year-olds. Males are more often affected than females. Worldwide reported incidence varies widely, but is highest in developed countries. The current annual UK incidence rate is 1.0 per 100,000 population. Although reported childhood rates increased before the 1970s, probably owing to improved diagnosis, there is no convincing evidence of a change in reported rates for any age group in more recent years. The favoured aetiological hypothesis involves atypical responses to infection as a result of delayed antigenic exposure in childhood, but this has proved hard to test in epidemiological studies. Human T-cell lymphoma/leukaemia virus-1 is a risk factor for T-cell ALL. Other potential risk factors include exposure to radiation or benzene and inherited syndromes.

Chronic myeloid leukaemia

Chronic myeloid leukaemia (CML) is characterized by the presence of the Philadelphia chromosome resulting in the expression of the *BCR/ABL* fusion gene. This gene codes for an abnormal cell-signalling protein, tyrosine kinase, which mediates sustained cell proliferation. The reported worldwide incidence varies (European incidence is 1.1 per 100,000 population), but is consistently reported more often in males. It is rare in childhood, with the peak incidence occurring in the 40- to 50-year-old age group. Overall, there appears to be a steady decline in the number of cases over time.

Myeloma

This is a malignant proliferation of plasma cells. Similar diagnostic difficulties occur in the elderly as occur for CLL, leading to problems in interpretation of routine incidence data and secular trends. Worldwide, reported rates vary widely, but most show an increasing incidence. It is thought that this represents improved diagnosis in the elderly, and more recent data suggest a levelling in incidence rates. Myeloma accounts for 1.5 per cent of all cancers and 1.6 per cent of cancer deaths. The aetiology of myeloma remains to be elucidated; however increasing age, male gender, black race, and obesity have all been associated with increased risk.

Hodgkin's disease

Hodgkin's disease (HD) is a lymphoma distinguished by the presence of the Reed–Sternberg cell, with subtypes recognized by the background cellular composition of involved lymph nodes. International rates vary widely, being lowest in the Far East and highest in Europe and America. The average annual European incidence is 2.5 per 100,000 population. In all areas there is a male excess. This disease has a typical age distribution, with a peak incidence in young adults, caused predominantly by the nodular sclerosing subtype. In the USA an increase in rates of HD in this young adult age group has been reported. In contrast, in the UK overall rates in males are reported to be declining, with no change in female rates over time. Some of this reduction may be due to changes in classification between HD and non-Hodgkin's lymphoma. The disparity in UK and USA trends has not been explained. Some cases have been linked to the Epstein–Barr virus, a ubiquitous herpes virus associated with glandular fever.

Non-Hodgkin's lymphoma

This is not a specific disorder but a collection of distinct disease entities characterized by a malignant proliferation of lymphocytes. Incidence rises with age, with a male excess in all age groups. The striking, ongoing increase in incidence of this group of disorders, dating from the 1950s, is apparent in high income countries with less convincing increases in ones with low and middle incomes. The annual worldwide incidence is 5.1 per 100,000. Increases have been apparent at all ages apart from younger age groups in whom the condition is rare. A rise in the number of cases of both high- and low-grade lymphoma has been reported. However, not all subtypes show a consistent increase in incidence: greater rises have been shown for extra-nodal disease, in particular for gastric and small bowel lymphoma, for B-cell skin lymphoma, and for CNS lymphoma.

Aetiological factors include infection, immunosuppression (incurred in tissue transplantation or infection with HIV, for example), antibiotic use, environmental exposure to agrichemicals, atmospheric pollution, and exposure to sunlight. Known risk factors for lymphoma do not account for the well-documented rise in incidence, particularly in females; to produce this consistent and universal increase, any alternative explanation would have to affect large numbers of people, which suggests that a ubiquitous environmental factor may be implicated.

Chronic lymphocytic leukaemia

Chronic lymphocytic leukaemia (CLL) is a malignant proliferation of mature lymphocytes which produces the most difficulty for epidemiologists because of an enormous variation in presentation (often asymptomatic), differences in diagnostic practice (blood film examination only), and advances in immunophenotypic sub-classification. It is commonly classified along with small lymphocytic leukaemia with annual European incidence rates of approximately five per 100,000. Reliable data do not exist for incidence or secular trends due to the potential asymptomatic nature of this cancer. Chronic lymphocytic leukaemia is predominantly a disease of older adults and is more common in males than females. Chemical exposure and a family history of hematologic malignancy are potential risk factors.

17.4 Risk factors

The pattern of cancer distribution differ markedly in the world regions as we saw in Fig. 17.2a–f, and, theoretically, this may be due to genetic or environmental factors, or a combination of both. Current evidence suggests that Mendelian inheritance accounts for only 5–10 per cent of cancers leading to intense interest in the past few decades in the role of environmental factors. Gene–environment interaction is a relatively recent mode of epidemiological investigation but is likely to form an important focus for new research.

Genetic factors

Many rare cancers such as retinoblastoma, Wilm's tumour, and high penetrance mutations such as *BRCA* in breast cancer, show clear evidence of Mendelian inheritance (see Chapter 19) but **epigenetic** mechanisms may also be relevant operating through oncogenes and tumour suppressor genes (Esteller 2008). Several tumours show evidence of familial aggregation (relative risk 2–4) including breast, prostate, colon, and lung (Boffetta and La Vecchia 2009).

A growing list of genetic markers is under epidemiological investigation in large cohort studies, which will allow the examination of gene–environment interactions for major cancers. Meanwhile, studies of twins have been used to provide estimates of heritability (see Chapter 19). Collaborative studies in Twin Registries indicate that for prostate cancer 42 per cent (95% CI 29–50 per cent) of the risk could be explained by genetic factors. Significant heritability was also reported for colorectal cancer, 35 per cent (95% CI 10–48 per cent), and breast cancer, 27 per cent (95% CI 4–41 per cent). Even in these cancers, however, environmental factors *not shared* between the twin pairs were estimated to account for between 58 per cent and 67 per cent of the risk (Lichtenstein *et al.* 2000).

Lifestyle and environmental risk factors

Many epidemiological studies have been conducted worldwide which have investigated the contribution of environmental factors, largely in high-income countries which can provide accurate mortality data, cancer registration, and detailed data on exposure to lifestyle or other environmental or occupational exposures. Based on such studies Fig. 17.3 shows the number and proportion of cancers in the UK which can be attributed to lifestyle and environmental risk factors. Note that fruit and vegetables, fibre, physical activity, and breastfeeding are protective risk factors. Worldwide, a comparative risk assessment has been made of nine behavioural and environmental risk factors (Danaei *et al.* 2005).

Tobacco

Smoking is a major risk factor for cancer, and is causally linked with cancer of the lung, larynx, mouth, oesophagus, kidney, bladder, pancreas, and cervix. In high income countries tobacco accounts for up to 30 per cent of all malignant tumours (Doll and Peto 2003). In the UK it has been causally linked with approximately 86 per cent of lung tumours, 79 per cent of laryngeal, 65 per cent of oesophageal and oral cavity/pharynx, 37 per cent of bladder, 29 per cent of pancreatic, 24 per cent of kidney, 23 per cent of liver, 22 per cent of stomach, eight per cent of colorectal, seven per cent of cervical, six per cent of leukaemia, and three per cent of ovarian cancers (Parkin 2011). Half of all regular cigarette smokers will eventually be killed by their habit (Doll *et al.* 2004). Stopping smoking reduces the risk of these cancers, but the risk does not return to that of a non-smoker for some years, and up to 30 years in the case of bladder cancer. Global marketing of tobacco has resulted in an increase in the number of people in low- and middle-income countries who are now smoking. Currently two out of three smokers live in these countries where the number of smokers is predicted to rise further, from current levels of 1.3 billion to 1.6 billion by 2025. Breathing other people's smoke has also been confirmed as a cause of lung cancer and other diseases; the excess risk for lung cancer of environmental tobacco smoke is 25 per cent (see Chapter 8). Lung cancer trends reflect changing patterns in tobacco consumption, with falling rates in men and steadily rising rates in women.

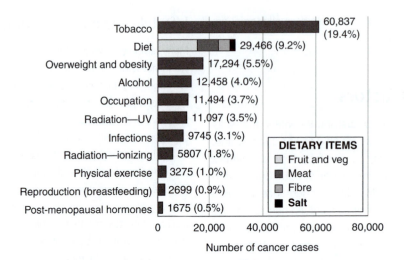

Figure 17.3 Attributable risk of cancer from lifestyle and environmental factors in the UK population 2010.
Reproduced from Parkin DM, Boyd L, and Walker LC (2011) 16. The fraction of cancer attributable to lifestyle and environmental factors in the UK in 2010. *British Journal of Cancer.* **105** Suppl 2, S77–81, with permission from Nature Publishing Group.

Prevention of lung cancer will be achieved by reducing tobacco use. The prevention of tobacco-related disease is further discussed in Chapters 8 and 20.

Alcohol

Heavy alcohol consumption is closely associated with cancer of the oral cavity, pharynx, larynx, and oesophagus, mainly acting synergistically with tobacco smoking. These cancers are rare in non-smokers and non-drinkers, but, as the habits are linked, assessment of the contribution of the individual risk factors poses difficulties. Nevertheless, the contribution of alcohol to risk of cancer can be assessed from well-designed cohort studies, and summary results for colon and breast cancer are shown in Chapter 20 (Table 20.2). Alcohol also causes cancer of the liver, particularly in areas where hepatitis B virus is uncommon, and often in combination with smoking. It has been estimated that alcohol causes between four and eight per cent of cancer deaths (Doll and Peto 2003). In Europe the contribution of alcohol consumption (both current and former) to total cancers has been recently reported using data from cohorts from eight countries (total number of participants 360,000) (Schütze *et al.* 2011). For all cancers the contribution

of alcohol was 10 per cent (95% CI 7–13 per cent) and in women three per cent (95% CI 1–5 per cent). For men attributable proportions were 44 per cent for cancers of the oropharynx and oesophagus, 33 per cent for liver cancer, 17 per cent for colorectal cancer; in women attributable proportions were about half those for men for oropharyngeal/oesophageal and liver cancers and four per cent for colorectal cancer and five per cent for breast cancer.

Alcohol has a direct, but mild, carcinogenic action, although some alcoholic drinks may contain more potent carcinogenic contaminants such as nitrosoamines, polycylic aromatic hydrocarbons, mycotoxins, esters, and phenols from the raw material and the production processes (World Cancer Research Fund 1997). Alcohol also acts as a solvent facilitating the penetration of cells by carcinogens.

Overweight and obesity

The population attributable risk of cancer in males and females with excess body mass indices are estimated at 2.5 per cent and 4.1 per cent in Europe (Renehan *et al.* 2010) and 4.1 per cent and 6.9 per cent respectively in the UK (Parkin *et al.* 2011), although an overall estimate of 14–20 per cent has been quoted for the USA (Calle *et al.* 2003; Kushi *et al.* 2012). Excess weight is particularly associated with endometrial, postmenopausal breast, and colorectal cancers. Risk of endometrial cancer increases threefold in the range of body mass index 20 to 35 kg/m². There is a consistent but weaker association between overweight and postmenopausal breast cancer. These effects are probably mediated by increased serum concentrations of bioavailable oestrogens. A causal relation between overweight and colorectal cancer has been reported, and some evidence for increased risk of thyroid, renal, hematopoietic malignancies and prostate cancer in people who are overweight or obese (Renehan *et al.* 2008). Evidence is increasing that obesity is a risk factor for oesophageal adenocarcinoma. Population trends in obesity may be contributing to recent rapid increases in the incidence of this cancer in high income countries. Global trends in overweight and obesity are predicted to increase the incidence of several cancers in low-, middle-, and high-income countries.

Physical activity

Regular physical activity is associated with a reduced risk of colon cancer (by 40–50 per cent) (Colditz *et al.* 1997). Physical activity helps prevent obesity and cancers related to it; in addition, moderate physical activity bolsters the immune system and reduces bowel transit time. A summary report (World Cancer Research Fund 2007) suggests that the evidence of an independent association with physical activity is strong for colon cancer and probable for endometrial and postmenopausal breast cancer. Evidence is suggestive for premenopausal breast cancer, lung, and pancreatic cancer (World Cancer Research Fund 2007).

Dietary factors

Diet and nutrition play a very complex role in the modification of cancer risk and, although the mechanisms of action may not be fully understood, there is sufficient evidence, largely from observational epidemiological studies, to identify and recommend dietary practices that decrease cancer risk. These recommendations, if fully implemented, would also reduce risk of other major chronic disease, such as cardiovascular diseases and diabetes. Dietary factors that have been studied most frequently include: energy intake (overweight and obesity), fruit, vegetable, and fibre consumption, and the intake of micronutrients and bioactive compounds. This body of literature has been reviewed and published by the World Cancer Research Fund with the American Institute of Cancer Research in 1997 and again in 2007. Evidence was obtained for all relevant foods, drinks, and supplements available across the globe and evidence for some common nutrient groups is reported here.

Fruit and vegetable consumption

There is weak-to-moderate evidence for a protective effect of fruit and vegetable consumption against colorectal, stomach, and breast cancers (World Cancer Research Fund 1997). Diets that are high in fruit and vegetables may protect against these cancers because they are rich in fibre and antioxidants or other metabolically active compounds, or because people with diets high in fruit and vegetables also tend to consume less meat and fat, and may be leaner. A recent review of four large cohort studies in high income countries suggest a modest and variable association between fruit and vegetable consumption and the risk of cancer (Key 2011).

Micronutrients and bioactive compounds

Oxidative DNA damage by free radicals may predispose to cancer. Therefore, high intakes of antioxidants, such as vitamins C and E, carotenoids, and selenium, can be expected to reduce cancer risk. There is evidence from observational studies that higher intake of antioxidants is associated with reduced risk of breast, colorectal, lung, stomach, oesophageal, and cervical cancers. However, intervention studies showed that dietary supplementation with carotenoids increased the risk of lung cancer (Bowen *et al.* 2003) especially in individuals who continued to smoke. Dietary supplementation with antioxidants is not recommended as a means of reducing cancer risk; instead dietary intake of these micronutrients should be increased by greater consumption of fruit and vegetables.

Box 17.2 Foods with potential cancer prevention activity

Mode of action

I Drug detoxification: broccoli, cucumber, squash, parsley, carrots, lemon oil, peaches, apples, cranberry, garlic, beets.

III Anti-inflammatory effects: melon, shitake mushrooms, oats, liquorice, ginseng, parsley, fish.

IV Antibacterial/antifungal effects: garlic, onions, cranberry, green tea, black tea, chocolate.

V Antioestrogenic effects: soybean, fennel, anise, carrots.

Folate plays an important role in DNA methylation, synthesis, and repair, and several prospective studies have shown low folate consumption to be associated with increased risk of colorectal cancer (Key et al. 2002). High intakes of calcium and vitamin D may also protect against colorectal cancers. There are many other bioactive compounds that are naturally present in plants that may offer protection against cancer. These include phyto-oestrogens (isoflavones, lignans), flavonoids, resveratrol, lycopene, and organo-sulphur compounds (Kris-Etherton et al. 2002; Anand et al. 2008). Much research is ongoing into the biological activities of these compounds and foods, such as those shown in Box 17.2, which have the potential for cancer prevention.

Meat consumption

Evidence for an association between meat consumption and cancer is most convincing for colorectal cancer; a large, recently reported cohort study found that consumption of red and processed meats was associated with higher risk, and that consumption of poultry and fish was protective (Chao et al. 2005). Meat consumption may increase colorectal cancer risk by increasing the levels of carcinogens within the bowel. These carcinogens include dietary haem found in red meat, nitrosamines and salt in processed foods, and compounds produced in smoked meats. There is also weak evidence supporting a causal relation between meat consumption and pancreatic, breast, and prostatic cancers.

Fibre consumption

Data from the large European Prospective Investigation into Cancer and Nutrition (the EPIC Study) have confirmed a substantial, dose-dependent reduction in the risk of colorectal cancer among people who have a high fibre intake (Murphy et al. 2012). Fibre may decrease colorectal cancer by bulking stools and decreasing transit time, allowing carcinogens in faeces less contact time with colonic mucosa. High fibre consumption may also increase fermentation in the bowel, with higher production of butyric acid, which appears to have antimitotic effects. There is also inconsistent evidence of a protective effect of a high-fibre diet against breast cancer.

Dietary recommendations for reducing cancer risk

Current American Cancer Society Guidelines (Kushi et al. 2012), which could be applied to the majority of high income countries stress the importance of:

maintaining a healthy body weight (a body mass index of less than 25 kg/m²), regular physical activity, adoption of a healthy diet including an emphasis on plant foods, fruit and vegetables, low consumption of processed and red meat, and an average consumption of two alcoholic drinks per day or less for men and one per day for women.

Occupational and environmental carcinogens

Many occupations and some specific chemicals are associated with increased risk of cancer. Most occupational carcinogens have been eliminated from, or are closely controlled, in the workplace, but some past exposures carry a significant burden. For example, although the use of asbestos was banned in the 1990s, the incidence of mesothelioma is still increasing in the UK, and may not peak for some years to come (Peto 2001). The lengthy incubation period or lag time (up to 40 years) from exposure to the clinical presentation of this cancer is characteristic of this tumour and several others associated with industrial exposures. It has been estimated that occupational exposures account for two to three per cent of fatal cancers in the UK, although in low- and middle-income countries this figure may be higher (see also Chapter 8). A recent detailed review of environmental and occupational causes of cancer worldwide suggests that these may be underestimates since chronic exposures to low doses of potential carcinogens are excluded from these estimates (Clapp et al. 2008).

By 2012 the International Agency for Research on Cancer (IARC) has classified 108 agents as carcinogenic to humans, a further 64 as probably carcinogenic, and 271 as possibly carcinogenic, based on evidence from epidemiological studies in humans and experimental studies in animals. A further 508 agents, which include chemicals, mixtures, beverages, biological and physical agents, and cultural habits, have been evaluated, which show some limited evidence of carcinogenicity (IARC 2012).

Radiation

Exposure to ionizing radiation, natural as well as that from industrial, medical, and other sources, can cause a variety of neoplasms including leukaemia, breast, and thyroid cancer.

Overall, ionizing radiation may account for up to 19 per cent of cancers. Much of the epidemiological information has been gleaned from studies of the survivors in the Japanese cities devastated by atomic explosions in 1945, and from patients given relatively high doses of radiotherapy several decades ago. A dose-dependent linear relation with no threshold is observed for most cancers, but for leukaemia, at higher levels of radiation, the risk is associated with the square of the dose, a proportionately higher risk. By 2006, 20 years after the nuclear meltdown at Chernobyl there were 5000 cases of thyroid cancer in young adults, largely as a result of drinking milk contaminated with radioactive fallout (WHO 2006).

A recent study of a large cohort of airline pilots from Nordic countries, who are exposed to higher than average levels of cosmic radiation, showed higher levels of skin cancers but no overall increase in cancer incidence. Radon, a radioactive gas associated with granite, may contribute to up to six per cent of all lung cancer cases in the UK and 12 per cent in the USA (Doll and Peto 2003).

Infections

A range of infectious agents are causally associated with cancers in humans and in animals: these are predominantly viral (oncoviruses), but in humans *Helicobacter pylori* and some tropical parasitic infections such as liver fluke and schistosomiasis are closely associated with specific cancers. Globally it has been estimated that infections account for 18 per cent of total cancers with a higher proportion in low- and middle-income countries (26 per cent) and eight per cent in high-income countries (Parkin 2006). In China which has a high prevalence of infection with *H. pylori* and with hepatitis B it has been estimated that 29 per cent of cancers are caused by infections (Wang et al. 2012). Five DNA viruses and three RNA viruses are associated with common cancers (see Table 17.3).

With the exception of the hepatitis C virus, the other cancer-associated RNA viruses are retroviruses. In immunodeficiency or in immunosuppression three DNA viruses (Epstein–Barr virus (EBV), human herpes virus 8, human papilloma virus (HPV), and Merkel cell carcinoma virus) spread more widely through body tissues and cause cancers opportunistically.

Epstein–Barr virus is associated with Hodgkin's disease, and in Africa with Burkitt's lymphoma where the disease is endemic. In many African countries the immune system is weakened by poor nutrition and malarial infection and EBV is facilitated to promote the growth of this lymphoma. Epstein–Barr virus is also implicated in the pathogenesis of nasopharyngeal cancer (Kieff 1995).

In addition to its strong association with cervical cancer HPV has also been associated with anal, vulval, vaginal, penile, and oropharyngeal cancers. A possible role for HPV in other cancers including breast and bladder cancer is under investigation (Li et al. 2011; Simoes et al. 2012).

Table 17.3   Viruses that cause cancer in humans

Virus	Disease
RNA viruses	
Human T-cell leukaemia virus type 1 (HTLV-I)	Adult T-cell leukaemia
Human T-cell leukaemia virus type II (HTLV-II)	Hairy cell leukaemia
Hepatitis C virus	Primary liver cancer, non-Hodgkin lymphoma
DNA viruses	
Hepatitis B virus	Primary liver cancer
Human papillomaviruses particularly HPV 16, and 18	Cervical, anal, vulval, vaginal, penile, and oropharyngeal cancer
Epstein–Barr virus	Burkitt lymphoma, nasopharyngeal carcinoma, Hodgkin lymphoma, post-transplant lymphomas
Human herpes virus 8	Kaposi's sarcoma
Merkel cell carcinoma virus	Merkel cell carcinoma

A summary of risk factors for common cancers, and the estimated strength of the relationship from current evidence, is shown in Table 17.4.

Table 17.4   Risk factors for the most common cancers worldwide

Cancer	Risk factors (strength of relationship)*
Lung	Tobacco smoke+++, asbestos+++, radon gas +++, tuberculosis +, herbicides/insecticides +
Skin (non-melanoma)	Solar radiation+++, fair skin +++, occupational carcinogens+++, human papillomavirus ++
Breast	Hormone replacement therapy+, oral contraceptive pill+, night time shift work+, physical inactivity+, obesity++, dietary fat++, nulliparity+++, age at menarchy +++, breastfeeding +++, age at menopause +++, breast density+++, ionizing radiation+++
Colorectal	Fat/meat consumption++, vitamin D+, sedentary behaviour++, obesity++, alcohol+, smoking+, colorectal polyps +++, inflammatory bowel disease+++, familial adenomatous polyposis++, Lynch syndrome++
Prostate	Black race++ , diet deficient in lycopene+
Bladder	Tobacco smoke+++, occupational carcinogens++, hormonal factors+, Schistosomiasis++
Stomach	*H. pylori*+++, diet deficient in fruit and vegetables++, salty foods+++, nitrosamines+, smoking+, radiation++
Ovary	Nulliparity++, infertility+, hormone replacement therapy++, smoking++, body mass index+, asbestos++
Skin (melanoma)	Solar radiation+++, fair skin +++, moles++
Cervix	Multiple sexual partners+++, human papillomavirus+++, smoking++

*+ weak; ++ moderate; +++ strong.

17.5 Prevention of cancer

It represents a challenge for epidemiologists, clinicians, and basic scientists to achieve for cancer prevention what seems to have been accomplished for cardiovascular disease in the past few decades (see Chapter 7). Opportunities exist at the three stages of prevention.

Primary Major opportunities exist for the primary prevention of some cancers, such as respiratory cancers, where the attributable fraction for tobacco smoking is close to 90 per cent in developed countries (see Chapter 8). As noted in section 17.4 smoking may account for about 30 per cent of all cancers, alcohol for four to eight per cent, occupational exposures for two to three per cent of fatal cancers, and domestic radon for six per cent of lung cancer in the UK. Current immunization strategies in many developed countries for HPV could prevent approximately 70 per cent of all cervical cancers. Effective childhood immunization programmes with Hepatitis B vaccine may eventually reduce the global burden of liver cancer. In Taiwan a national programme of antibiotic treatment to eradicate chronic infection with *H. pylori* in those over 30 years of age is reported to have reduced the incidence of gastric cancer by 25 per cent and peptic ulcer by 67 per cent (Lee *et al.* 2012) although there is only limited evidence from controlled trials that eradication of this organism can effectively reduce this cancer (Wong 2004). Reduction in population levels of overweight, obesity, and sedentary behaviour could also decrease the incidence of certain cancers, such as endometrial, colorectal, and breast cancers, but the public health reality is that the obesity epidemic is likely to get worse before it gets better. Appropriate behavioural interventions and policy initiatives which facilitate the maintenance of a healthy body weight and regular physical activity are urgently required globally, and apply equally to the prevention of cardiovascular disease and many other age-related diseases. Opportunities also exist for research into specific foods and micronutrients, but with the current levels of evidence, the American Cancer Society guidelines (Kushi *et al.* 2012) outlined above to reduce the population levels of cancer risk, seem uncontroversial.

Secondary Currently population-based screening is common for cervical, breast, and colorectal cancers in most high-income countries including the UK. Early detection of cancers by the use of population or selective screening programmes may offer future prospects for cancer prevention (secondary prevention), particularly in the development of molecular assays for biomarkers in clinical samples such as saliva, sputum, urine, or faeces (Caldas 1998). As noted in Chapter 5, however, these programmes require careful evaluation by large-scale controlled trials before their introduction into routine practice. Recent results from the USA of trials among populations of more than 150,000 men and women for prostate and ovarian cancers which were begun in 1993 have shown no evidence of mortality benefit (Andriole *et al.* 2012; Buys *et al.* 2011).

Tertiary Finally, improvements have been made, and are likely to continue to be made, in the treatment of cancer, improvements both in five-year survival and quality of life. Updated evidence on the effectiveness of cancer treatments is available from web sources such as the National Cancer Institute (USA) and Cancer Research UK (see 'Web addresses').

In conclusion, it is clear that both epidemiological and basic research are required in parallel to improve our understanding of the causes of cancer. Further development of tumour markers should assist in detecting important gene–environment interactions, and enhance the prospects for cancer control.

Web addresses

Cancer Research UK Factsheets
www.cancerresearchuk.org/aboutcancer/statistics/factsheets

Cancer Back Up: Information source for cancer patients (and professionals)
cancerbackup.org.uk/home

International Agency for Research on Cancer: Monographs on the evaluation of carcinogenic risks to humans
www-cie.iarc.fr/monoeval/cie.html

National Cancer Institute USA
www.nci.nih.gov/

Further reading

Boffeta P and La Vecchia C (2009) Neoplasms. In: Detels R, Beaglehole R, Lansang MA, and Gulliford M (eds) *Oxford Textbook of Public Health*, 5th edn, pp. 957–1020. Oxford: Oxford University Press.

Doll R and Peto R (2003) Epidemiology of Cancer. In: Warrell DA, Cox TM, Firth JD, and Benz EJ Jr (eds) *Oxford Textbook of Medicine*, pp. 193–218. Oxford: Oxford University Press.

Nasca PC and Pastides H (2001) *Fundamentals of Cancer Epidemiology*. Gaithersburg, MD: Aspen Publishers.

World Cancer Research Fund/ American Institute for Cancer Research (2007) *Food, Nutrition, Physical Activity and the Prevention of Cancer: A Global Perspective*. Washington DC: American Institute for Cancer Research.

References

American Cancer Society (2012) *Cancer basics*. http://www.cancer.org/Cancer/CancerBasics/lifetime-probability-of-developing-or-dying-from-cancer.

Anand P, Kunnumakkara AB, Kunnumakara AB, Sundaram C, *et al.* (2008) Cancer is a preventable disease that requires major lifestyle changes. *Pharmaceutical Research* **25** (9), 2097–116.

Andriole GL, Crawford ED, Grubb RL, Buys SS, *et al.* (2012) Prostate cancer screening in the randomized Prostate, Lung, Colorectal, and Ovarian Cancer Screening Trial: mortality results after 13 years of follow-up. *Journal of the National Cancer Institute* **104** (2), 125–32.

Barnes BBE, Steindorf K, Hein R, Flesch-Janys D, *et al.* (2011) Population attributable risk of invasive postmenopausal breast cancer and breast cancer subtypes for modifiable and non-modifiable risk factors. *Cancer Epidemiology* **35** (4), 345–52.

Berrino F, De Angelis R, Sant M, Rosso S, *et al.* (2007) Survival for eight major cancers and all cancers combined for European adults diagnosed in 1995–99: results of the EUROCARE-4 study. *The Lancet Oncology* **8** (9), 773–83.

Boffeta P and La Vecchia C (2009) Neoplasms. In:Detels R, Beaglehole R, Lansang MA, and Gulliford M (eds) *Oxford Textbook of Public Health*, 5th edn, pp. 957–1020. Oxford: Oxford University Press.

Bowen DJ, Thornquist M, Anderson K, Barnett M, *et al.* (2003) Stopping the active intervention: CARET. *Controlled Clinical Trials* **24** (1), 39–50.

Buys SS, Partridge E, Black A, Johnson CC, *et al.* (2011) Effect of screening on ovarian cancer mortality: the Prostate, Lung, Colorectal and Ovarian (PLCO) Cancer Screening Randomized Controlled Trial. *JAMA* **305** (22), 2295–303.

Caldas C (1998) Molecular assessment of cancer. *BMJ (Clinical Research Ed)* **316** (7141), 1360–3.

Calle EE, Rodriguez C, Walker-Thurmond K, and Thun MJ (2003) Overweight, obesity, and mortality from cancer in a prospectively studied cohort of U.S. adults. *The New England Journal of Medicine* **348** (17), 1625–38.

Cartwright RA, Gilman EA, and Gurney KA (1999) Time trends in incidence of haematological malignancies and related conditions. *British Journal of Haematology* **106** (2), 281–95.

Chao A, Thun MJ, Connell CJ, McCullough ML, *et al.* (2005) Meat consumption and risk of colorectal cancer. *JAMA: The Journal of the American Medical Association* **293** (2), 172–82.

Clapp RW, Jacobs MM, and Loechler EL (2008) Environmental and occupational causes of cancer: new evidence 2005–2007. *Reviews on Environmental Health* **23** (1), 1–37.

Clifford GM, Gallus S, Herrero R, Muñoz N, *et al.* (2005) Worldwide distribution of human papillomavirus types in cytologically normal women in the International Agency for Research on Cancer HPV prevalence surveys: a pooled analysis. *Lancet* **366** (9490), 991–8.

Colditz GA, Cannuscio CC, and Frazier AL (1997) Physical activity and reduced risk of colon cancer: implications for prevention. *Cancer Causes & Control: CCC* **8** (4), 649–67.

Croce CM (2008) Oncogenes and cancer. *The New England Journal of Medicine* **358** (5), 502–11.

Danaei G, Vander Hoorn S, Lopez AD, Murray CJL, *et al.* (2005) Causes of cancer in the world: comparative risk assessment of nine behavioural and environmental risk factors. *Lancet* **366** (9499), 1784–93.

Doll R and Peto R (2003) Epidemiology of Cancer. In: Warrell DA, Cox TM, Firth JD, and Benz EJ Jr (eds) *Oxford Textbook of Medicine*, pp. 193–218 Oxford: Oxford University Press.

Doll R, Peto R, Boreham J, and Sutherland I (2004) Mortality in relation to smoking: 50 years' observations on male British doctors. *BMJ (Clinical Research Ed)* **328** (7455), 1519.

Esteller M (2008) Epigenetics in cancer. *The New England Journal of Medicine* **358** (11), 1148–59.

Gunter MJ, Hoover DR, Yu H, Wassertheil-Smoller S, *et al.* (2009) Insulin, insulin-like growth factor-I, and risk of breast cancer in postmenopausal women. *Journal of the National Cancer Institute* **101** (1), 48–60.

IARC (2012) *Agents classified by the IARC Monographs, volumes 1–105*. Available from: http://monographs.iarc.fr/ENG/Classification/

IARC (2008a) Globocan. Available from: http://globocan.iarc.fr/factsheets/populations/

IARC (2008b) *World Cancer Report 2008*. Available from: http://www.iarc.fr/en/publications/pdfs-online/wcr/2008/

Key TJ, Allen NE, Spencer EA, and Travis RC (2002) The effect of diet on risk of cancer. *Lancet* **360** (9336), 861–8.

Key TJ (2011) Fruit and vegetables and cancer risk. *British Journal of Cancer* **104** (1), 6–11.

Kieff E (1995) Epstein–Barr virus—increasing evidence of a link to carcinoma. *The New England Journal of Medicine* **333** (11), 724–6.

Kris-Etherton PM, Hecker KD, Bonanome A, Coval SM, *et al.* (2002) Bioactive compounds in foods: their role in the prevention of cardiovascular disease and cancer. *The American Journal of Medicine* **113** Suppl. 9B71S–88S.

Kushi LH, Doyle C, McCullough M, Rock CL, *et al.* (2012) American Cancer Society Guidelines on nutrition and physical activity for cancer prevention: reducing the risk of cancer with healthy food choices and physical activity. *CA: A Cancer Journal for Clinicians* **62** (1), 30–67.

Lee Y-C, Chen TH-H, Chiu H-M, Shun C-T, *et al.* (2012) The benefit of mass eradication of Helicobacter pylori infection: a community-based study of gastric cancer prevention. *Gut* [Epub 2012 14 June].

Li N, Bi X, Zhang Y, Zhao P, *et al.* (2011) Human papillomavirus infection and sporadic breast carcinoma risk: a meta-analysis. *Breast Cancer Research and Treatment* **126** (2), 515–20.

Lichtenstein P, Holm NV, Verkasalo PK, Iliadou A, *et al.* (2000) Environmental and heritable factors in the causation of cancer—analyses of cohorts of twins from Sweden, Denmark, and Finland. *The New England Journal of Medicine* **343** (2), 78–85.

Merry AHH, Schouten LJ, Goldbohm RA, and van den Brandt PA (2007) Body mass index, height and risk of adenocarcinoma of the oesophagus and gastric cardia: a prospective cohort study. *Gut* **56** (11), 1503–11.

Murphy N, Norat T, Ferrari P, Jenab M, *et al.* (2012) Dietary Fibre Intake and Risks of Cancers of the Colon and Rectum in the European Prospective Investigation into Cancer and Nutrition (EPIC). *PloS One* **7** (6), e39361.

Parkin DM (2006) The global health burden of infection-associated cancers in the year 2002. *International Journal of Cancer* **118** (12), 3030–44.

Parkin DM (2011) Tobacco-attributable cancer burden in the UK in 2010. *British Journal of Cancer* **105**, S6–S13.

Parkin DM, Boyd L, and Walker LC (2011) The fraction of cancer attributable to lifestyle and environmental factors in the UK in 2010. *British Journal of Cancer* **105**, Suppl. 2S77–81.

Perez-Perez GI, Rothenbacher D, and Brenner H (2004) Epidemiology of Helicobacter pylori infection. *Helicobacter* **9** Suppl. 11–16.

Peto J (2001) Cancer epidemiology in the last century and the next decade. *Nature* **411** (6835), 390–5.

Pohl H and Welch HG (2005) The role of overdiagnosis and reclassification in the marked increase of esophageal adenocarcinoma incidence. *Journal of the National Cancer Institute* **97** (2), 142–6.

Reeves GK, Pirie K, Beral V, Green J, *et al.* (2007) Cancer incidence and mortality in relation to body mass index in the Million Women Study: cohort study. *BMJ (Clinical research Ed)* **335** (7630), 1134.

Renehan AG, Soerjomataram I, and Leitzmann MF (2010) Interpreting the epidemiological evidence linking obesity and cancer: A framework for population-attributable risk estimations in Europe. *European Journal of Cancer* **46** (14), 2581–92.

Renehan AG, Tyson M, Egger M, Heller RF, *et al.* (2008) Body-mass index and incidence of cancer: A systematic review and meta-analysis of prospective observational studies. *Lancet* **371** (9612), 569–78.

Sant M, Aareleid C, Santaquilani M, *et al.* (2009) EUROCARE-4: Survival of Cancer Patients Diagnosed in 1995–1999—Results and Commentary. *European Journal of Cancer* **45** (6), 931–91.

Schütze M, Boeing H, Pischon T, Rehm J, *et al.* (2011) Alcohol attributable burden of incidence of cancer in eight European countries based on results from prospective cohort study. *BMJ (Clinical Research Ed)* **342**, d1584.

Simões PW, Medeiros LR, Simões Pires PD, Edelweiss MI, *et al.* (2012) Prevalence of human papillomavirus in breast cancer: a systematic review. *International Journal of Gynecological Cancer* **22** (3), 343–7.

Tay S-K (2012) Cervical cancer in the human papilloma-virus vaccination era. *Current Opinion in Obstetrics & Gynecology* **24** (1), 3–7.

Wang JB, Jiang Y, Liang H, Li P, *et al.* (2012) Attributable causes of cancer in China. *Annals of Oncology* **23** (1), 2983–9.

Wong BC-Y (2004) Helicobacter pylori eradication to prevent gastric cancer in a high-risk region of China: a randomized controlled trial. *JAMA: The Journal of the American Medical Association* **291** (2), 187–94.

World Cancer Research Fund/ American Institute for Cancer Research (1997) *Food, Nutrition, Physical Activity and the Prevention of Cancer: A Global Perspective.* Washington DC: American Institute for Cancer Research.

World Cancer Research Fund/ American Institute for Cancer Research (2007) *Food, Nutrition, Physical Activity and the Prevention of Cancer: A Global Perspective.* Washington DC: American Institute for Cancer Research.

WHO (2006) *Health Effects of the Chernobyl Accident and Special Health Care.* Available from: http://whqlibdoc.who.int/publications/2006/9241594179_eng.pdf

Wiemels J (2012) Perspectives on the causes of childhood leukemia. *Chemico-Biological Interactions* **196** (3), 59–67.

Model answer

Question 1

(a) In general terms investigators should attempt to determine whether the level of **ascertainment** (the level of case detection) is comparable in the World Regions. IARC data are based on cancer registries, and in low-income countries registry populations may be unrepresentative of the country population, and also some cancers carrying a high mortality may be under-represented. Conversely, in high-income countries with well-developed screening programmes some cancers may be over-represented.

(b) For specific cancers possible environmental, occupational, and infectious causes can be investigated in case-control studies in the first instance. Family studies help identify genetic causes and migrant studies may suggest that environmental factors may be relevant. If resources permit, large cohort studies can be conducted to examine dietary and other environmental causes. Nested case-control studies, using stored biological materials, have been used to investigate the associations between some infectious agents and the development of certain cancers. Molecular epidemiological studies using such approaches may contribute to the understanding and prevention of cancer in the coming decades.

18 Infectious diseases

BRIAN SMYTH, ADRIANO DUSE, RICHARD SMITHSON, MAUREEN MCCARTNEY, LORRAINE DOHERTY, AND JOHN YARNELL

CHAPTER CONTENTS

This chapter reviews the epidemiology of infectious disease and the global influences on patterns of spread. Surveillance of infectious diseases and the emergence of new diseases are covered, as is the prevention of infectious diseases by immunization, infection control, and management of outbreaks. Examples of epidemiological studies during outbreaks are provided at the end of the chapter.

Introduction

Understanding infectious diseases, their patterns of transmission and control, requires an increasingly global perspective, one in which individuals and populations interact with each other and with broader ecosystems. Three aspects of these systems conspire to produce epidemics of disease: the **agent**, the **host**, and the **environment**. In most countries, the pace of environmental change promotes the spread of old infections and encourages micro-organisms to evolve into human environments. Human travel, migration, armed conflict, and the global trade in foodstuffs, plants, and animals all impact on infectious disease transmission and spread. This dynamic global situation requires continuous surveillance and responsive international control measures. Recent examples are the emergence of HIV/AIDS in Africa and the USA in the 1970s and 80s and of the influenza H1N1 pandemic in 2009.

18.1 Epidemiology of infectious disease

For most of the 180,000 years of modern man's existence, it was only a minority of each generation that reached adulthood, if they managed to avoid or survive the physical hazards, starvation, or infection that prevailed upon the rest. The rise of agriculture and the domestication of several animal species provided new opportunities for the formation of human settlements and exposure to a wider range of potentially pathogenic organisms. Pathogens include protozoa, fungi, bacteria, and viruses; more recently 'slow viruses', more appropriately described as prions (proteinaceous particles) have passed from cattle to man (bovine spongiform encephalopathy—BSE). Detailed consideration of biological principles in human infectious disease is beyond the scope of this text but a basic understanding of the wide ranges of *infectivity, pathogenicity, modes of transmission, virulence, immunogenicity,* and

Table 18.1 Biological definitions in infectious disease

Infectivity	The capacity of an organism to multiply in the host	Also defined as the proportion of exposures that results in infection
Pathogenicity	The capacity of an organism to cause disease in an infected host	Smallpox shows high pathogeneity: polio virus low pathogeneity (many infected individuals are asymptomatic)
Virulence	The degree of pathogeneity of an organism	Virulence may vary by strain, 'wild' strains of measles and polio. Virulence may vary over time, e.g. *Streptococcus*
Immunogenicity	The capacity of an organism to induce specific and lasting immunity in the host	Generalized systemic infections usually produce a strong, lasting immune response in contrast to localized infections
Antigenic variability	The capacity of an organism to exist or evolve different antigenic forms	Influenza is unstable and rhinoviruses exist in many antigenic forms
Host specificity	The lack of capacity of an organism to infect more than one animal species	Smallpox or measles specific to humans. TB and brucella in many animal species.

Modified from Farmer *et al.* (1996).

antigenic variation in infectious agents is important for an understanding of the principles of spread and control of epidemics (see Table 18.1).

The emergence of infections, such as smallpox, plague, cholera, measles, pertussis, meningococcal meningitis, gonorrhoea, and syphilis around 10,000 years ago, depended as much on population dynamics as on any inherent pathogenicity of the organisms themselves. The creation of villages, then towns and finally cities, provided the opportunity for the emergence and spread of the major epidemic diseases. Table 18.2 shows the main modes of transmission of common communicable diseases.

The spread of communicable disease Infection is considered directly transmitted when passed by direct contact with an infected person. In indirect transmission the agent has passed into the wider environment and may be passed on through water, air, food, insect, or animal vectors, or through the soil. Person-to-person transmission is governed by a factor known as the reproductive rate which depends on host, agent, and population factors (see Box 18.1).

If each infected person during the course of their infection infects only one other person on average the reproductive rate (Ro) is 1; the disease exists in a steady state and is said to be **endemic** in the population. If an infected individual infects more than one individual the number of cases builds up and the disease becomes **epidemic** (Ro >1). Assuming the disease produces immunity then gradually the proportion of susceptible individuals in the population will fall; Ro <1 and eventually the disease will die out. Artificial creation of **herd immunity** is the aim of the majority of immunization programmes. Recent outbreaks of measles and mumps in parts of the UK and in Europe reflect decreasing herd immunity because of poor uptake of combined measles, mumps and rubella (MMR) vaccine. Modelling studies based on WHO figures suggested a herd immunity effect above 80 per cent coverage of infants and a powerful effect of supplementary immunization activities in children under nine years of age in defined geographic regions within countries (Hall and Jolley 2011). Herd immunity effects have also been suggested in immunization against

Table 18.2 Directly and indirectly transmitted infections

Direct	Indirect
Droplets	*Water*
Influenza, coryza, measles, SARS	Hepatitis A and probably E, polio, cholera, typhoid, cryptosporidiosis
Blood and other body fluids	*Air*
Hepatitis B, C, HIV	Chickenpox, anthrax, aspergillosis, legionella
Transplacental	*Food*
Toxoplasmosis	*Campylobacter, Salmonella, Staphylococcus* toxin, *E. coli* strains
Epidermal	*Vectors*
Herpes type 1	Malaria, yellow fever, sleeping sickness, West Nile fever
Mucous membrane	*Soil*
STDs, HIV	Tetanus, anthrax

Box 18.1 Determinants of the spread of infection in a population (reproductive rate)

Infectivity of agent

- Frequency and type of contacts in the population
- Period of infectivity in each infected individual
- Proportion immune in the population

Reproduced from Giesecke J *Modern Infectious Disease Epidemiology* 2001, with permission from Taylor & Francis.

meningococcus type C (Ramsay *et al.* 2003), and in current human papilloma vaccination programmes (Brisson *et al.* 2011).

It is well recognized that global travel facilitates the spread of infectious diseases and long distance air travel means that humans can reach almost any part of the earth today within the incubation period for most microbes that cause disease in humans (Institute of Medicine 2010).

In the past three decades over 30 newly identified infections have emerged, some of major public health importance such as HIV and Hepatitis C. The global human population is now the largest ever recorded and so also is the population of food animals. Increasingly, people live in densely populated urban areas but may also frequently visit rural areas in their own country and a wider range of other countries across the world. Human and animal populations co-exist in many rural areas, and also in densely populated slum areas which may lack consistent access to clean water and sanitary facilities. In the 1990s over two-thirds of emerging infections have been closely linked with animals, both wild and domestic. New strains of influenza virus have occurred in those farming geese, chickens, ducks (avian influenza H5N1), and pigs, and more recently the virus causing severe acute respiratory syndrome (SARS) was discovered in live animal markets in Asia (Webster 2004). The rapid global spread of swine influenza H1N1 in the human population was facilitated by air travel resulting in the first influenza pandemic of the 21st century in 2009. Outbreaks of serious food-borne infections continue to be linked with faulty food-processing practices (*E. coli* 0157, BSE, and variant Creutzfeldt–Jakob disease). The continued emergence of such diseases emphasizes the need for an international surveillance network and a rapid and efficient outbreak investigation system. The biology of newly emerging organisms and epidemics are discussed in detail elsewhere (Antia *et al.* 2003).

18.2 Major global infections

Tuberculosis

Tuberculosis (TB) is one of the oldest infectious diseases infecting both animals and humans, and claims at least 1.8 million lives annually. Tuberculosis is caused by organisms belonging to the *Mycobacterium tuberculosis* complex which includes *M. tuberculosis, M. bovis* (causing both bovine and human TB), *M. africanum* (causing TB in West Africa), and *M. microti* (a pathogen of voles). Until the advent of anti-TB drugs in the mid 20th century tuberculosis was thought to be an incurable disease. Regrettably, optimism regarding the conquest of tuberculosis has been shattered by, not only the re-emergence of tuberculosis worldwide that has been largely fuelled by the HIV pandemic, but also by the burgeoning problem of the emergence of multidrug-resistant TB (MDR-TB) and, more recently, of extensively drug-resistant TB (XDR). Multidrug-resistant TB is defined as tuberculosis caused by *M. tuberculosis* strains that are resistant to at least two first-line therapeutic agents; isoniazid and rifampicin. Extensively drug-resistant TB refers to tuberculous infection where the organisms are MDR plus resistant to any fluoroquinolone and at least one of three injectable aminoglycosides. Multidrug-resistant TB- and XDR-TB should be considered a 'man-made' problem, as it is a consequence of the non-compliance by patients with treatment (which may be related to its cost in some countries), inappropriate prescribing by physicians, and inadequacy of provision of good quality care, as well as the development of novel, anti-TB drugs. Tuberculosis, but most especially MDR-TB and XDR-TB, are posing a major global threat to the targets set by the Millennium Development Goals (MDG) and the Stop TB Partnership of controlling and eliminating TB by 2050. Multidrug-resistant TB and XDR-TB are also posing serious challenges to programmes for the control of the HIV and TB co-epidemics and are becoming an increasing challenge in Asia, Eastern Europe, sub-Saharan Africa, and South America.

It is estimated that approximately one-third of the world's population is infected with *M. tuberculosis* and new infections are occurring at a rate of one per second. The majority of infections are asymptomatic in immune-competent individuals, but up to 15 per cent of infections eventually progress to active disease which, left untreated, can result in the death of more than half of those infected. Smokers are at increased risk of developing active disease. The characteristic symptom cluster of pulmonary TB includes chronic cough, haemoptysis, fever, night sweats, and weight loss. Extra-pulmonary disease can also occur, particularly in immune-compromised patients with underlying HIV infection.

The cornerstone of diagnosis of TB in many low- and middle-income countries has been to test smears from patient samples (e.g. sputum) for acid-fast bacilli. However, this has relatively low sensitivity, particularly in paediatric populations and HIV-infected individuals, and as *M. tuberculosis* is a slow-growing organism, conventional diagnostic culture methods can take in excess of six weeks to yield a positive result. Interferon-gamma release assays are *in vitro* blood tests that are more sensitive and produce fewer false-negative results than the tuberculin skin test for the diagnosis of latent TB infection. Since early diagnosis and treatment of TB are crucial to decreasing the infectious pool of infected (and thus infectious) individuals, newer rapid and accurate molecular-based assays and line probe assays have greatly improved TB diagnostics.

The treatment of active tuberculosis usually requires six months for pulmonary TB and up to 24 months for certain complicated or extra-pulmonary infections to cure the infection. For active tuberculosis multi-drug therapy with agents that include rifampicin and isoniazid is required to decrease the risk of the development of antibiotic resistance. Whereas primary drug resistance occurs in a patient that is infected *de novo* with a resistant strain of TB, secondary resistance which is acquired during therapy is a consequence of inadequate treatment, non-compliance with therapy, lack of access to anti-TB drugs, and taking poor quality or counterfeit drugs. The DOTS programme (Directly Observed Treatment, Short-course) was established by WHO in 1995 to overcome some of these problems and is reported to have saved seven million lives between 1995 and 2010 with 46 million patients treated successfully, but with an unacceptably high relapse or failure rate in a further nine million (WHO 2011a). Five of the WHO world regions are on track to halving the prevalence rates of TB by 2015 compared to those in 1990, but this is not the case for the African region, and elsewhere it is essential to monitor the emergence of drug resistance.

In order to prevent and control TB it is essential to identify infected individuals and their contacts. As nosocomial transmission of TB has been well documented, appropriate infection prevention and control measures must be instituted. Vaccination against tuberculosis using the Bacillus Calmette-Guérin (BCG) is given to infants in many countries. Although BCG protects against severe forms of paediatric TB (e.g. TB meningitis), it does not reliably protect against pulmonary tuberculosis. Several candidate vaccines against TB are being developed. Phase I clinical trials using H56, a vaccine that promotes a polyfunctional CD4+ T cell response against *M. tuberculosis* protein components, are underway in South Africa.

HIV/AIDS

In contrast to the tubercle bacillus the human immunodeficiency virus (HIV) is a recently emerging retrovirus in the human population. Lineage studies in molecular epidemiology indicate that it passed from the simian retrovirus (SIV) in central Africa into the human population some time during the latter part of the 19th century (Gilbert *et al.* 2007). The main types are: HIV-1, which is virulent and more readily transmitted, and its commonest group (M) is responsible for about 33 million prevalence cases worldwide; and HIV-2 which is less transmissible and largely confined to West Africa. There is now considerable genetic diversity worldwide with many subtypes, which are often associated with particular world regions and are helpful in tracking the evolution of the pandemic (Shao and Williamson 2012). Infection of thymocytes leads to gradual decline of the immune system of infected individuals, leading to greater susceptibility to infections and some cancers. After a period of 10–15 years, without treatment, individuals become infected with opportunistic pathogens, such as cryptococcosis and *Pneumocystis jirovecii*

pneumonia, which are uncommon in people with intact immune systems. The development of these opportunistic infections, or certain cancers such as Kaposi's sarcoma, defines acquired immunodeficiency syndrome (AIDS) in those with HIV. People infected with HIV are also more susceptible to infections common in HIV-negative people, such as tuberculosis and pneumococcal pneumonia.

AIDS first became apparent in the early 1980s in the USA in young homosexual men, although the disease termed 'slim disease' with diarrhoea and weight loss had been spreading in central Africa for decades in the heterosexual population and through sex workers. With intensive investigation of this devastating disease came the recognition of an infective cause, the realization that this was a sexually-transmitted/blood-borne disease, and the identification of the causative virus in 1983 (Barré-Sinoussi *et al.* 1983). The long incubation period of up to 10 years, and its emergence in an area of the world without well-developed surveillance or health care systems allowed the virus to spread widely before the disease was adequately described and the cause identified. HIV has been identified in a frozen blood sample (1959) and a lymph node (1960) from two patients who were treated at Kinshasa in Central Africa. By 1980 the virus had spread to North America, South America, Europe, Australia, and many other countries in Africa. Twenty-five million people are estimated to have died of HIV/AIDS since 1980. Different world regions, and, within those areas, have varying prevalence rates and populations at highest risk. In 2010, 22.5 million people in sub-Saharan Africa were living with HIV (68 per cent of the world total, with four million in South and South East Asia, and 1.4 million in Eastern Europe and Central Asia, and in Central and South America, respectively. Three million cases are in the high-income countries of Europe, North America, and Australasia. The main transmission routes are shown in Box 18.2 and different modes of transmission are responsible for the spread of infection in different parts of the world. For example, in 2007 in Eastern Europe 27 per cent of the three and a half million users of intravenous drugs were estimated to be infected with HIV; in Latin America this was 29 per cent of two million users, and in Western Europe there

Box 18.2 Modes of transmission of HIV

HIV is transmitted via close contact with body fluids such as blood, semen and vaginal secretions, and breast milk. The most important routes of infection are:

- unprotected sexual intercourse (vaginal or anal) or oral sex with an infected person;
- receiving contaminated blood or blood products;

- sharing needles or other injecting equipment during injecting drug use;
- unsterile cutting or piercing procedures;
- transmission from mother to baby during pregnancy, childbirth, and breastfeeding.

Reproduced with permission from 'Recommended Routine Immunization', WHO 2012.

---

were one million users and 11 per cent infected (Shao and Williamson 2012). Figures suggest that worldwide the pandemic peaked in 1999 though the incidence continues to increase in Eastern Europe and in Central Asia (UNAIDS 2010).

Key prevention strategies Social and political factors are particularly important in HIV/AIDS. Stigma and discrimination, along with the lack of effective treatments before the 1990s, lead to reluctance to be tested. In addition, some political leaders have denied the existence of HIV or its modes of transmission. Gender inequality is a significant factor in some countries, with women finding it difficult to protect themselves from being infected. HIV/AIDS also is more prevalent in some marginalized groups such as injecting drug users and sex workers, who are more difficult to reach with prevention activities and treatment.

Education about HIV/AIDS and 'safer sex' messages have been vital in reducing the rates of infection. Other key strategies include:

- Minimizing the number of sexual partners and using male and female condoms consistently.
- Harm reduction measures for people who inject drugs.
- Antenatal testing and treatment to prevent mother-to-child transmission at childbirth and during breastfeeding.
- Male circumcision.
- Testing for HIV if at risk so that transmission reduction and treatment can be started early.
- Treatment of HIV-positive individuals.

Early identification and treatment of HIV-positive individuals with highly active antiretroviral treatment has extended lifespans by greatly reducing the rate of progression from initial infection to AIDS, and also importantly reduces transmission of HIV from infected individuals. Treatment is expensive and requires significant political engagement and investment in infrastructure and drugs. UNAIDS was founded in 1995 to bring together 10 UN agencies in the fight against HIV/AIDS worldwide. In 2001 this received significant international funding to monitor country trends and improve prevention and treatment initiatives; progress and lessons learned have been discussed by UNAIDS first executive director and colleagues (Piot *et al.* 2009). Treatment availability has improved worldwide which, along with prevention activities, such as advice about safe sex, availability of condoms, and increasing the safety of blood products, has led to the decrease in the numbers being infected. In 33 countries, including 22 countries in sub-Saharan Africa, the incidence decline exceeded 25 per cent between 1999 and 2009; but the incidence continues to rise in Eastern Europe and Central Asia, principally fuelled by a high incidence in injecting drug users (UNAIDS 2010). The incidence is also increasing in some high-income countries such as UK, Germany, and Switzerland in men who have sex with men. In low- and middle-income countries, of the estimated 15 million eligible for treatment, only about one-third is receiving treatment. Multi-disease prevention may provide a cost-effective approach in low-income countries (Kahn *et al.* 2012).

Malaria

Malaria is a vector-borne (*Anopheles* mosquitoes) infection of humans and animals caused by protozoa belonging to the genus *Plasmodium*. There are five species of *Plasmodium* that can cause disease in humans. *Plasmodium falciparum* accounts for 95 per cent of malaria cases in Africa and is the organism that most commonly causes severe and fatal malaria. The severity of disease caused by *P. falciparum* infection is due to: (1) invasion of erythrocytes of all ages thus producing higher parasitaemias, and (2) the phenomenon of 'rosetting' (clumping of uninfected erythrocytes to knobs on the surface of infected erythrocytes) that, together with increased endothelial cytoadherence, results in occlusion of the microvasculature. Other species, causing less severe and generally uncomplicated infections, include *P. vivax*, *P. ovale*, and *P. malariae*. Both *P. vivax and P. ovale* infect reticulocytes and have a latent liver stage responsible for the phenomenon of relapsing malaria. *P. malariae* only infects older erythrocytes and can cause low-grade, chronic infections. *P. knowlesi*, found in South East Asia, is predominantly a pathogen of macaque monkeys, but has been described as a cause of human infections. Malaria is an ancient disease and in Africa the distribution of sickle cell trait, which provides some degree of protection against the most severe consequences of infection, tracks the distribution of endemic malaria (Rosenthal 2011). Blood group O also confers a degree of protection but group B exhibits greater risk of severe disease (Amodu *et al.* 2012).

Malaria should be suspected in any patient or traveller with fever residing in or returning from a malaria endemic area. The majority of cases present with fever, headache, chills, myalgias, and arthralgias. Gastrointestinal symptoms (diarrhoea, nausea, and vomiting) may occur in up to 50 per cent of cases. In severe malaria (mostly *P. falciparum*) cerebral involvement, severe anaemia, renal failure, blackwater fever, respiratory distress, jaundice and liver dysfunction, acidosis, hypoglycaemia, and haemorrhaging may occur. The progression of severe malaria can be extremely rapid causing death, despite intensive care, within hours or days. Early diagnosis and management of this disease are therefore of paramount importance. Microscopy of Giemsa-stained smears of peripheral blood films remains the gold standard for the identification of malarial species as well as for the determination of parasite load. It also has the advantage of enabling the detection of other parasites (e.g. *Babesia*, *Trypanosoma*, and filariae) in peripheral blood. Severe malaria caused by *P. falciparum* necessitates treatment with parenterally-administered antimalarial agents. These include quininine (conventional treatment) with or without the addition of either doxycycline or clindamycin and, more recently, artemisin-combination therapy (ACT), aimed at delaying the development of resistance to artemisin-based drugs. Furthermore, whereas the artemisins are short-acting and highly effective in rapidly reducing the parasite load, the second antimalarial in the combination eliminates residual parasites. More recently, artesunate has been found to be superior to quinine in the treatment of both adult and paediatric infections. Intensive care, supportive therapy, and careful monitoring and management of complications are important to improve patient survival from severe malaria.

Malaria remains a global public health problem. Approximately 50 per cent (more than 3.3 billion humans) of the world's population is at risk, more than 250 million people are infected yearly, and malaria claims one to two million lives each year. Although malaria occurs in a broad band around the equator, parts of America, and Asia, it is in sub-Saharan Africa where more than 90 per cent of deaths occur (it is estimated that every 30 seconds a child dies from malaria in this region). A decade ago, with the emergence of antimalarial drug resistance, insecticide resistance, failure of national programs, increasing human migration and tourism, the dream of eliminating malaria became elusive. However, more recently, following initiatives by the Gates Foundation, WHO, and many other stakeholders, the prospect of elimination of malaria is more realistic. Political commitment, allocation of financial and other resources, the availability of artemisin-based combination treatment, insecticide-impregnated bed nets, integrated vector control, intermittent presumptive treatment, and vaccine strategies are all crucial for the elimination of this disease. Integrated vector control, crucial to the control of malaria, involves the following: DEET-containing mosquito repellents, indoor residual spraying, insecticide-impregnated bed nets, destroying larvae, drainage, screening, and the release of sterile male mosquitoes. Preliminary trials of the latter have produced ambiguous results. Details of control measures and country reports are to be found in the World Malaria Report (WHO 2011b).

Partial immunity to malaria occurs in response to repeated infection with multiple strains of malarial parasites. Upon leaving a malaria-endemic area, however, this immunity is rapidly lost. There is currently no available vaccine that is completely effective against malaria. Trials in the 1990s using SPf66 in endemic areas showed disappointing results. More recently, vaccines based on the RTS, S antigen, targeting the pre-erythrocytic stage of the parasite's life cycle, have shown the most promising results.

Pandemic influenza

Influenza viruses circulate globally in animal and human populations. Influenza A is widely distributed in birds, mammals, and in humans, has the ability to mutate relatively rapidly, and is responsible for seasonal influenza (flu) epidemics that typically kill up to half a million people (often the frail and elderly) worldwide every year. Influenza B is largely confined to human populations and mutates sufficiently slowly that it is unlikely to cause pandemics. Influenza C infects humans, dogs, and pigs and can cause local epidemics and severe illness. Influenza viruses are estimated to cause severe illness in up to five million people annually.

Influenza A subtypes are identified by surface receptors called haemagglutinin (the H component) and neuraminidase (the N component). Subtypes are largely species-specific and usually only efficiently infect, and spread between, one species. The virus changes by small increments *frequently* (antigenic drift within a strain), and by large amounts *infrequently* (antigenic shift to a new strain). Mixing of avian, swine, and human viruses in the same host can result in the incorporation of virus genes resulting in a shift to a new

strain (re-assortment). Direct transmission of avian viruses may also occur. As immunity to flu is specific to a particular strain most people will have little or no immunity to a new virus and will be susceptible to infection. This, allied to the short incubation period of flu, allows the virus to spread rapidly. A new strain may appear at any time of the year and spread worldwide from the original source in approximately six months, although this time may be greatly reduced if the new strain arises in an area with a high volume of international travel. Pandemics often come in waves of infection, with second and third waves potentially more severe than the first. Pandemic flu strains infect many more people and can cause considerably more morbidity and mortality, but differ in the severity of disease they cause, the age-group most affected, and the attack rate.

20th-century pandemics

Intervals between previous known pandemics have varied from 11 to 42 years with no recognizable pattern. It is not possible to predict when the next pandemic will occur, but surveillance is vital in allowing identification of flu with pandemic potential, particularly in animals, and emergence of new strains in humans. Some of the major pandemics include:

1918–1919 'Spanish flu' This was caused by direct transmission of an avian strain of H1N1 influenza. The first outbreaks were noted in USA from where it spread worldwide within six months and, over several waves of infection in two years, killed an estimated 50–100 million people. The approximate mortality rate was 2.5 per cent in those infected, with young adults particularly susceptible.

1957–1958 'Asian flu' First identified in China, this H2N2 virus caused approximately two million deaths worldwide, mainly in elderly people. The virus is thought to have emerged after an H1N1 strain re-assorted with an H2N2 avian strain. This strain was replaced by the 1968–69 pandemic strain and has not circulated since then, so immunity to 'Asian flu' is restricted to those born before 1968.

1968–1969 'Hong Kong flu' This pandemic was first detected in Hong Kong, but originated in China, and was caused by a genetically re-assorted H3N2 virus. Around one million people died, and again those over 65 years of age had the highest mortality rate. Similar (drifted) H3N2 strains remain in circulation.

The 2009 pandemic On 11 June 2009 WHO formally confirmed the first pandemic of influenza for 40 years. The novel pandemic A (H1N1) (swine flu) virus probably originated in a town called La Gloria in Veracruz, Mexico in mid-February 2009. It had already spread widely in Mexico by the time it was recognized as a new virus in the USA in April 2009. The virus genes were a unique combination most closely related to North American swine-lineage H1N1 and Eurasian lineage swine-origin H1N1 influenza viruses. By June 2009 the virus had infected people in many countries worldwide, and by the time WHO declared the pandemic over in August 2010 almost 19,000 deaths were recorded in laboratory-confirmed cases worldwide; but this will be a great underestimation of overall mortality as many people will not have been tested. Nonetheless this is considered a mild pandemic. Elderly people were less likely to be infected with the new virus, presumably because of pre-existing immunity to H1N1 viruses circulating from the 1918 pandemic. Although illness was mild in the majority of people infected, severe illness was more common in those with co-morbidities such as asthma and diabetes, elderly people, and pregnant women. In England it was estimated that 30 per cent of children aged 5–14 years were infected compared to 11 per cent of the general population (Presanis *et al.* 2011). Following a pandemic, the pandemic strain often replaces the influenza A strains which were previously circulating. This has not happened to date with the 2009 pandemic strain, as a mixture of pandemic and pre-existing H3N2 strains continues to circulate with different proportions evident in different countries in subsequent seasons. The evolution of the pandemic and vaccine development is summarized elsewhere (CDC 2010).

Avian and swine influenza

Avian influenza virus subtypes H5N1, H7N7 and H9N2, and swine subtypes H1N1 and H3N2 have the most potential to infect humans and are therefore currently of most concern. Avian H7N7 infected 89 people and caused the death of one veterinarian in a poultry outbreak in the Netherlands in 2003. There have also been reports in the USA of human infections in 2011 with novel viruses which have evolved from re-assortments between a swine-origin influenza A (H3N2) virus circulating in North American swine and a 2009 influenza A (H1N1) virus (Anon 2011). Recent concern has centred on a strain of H5N1 which first emerged in 1996. The first outbreak in Hong Kong killed six of 18 people infected. The Hong Kong authorities acted swiftly to stamp out poultry flocks which had the potential to be a reservoir of disease. However this lineage of H5N1 re-emerged in 2002, and has circulated in Asia and Europe since then. It has caused widespread outbreaks in poultry, infecting millions of birds, and also circulates in wild birds. H5N1 continues to mutate with new clades (branches) identified periodically. Widespread vaccination of poultry in H5N1-endemic countries has controlled spread where systematically applied, but may have accelerated mutation of the virus where vaccination has been sub-optimal. Few human infections have been identified to date, and these have occurred in people with very close contact with infected birds, almost always domestic fowl, with almost no spread from person-to-person. Up to 6 July 2012, WHO had received reports of 606 human infections, with 357 deaths, occurring mainly in Egypt, Indonesia, Vietnam, and China. This very high mortality rate (59 per cent) increases concern about the possibility of this virus becoming transmissible between humans, although it is impossible to predict this or the associated mortality rate. The present high mortality rate seems to be due to an excessive host immune response. Recent research has shown that H5N1 can, under research conditions, become airborne and cause ferret to ferret transmission, and that a 'reassortant' virus, H5 HA/H1N1, can be transmitted by droplets (Herfst *et al.* 2012; Imai *et al.* 2012), indicating a strong possibility of potential mutation of this virus to enable human to human transmission (Russell *et al.* 2012).

Surveillance and the emergence of pandemics Syndromic and virological surveillance (see section 18.4) is key to recognizing the emergence of a novel influenza strains. The WHO Global Influenza Surveillance and Response System (WHO 2012a) collects information from National Influenza Centres to:

- monitor the evolution of influenza viruses;

- provide recommendations in areas including laboratory diagnostics, vaccines, antiviral susceptibility, and risk assessment;

- serve as a global alert mechanism for the emergence of influenza viruses with pandemic potential.

Very rapid recognition of a newly emerging virus close to the source might allow an attempt to eradicate the new strain with widespread treatment and prophylaxis close to the source. Both the difficulty of recognition of a new strain and the delivery of the response required to arrest spread, means that this is unlikely to be successful. This is likely to be particularly true if the pandemic strain is mild overall, as many cases may have occurred before the situation is recognized. This was certainly true of the 2009 pandemic.

Pandemic planning and vaccination Planning for a future influenza pandemic at country and region wide level is strongly recommended by WHO, which has a range of tools to assist in this. Social distancing, respiratory hygiene measures, use of antiviral medication for treatment and prophylaxis, and vaccination, may all be strategies of value during a pandemic. All of these require careful advance planning, which may include stockpiling of antivirals and other clinical countermeasures. Pre-existing seasonal flu vaccines will not give protection against a new pandemic virus, so an early priority when a new strain is identified is to develop a new, usually monovalent, vaccine. Current production methods take around six months for development from the time of a new strain being identified. Production is also likely to be limited initially, which means that prioritization may be necessary. There may also be competition between countries for supply, and difficulties with affordability for developing countries. This occurred during the 2009 pandemic and in response WHO developed a Pandemic Influenza Preparedness Framework with the objective of improving the sharing of H5N1 and other influenza viruses with human pandemic potential, access to vaccines, and sharing of other benefits (Fidler and Gostin 2011). Recent work may indicate

that a 'universal' flu vaccine, which is cross-reactive against all subtypes of influenza, is a possibility in the future.

In summary, increased globalization of human populations and trade in live and dead animal sources of infection underline the importance of continuing surveillance in human and animal populations, development of vaccination strategies, and planning for future pandemics.

Gastroenteritis and hepatitis

Gastroenteritis can be caused by infective and non-infective causes. Infective causes include bacteria (e.g. *Salmonella*, *Shigella*, *Campylobacter*, *E. coli* 0157), viruses (e.g. norovirus and rotavirus), and protozoa (e.g. gardia and cryptosporidia). Some of these organisms produce large quantities of toxins which often cause vomiting, diarrhoea, and, in severe cases, shock. On a global scale rotavirus has the most significant impact as it is the commonest cause of severe diarrhoea in children and is estimated to cause over half a million deaths each year in children under five years of age and 37 per cent of all child deaths due to diarrhoea. The majority of these deaths have been in malnourished or poorly nourished children. More than half of all deaths attributable to rotavirus occurred in five countries; three of these are in Africa, and 22 per cent of deaths occurred in India (Tate *et al.* 2012).

There has been an overall decline in deaths due to gastroenteritis from 1.8 million in 2003 to 1.3 million in 2008. This may be due to improvements in sanitation and hygiene with a decrease in bacterial and parasitic infections spread by water and food. In contrast rotavirus is spread by person-to-person (faeco-oral) contact (Tate *et al.* 2012) and it is estimated that all children worldwide will become infected with rotavirus before their fifth birthday (Grimwood *et al.* 2010). Rotavirus vaccination has been introduced following appropriate trials in some high-income countries such as the USA and Australia, and in some mid-income countries such as Mexico and Brazil. In the USA one report has estimated that during the period 2007–2009 there was a reduction of almost 65,000 hospital admissions in children and a saving of $278 million in treatment costs (Cortes *et al.* 2011). In Brazil a reduction of 22 per cent in diarrhoea-associated mortality in children under five years of age was reported following introduction of the vaccine in 2006 (do Carmo *et al.* 2011). Successful trials have been conducted in Asia and in Africa and a review of cost-effectiveness studies concluded that introduction of rotavirus vaccine into low-income countries in these regions, as recommended by WHO, is cost-effective; but the current cost of the vaccines is a limiting factor at present (Tu *et al.* 2011).

Shigella species are the second most common cause of infant and child gastroenteritis worldwide (25–30 per cent) but outbreaks frequently occur in adults also. Typhoid fever (*Salmonella typhi*) does not cause diarrhoea but significant outbreaks occur worldwide with 22 million cases annually and more than 200,000 deaths (Neil *et al.* 2012). Cholera is classed as a pandemic disease and causes sporadic epidemics, recently in Zimbabwe (2008) and Haiti (2009). In 2009 there were more than 200,000 cases reported worldwide (with strong evidence of under-reporting), and almost 5000 deaths (Morris 2011).

Hepatitis A virus can be acquired through contaminated food or water and causes nausea, fever, and jaundice; it is endemic in low- and middle-income countries, routinely acquired in childhood without significant morbidity. Hepatitis E is also endemic in low- and middle-income countries, spread by the faeco-oral route and carries a higher rate of significant morbidity and mortality than Hepatitis A. Hepatitis B is endemic in Asia, parts of the Middle East and South America, and in sub-Saharan Africa; chronic long-term infection and carriage is common. Transmission is usually from mother to infant at birth or between children in low- and middle-income countries, but in high-income countries sexual intercourse and needle-sharing in injecting drug users are the most common modes of transmission. Use of unsterilized needles for tattooing, acupuncture, or similar procedures is associated with increased risk. Hepatitis C which is less common but more widely distributed is believed to be mainly transmitted by unsterile needles or instruments or contaminated blood transfusions. It is estimated that up to 80 per cent of infected individuals develop chronic

disease. Hepatitis D occurs only in conjunction with Hepatitis B, but is less widely distributed. Hepatitis E is endemic in many low and middle income countries causing significant morbidity and mortality, and is associated with inadequate sanitation and contaminated water.

A wide range of toxins can also cause significant disease. Botulism results from the ingestion of foods such as home preserved meat or vegetables containing a preformed neurotoxin from *C. botulinum* spores causing nervous system dysfunction with blurred vision, muscle weakness, and potentially, respiratory failure. Food poisoning can also be caused by chemicals. For example scombrotoxin poisoning is caused by excess histamine found in inadequately refrigerated tuna and mackerel and is associated with diarrhoea, facial flushing, headache, and sweating within two hours of ingesting the contaminated food. Shellfish and certain mushrooms can also be associated with chemical food poisoning.

Most infectious intestinal disease is not preventable by vaccination and prevention is therefore based on reducing microbiological exposure. These control measures include: safe drinking water; adequate sanitation; minimizing contamination of meat at slaughter; pasteurization or sterilization of milk; the hygienic processing, storage, and distribution of foodstuffs; the prevention of cross-contamination when preparing food; and good personal hygiene—a key component of which is thorough hand washing after using the toilet and before handling or eating food. In 2005 it was estimated that 1.1 billion of the world's population did not have sustainable access to improved water sources and a further 2.6 billion lacked adequate sanitation. Cost-benefit analysis suggested that investment of one US$ would produce an investment return of between US$5–46 in terms of economic and health benefit in low and middle income countries (Hutton *et al.* 2007). Chapter 6 (Scenario 2) provides an example of the effectiveness of solar disinfection of water supplies in a cluster randomized trial in Bolivia. A systematic review and meta-analysis of studies in high-income countries suggest that training and re-training of food handlers improves hand hygiene knowledge and self-reported practice (Soon *et al.* 2012).

Viral haemorrhagic fevers

Viral haemorrhagic fevers (VHFs) are caused by RNA viruses belonging to four families: *Arenaviridae, Bunyaviridae, Filoviridae*, and *Flaviviridae*. These viruses are highly infectious and cause a syndrome that may be fatal characterized by fever, malaise, myalgia, pharyngitis, vomiting and diarrhoea, bleeding, hypotension, and multi-organ failure. Table 18.3 summarizes the common VHF aetiological agents belonging to each of these families as well as their geographical distribution, reservoirs, and available prophylaxis and treatment. It is important to note that although the current geographical distribution of VHF viruses appears reasonably well-defined, changing climatic factors, migration of humans and animals, as well as movements of vectors and animal reservoirs could result in significant changes in the future distribution of some of these infections. In the case of dengue and severe dengue (haemorrhagic) fever this has already occurred; before the 1970s it caused significant disease in only nine countries but is now present in more than 100 countries with 50–100 million cases per year, 500,000 hospitalized cases and an estimated 12,000 deaths. *Aedes aegypti* is the main mosquito vector, thrives in urban habitats, and bites its human prey during the daylight hours in contrast to the *Anopheles* mosquitoes responsible for malaria, which bite at night.

Although some VHF agents (e.g. Rift Valley Fever virus) cause relatively mild disease in the majority of infected cases, severe illness leading to death may occur. VHF agents such as Marburg and Ebola viruses, however, are among the most virulent pathogens known and generally cause severe life-threatening disease associated with high fatality rates. Lujo virus, a novel Old World arenavirus, is the most recently described VHF agent that caused a nosocomial outbreak in a South African health care facility in 2008 involving five health care-associated workers (Paweska *et al.* 2009). The source of the outbreak was a critically ill patient who underwent emergency air evacuation from Zambia and was transferred to a private medical facility in Johannesburg. Air evacuation of critically ill patients to countries with well-equipped hospitals and sophisticated intensive care units as well as the

increase in, and ease of, human international travel means that VHF infections can present in non-endemic areas anywhere in the world. It is therefore essential that all health care professionals continuously update themselves on the current epidemiology of VHFs and maintain a high index of suspicion for patients from VHF endemic areas that present with fever and bleeding. However, in non-endemic areas, VHFs are a rare cause of fever and bleeding. The differential diagnosis is broad and includes diseases caused by bacteria (e.g. meningococcal infection and typhoid), rickettsias (e.g. tick-bite fever), spirochaetes (e.g. leptospirosis), parasites (e.g. malaria), viruses other than VHF agents (e.g. HIV, herpes and hepatitis virus infections), as well as non-infectious causes (e.g. poisons, traditional medicines or idiopathic thombocytopaenic purpura). The laboratory confirmation of a VHF takes time and it is important that if the diagnosis is suspected strict adherence to infection prevention and control precautions is maintained at all times. With the exception of Rift Valley fever, nosocomial transmission and outbreak amplification of most VHF agents among health care workers is a well-described phenomenon. Box 18.3 provides a summary of the infection prevention and control precautions required for the management of suspected/confirmed VHF cases.

As VHFs such as Ebola and Marburg pose a serious public health problem, cause considerable panic, and can result in disruption of normal hospital services, it is essential to set up a representative and suitably qualified outbreak response team to ensure that national, regional, and local experts work together. Contact tracing and identification of high-, medium-, and low-risk contacts must be carried out and high-risk contacts must be counselled and monitored for a period of 21 days after the last contact they had with a confirmed case. Education of the general public and engaging the press with honesty and transparency is of paramount importance.

Prion diseases

Prion diseases show many of the characteristics of infectious diseases but the responsible agents lack DNA or RNA. Prion diseases occur in animals (scrapie

Table 18.3 Viruses causing haemorrhagic fevers

Virus family and genus	Virus	Disease	Geographical distribution	Reservoir	Antiviral Treatment	Vaccine currently available for human use
Arenaviridae						
Arenavirus	Lassa	Lassa fever	Africa	Rodent	Ribavirin*	No
	Lujo	Lujo HF	Africa	Rodent		No
	Junin	Argentine HF	South America	Rodent		Yes**
	Machupo	Bolivian HF	South America	Rodent		
	Sabia	Brazilian HF	South America	Rodent		
	Guanarito	Venezuelan HF	South America	Rodent		
Bunyaviridae						
Hantavirus		HF with renal syndrome (HFRS), Hantavirus pulmonary syndrome (HPS)	Asia, Europe, Worldwide	Rodent	Ribavirin	Yes
Nairovirus	Crimean-Congo HF virus	Crimean-Congo HF	Africa, Asia, Europe	Hard ticks	Ribavirin	No
Phlebovirus	Rift Valley fever	Rift Valley fever	Africa, Arabian peninsula (Yemen and Saudi Arabia)	Mosquito	None	Yes
Filoviridae						
Filovirus	Marburg	Marburg HF	Africa	Bats	None	No
	Zaire ebolavirus	Ebola HF	Africa	Bats	None	No
	Sudan ebolavirus					
	Cote d'Ivoire ebolavirus					
	Budinbugyoebolavirus					
Flaviviridae						
Flavivirus	Yellow fever	Yellow fever	Tropical Africa, South America	Mosquito	None	Yes
	Dengue	Dengue HF	Africa, Americas, Asia	Mosquito	None	No

* Administration of ribavirin may be useful in other infections caused by the Arenaviridae. Furthermore, it may be effective for post-exposure prophylaxis for some arenavirus and bunyavirus infections.
** Argentine HF (Junin) vaccine may also protect against Bolivian HF.
Adapted from: **http://emedicine.medscape.com/article/830594-overview**.

Box 18.3 Infection prevention and control viral haemorrhagic fever (VHF) precautions in a nutshell.

- Notification of the suspected/confirmed VHF to health authorities and to all medical and allied health care personnel (including the laboratory)
- Limiting health care worker and family member exposures as far as possible
- Isolation of the patient; cohorting of multiple patients. A negative pressure room, *if available*, is ideal
- Strict enforcement of enhanced standard and contact precautions and protection against aerosols: hand hygiene, double gloves, impervious gown, shoe and leg covers, FFP3 (UK) or N95 respirator, protective eyewear (goggles or face-shield). Thorough training of all personnel in the correct procedures for donning and doffing of PPE
- Identification, classification, counselling, and monitoring of contacts
- Safe disinfection of all fluid spills, equipment and supplies (hypochlorites frequently used for this purpose)
- Monitoring of the safe disposal of medical hazardous waste
- Safe handling and burial of corpses
- Education and counselling to family members

in sheep, bovine spongiform encephalopathy (BSE) in cattle, and chronic wasting disease in deer) and in humans (kuru, Creutzfeldt–Jakob disease (CJD), variant CJD (vCJD), and some rare inherited syndromes). CJD also occurs in families and inherited prion disease accounts for up to 15 per cent of human prion disease, although relevant mutations of the gene encoding the prion particle PRNP (PRioN protein) has also been demonstrated in familial early onset dementia (Mead 2006). Several questions remain to be answered about these agents which are misfolded and aggregated isoforms of proteins from this gene but like viruses can be transmitted orally, parenterally, by direct surgical or other contact with the brain, and in the laboratory by aerosols (Aguzzi and Zhu 2012).

The story of BSE in the UK is salutary for public health as it illustrates the close relationships between farming practice and veterinary and public health. BSE was first described in the UK as a rapidly progressive neurodegenerative disease in cattle in 1986. By 1992 there had been almost 160,000 confirmed cases despite the introduction of widespread culling of cattle early in the epidemic (Nathanson *et al.* 1997). The economic cost to the UK and other affected countries ran into billions of pounds. A National CJD Research and Surveillance Unit was established 'to identify any change in the pattern of CJD that might be attributable to human infection with the agent responsible for the emergence of BSE in cattle.'

Variant CJD was first described in 1996 (Will *et al.* 1996) when ten UK cases of CJD were reported with a new neuropathological profile. These cases were also younger (median age at death being 29 years) and had a different clinical profile compared to other cases of CJD (average age 65 years). Since then, to December 2012, the UK CJD Surveillance Unit (CJD 2012) has reported 176 cases of vCJD, all having died. France reported 25 cases but only a handful of cases have been reported elsewhere. Modelling studies indicate that vCJD peaked in the UK in 2000 when there were 27 cases diagnosed and 28 deaths, and these have now fallen to approximately one diagnosis/death annually. Extensive epidemiological studies have concluded that most cases of vCJD were considered to be due to the acquisition of abnormal prion protein (PrP) through eating beef and beef products from cattle infected with BSE. A small number of cases are thought to have acquired infection through blood transfusions and plasma products sourced in the UK from donors who were diagnosed with vCJD after donating blood. Risk factors for vCJD include age, living in the UK, and methionine homozygosity at codon 129 of the PRNP gene. PrP are very resistant to the usual methods of inactivating micro-organisms. Autoclaving cannot be relied on to denature PrP—contaminated surgical instruments following use on CJD patients and special precautions and procedures are therefore required. A range of control measures has been introduced in the UK. These include:

- banning the consumption of potentially infected feed to cattle;

- avoiding human consumption of nervous and lymphoreticular tissues from ruminants;

- safe preparation of carcasses and slaughter of infected herds;

- removal of white blood cells (leucodepletion) from all blood used for transfusions;

- use of non-UK sourced plasma and blood products;

- not using transplant, tissue donations, and blood transfusions from certain high-risk groups;

- using single-use disposable surgical instruments where possible and destruction of surgical instruments used on definite and probable vCJD cases;

- improving the standards and processes for decontaminating instruments.

Health care-associated infections

In high-income countries up to 10 per cent of patients acquire infections in hospital and low- and middle-income countries up to 25 per cent (Damani 2012; Allegranzi and Pittet 2009). In the USA it has been estimated that 90,000 patients die prematurely from these infections and that the economic cost in 2008 was about $30 billion (Damani 2012). Infections are particulary prevalent in intensive care units but are also common in general wards, outpatients, and in long-term care facilities. The commonest overall sites are the urinary and lower respiratory tracts (ca. 23 per cent) but infections are also common in surgical wounds (11 per cent), on skin (10 per cent), and in the bloodstream (six per cent). Many organisms such as *Staphylococcus aureus* and enterococci have acquired antibiotic resistance, e.g. methicillin-resistant *Staphylococcus aureus* (MRSA), and VRSA (resistant to vancomycin). If these become endemic in hospitals they are difficult to eradicate and contribute significantly to morbidity in the hospital population. Other organisms such as *Clostridium* species, *Salmonella*, *Shigella*, and viruses such as rotavirus or norovirus are also 'alert' organisms (Darmani 2012). Fig. 18.1 shows the distribution of infections in English hospitals in 2007.

Prevention and control are essential to prevent a rising tide of antibiotic resistance and other health care-related infection. Key elements in these twin strategies are: surveillance, antibiotic policy, hand hygiene, aseptic technique, and decontamination of equipment, disposal of waste, and cleaning of theatres, wards, and all relevant microenvironments, isolation of infected patient, and use of personal protection (Damani 2012). WHO has recently produced a report on hospital infections worldwide and guidelines for the implementation of improved hand hygiene measures in health care environments (WHO 2009).

18.3 Immunization

Immunization and vaccination against an increasing range of bacteria, their toxins and viruses have been a global public health success and are among the most cost-effective health interventions. Through programmes coordinated by WHO smallpox was declared eradicated in 1980; building on this programme WHO introduced its Expanded Programme in 1974 to promote the goal of universal coverage of essential immunizations in children in all countries, particularly in resource-poor countries (WHO 2012b). WHO recommendations for all countries are shown in Table 18.4, although this varies in practice, particularly in high income countries where different socio-economic conditions exist with different profiles of infectious disease. The Global Alliance for Vaccines and Immunizations (GAVI), a public-private initiative, launched in 2000 with support from the Gates Foundation enabled further expansion of the WHO programme. It is estimated that vaccination of children in low-income countries has saved 2.5 million lives annually since the year 2000. Since 1988 poliomyelitis cases have declined by 99 per cent to 1352 cases in 2010; it remains endemic in only three countries (Afghanistan, Nigeria, and Pakistan), although outbreaks have occurred in up to 18 countries from cases imported from endemic countries. Measles mortality has reduced by 74 per cent in a decade to less than 14,000 in 2010 and current evidence suggests that the disease may have been eliminated from the Americas.

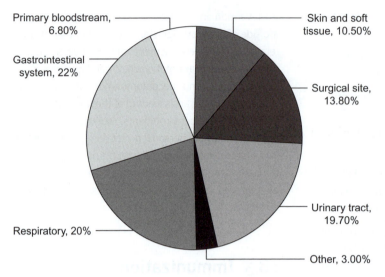

Primary bloodstream, 6.80%

Skin and soft tissue, 10.50%

Gastrointestinal system, 22%

Surgical site, 13.80%

Urinary tract, 19.70%

Respiratory, 20%

Other, 3.00%

Figure 18.1 Health care associated infections by body system for the UK. Source: *Summary of Preliminary Results of the Third Prevalence Survey of Healthcare Associated Infections in Acute Hospitals 2006*. England: Hospital Infection Society and Infection Control Nurses Association, 27 February 2007.

It is estimated that 1.7 million children still die every year from diseases preventable by vaccines currently recommended by WHO. Pneumococcal disease and rotavirus are now the biggest causes of vaccine preventable deaths each accounting for just over half a million deaths (WHO 2010). Vaccines to protect against these diseases have been introduced only in recent years. The case for HPV vaccine is also strong as there are more than half a million cases of cervical cancer and a quarter of a million deaths worldwide, 85 per cent in low- and middle-income countries (Tay 2012). HPV vaccine contains two strains of HPV (16 and 18) which cause 70 per cent of cervical cancers.

Many other vaccines and immunizations are available for use by travellers to countries where a number of serious diseases remain endemic. As illustrated in the case of the H1N1 influenza pandemic vaccines can be produced within a few months if there is a threat of a global epidemic; smallpox vaccines remain stockpiled in secure locations against the possibility of bioterrorism. Further information on specific diseases and available immunizations is to be found elsewhere (WHO 2012b). Vaccines against malaria, HIV, and dengue, and improved vaccines for TB would greatly advance global health, but these remain in the early stages of development.

Benefits versus hazards of vaccination: Public health immunization programmes worldwide need to retain public and professional confidence in both the efficacy of the programme and the perceived safety of the vaccines. Smallpox has been eradicated and routine vaccination was discontinued in the post smallpox era when the hazards of continued vaccination were evaluated (Ada 2001). For the majority of vaccines, however, the infectious agents persist in the population or in other parts of the world and continued immunization programmes are necessary. As the diseases become rare or are eliminated from countries then the perceived risk of the disease falls and any real or suggested risks from the vaccine seem higher in comparison. Reports and subsequent publicity about the risk associated with pertussis vaccine in the 1970s, and combined measles, mumps, and rubella (MMR) vaccine in the 1990s, led to a loss in public confidence in this vaccine and a fall in uptake rates. In 2011 there were measles outbreaks across Europe, most notably in France which reported 14,000 cases in the first six months.

All vaccines are fully tested in animal studies, human volunteers, and in field trials before being licensed for general use. Safety trials on vaccines have to be particularly rigorous as vaccines are often given in large

Table 18.4 WHO recommendations for routine immunizations

Antigen	Children	Adolescents	Adults	Considerations
Recommendations for all				
BCG	1 dose			Exceptions HIV
Hepatitis B	3–4 doses	3 doses (for high-risk groups if not previously immunized)		Birth dose; Premature and low birth weight; Co-administration and combination vaccine; Definition high-risk
Polio	3 doses, with DTP			OPV birth dose; Transmission and importation risk criteria; Type of vaccine
DTP	3 doses Booster (DTP) 1–6 years of age	Booster (Td)	Booster (Td) in early adulthood of pregnancy	Delayed/interrupted schedule; Combination vaccine
Haemophilus influenzae type b	3 doses, with DTP			Single dose if 12–24 months of age; Delayed/interrupted schedule; Co-administration and combination vaccine
Pneumococcal (Conjugate)	Option 1: 3 doses, with DTP Option 2: 2 doses before 6 months of age, plus booster dose at 9–15 months of age			Vaccine options; Initiate before 6 months of age; Co-administration; HIV+ and preterm neonates booster
Rotavirus	Rotarix: 2 doses with DTP RotaTeq: 3 doses with DTP			Vaccine options
Measles	2 doses			Combination vaccine; HIV early vaccination; Pregnancy
Rubella	1 dose	1 dose (adolescent girls and/or child bearing aged women if not previously vaccinated)		Achieve and sustain 80% coverage; combination vaccine and co-administration; Pregnancy
HPV		3 doses (girls)		Vaccination of males for prevention of cervical cancer is not recommended at this time

Reproduced from Recommended Routine Immunization, WHO 2012, with permission.

numbers to healthy people, most frequently children. Even very small risks of serious side effects are therefore not tolerated. Further details on individual vaccine safety and side effects are to be found on the relevant WHO website (WHO 2012b). The use of epidemiological methods in the evaluation and surveillance of immunization programmes is discussed in detail elsewhere (Chen and Orenstein 1996).

18.4 Surveillance of communicable disease

Communicable disease surveillance has been described as:

> **the continued watchfulness over the distribution and trends of incidence through the systematic collection, consolidation and evaluation of morbidity and mortality reports and other relevant data. Intrinsic in the concept is the regular dissemination of the basic data and interpretations to all who have contributed and to all others who need to know (Langmuir 1963).**

Surveillance is therefore information for action. Surveillance systems should ideally be: simple to use; flexible to adapt to changing circumstances; have complete and accurate data; acceptable to participants; sensitive with a high positive predictive value; representative of a population/event; timely with a short interval between onset and report to the surveillance system, in order to facilitate early, appropriate action; and capable of being sustained over time (Anon 1988).

Passive surveillance describes most routine systems in which doctors and others report diseases while **active surveillance** implies that a health authority or surveillance centre actively seeks out such reports. Surveillance systems should enable: the establishment of baseline trends in the incidence and demography of a disease or event; the early recognition of an outbreak or a new infection/syndrome; the identification of those at risk; the evaluation of controls and other interventions; and, the development of policies, action plans, priority setting, and research. Traditionally, surveillance systems for

communicable disease are based on the outcomes of interactions with health services. However there are a number of influences which will impact on individual health-seeking behaviour and need to be recognized particularly when studying long-term trends on communicable disease or international data. Besides ensuring comparable case definitions these include: duration, nature and severity of symptoms; disruption to daily living; geographical factors such as mobility, distance and ease of travel to the relevant health facility; organization of health care; and cultural issues. In some countries monetary cost is a major factor on an individual's decision to access health care. The media and public opinion can also influence health-seeking behaviour.

The two main components of routine surveillance in most high income countries are: (a) statutory infectious diseases notification and (b) laboratory reporting of infectious agents.

Notifications Most countries have a list of communicable diseases which doctors are legally required to report or notify to the appropriate authority (Hawker *et al.* 2005). These notifications of infectious disease are the historical bedrock of surveillance and have been in existence in the UK for over a century. Notification prompts local investigation and appropriate action to control the disease. There are currently 31 diseases notifiable in England and Wales (see website in 'Web addresses'). They comprise most of the vaccine-preventable infections while others such as SARS and smallpox are included to facilitate reporting to WHO under International Health Regulations (2005).

These regulations also require the medical practitioner to notify an infection which presents or could present significant harm to human health; or the patient is contaminated with toxic material which presents or could present significant harm to human health. This new legislation enables notification of newly emerging infections or of individuals contaminated with toxic or radiological substances.

Certain enforcement powers can be applied to an individual with a notifiable disease such as: compulsory medical examination; removal to—and detention in—hospital, although treatment is not compulsory; restriction on movements or work; and use of infected premises. Notifications can be used for:

- baseline surveillance;
- assessing the efficacy of the childhood vaccination programme;
- initiating an investigation, e.g. food poisoning;
- initiating contact tracing to identify and protect others at risk, e.g. in tuberculosis and meningococcal infection.

Doctors are required to notify on the basis of clinical suspicion—laboratory confirmation is not required in order that public health action can be initiated at the earliest opportunity. This should be within three days or earlier if thought urgent. However, although it is a legal requirement to notify (and a modest fee is paid) many doctors either fail to notify at all or do not notify in a timely manner to enable public health action or tend only to notify certain infections. This may reflect a lack of understanding of the purposes of notification, which also has no perceived benefit to their patient.

Laboratory surveillance Laboratory reporting of organisms of public health interest is now the cornerstone of communicable disease surveillance. Until recently this was undertaken on a voluntary basis but new regulations (2010) now make it a requirement in England for diagnostic laboratories to notify causative agents from human samples to the Health Protection Agency. However, even with complete laboratory reporting, the incidence of many infections remains underestimated. To be reported in the national database requires:

- The individual to seek medical attention. This will be influenced by the severity, nature and duration of symptoms.
- The doctor to initiate appropriate investigations. This will also be influenced by the patient's history and clinical examination, and the patient's willingness to provide a laboratory sample.
- The laboratory to perform the appropriate analysis. Laboratory practice using specific enrichment media or referral to a reference laboratory may depend on the clinical information on the request form.
- The laboratory to inform the national surveillance centre.

Some common infections of public health concern may not be notifiable or not routinely subject to laboratory investigation; for example, influenza and viral gastroenteritis. Therefore alternative surveillance arrangements are required. Throughout the UK there are networks of **sentinel general practices** which report the number of consultations for influenza or influenza-like illness in the preceding week as a proportion of the practice population. Aggregation of these data provides age-specific consultation rates for a region which, combined with the laboratory analysis of nasopharyngeal swabs from such patients, can provide early warning of the emergence of influenza virus in the community before it would be normally noted from rises in hospital admissions or positive laboratory reports from hospitalized patients.

Influenza is primarily a clinical diagnosis and it would be unusual for a GP to seek laboratory confirmation. In addition, those with influenza or influenza-like illness are actively discouraged from visiting their GP unless their symptoms are severe or prolonged. In the case of food poisoning in the UK it was estimated that for every 1000 cases of infectious intestinal disease in the community, 160 presented to their general practitioner, 45 had a stool sample sent routinely for microbiological examination, ten had a positive laboratory result and only seven were reported to national surveillance. This under-ascertainment varied by organism with three cases of salmonella infection in the community for each case reported nationally compared with a ratio of approximately 1500: 1 for norovirus.

Therefore surveillance systems need flexibility and the opportunities provided through the increased use of electronic datasets. One example is using data from nurse-led telephone helplines that now operate in Britain. Data on ten symptoms/syndromes are received electronically from call centres and analysed on a daily basis; cough, cold/flu, fever, diarrhoea, vomiting, eye problems, double vision, difficulty breathing, rash, and lumps. Significant statistical excesses in calls for any of these symptoms are automatically highlighted and assessed by a multidisciplinary team. The aim is to identify an increase in symptoms indicative of the early stages of illness caused by the deliberate release of a biological or chemical agent, or more common infections (Baker *et al.* 2003).

Sexually-transmitted diseases also require special monitoring and anonymized data for infections such as syphilis, gonorrhoea, chlamydia, and HIV are obtained from genito-urinary (GU) clinics throughout the UK. HIV surveillance also includes confidential reporting by clinicians of diagnoses of HIV, AIDS, and HIV-related deaths to the national surveillance centres, and the unlinked anonymous surveys of all attendees at GU clinics, as well as injecting drug users attending specialist treatment/support services.

Some communicable diseases are under enhanced surveillance in order to capture additional information on risk factors/lifestyle. Extra effort and resources are required and, in the UK, diseases under enhanced surveillance include tuberculosis and *E. coli 0157*.

••

Question 1

HIV infections can be passed from mother to baby before, during, and after birth. Breastfeeding can pass on HIV infection. What surveillance systems and control measures would be appropriate?

••

WHO has a major role in coordinating international surveillance and outbreak response (Global Alert and Response (GAR): WHO 2012c). Recent developments in Europe have included the establishment in 1995 of the European Centre of Disease Prevention and Control (ECDC) (see website in 'Web addresses') to strengthen Europe's defences against infectious disease. It works to identify, assess, and communicate current and emerging infectious threats to human health by working with health protection bodies in each Member State. It also operates an early warning and response system to alert public health authorities, Member States, and the Commission on outbreaks with EC implications, to enable coordinated Community action. In the US the Centers for Disease Control coordinates surveillance across the USA and works in conjunction with WHO.

18.5 Outbreak investigation

An outbreak of infection is said to have occurred when the number of observed cases exceeds that which is expected in a particular population. It can also be defined as two or more individuals with the same infection or symptoms and linked through common exposure, personal characteristics, time or place. There is no specific number of cases to constitute an outbreak. For example, a single case of a rare or highly virulent infection such as smallpox, diphtheria, or polio in the UK would be regarded as an outbreak with international consequences. Box 18.4 describes a small outbreak and illustrates some of the key aspects of outbreak investigation.

A reference laboratory may note increasing cases nationwide as in the case of the *Salmonella agona* outbreak shown in Box 18.4. Clinicians may report seeing an unusually high number of patients with diseases such as acute gastroenteritis, severe 'flu-like illness, or an atypical clinical syndrome such as tetanus in injecting drug users. The public or media may contact the local environmental health department to report illness after a particular function or associated with an institution such as a school. Further enquiries include: contacting neighbouring districts and microbiologists and checks are made to ensure no recent change in laboratory practice or catchment area, which could explain increased laboratory reporting. In the USA HIV/AIDS was first discovered by increased laboratory reports of atypical pneumonia.

If initial suspicions of an outbreak are confirmed, a decision is required as to whether it should be investigated. Factors to consider include: initial information on morbidity and mortality; the vulnerability of the population at risk; association with a high risk facility, e.g. a hospital or food premises; its transmissibility; the likelihood of continuing exposure to the suspected source; national and international implications through human travel or distribution of a particular food product; and potential media and political interest. Usually the need for an outbreak investigation is self-evident and a pre-prepared outbreak plan is activated. This initiates a sequence of events and may involve a large number and range of individuals and agencies, postponing routine work. An incident room with dedicated staff, communications, and laptops may be required to facilitate coordination of the management of the outbreak. An outbreak control team (OCT) is established which: coordinates the investigation; ensures sufficient resources are made available to control the outbreak; ensures appropriate

Box 18.4 International outbreak of *Salmonella agona*: the importance of national laboratory surveillance and international cooperation.

Between 5 December 1994 and 30 January 1995, 27 isolates of *S. agona* were identified in England and Wales by the Salmonella Reference Laboratory of the Public Health Laboratory Service (now the Health Protection Agency). This was in contrast to 12 isolates in the same period in the previous year. Many of the cases were children, there was geographical clustering and many of the children had Jewish surnames. From initial interviews with eight primary cases, four had eaten a peanut flavoured ready-to-eat snack made of maize and imported from Israel. Case finding was not restricted to the UK but included Europe using Salm-Net, a network for the surveillance of salmonella in Europe. Other countries including Israel, the USA and Canada were also alerted (Killalea *et al.* 1996).

A case-control study subsequently confirmed a strong association between infection with the outbreak strain of *S. agona* and consumption of the snack food. The outbreak strain was identified in 83 per cent (44/53) of packets obtained from retailers and manufactured on a certain day. Approximately 20,000 packets from this batch had been distributed throughout the UK. At the same time Israeli authorities were investigating a large outbreak of *S. agona* and, with information from the UK, were able to ascertain that the savoury snack was the source of their outbreak (Shohat *et al.* 1996). Individuals with the outbreak strain were also identified in North America. However none of the European members of Salm-Net reported any increase of *S. agona* isolates.

This study therefore highlights the role of national laboratory based surveillance and the benefits of international cooperation in outbreak investigation particularly with a widely distributed food product.

Table 18.5 Association between illness due to *S. agona* phage type 15 and consumption of the kosher savoury snack

	Cases			Controls			Odds ratio (95% confidence interval)	P value (Fisher's exact test)
	Ate snack	Did not eat snack	Not sure	Ate snack	Did not eat snack	Not sure		
All cases	13	1	2	4	27	1	87.8 (7.5 to 2400)	<0.0001
Subset of cases*	6	0	2	4	27	1	∞ (14.6† to ∞)	0.0002

*Cases from preliminary inquiry excluded
†Lower limit by profile likelihood approach
British Medical Journal (1996), 313: 1109, reproduced with permission from the BMJ Publishing Group.

care for those who are ill; identifies the cause; initiates and evaluates the efficacy of control measures in preventing spread to others; and compiles a formal report. Membership will reflect those agencies involved or likely to be involved in investigating and controlling the outbreak, including environmental health, the local microbiologist, a clinician, particularly if cases are hospitalized, and a public relations officer. In zoonotic outbreaks, farm or animal investigations may be necessary and veterinary officers would attend.

Similarly in a legionnaires' disease outbreak involving industrial premises officials from the Health and Safety Executive would be involved.

When appropriate the OCT will initiate a **descriptive study** (see Chapter 3) to identify the characteristics of those affected, from which hypotheses are developed for testing in an **analytical study**. A case is defined in terms of time, place and person (Box 18.4 and Table 18.5). The initial **case definition** may be relatively broad in order to identify as many potentially affected subjects as possible, i.e. highly **sensitive** but not necessarily wholly **specific**. There may be a clinical case definition which is based on the presenting symptoms and signs found in the initial reported cases. *Confirmed cases* will be those matching the case definition with subsequent laboratory confirmation (see Box 18.4). A detailed interview of the initial cases is undertaken to ascertain the relevant symptoms and signs and risk factors/exposure histories, i.e. household and other contacts; travel history; occupational details; lifestyle factors; and knowledge of others similarly affected. In food poisoning investigations the history is usually confined to events or exposures in the 72 hours preceding illness. This period must reflect the incubation period of the anticipated organism. The initial interview is important and, on occasions, may take several hours of careful questioning to gather all relevant information. Based on these initial interviews a questionnaire is devised to capture details on all further reported cases. The investigators then need to identify other individuals who may have been infected (**case finding**). This allows the extent of the outbreak to be quantified and provides a more accurate presentation of presenting symptoms. This can include alerting local GPs, emergency departments, out of hours centres, laboratories, other consultants, and liaising with function organizers when appropriate. If cases are suspected throughout the country a national alert would be sent electronically to clinicians and infectious diseases consultants advising how suspected cases should be reported, and international liaison with ECDC and WHO may also be required.

Questionnaires may be administered by telephone, face-to-face interview, by post or e-mail. Telephone interviews are quick, cheap, and usually associated with higher response rates. Data from completed questionnaires are coded and entered into an appropriate epidemiological software package. Tables are constructed classifying the cases by age, gender, date of onset of illness, and by exposure to the main risk factors. Graphs of the occurrence of cases over time (the **epidemic curve**) can provide valuable information on the incubation period and whether the outbreak is a *point source*, e.g. a food poisoning in a hotel outbreak with a short exposure period, or a *continuing source* indicating serial transfer from the infective source. The epidemic curve can also assist monitoring the impact of control measures. Box 18.5 and Figure 18.2 describe the epidemic curve in the 2002/3 SARS outbreak and its shape is typical of a continuing source with person-to-person spread.

If a *Salmonella* outbreak is mainly in young children it could suggest a food or drink usually consumed by this group. Mapping reports of cryptosporidiosis or legionnaires' disease may reveal clusters in the distribution of a particular water supply or near a cooling tower, air-conditioning unit, or showers, taps or other sources of water aerosols in hospitals or hotels. Thus, if the preliminary, descriptive studies have revealed particular characteristics, or locations of affected individuals, further studies can be done to test particular hypotheses. The case definition may need to be reviewed and revised before commencing an analytical study, and sample size calculations are needed to ensure the study has sufficient statistical power. A **cohort study** is typically undertaken when the population at risk can be readily identified. For example at a wedding reception, all on the guest list would be contacted and details sought on the food and drinks they consumed, and whether or not they had become ill. A table is constructed comparing the number (and proportion) of those who ate a particular food item and became ill (the **attack rate**) with the number of those who did not eat the food item but who also became ill. This allows comparison of the attack rates among different groups and calculation of the relative risk of illness for each food item (Box 18.6 and Table 18.6).

A **case-control study** is performed when the population at risk is not known or it is impractical to follow up the whole population at risk. Controls should have the same chance of being exposed to the risk factor as the case. Controls could be nominated by cases, selected from general practitioner patient lists or at random from telephone records.

All studies should be supported by an environmental investigation whenever relevant and practicable. In a food poisoning outbreak this will include an inspection of the food preparation area, assessing kitchen practice

Box 18.5 Severe acute respiratory syndrome (SARS): case definitions

Clinical case

Fever of ≥ 38°C (documented or reported)

And one or more symptoms of lower respiratory tract illness (cough, difficulty breathing, shortness of breath)

And radiographic evidence of lung infiltrates consistent with pneumonia or respiratory distress syndrome (RDS) or autopsy findings consistent with the pathology of pneumonia or RDS without an identifiable cause

And no alternative diagnosis to fully explain the illness

Possible case

Meets clinical case definition

And within 10 days of onset of illness traveled to a zone of potential SARS re-emergence (currently mainland China and Hong Kong)

Or within 10 days of onset of illness a history of exposure to laboratories or institutes which have retained SARS virus isolates and/or diagnostic specimens from SARS patients

Probable case

An individual with symptoms and signs consistent with clinical SARS ('Possible case') and with preliminary laboratory evidence of SARS CoV infection based on the following:

Either Single positive antibody test for SARS CoV

Or Positive PCR for SARS CoV on a single clinical specimen and assay

Confirmed case

An individual with symptoms and signs consistent with clinical SARS ('Possible case') and with preliminary laboratory evidence of SARS CoV infection based on one or more of the following:

a) *PCR positive for SARS-CoV using a validated method from:*

At least two different clinical specimens (e.g. nasopharyngeal and stool) OR

The same clinical specimen collected on two or more occasions during the course of the illness (e.g. sequential nasopharyngeal aspirates) OR

Two different assays or repeat PCR using a new RNA extract from the original clinical sample on each occasion of testing.

b) *Seroconversion by ELISA or IFA*

Negative antibody test on acute serum followed by positive antibody test on convalescent phase serum tested in parallel OR

Fourfold or greater rise in antibody titre between the acute and convalescent phase sera tested in parallel

Reproduced from 'WHO consensus document on the epidemiology of SARS', 2003, with permission from WHO.

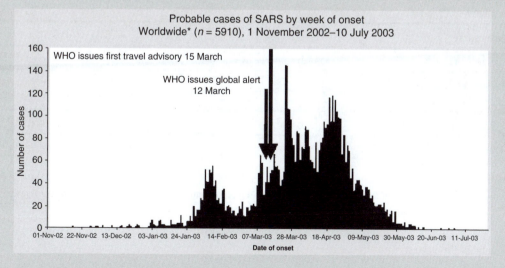

Figure 18.2 Probable cases of SARS by week of onset worldwide*. (n=5910), 1 November 2002–10 July 2003. *This graph does not include 2527 probable cases of SARS (2521 from Beijing, China), for whom no dates of onset are currently available.

Box 18.6 Cohort study of food poisoning incident.

Nine out of 24 guests at a wedding party developed gas-troenteritis between one and three days later. The menu consisted of a starter from a seafood platter or melon and strawberries. The main course consisted of duck or vegetable lasagne. A retrospective cohort study was undertaken of all the guests using a postal questionnaire containing the food items served at the party.

Twenty questionnaires were returned (87 per cent response rate). Analysis of food-specific attack rates showed that illness was significantly associated with eating items from the seafood platter. Nine of the 11 consuming raw oysters were ill compared with none of the nine who did not eat oysters. Small round-structured virus (SRSV) infection was confirmed in two cases.

Raw oysters have been frequently associated with SRSV outbreaks. In this incident it is likely that those eating oysters consumed other types of seafood from the platter.

Table 18.6 Food-specific attack rates among wedding guests

Food eaten	Ate food			Did not eat		Attack rate %	p value*
	Ill	Not ill	Attack rate %	Ill	Not ill		
First course							
Oysters	9	2	82	0	9	0	0.0003
Smoked salmon	9	3	75	0	8	0	0.001
Crab sticks	9	3	75	0	7	0	0.001
Prawns	9	4	69	0	6	0	0.005
Lettuce garnish	8	4	69	0	6	0	0.005
Melon	0	2	0	9	56	0.47	
Raspberries	1	4	25	8	6	71	0.30
Main course							
Duck with orange sauce	9	10	47	1	0	100	0.47
Mashed potato with spring onion ('champ')	5	5	50	1	5	57	0.31
Vegatable lasagne	1	0	100	8	10	44	0.47
Mixed vegetables	–	–	–	0	1	0	1.00

*Fisher's exact test.

and hygiene, and may involve study of the food supply chain. Environmental swabs and samples of remaining food items would be taken to provide additional evidence on the cause of the outbreak. In a Legionnaires' investigation an environmental assessment would be made of large air-conditioning systems and aerosol generating processes located in the vicinity of the outbreak, and appropriate water samples taken in order to detect the presence of *Legionella* which could then be compared with patient samples.

Control measures to prevent further cases should be introduced as soon as a suspect source is identified, often while awaiting the outcome of analytical studies. These include: controlling the source of infection by withdrawing infected food from sale; interrupting transmission by excluding a food handler with gastroenteritis from work; protecting others at risk by closure of a food premise pending refurbishment or deep cleaning; shut down and disinfection of an air-conditioning system; and issuing a 'boil water' notice. The impact of control measures can be monitored through the epidemic curve.

Outbreaks increasingly attract public, political, and media interest and responding to this is an ongoing challenge to the outbreak investigators. In the midst of a large outbreak it is essential to have clear lines of communication between all agencies involved, ensuring that key stakeholders and local opinion makers are regularly briefed. Surveillance for new cases should continue until the outbreak is declared over. The outbreak may be followed by legal proceedings if patients seek financial compensation for their illness and loss of earnings. The investigators' report is therefore an important document that should describe the outbreak chronology, investigations and results, control measures applied, lessons learned, including how the outbreak occurred, and how to prevent a recurrence.

Outbreak training and field epidemiology

The Centers for Disease Control, USA and the European Centres for Disease Control in Stockholm, both lead and coordinate programmes of interventional field epidemiology training, and have trained a cadre of specialist epidemiologists over many years.

Similarly, other countries in Europe, the Americas, and Asia have established field epidemiology training programmes. This strengthens the global resource available for undertaking rapid epidemiological investigations in the field, and initiating an appropriate response. WHO's Global Outbreak Alert and Response Network (GOARN) recognizes the strength of collaboration between countries and institutions for the rapid identification and response to outbreaks of international importance. Countries work in partnership to undertake these investigations in the field and limit the spread of infectious diseases internationally.

Web addresses

Notifiable diseases England and Wales 2011

http://www.legislation.gov.uk/uksi/2010/659/schedule/1/made

European Programme for Disease Prevention and Control

www.epiet.org

Centers for Disease Control: Control-Epidemiology Intelligence Service

www.cdc.gov/eis

WHO Outbreak Network

www.who.int/csr/outbreaknetwork

European Centre for Disease Prevention and Control

http://www.ecdc.europa.eu/en/Pages/home.aspx

References

Ada G (2001) Vaccines and vaccination. *The New England Journal of Medicine* **345** (14), 1042–53.

Aguzzi A and Zhu C (2012) Five questions on prion diseases. *PLoS Pathogens* **8** (5) e1002651. Epub 2012 May 3.

Allegranzi B and Pittet D (2009) Role of hand hygiene in healthcare-associated infection prevention. *The Journal of Hospital Infection* **73** (4), 305–15.

Amodu OK, Olaniyan SA, Adeyemo AA, Troye-Blomberg M, *et al.* (2012) Association of the sickle cell trait and the ABO blood group with clinical severity of malaria in southwest Nigeria. *ActaTropica* **123** (2), 72–7.

Anon (1988) Guidelines for evaluating surveillance systems. *Morbidity and Mortality Weekly Report* **6** 37 Suppl. 51–8.

Anon (2011) Limited human-to-human transmission of novel influenza A (H3N2) virus—Iowa. *Morbidity and Mortality Weekly Report* **60** (47), 1615–17.

Antia R, Regoes RR, Koella JC, and Bergstrom CT (2003) The role of evolution in the emergence of infectious diseases. *Nature* **426** (6967), 658–61.

Ang LH (1998) An outbreak of viral gastroenteritis associated with eating raw oysters. *Communicable Disease and Public Health / PHLS* **1** (1), 38–40.

Baker M, Smith GE, Cooper D, Verlander NQ, *et al.* (2003) Early warning and NHS Direct: a role in community surveillance? *Journal of Public Health Medicine* **25** (4), 362–8.

Barré-Sinoussi F, Chermann JC, Rey F, Nugeyre MT, *et al.* (1983) Isolation of a T-lymphotropic retrovirus from a patient at risk for acquired immune deficiency syndrome (AIDS). *Science (New York, NY)* **220** (4599), 868–71.

Brisson M, van de Velde N, Franco EL, Drolet M, *et al.* (2011) Incremental impact of adding boys to current human papillomavirus vaccination programs: role of herd immunity. *The Journal of Infectious Diseases* **204** (3), 372–6.

CDC (2010) *The 2009 H1N1 Pandemic: Summary Highlights, April 2009–April 2010.* Available at: http://www.cdc.gov/h1n1flu/cdcresponse.htm

Chen RT and Orenstein WA (1996) Epidemiologic methods in immunization programs. *Epidemiologic Reviews* **18** (2), 99–117.

CJD Research and Surveillance Unit (2008) *Creutzfeldt-Jakob disease in the UK. Seventh annual report 2008.* Available from: www.cjd.ed.ac.uk

Cortes JE, Curns AT, Tate JE, Cortese MM, *et al.* (2011) Rotavirus vaccine and health care utilization for diarrhea in U.S. children. *The New England Journal of Medicine* **365** (12), 1108–17.

Damani NN (2012) *Manual of Infection Control Procedures*, 3rd edn. Oxford: Oxford University Press.

do Carmo GMI, Yen C, Cortes J, Siqueira AA, *et al.* (2011) Decline in diarrhea mortality and admissions after routine childhood rotavirus immunization in Brazil: a time-series analysis. *PLoS Medicine* **8** (4), e1001024.

Farmer RDT, Miller D, and Lawrenson R (1996) *Lecture Notes on Epidemiology and Public Health*, 4th edn. Oxford, Blackwell.

Fidler DP and Gostin LO (2011) The WHO pandemic influenza preparedness framework: a milestone in global governance for health. *JAMA* **306** (2), 200–1.

Giesecke J (2001) *Modern Infectious Disease Epidemiology*. London: Taylor & Francis.

Gilbert MTP, Rambaut A, Wlasiuk G, Spira TJ, *et al.* (2007) The emergence of HIV/AIDS in the Americas and beyond. *Proceedings of the National Academy of Sciences of the United States of America* **104** (47), 18566–70.

Grimwood K, Lambert SB, and Milne RJ (2010) Rotavirus infections and vaccines: burden of illness and potential impact of vaccination. *Paediatric Drugs* **12** (4), 235–6.

Hall R and Jolley D (2011) International measles incidence and immunization coverage. *The Journal of Infectious Diseases* **204** Suppl. 1S158–63.

Hawker J, Begg N, Blair I, Reintjes R, *et al.* (2005) *Communicable Disease Control Handbook*, 2nd edn. Oxford: Blackwell Publishing.

Health Protection Agency (2011) *Surveillance of Influenza and Other Respiratory Viruses in the UK: 2010–2011 Report*. London: Health Protection Agency.

Herfst S, Schrauwen EJA, Linster M, Chutinimitkul S, *et al.* (2012) Airborne transmission of influenza A/H5N1 virus between ferrets. *Science (New York, NY)*. **336** (6088), 1534–41.

Hutton G, Haller L, and Bartram J (2007) Global cost-benefit analysis of water supply and sanitation interventions. *Journal of Water and Health* **5** (4), 481–502.

Imai M, Watanabe T, Hatta M, Das SC, *et al.* (2012) Experimental adaptation of an influenza H5 HA confers respiratory droplet transmission to a reassortant H5 HA/H1N1 virus in ferrets. *Nature* **486** (7403), 420–8.

Institute of Medicine (2010) (US) *Forum on Microbial Threats. Infectious Disease Movement in a Borderless World: Workshop Summary*. Washington, DC: National Academies Press (US). Available from: http://www.ncbi.nlm.nih.gov/books/NBK45724/?report=printable

Kahn JG, Muraguri N, Harris B, Lugada E, *et al.* (2012) Integrated HIV testing, malaria, and diarrhea prevention campaign in Kenya: modeled health impact and cost-effectiveness. *PLoS One* **7** (2), e31316.

Killalea D, Ward LR, Roberts D, de Louvois J, *et al.* (1996) International epidemiological and microbiological study of outbreak of Salmonella agona infection from a ready to eat savoury snack—I: England and Wales and the United States. *BMJ (Clinical Research Ed)* **313** (7065), 1105–7.

Langmuir AD (1963) The surveillance of communicable diseases of national importance. *The New England Journal of Medicine* **268**, 182–92.

Mead S (2006) Prion disease genetics. *European Journal of Human Genetics: EJHG* **14** (3), 273–81.

Morris JG Jr (2011) Cholera—modern pandemic disease of ancient lineage. *Emerging Infectious Diseases* **17** (11), 2099–104.

Nathanson N, Wilesmith J, and Griot C (1997) Bovine spongiform encephalopathy (BSE): causes and consequences of a common source epidemic. *American Journal of Epidemiology* **145** (11), 959–69.

Neil KP, Sodha SV, Lukwago L, O-Tipo S, *et al.* (2012) A large outbreak of typhoid fever associated with a high rate of intestinal perforation in Kasese District, Uganda, 2008–2009. *Clinical Infectious Diseases* **54** (8), 1091–9.

Paweska JT, Sewlall NH, Ksiazek TG, Blumberg LH, *et al.* (2009) Nosocomial outbreak of novel arenavirus infection, southern Africa. *Emerging Infectious Diseases* **15** (10), 1598–602.

Piot P, Kazatchkine M, Dybul M, and Lob-Levyt J (2009) AIDS: lessons learnt and myths dispelled. *Lancet* **374** (9685), 260–3.

Presanis AM, Pebody RG, Paterson BJ, Tom BDM, *et al.* (2011) Changes in severity of 2009 pandemic A/H1N1 influenza in England: a Bayesian evidence synthesis. *BMJ (Clinical Research Ed)* **343**, d5408.

Ramsay ME, Andrews NJ, Trotter CL, Kaczmarski EB, *et al.* (2003) Herd immunity from meningococcal serogroup C conjugate vaccination in England: database analysis. *BMJ (Clinical Research Ed)* **326** (7385), 365–6.

Rosenthal PJ (2011) Lessons from sickle cell disease in the treatment and control of malaria. *The New England Journal of Medicine* **364** (26), 2549–51.

Russell CA, Fonville JM, Brown AEX, Burke DF, *et al.* (2012) The potential for respiratory droplet-transmissible A/H5N1 influenza virus to evolve in a mammalian host. *Science (New York, NY)* **336** (6088), 1541–7.

Shao Y and Williamson C (2012) The HIV-1 epidemic: low- to middle-income countries. *Cold Spring Harbor Perspectives in Medicine* **2** (3), a007187.

Shohat T, Green MS, Merom D, Gill ON, *et al.* (1996) International epidemiological and microbiological study of outbreak of Salmonella agona infection from a ready to eat savoury snack—II: Israel. *BMJ (Clinical Research Ed)* **313** (7065), 1107–9.

Soon JM, Baines R, and Seaman P (2012) Meta-analysis of food safety training on hand hygiene knowledge and attitudes among food handlers. *Journal of Food Protection* **75** (4), 793–804.

Tate JE, Burton AH, Boschi-Pinto C, Steele AD, *et al.* (2012) 2008 estimate of worldwide rotavirus-associated mortality in children younger than 5 years before the introduction of universal rotavirus vaccination programmes: a systematic review and meta-analysis. *The Lancet Infectious Diseases* **12** (2), 136–41.

Tay S-K (2012) Cervical cancer in the human papillomavirus vaccination era. *Current Opinion in Obstetrics & Gynecology* **24** (1), 3–7.

Tu H-AT, Woerdenbag HJ, Kane S, Rozenbaum MH, *et al.* (2011) Economic evaluations of rotavirus immunization for developing countries: a review of the literature. *Expert Review of Vaccines* **10** (7), 1037–51.

UNAIDS (2010) *Global Report for 2010.* Available at: http://www.unaids.org/en/media/unaids/contentassets/documents/unaidspublication/2010/20101123_globalreport_en%5B1%5D.pdf

Webster RG (2004) Wet markets—a continuing source of severe acute respiratory syndrome and influenza? *Lancet* **363** (9404), 234–6.

WHO (2005) *International Health Regulations. 2nd edn.* Geneva: World Health Organization.

WHO (2009) Healthcare Infections. Available at:http://www.who.int/gpsc/en/.

WHO (2010) Global Immunization Data. World Health Organization. Available at: http://www.who.int/immunization_monitoring/Global_Immunization_Data.pdf on 08/11/11

WHO (2011a) *Global Tuberculosis Control: WHO Report 2011.* Geneva: World Health Organization.

WHO (2011b) *World Malaria Report 2011.* Geneva: World Health Organization.

WHO (2012a) Global Influenza Surveillance and Response System (GISRS). Available at: http://www.who.int/influenza/gisrs_laboratory/en/.

WHO (2012b) *Immunizations.* Geneva: World Health Organization.

WHO (2012c) Global Alert and Response (GAR). Available at: http://who.int/csn/en/.

Will RG, Ironside JW, Zeidler M, Cousens SN, *et al.* (1996) A new variant of Creutzfeldt-Jakob disease in the UK. *Lancet* **347** (9006), 921–5.

Model answer

Question 1

In the UK and most high-income countries screening for HIV infection is available antenatally. At booking clinic (the initial antenatal appointment in the UK), this will be done with the informed consent of the mother. In HIV-positive cases early treatment in pregnancy reduces the likelihood of the virus being passed to the fetus. In HIV-positive cases breastfeeding is contraindicated. In low-income countries sentinel surveillance is conducted at antenatal clinics where resources are available and this is widely used by UNAIDS to monitor trends in the prevalence of HIV.

19 Genetic epidemiology

AMY JAYNE MCKNIGHT AND PETER MAXWELL

CHAPTER CONTENTS

In this chapter the molecular basis of genetic disease is outlined with an explanation of the key differences between monogenic, polygenic, and multifactorial diseases. A background understanding of basic genetics is assumed. Study designs and techniques used in genetic epidemiology are discussed alongside strategies for identifying risk loci involved in specific diseases or biological pathways. Finally pharmacogenetics and the complex ethical issues concerning genetic testing and screening are briefly reviewed.

Introduction

Genetic epidemiology focuses upon the role of inherited factors in disease aetiology, with the aims of establishing:

1 whether there is a genetic contribution to disease;

2 the relative size of the genetic effect;

3 if inherited risk factors contribute to disease susceptibility;

4 better tools for disease prediction, prevention, and treatment.

Genetic epidemiology has been defined as: 'the study of the joint actions of genes and environmental factors in causing disease in human populations and their patterns of inheritance in families' (Morton 1982).

Genetic epidemiology research strategies may also help to pinpoint specific molecular pathways implicated in a disorder. It has been stated that, 'except for some cases of trauma, it is fair to say that virtually every human illness has a hereditary component' (Collins 2011). Genetic epidemiology therefore encompasses a very broad range of clinical disorders. Considerable success has been achieved identifying disease-causing mutations for a wide variety of **Mendelian** ('single-gene' or monogenic) **disorders**, but there has been much slower progress unravelling the interactions between inherited and environmental factors that contribute to **multifactorial**, common complex diseases such as diabetes mellitus, cardiovascular disease, and cancer. Some basic terms used in this chapter are summarized in Box 19.1.

19.1 Genetic information: understanding the language

Understanding the role of genetics in disease causation requires a working knowledge of the principles governing Mendelian inheritance. Genetic information is stored in chromosomes and encoded

Box 19.1 Glossary of basic terms

alleles Alternative forms of the same gene occurring at a specific locus. One allele is inherited from the father and the other from the mother.

allelic heterogeneity Where the same phenotype results from different mutations in the same gene in separate individuals. For example, autosomal dominant polycystic kidney disease.

aneuploidy A chromosome complement with one or more chromosomes extra or missing.

association A statistical observation where disease and a genetic marker occur together more frequently than would be expected by chance.

autosomes Any chromosome other than the sex (X or Y) chromosomes.

base Chemical building block of DNA—A (adenine), T (thymine), C (cytosine), and G (guanine).

base-pairs Bases on opposite strands of DNA in the double helix. Permitted base pairings are AT and GC.

chromosome abnormality Disruption of the normal chromosome content; typically a duplication but can refer to any abnormality in chromosomal structure.

co-dominant Alleles that are both expressed in the heterozygote (e.g. ABO blood groups).

codon The sequence of nucleotide triplet, which determines what specific amino acid will be inserted into a polypeptide chain.

common disease-common variant A hypothesis that predicts that common genetic variants will be found in a population suffering from a common disease.

concordance The degree of similarity between individuals for a particular trait.

copy number variation Different numbers of copies of specific genetic regions between individuals.

cytogenetics The scientific study of chromosome structure and function.

degenerate Different nucleotide trios can encode the same amino acid.

deletion Loss of a segment of genetic material from a chromosome.

dizygotic Twins arising from two eggs separately fertilized by two sperm.

dominant The trait which is expressed in the heterozygous state.

duplication Addition of genetic material where a chromosome segment occurs more than once in the haploid genome.

epigenome Represents those structural modifications to DNA (such as methylation) or histone proteins which are potentially modifiable.

epistasis The alteration of expression of a gene by the effect of another gene.

epigenetic Heritable feature that is not transmitted by a change in DNA sequence; for example, DNA methylation.

exon Segment of gene retained during splicing, includes the protein coding DNA sequence of a gene.

familial trait A characteristic that occurs within families more often than expected by chance and which is often suspected to be genetic in nature.

gene Functional unit of heredity.

genetic association The occurrence, more often than can be readily explained by chance, of genotypes occurring with disease in a population.

genetic marker Any variation in DNA, typically used to investigate specific regions of chromosomes.

genome-wide association study Common approach to investigate genetic susceptibility to complex diseases.

genotype A description of the base pairs for a particular individual.

genotype–phenotype correlation The relationship by which genotype can predict the phenotype. Suboptimal correlation, particularly for complex diseases, makes genetic testing and counselling difficult.

haplotype A series of alleles from two or more linked loci on a single chromosome.

heritability The proportion of a disease or trait which can be attributed to genetic causes by regression/correlation analysis among twins or other close family members.

human genome The total content of DNA in each individual. The human genome comprises a mitochondrial chromosome, plus 22 autosomes, plus two sex chromosomes.

imprinting The phenomenon of differential expression of genes according to whether they are inherited from the father or mother.

incomplete penetrance Not all individuals with a mutation will develop the relevant phenotype.

intron Segment of gene removed during splicing; may contain important regulatory elements.

karyotype The chromosome complement of a cell; often represented by an arrangement of metaphase

(continued)

chromosomes according to their lengths and to the positions of their centromeres.

linkage The association of genes on the same chromosome.

linkage analysis A statistical analysis which is used to estimate distances between genes along particular chromosomes following recombination. Typical measure of the likelihood of linkage is the **LOD score**.

linkage disequilibrium Non-random association of alleles within a randomly mating population.

locus Unique chromosome location describing the position of a genetic feature.

Mendelian disorder A disorder or trait inherited in a Mendelian manner such as cystic fibrosis; typically due to a major single gene effect.

Mendelian randomization Approach to evaluate a causal genetic effect in the presence of confounding.

mitochondrial DNA (mtDNA) DNA contained in mitochondria that consists of a single circular DNA molecule.

monozygotic A member of a twin pair or multiple birth group derived from the same fertilized ovum.

multifactorial When used in genetics, this usually refers to characteristics caused by a combination of genetic and environmental factors, such as hypertension. Also refers to 'complex' diseases.

next-generation resequencing A high-throughput, massively parallel DNA sequencing approach.

pedigree A family tree which assists the detection of inherited traits and the mode of inheritance.

phenotype The observable characteristics exhibited by an individual.

pleiotropic Multiple characteristics resulting from variation in a particular gene.

polygenic Characteristics derived from the combined action of several genes.

polymerase chain reaction Repeated cycles of DNA denaturation, annealing of primer sequences, and replication, resulting in exponential growth in the number of copies of the DNA sequence located between a pair of primers.

polymorphism A term often used to indicate any genetic variation but strictly the occurrence of two or more variants at a frequency ≥ 1 per cent in a population. Single nucleotide polymorphisms (SNPs) are a specific class of polymorphism studied by molecular geneticists and may be pathogenic.

population stratification The existence of genetically different groups within a population supposed to be homogeneous; systematic ancestry differences between cases and controls.

quantitative trait locus (QTLs) A chromosome location that affects a continuous characteristic measured on a quantitative (linear) scale.

recessive The trait which is expressed only in the homozygous state.

recombination Normally occurs during meiosis where breaks in homologous chromosome pairs allow for the reciprocal exchange of chromosome segments.

segregation analysis The general statistical methodology for determining a pattern of inheritance.

splicing Processing of genetic material whereby the introns are removed and exons are joined together for a given gene.

systems biology An inter-disciplinary field of research that examines the complex interactions between different biological systems.

transcription The synthesis of RNA from a DNA template.

translation The synthesis of protein from messenger RNA template.

translocation Transfer of chromosome segments between non-homologous chromosomes.

twin/adoption study Study based on monozygotic and dizygotic twins which aim to distinguish genetic and environmental causes of disease. Studies of adopted twins raised in different environments represent an extension of this approach.

whole-exome sequencing A laboratory method to determine the DNA sequence of protein coding regions (exons) within genes.

whole-genome sequencing: A laboratory method to determine the entire DNA sequence of an organism or individual.

X-linked Characteristics that are transmitted with the X chromosome. For example, a father (XY) with an X-linked dominant disorder such as vitamin D-resistant rickets will pass this onto his daughter (XX), but never to his son (XY).

by double-stranded deoxyribose nucleic acid (DNA) which is made up of a sugar, a phosphate, and a base. Each human cell typically contains 23 chromosome pairs of which 22 are termed **autosomes** (numbered 1–22 according to size), plus one pair of **sex (X or Y) chromosomes** where females have XX and males XY paired chromosomes. The particular sequence alignment of the various DNA bases—adenine (A), guanine (G), cytosine (C), thymine (T) on each chromosome, determines the specific genetic information for an individual. **Base-pairs** are linked across the two adjacent, but separate strands of the DNA double helix molecule. Base-pairs are limited in that **base** A can only pair with T, and G can only pair with C. During cell division the entire DNA of the cell is copied: DNA strands separate, complementary strands are synthesized, and two duplicate DNA sequences are produced. During **transcription**, DNA is copied into single-stranded ribonucleic acid (RNA), which is similar to DNA, but base T is replaced by U (uracil), after which three-base units, together with the sugar and phosphate component (**codons**) form the template molecule known as messenger RNA (mRNA). **Translation** describes the process of protein assembly from this mRNA template. Several triplet codons can code for the same amino acid and this codon redundancy is said to be **degenerate**. A **gene** is a DNA sequence that represents a functional unit of hereditary; genes often encode proteins, but non-protein coding genes also perform important regulatory roles (Guttman 2009). **Exons** are the parts of a gene typically translated into protein whereas **introns** are the sections that are removed (by **splicing**) during translation of mRNA to protein. Fig. 19.1 shows the essential elements of genetic structure as the DNA double helix, an annotated chromosome and gene structure respectively.

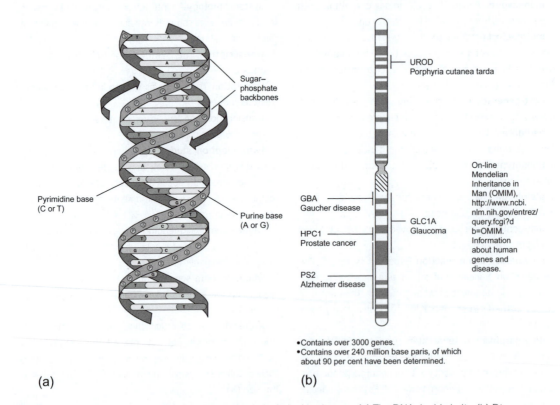

(a)

(b)

Figure 19.1 Genes are stored in chromosomes and may be linked to disease. (a) The DNA double helix. (b) Diseases mapped to chromosome 1.

Source: (a) Mange and Mange (1999). (b) U.S. Department of Energy Genomic Science program,
http://genomicscience.energy.gov.

Version 37.3 of the **human genome** contains approximately 36,000 genes and more than 50 million genetic differences between individuals have been annotated within the three billion bases that comprise the human genome.

Genetic variation may be large-scale involving chromosome sets (**polyploidy**), whole chromosomes (**aneuploidy**), or rearrangement of chromosome segments (**translocation, deletion, duplications** and **inversions**). Each individual human genome contains large numbers of smaller changes within DNA sequences, e.g. single base substitutions, insertions or deletions that are known as **single nucleotide polymorphisms (SNPs)**. Single nucleotide polymorphisms may directly affect gene function or act as **genetic markers** that are correlated with particular characteristics (**phenotypes**) including diseases and drug responses. **Non-synonymous SNPs** are genetic variants that occur within exons resulting in a change in the expected amino acid sequence of a protein. Other SNPs occur in non-protein coding regions of DNA, but these may also affect protein synthesis and function by influencing the regulation of nearby genes. Common SNPs (present at greater than five per cent in the general population) may be associated with only a modest increase in disease risk, however because of their higher frequency in the population, these **polymorphisms** can have a large **population attributable risk** and consequently a significant impact on disease burden.

Mutations in DNA can result from replication errors during cell division, exposure to ionizing radiation, exposure to chemicals called mutagens, or infections. Germ line mutations occur in the gametes (eggs and sperm) and are transmitted to offspring. In contrast, somatic mutations occur in body cells and are not heritable, although these are passed through successive generations of cells in cancer and other diseases. **Epigenetics** is a rapidly evolving discipline which studies such mechanisms involving somatic alterations in gene expression and are particularly important in cancer studies where hypermethylation of DNA can result in the silencing of tumour-suppressing genes and hypomethylation can result in the activation of oncogenes (Handel *et al.* 2010). The science of epigenetics

is likely to become increasingly important for epidemiology; a number of diseases are potentially epigenetic in nature resulting from gene–environmental interactions including cancers, psychoses, depression, multiple sclerosis, COPD, asthma and obesity (Handel *et al.* 2010). The potential use of DNA methylation in white blood cells as a biomarker for environmental exposures is discussed in detail elsewhere (Terry *et al.* 2011).

The human genome is also affected by **copy number variation (CNV)** whereby individuals have different numbers of copies of specific genetic regions within their genome; it is believed that more genetic variation is due to copy number variation than single base changes (Alkan *et al.* 2011). An **allele** is one of two or more alternative forms of a defined DNA sequence. For example, most persons have two functional (normal) alleles of the phenylalanine hydroxylase (*PAH*) gene, whereas asymptomatic carriers of phenylketonuria (PKU) have one functional allele and one mutant allele. Classical PKU is an autosomal **recessive** condition so that individuals with the disease have two mutant alleles, i.e. they have inherited a mutant allele from each parent. More than 500 individual disease-causing mutations in the *PAH* gene have been identified illustrating that a clinical disorder can be caused by different mutations within the same gene. The **genotype** is the composition of alleles present in an individual at a given position. A **phenotype** refers to clinically observable characteristics that are often influenced by a specific genotype. The phenotype can be a trait such as eye colour, a physiological variable such as serum cholesterol or blood pressure, or a disease such as PKU or diabetes. Diseases inherited in a Mendelian manner are typically rare, occurring in less than one in 200 births. **Incomplete penetrance** of a single gene mutation (variation in the extent of the gene's expression in the phenotype) can complicate the interpretation of the pattern of inheritance. **Mendelian disorders** which are not completely penetrant may appear to be non-Mendelian when examined in a family pedigree. Mendelian disorders may be caused by multiple mutations in the same gene, multiple mutations in the same biological pathway, or inherited variation in modifier genes that impact upon the primary disease-causing mutation. For example, cystic fibrosis (CF) is caused

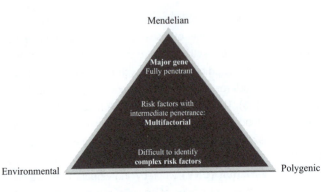

Figure 19.2 Genetic and environmental contributions to inherited disease.
Adapted from Strachan T and Read A P (2004). *Human and Molecular Genetics*, 3rd edn, with permission from Garland Science.

by mutations in the cystic fibrosis transmembrane conductance regulator (*CFTR*) gene; however several additional genes are proposed to modify CF disease severity (Witt 2011). Complex inherited diseases may be multifactorial and/or polygenic, influenced by gene–environment interactions involving more than one gene. The complexity of inherited and environmental factors is illustrated in Fig. 19.2.

Techniques to identify genetic variation

Cytogenetics encompasses methods for the direct visualization and evaluation of chromosome number, structure, and abnormalities. Historically, chromosomes were investigated by means of a **karyotype** analysis where cytogenetic dyes were added to track genetic regions on chromosomes. Chromosome pairs are aligned to ensure that no genetic material has been deleted, duplicated, or rearranged. Numerical and structural changes are increasingly being evaluated using microarrays and 'next-generation' sequencing technologies which are faster and typically provide more information than a traditional karyotype. To identify small to moderate genetic variation, specific regions of DNA can be amplified (copied) using a technique known as **polymerase chain reaction (PCR)**. Single nucleotide polymorphisms may be investigated using enzyme or dye-based experiments that assay known single base changes at a precise positions (*uniplex assays*). *Multiplex assays* examine combinations of small genetic variants (SNPs and CNVs) and the assays may be based on

mass spectrometry (up to 40 SNPs) or array hybridization (hundreds to millions of SNPs). Further development of these microarray techniques has enabled the rapid genotyping of up to five million common and rarer genetic variants from a single DNA sample. Technological advances have also made it possible to identify the complete base sequence for each individual's entire genome by comprehensive **next-Generation resequencing**.

19.2 Mendelian disorders

The simplest genetic disorders are those which depend on the genotype at a single site (also known as a **locus**). This altered genotype may be **necessary** and **sufficient** for the character or trait to be expressed. Such characters, traits, and diseases follow the patterns of inheritance first described for plants by Mendel. These diseases are usually rare, conferring a small population-attributable risk. Essential sources of reference include the Online Mendelian Inheritance in Man (OMIM) and Orphanet resources (see 'Web addresses' section at the end of the chapter). Such diseases may have different family **pedigree** patterns of inheritance. If the mutant allele results in the same phenotype irrespective of the second allele, the mutant allele is said to be **dominant** (e.g. Huntington's disease). If the mutant allele is required in both chromosomes (homozygous) to yield the phenotype, then it is termed **recessive** (e.g. cystic fibrosis). If the phenotype for the heterozygous genotype is intermediate, displaying characteristics of each allele, then the alleles are **co-dominant** (e.g. ABO blood groups).

X-linked disorders such as colour blindness carry the mutation on the X chromosome and are often recessive, thus conferring carrier status on females who have the mutation on one of their two X chromosomes, but causing disease in males who have only one X chromosome. Diseases caused by mutations in **mitochondrial DNA (mtDNA)** typically demonstrate variable expression of the clinical phenotype and are transmitted through the maternal line in the egg's cytoplasm. Mitochondria are specialized cellular structures that generate energy; these contain additional DNA (mtDNA) which is approximately 16.5 kb long, contains 37 essential genes, and is stored as a single chromosome.

19.3 Multifactorial disorders

Multifactorial diseases have complex inheritance patterns. For dichotomous traits (present/absent) the underlying genetic loci are designated *susceptibility loci*, while for quantitative or continuous traits they are termed *quantitative trait loci (QTL)*. If there are also important environmental factors contributing to risk, the disease is considered to be **multifactorial**. For many common diseases, (e.g. hypertension, coronary artery disease, diabetes, and most cancers) known genetic risk factors appear to account for only a fraction of the estimated genetic component or heritability of the disease. This may be because current knowledge does not explain several characteristics of 'genetic' diseases, including age of onset, sex-specific effects such as **imprinting** (in the child a gene originating from the father may be expressed differently to the same gene coming from the mother), interactions between multiple genes and the environment, the impact of differential DNA methylation patterns or small non-coding RNAs on gene expression, and secular trends in disease presentation. Extensive, multidisciplinary, collaborative research is unravelling the complexity of the genetic architecture for multifactorial diseases.

The **heritability** (genetic risk) of asthma provides a good example of some practical challenges in understanding the genetic epidemiology of a multifactorial disorder. The estimated heritability was reported to be 50 per cent based on studies conducted in the 1970s. Recent data from Nordic countries revised the estimated heritability figure upwards to 70 per cent. Asthma prevalence has rapidly increased in some areas of the world, e.g. Africa and Eastern Europe whilst in other locations asthma prevalence has increased in the past, but more recently has remained static or even decreased, e.g. Western Europe (Pearce *et al.* 2007). The relative frequency of gene variants conferring an inherited susceptibility to asthma cannot change much in one or two generations. Epigenetic changes in the immune response following environmental triggers from respiratory viruses and subsequent exposure to other allergens have been proposed as the important determinants of asthma (Kumar *et al.* 2009), which suggests a changing pattern of exposure to environmental allergens.

Genes may also have multiple (**pleiotropic**) effects. This is exemplified by the apolipoprotein E (*APOE*) gene which has a modest effect on determining serum cholesterol levels. It has been suggested that lipids and lipoproteins may have roles as natural antiviral agents. If so, variation in a gene that affects cholesterol levels, such as *APOE*, could have been 'selected for' due to beneficial antiviral effects. Nevertheless, the specific *APOE**E4 allele is associated with a greatly increased risk of Alzheimer's disease. Hence a gene whose primary effect is on lipid metabolism may have pleiotropic effects which can result in pathological changes in the brain of older adults. Similarly, gene mutations that lead to thalassaemia and sickle cell disease are relatively common in some populations as the heterozygous carrier status for a mutant allele provided natural protection against malaria. There was evolutionary selection pressure for this 'genetic advantage' as resistance to malaria was more beneficial to the population albeit at the expense of some individuals, homozygous for the mutant alleles, dying from a blood disorder.

19.4 Methods in genetic epidemiology

The major study designs currently used in genetic epidemiology are introduced in Table 19.1. Descriptive

Table 19.1 Study designs in genetic epidemiology of complex disorders

Design	Advantages	Limitations
Descriptive		
Ecological	Simple to conduct	Subject to confounding
Migrant	Simple to conduct	Migrant selection bias may operate
Familial aggregation		
Family	Relatively simple to conduct	Uncertain genotypic prediction
Twin	High level of genotypic accuracy if	Accurate twin registers required
Twin adoption	monozygotic or dizygotic twin status	Confidentiality and ethical issues
	correctly identified	restrict utility
	As above	
Population-based studies		
Case-control	Simple to conduct	Selection biases are likely
Cohort	Minimal selection bias; exposures	Expensive and difficult to mount
	examined prospectively	

studies have tended to fall into the domain of classical epidemiology, whereas family and population-based studies are largely conducted by epidemiologists and biostatisticians specializing in genetics.

Descriptive epidemiology

Genetic and environmental clues to disease aetiology can be gleaned from classical epidemiological studies. The pattern of international variation in disease, changes in disease risk among migrants, and also temporal, racial, and sociodemographic variations often yield valuable insights. For example breast cancer incidence varies more than 10-fold between countries implying that there are differences in genetic or environmental exposures, or both. Ecological comparisons of sex hormone levels among low-risk Chinese compared to (high-risk) Western populations, suggest that, given differences in the prevalence of polymorphisms in genes controlling hormone metabolism, a genetic component to breast cancer is probable. Nevertheless, breast cancer incidence has been observed to increase in women migrating from relatively low breast cancer incidence countries to high-risk countries, confirming also the importance of environmental risk factors (Ziegler et al. 1993).

Familial aggregation

If a genetic contribution to a particular disease is suspected then efforts are made to estimate the risk of transmission in families. The disease risk (or strength of familial aggregation/degree of clustering) in relatives of an affected individual, is compared with the general risk of this disease in the population. This risk is termed the recurrence risk or familial risk ratio (λ). Early examples of familial risk of some congenital malformations are shown in Table 19.2, and strongly suggest a genetic component. Familial aggregation of disease may also indicate shared environmental risk factors, but the larger the gradient from identical twins to first and second degree relatives, the more likely the pattern is due to major genetic factors. Congenital abnormalities are further discussed in Chapter 16.

Case-control comparisons of family history or **twin/ adoption studies** are most useful, but **cohort studies** can also be informative for common diseases. Alternatively, a **familial trait** may be investigated by estimating **heritability (h^2)**, which is the proportion of the total variance in a trait that can be explained by genetic effects. Heritability only applies to the population on which observations are made and cannot be used to explain differences between populations, since

Table 19.2 Familial patterns in congenital malformation

Congenital abnormalities	'Incidence' relative to the general population			
	Monozygotic twins	First-degree relatives	Second-degree relatives	Third-degree relatives
Cleft lip (± cleft palate)	x 400	x 40	x 7	x 3
Club foot	x 300	x 25	x 5	x 2
Neural tube defects		x 8		x 2
Congenital dislocation of hip (females)	x 200	x 25	x 3	x 2
Pyloric stenosis (males)	x 80	x 10	x 5	x 1.5

Sources: Carter (1968); Smith and Aase (1970).

populations may differ in their allele frequencies and/or in the environmental exposures.

Twin studies play an important role in probing the genetic component of disease causation. A high **concordance** rate in **monozygotic** (MZ) twins (whose genetic identities are the same) compared to that in **dizygotic** (DZ) twins, (who share 50 per cent of their genes and are no more like than non-twin siblings), provides evidence that genes contribute significantly to familial aggregation for a particular disease. Concordance, however, may be prone to **ascertainment bias** since affected co-twins will be more likely to join a volunteer study. In addition, the twin design assumes that the degree of sharing of their environment is the same for both types of twins and, in general, an increased risk in family members does not necessarily indicate that the disease has an inherited component, but may be related to a shared environment which may include behavioural, biological, and physical components (e.g. smoking, diet, physical activity, infections, climate, and housing). For example, MZ twins tend to select similar habits and micro-environments more commonly than DZ twins. However, as noted in Table 19.3, stratification of risk by degree of relatedness (first-degree versus second-degree relatives), and comparisons with unrelated individuals living in the same household (typically spouses), can assist in distinguishing genetic and non-genetic familial effects, while a detailed extended family history may provide crucial information about the level of genetic risk.

Among over 4000 twin pairs from six European countries and Australia, heritabilities were 52–66 per cent for systolic blood pressure and 44–66 per cent for diastolic blood pressure, with little to no evidence of a significant contribution from a shared family environment. This suggests that the remainder of the contribution to these traits is due to individual, non-shared behaviours and/or environments (Evans et al. 2003; see Table 19.3). Genetic heterogeneity exists for blood pressure where multiple variants in several genes interact with environmental stimuli; it is believed rare genetic variants contribute substantially to risk within individual families although not at a population level.

Twin studies, therefore, can assist in partitioning the three types of influence on a particular trait: genetic (heritability), shared environment (family members), non-shared environment (individual). However, in adoption studies, correlation of a phenotype between adoptive siblings can only be due to shared environment. The correlation of a phenotype between adoptive and biological siblings can be used to estimate a genetic component, and shared and non-shared environmental components. Combinations of designs, such as the inclusion of parents and siblings in twin studies, can permit more incisive estimation of the role of genetic factors by taking account of systematic genetic differences (**population stratification**) between unrelated case-control groups.

Table 19.3 Twin correlations (r) and heritability (h^2) with 95% confidence intervals (CI), based on age and sex adjusted data

	MZm	DZm	MZf	DZf	Heritability	
	r	r	r	r	h^2	(95% CIs)
Systolic blood pressure						
Australia	0.47	0.15	0.55	0.28	0.52	(0.44, 0.59)
Denmark	0.60	0.32	0.70	0.46	0.66	(0.60, 0.71)
Finland	0.45	0.33	0.50	0.43	0.53	(0.46, 0.60)
Netherlands	0.50	0.25	0.47	0.36	0.54	(0.44, 0.62)
Sweden	0.51	0.28	0.51	0.28	0.54	(0.41, 0.65)
UK	–	–	0.56	0.27	0.53	(0.48, 0.58)
Diastolic blood pressure						
Australia	0.47	0.23	0.53	0.39	0.51	(0.44, 0.58)
Denmark	0.63	0.31	0.71	0.43	0.66	(0.60, 0.71)
Finland	0.40	0.29	0.50	0.38	0.47	(0.39, 0.54)
Netherlands	0.51	0.28	0.46	0.30	0.53	(0.44, 0.61)
Sweden	0.24	0.31	0.50	0.16	0.44	(0.29, 0.56)
UK	–	–	0.49	0.23	0.48	(0.42, 0.53)

MZm/f—monozygotic male/female
DZm/f—dizygotic male/female.
Reproduced from Evans A *et al*, The genetics of coronary heart disease: the contribution of twin studies, *Twin Research* **6** (5), 432–41, 2003, with permission from Cambridge University Press.

Segregation analysis

Before the advent of routine molecular techniques, the genetic component of a particular disease was usually examined by **segregation analysis**; this determined whether the pattern of disease observed among relatives was compatible with one or more major genes or several minor genes. Segregation analysis is typically employed to identify inheritance mechanisms, to evaluate the pathogenicity, penetrance, and expression of mutations, and to facilitate CNV analysis. Fig. 19.4 highlights segregation analysis used to examine genetic inheritance in 1500 families affected by breast cancer. This analysis indicated that four to five per cent of cases may be consistent with a dominant allele for disease susceptibility. A summary of genetic approaches leading to the identification of candidate genes in complex disorders is shown in Fig. 19.3.

Identifying candidate genes

Animal studies can be used to help identify human candidate genes. Strains of various animals have been widely used to study complex phenotypic traits such as hypertension. In breeding experiments a particular phenotype is selectively bred. *Transgenic* or *knock-out models* in which the gene of interest is deleted (or another inserted, or both) at the embryonic stage of development are widely used, and the resulting phenotype is examined. Such methods are clearly inappropriate in human studies. *Chromosome abnormalities* in humans, such as

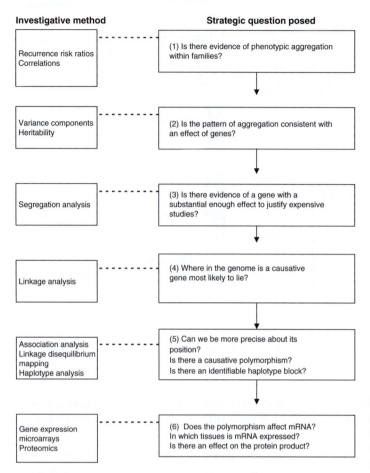

Investigative method	Strategic question posed
Recurrence risk ratios Correlations	(1) Is there evidence of phenotypic aggregation within families?
Variance components Heritability	(2) Is the pattern of aggregation consistent with an effect of genes?
Segregation analysis	(3) Is there evidence of a gene with a substantial enough effect to justify expensive studies?
Linkage analysis	(4) Where in the genome is a causative gene most likely to lie?
Association analysis Linkage disequilibrium mapping Haplotype analysis	(5) Can we be more precise about its position? Is there a causative polymorphism? Is there an identifiable haplotype block?
Gene expression microarrays Proteomics	(6) Does the polymorphism affect mRNA? In which tissues is mRNA expressed? Is there an effect on the protein product?

Figure 19.3 Framework for the investigation of genetic contribution to complex disease. Reproduced from Burton *et al.*, 'Key concepts in genetic epidemiology', *Lancet* **366** (9489), with permission from Elsevier.

translocation of chromosome 22 to the long arm of chromosome 9 (the Philadelphia chromosome, only found in tumour cells of chronic myeloid leukaemia), and trisomy of chromosome 21 (accounting for the majority of cases of Down's syndrome) serve as examples of (macro) genetic faults which can be easily identified in humans and can also be used to inform candidate gene selection.

Linkage analysis and genetic markers

Linkage studies are often conducted in multigenerational families and aim to discover the approximate location of disease genes (*positional mapping*) relative to a genetic marker whose position is already known. The principle of linkage analysis relies on the knowledge that while each pair of chromosomes contains the

same genes in the same order, the sequences are not identical at many loci due to mutations and *recombination*. Recombination normally occurs during meiosis where breaks in homologous chromosome pairs allow for the reciprocal exchange of chromosome segments known as *crossing over*.

After recombination, the chromosomes contain a mixture of alleles with different parental origins. If there is a large distance between two DNA sequences on a chromosome, it is highly probable that recombination will occur between them. In contrast, if two DNA sequences are very close together, crossing over and hence recombination will be less common so that typed markers and phenotypic determinants *co-segregate*. Recombination 'hotspots' exist whereby recombination is more likely to occur at these points

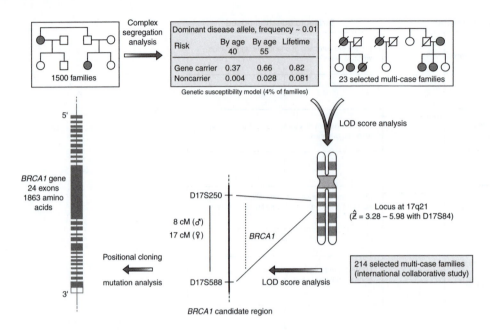

Figure 19.4 Discovering the *BRCA1* gene.
Reproduced from Strachan T and Read AP (2004) *Human and Molecular Genetics*, 3rd edn, with permission from Garland Science.

and blocks between these hotspots are inherited with relatively little recombination. Such sets of alleles, on the same small segment of chromosome, tend to be transmitted together and are termed **haplotypes** that can subsequently be tracked through **pedigrees** and populations. The results of linkage analyses are usually expressed in terms of a **LOD score** (often denoted as **Z**), where a LOD score of three or more (representing odds of 1000 : 1 ($\log_{10}(1000) = 3$) or greater in favour of linkage is used to indicate statistically significant linkage. A LOD score of minus two or less indicates that linkage is unlikely. In the example shown for *BRCA1* in Fig. 19.4 a significant range of values for the LOD score was calculated.

In a search for a disease gene, the alternative alleles at any locus will be the normal allele and the disease (or mutant) allele, and they can be distinguished by looking for the disease expressed phenotypically in a family tree or pedigree. Genetic markers, used for the mapping of disease genes, need to show a degree of polymorphism (variations in length or DNA sequence), which can be identified (*typed*) using techniques such as those described previously. Disease genes are

mapped by measuring recombination against a panel of different markers spread over the entire genome. Denser linkage panels (more markers typed) mean that the genetic region harbouring a disease gene (*candidate region*) can be more narrowly defined. In most cases, recombination will occur frequently, indicating that the disease gene and marker are far apart (*exclusion mapping*). Some markers, however, will tend not to show recombination with the disease gene and these are said to be linked to it. In a genome-wide *linkage analysis scan*, markers at regular intervals covering the whole genome are typed. Linkage analysis may be parametric, where the genetic model is known or non-parametric (model-free). Chromosome segments are sought that are shared by affected individuals more often than predicted by random Mendelian segregation. Family-based linkage studies initially dominated the search for disease genes with significant success for major genes causing Mendelian diseases. It has proved challenging to achieve similar progress for diseases with complex, multifactorial aetiology. **Association** studies have been more successful than linkage studies for identifying genetic risk factors implicated in common complex multifactorial diseases such as diabetes or ischaemic heart disease. The transition in research methods from historical linkage studies to association-based analyses that have more statistical power to identify small to moderate effects on disease was driven by Risch and Merikangas' influential paper (Risch and Merikangas 1996). Fig. 19.4 shows the sequence of events leading to the discovery of the *BRCA1* gene and clinical testing approaches.

A large-scale segregation analysis of 1500 families affected with early onset breast cancer performed in 1988 suggested approximately four per cent of breast cancer cases (especially those with early onset) could be attributed to inherited factors (top left and central panel, Fig. 19.4). Some families demonstrated a pattern of inheritance similar to a Mendelian disorder. Subsequent linkage analysis showed that a susceptibility locus (designated *BRCA1*) could be mapped to chromosome 17q. This was confirmed in a large-scale international study and the *BRCA1* gene was isolated shortly afterwards, and genetic testing for *BRCA1* mutations is now available for individuals in affected families.

Candidate gene association studies

Association studies are commonly used to map disease susceptibility genes in complex disorders where several genes are suspected to influence the onset and progression of a disease. *Candidate genes* are typically selected due to their location in a genetic region prioritised from genome-wide studies (*positional*) or based on knowledge of their function from experimental or computational studies (*biological*). Candidate genes may either be directly sequenced to identify novel genetic variation or the known genetic markers within these genes may be identified from online catalogues of DNA polymorphisms such as dbSNP (see Web addresses). These genetic markers, within candidate genes, are typed and compared between population-based cases (affected) and controls (ideally matched for environmental risk factors, but unaffected), or the transmission of alleles is compared

between affected and unaffected individuals in pedigrees. Where a genetic marker appears more frequently in cases than in controls, this is considered to be a possible risk (or protective) factor for genetic susceptibility to disease. **Genetic association** is a statistical statement describing the co-occurrence of a genetic profile with a phenotype and does not necessarily signify causation. The strength of association is typically presented in terms of relative risk or odds ratios where a value of one suggests no difference in risk. Case-control association studies can be confounded by **population stratification** where several genetically distinct subpopulations with different disease prevalence and different allele frequencies exist. Ancestry may act as a hidden confounder; consider Lander and Schork's example in which Chinese cases are compared with White controls when investigating the ability to eat with chopsticks in a San Francisco population. The HLA*A1 allele would be significantly associated with chopstick ability as this allele is more commonly observed in Asian individuals than in those with White ethnicity (Lander and Schork 1994).

Linkage disequilibrium (LD), where combinations of related alleles occur more or less frequently than expected based on individual allele frequencies in a population, is a phenomenon that is often exploited in association studies. This relationship between genetic markers is particularly useful for SNPs because an individual's genome can be investigated by genotyping only an informative subset of SNPs rather than all of those currently identified. SNPs in close proximity on a chromosomal segment that are inherited together may form haplotypes from which informative 'tag' SNPs are selected for genotyping (Fig. 19.6).

Some populations exhibit a high level of linkage disequilibrium; e.g. genetically-isolated populations such as those in regions of Sardinia and Finland that have experienced little admixture from immigrant populations for several centuries. The *International HapMap project* (Altshuler *et al.* 2010) developed a public resource describing patterns of LD across multiple worldwide populations and this information facilitated genome-wide association studies.

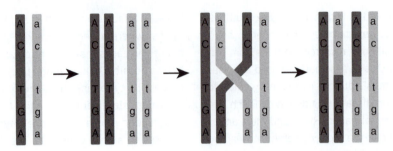

Figure 19.5 Recombination. DNA replication of maternal and paternal chromosomes leading to pairing of homologous chromosomes with genetic markers represented by letters. During recombination, chromosomes physically cross over and are resolved into recombined chromosomes. If T is a disease-causing gene, then recombination is more likely to occur between T and C than T and G; this is the principle of linkage studies.

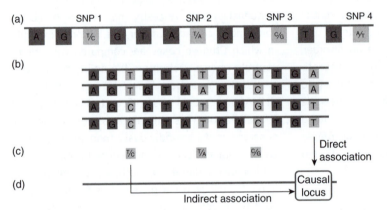

Figure 19.6 The principle of tag single nucleotide polymorphisms (SNPs) selection. (a) SNPs: individual bases within a given sequence; (b) Genotyped tag SNPs: SNPs that can 'tag' (differentiate) between haplotypes and act as proxies to estimate genotypes at related SNP loci (SNP1 is a proxy for SNP4); (d) direct or indirect association with disease.

Genome-wide association studies (GWAS)

Early association studies were limited by small sample sizes (underpowered), inadequate matching of controls, and insufficient correction for multiple testing (markers and phenotypes), resulting in many published associations being false positives. To circumvent the problems with testing individual candidate genes, researchers began exploring genetic determinants associated with complex disease by simultaneously using thousands to millions of SNPs (Anon 2007). To improve sample sizes, many research groups interested in particular diseases or traits, formed consortia and took advantage of developments in genotyping technologies that enabled large numbers of genetic variants to be genotyped

quickly and efficiently. The National Human Genome Research Institute (NHGRI) maintains a catalogue of more than 1600 published GWAS for over 200 traits (see Web addresses). Genome-wide significance is typically considered to be $P < 10^{-8}$ in an effort to minimize the risk of false positive findings, and confirmation of significant genetic loci in an independent population is highly desirable. Analogous to GWAS, large-scale epigenetic studies (inherited changes not directly due to changes in base sequence but rather caused by altered chemical marks on the DNA helix; the **epigenome**) are revealing novel insights and offering attractive therapeutic targets for disease. Three main epigenetic mechanisms regulate gene expression: (1) DNA methylation which can inhibit gene expression; (2) histone modifications or altered chromatin structure; and

(3) RNA interference, which may repress transcription or increase mRNA degradation. For example, epigenetic changes have been extensively associated with neurodegenerative diseases (Qureshi and Mehler 2011).

Next-generation sequencing

Carefully designed GWAS offer unprecedented power to identify disease risks, however they are based on a **common disease-common variant** hypothesis and are limited to testing known variants. The genetic architecture of complex disease is being further elucidated by means of high-throughput sequencing approaches where the exact sequence of bases is identified, providing valuable information on multiple aspects of gene structure and function. Extensive datasets have been generated annotating common and rarer SNPs, copy number variation, gene expression levels, and epigenetic modifications. These resequencing strategies may be focused on targeted components of the genome such as the protein coding regions (also known as **whole-exome sequencing**) or an individual's entire genome (**whole-genome sequencing**). Large-scale population-based resequencing efforts are underway, including the 1000 Genomes Project which aims to identify the majority of SNPs with a minor allele frequency > 1 per cent, and the UK10K initiative which is sequencing the genome of one in 6000 individuals in the UK to uncover many rare genetic variants important for human disease (see 'Web addresses' section).

Further analysis of provisional 'hits' from linkage and association studies

As noted previously, the rapid evolution and accessibility of genomic technology has encouraged researchers to publish thousands of reports describing genetic associations with disease, but few of these have subsequently been replicated. This lack of replication is largely due to differences in biological exposures or study designs and guidelines have been promoted to improve consistency and enhance transparency when searching for genetic risk factors: STrengthening the REporting of Genetic Association studies (STREGA). Crucial issues for study design include comprehensively phenotyped individuals carefully allocated to comparison groups, consideration of potential confounders, the number and allele frequency of genetic variants typed, stringent quality control of data, and adjustment for multiple testing.

Genetic markers may be directly associated with a trait (disease-causing variant) or indirectly associated (tag SNP) where the marker associated with disease is in linkage disequilibrium with the disease-causing variant. Ideally all novel genetic linkage or association loci identified should be replicated in an independent, phenotypically similar population. If robustly replicated, then additional support for functionality is sought from *fine-mapping* the genetic region to identify other associated markers in the same region, *pathway analysis* to identify relevant biological mechanisms for disease and *in silico*, *in vivo*, and *in vitro* experiments. The magnitude of the effect of the various mutations in terms of relative and absolute risk is also assessed, i.e. the public health importance of the genetic risk factor is investigated. **Mendelian randomization** is an approach to verify that observed exposures are actually causal for disease, and has been equated to randomized controlled trials (Slieman and Grant 2010). Genes are randomly assigned during meiosis (hence the term Mendelian randomization), and the established relationship between a known genetic risk factor (instrumental variable) and particular exposure is exploited to determine if the exposure-disease relationship is causal. Inferring causality from observational studies may be difficult and the reliable identification of a modifiable risk factor on a disease could have important implications for public health intervention. However, this approach may be limited in the presence of small sample sizes, linkage disequilibrium, genetic heterogeneity, pleiotropy, population stratification, and lack of understanding of interacting confounders. Causal models in genetic epidemiology are discussed in further detail elsewhere (Thomas and Conti 2004). Table 19.1 summarizes a variety of study designs to identify genetic risk factors based on both epidemiological and genetic principles.

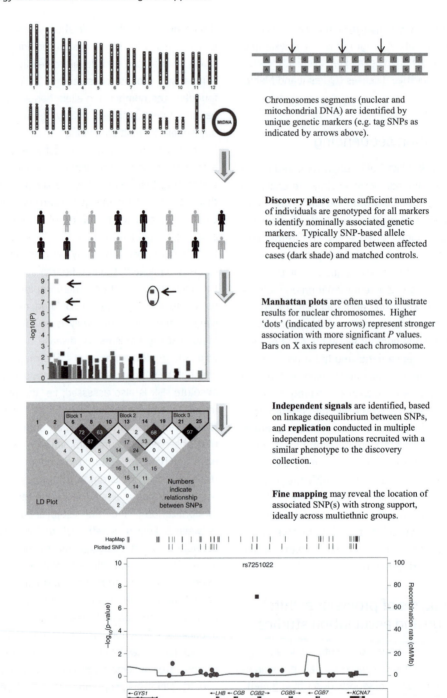

Chromosomes segments (nuclear and mitochondrial DNA) are identified by unique genetic markers (e.g. tag SNPs as indicated by arrows above).

Discovery phase where sufficient numbers of individuals are genotyped for all markers to identify nominally associated genetic markers. Typically SNP-based allele frequencies are compared between affected cases (dark shade) and matched controls.

Manhattan plots are often used to illustrate results for nuclear chromosomes. Higher 'dots' (indicated by arrows) represent stronger association with more significant *P* values. Bars on X axis represent each chromosome.

Independent signals are identified, based on linkage disequilibrium between SNPs, and **replication** conducted in multiple independent populations recruited with a similar phenotype to the discovery collection.

Fine mapping may reveal the location of associated SNP(s) with strong support, ideally across multiethnic groups.

Figure 19.7 Genetic association studies.

19.5 Genomic tests in public health and clinical medicine

Over the past two decades there has been a dramatic expansion in the number of clinically relevant genetic tests and it is critically important that laboratories maintain high standards of quality, utility, and data protection (UKGTN). Genetic tests may directly reflect the risk of developing a severe, highly penetrant disease (e.g. X-linked Alport syndrome) or facilitate the calculation of a genetic risk score for predisposition to diseases such as diabetes. Population-based genetic screening has traditionally focused on the identification of pre-symptomatic persons with certain Mendelian disorders to initiate early treatment that will minimize the impact of disease (e.g. screening of newborns for phenylketonuria), or the testing of selected populations for carrier status so that prospective parents can make informed choices for their planned offspring (e.g. Tay Sachs disease). There are now commercially available options that will evaluate a broad range of evidence-based, disease-causing mutations in a single test at low cost; e.g. Counsyl offers a non-invasive, saliva-based test for more than 100 Mendelian diseases across all major population groups (Srinivasan *et al.* 2010). Commercial organizations also offer high-throughput, direct-to-consumer genetic susceptibility testing worldwide without providing personal medical advice, counselling, or ensuring customers understand the implications of their results. Different companies may test different markers and often generate different risk prediction scores for the same disease in a single individual (Ng *et al.* 2009). Despite recent successes identifying genetic risk factors for complex diseases, few genetic risk profiles have been identified that provide robust and clinically relevant risk prediction. For example, genetic risk factors identified for cardiovascular disease from multiple GWAS resulted in a genetic risk score based on 101 SNPs ($P < 10^{-7}$) that was evaluated in more than 19,000 white women. The use of this combined genetic profile did not significantly improve on traditional risk factors for prediction of cardiovascular disease (Paynter *et al.* 2010).

Appropriate genetic testing and screening strategies have the potential to improve public health outcomes, but they involve significant Ethical, Legal, and Social Issues (ELSI)—a term emanating from the Human Genome Project. Some of these 'ELSI' challenges include the following questions:

- Should a genetic test always generate a definitive risk score?

- Should genetic testing be offered if no useful therapeutic intervention is possible?

- What happens if testing for one disease inadvertently reveals the risk of another disease?

- To whom should results be disclosed; health care workers, relatives?

- If testing an individual indirectly reveals a major risk to another person (e.g. identical twins, or revealing the status of a later onset condition such as Huntington's disease in a young person will also provide information on parental status), is there an obligation to reveal that information?

- Is it appropriate to select out embryos diagnosed pre-implantation with a late-onset condition for which screening and treatment are available?

Clearly accurate information regarding the utility, purpose, and appropriateness of testing should be understood before genetic tests are performed. Genetic counselling should be available while preservation of privacy, confidentiality, and data security are paramount.

Pharmacogenetics and personalized medicine

Investigating how individuals respond to drugs based on their genotype profile may lead to practical pre-treatment genetic testing and 'smart' drug development. The clinical finding that drug choice and dosages must be tailored for individual patients has been recognized for years, but progress has been challenging to implement clinically relevant testing. Success stories include FDA approval for genotype-specific dosage range for warfarin, and warnings on the label for genotype-based major adverse reactions to clopidogrel (see 'Web addresses' section).

Comprehensive genotyping is being increasingly implemented for the clinical assessment of individuals. For example, genotyping 2.6 million SNPs may reveal an individual's risk of myocardial infarction, diabetes, and cancer along with various drug responses (Ashley *et al.* 2010). Whole-genome sequencing has been employed to develop personalized blood tests to optimize treatment for cancer patients at Johns Hopkins Hospital, USA. Clearly many challenges remain before pharmacogenetics and personalized medicine reach their full potential, but research confirms that genotype profiles can yield informative data that are clinically relevant for individuals. Pharmacogenetics may also provide new insights into the biological mechanisms of drug action and redefine how drugs undergo clinical development by avoiding the recruitment of individuals whose genetic profile makes them susceptible to adverse drug reactions. Employing dedicated genotype profiles may also result in substantial reductions in requisite sample sizes for clinical trials investigating pharmacogenetic effects that are influenced by genetic variations.

CONCLUSIONS

Genetic epidemiology is concerned with understanding heritable aspects of disease risk, individual susceptibility to disease, and ultimately with contributing to a comprehensive molecular understanding of pathogenesis. Major research collaborations are required to ensure efficient uses of resources and the sharing of genetic data; locus-specific (LOVD, PKHD1), and disease-specific resources (ALZGENE, CORGI) are being developed to facilitate genetic research. The rapid generation of large volumes of biological information means that integrating complementary genetic (DNA), transcriptomic (RNA), proteomic (proteins), and other -omic datasets is a high priority. These valuable bioinformatics data are helping researchers to better understand pathways involved in mechanisms of disease. **Systems biology** is a multidisciplinary approach to combine quantitative experimental data and computational modelling to identify biological networks, biomarkers, and risk factors that inform genetic medicine. Practitioners in clinical medicine, public health, and basic science need

to ensure that the massive investment in human genetics and expansion of genetic epidemiological data are carefully integrated into their practice for the ultimate benefit of the whole population.

Web addresses

1000 Genomes Project resequencing individuals
www.1000genomes.org

NHGRI Catalogue of genome wide association studies
www.genome.gov/GWAStudies

dbSNP database for short genetic variations
www.ncbi.nlm.nih.gov/snp

Food and Drug Administration (US)—Table of Pharmacogenetic Biomarkers in Drug Labels
www.fda.gov/Drugs/ScienceResearch/ResearchAreas/Pharmacogenetics/ucm083378.htm

Foundation for Genomics and Population Health (PHG Foundation)
www.phgfoundation.org

GeneReviews
http://www.genereviews.org

Human Epigenome Atlas
http://www.genboree.org/epigenomeatlas/index.rhtml

Human Genetic Epidemiology (HuGENet) network
www.hugenet.org.uk

International HapMap Project for LD patterns in populations
http://hapmap.ncbi.nlm.nih.gov

Online Mendelian Inheritance in Man (OMIM)
www.omim.org

Orphanet information for rare diseases
www.orpha.net

UK10K Project for rare variant discovery
www.uk10k.org

Further reading

Handel AE, Ebers GC, and Ramagopalan SV (2010) Epigenetics: molecular mechanisms and implications for disease. *Trends in Molecular Medicine* **16** (1), 7–16.

Manolio TA (2010) Genomewide association studies and assessment of the risk of disease. *The New England Journal of Medicine* **363** (2), 166–76.

Read AP and Donnai D (2010) *New Clinical Genetics*, 2nd edn. Banbury, UK: Scion Publishing Ltd.

Strachan T and Read AP (2011) *Human Molecular Genetics*, 4th edn. New York: Garland Science/Taylor and Francis.

Tennessen JA, Bigham AW, O'Connor TD, Fu W, *et al.* (2012) Evolution and functional impact of rare coding variation from deep sequencing of human exomes. *Science (New York, NY)* **337** (6090), 64–9.

von Elm E, Moher D, and Little J (2009) Reporting genetic association studies: the STREGA statement. *Lancet* **374** (9684), 98–100.

Wang L, McLeod HL, and Weinshilboum RM (2011) Genomics and drug response. *The New England Journal of Medicine* **364** (12), 1144–53.

References

Alkan C, Coe BP, and Eichler EE (2011) Genome structural variation discovery and genotyping. *Nature reviews. Genetics.* **12** (5), 363–76.

Altshuler DM, Gibbs RA, Peltonen L, Altshuler DM, *et al.* (2010) Integrating common and rare genetic variation in diverse human populations. *Nature* **467** (7311), 52–8.

Anon (2007) Genome-wide association study of 14,000 cases of seven common diseases and 3,000 shared controls. *Nature* **447** (7145), 661–78.

Ashley EA, Butte AJ, Wheeler MT, Chen R, *et al.* (2010) Clinical assessment incorporating a personal genome. *Lancet* **375** (9725), 1525–35.

Carter CO (1969) Genetics of common disorders. *British Medical Bulletin* **25** (1), 52–7.

Collins FS (2011) *The language of life: DNA and the revolution in personalized medicine*. London: Harper Perennial.

Evans A, Van Baal GCM, McCarron P, DeLange M, *et al.* (2003) The genetics of coronary heart disease: the contribution of twin studies. *Twin research* **6** (5), 432–41.

Guttman M, Amit I, Garber M, French C, *et al.* (2009) Chromatin signature reveals over a thousand highly conserved large non-coding RNAs in mammals. *Nature* **458** (7235), 223–7.

Handel AE, Ebers GC, and Ramagopalan SV (2010) Epigenetics: molecular mechanisms and implications for disease. *Trends in Molecular Medicine* **16** (1), 7–16.

Kumar RK, Hitchins MP, and Foster PS (2009) Epigenetic changes in childhood asthma. *Disease Models & Mechanisms* **2** (11–12), 549–53.

Lander ES and Schork NJ (1994) Genetic dissection of complex traits. *Science (New York, NY)* **265** (5181), 2037–48.

Morton NE (1982) *Outline of Genetic Epidemiology*. London: Karger.

Ng PC, Murray SS, Levy S, and Venter JC (2009) An agenda for personalized medicine. *Nature* **461** (7265), 724–6.

Paynter NP, Chasman DI, Paré G, Buring JE, *et al.* (2010) Association between a literature-based genetic risk score and cardiovascular events in women. *JAMA* **303** (7), 631–7.

Pearce N, Aït-Khaled N, Beasley R, Mallol J, *et al.* (2007) Worldwide trends in the prevalence of asthma symptoms: phase III of the International Study of Asthma and Allergies in Childhood (ISAAC). *Thorax* **62** (9), 758–66.

Qureshi IA and Mehler MF (2011) Advances in epigenetics and epigenomics for neurodegenerative diseases. *Current Neurology and Neuroscience Reports* **11** (5), 464–73.

Risch N and Merikangas K (1996) The future of genetic studies of complex human diseases. *Science (New York, NY)* **273** (5281), 1516–17.

Sleiman PMA and Grant SFA (2010) Mendelian randomization in the era of genomewide association studies. *Clinical Chemistry* **56** (5), 723–8.

Smith DW and Aase JM (1970) Polygenic inheritance of certain common malformations. Evidence and empiric recurrence risk data. *The Journal of Pediatrics* **76** (5), 652–9.

Srinivasan BS, Evans EA, Flannick J, Patterson AS, *et al.* (2010) A universal carrier test for the long tail of Mendelian disease. *Reproductive Biomedicine Online* **21** (4), 537–51.

Strachan T and Read AP (2004) *Human and Molecular Genetics*, 3rd edn. London: Garland Science.

Terry MB, Delgado-Cruzata L, Vin-Raviv N, Wu HC, *et al.* (2011) DNA methylation in white blood cells: association with risk factors in epidemiologic studies. *Epigenetics* **6** (7), 828–37.

Thomas DC and Conti DV (2004) Commentary: the concept of 'Mendelian Randomization'. *International Journal of Epidemiology* **33** (1), 21–5.

Witt, H. (2011) New modifier loci in cystic fibrosis. *Nature Genetics* **43** (6), 508–9.

Ziegler RG, Hoover RN, Pike MC, Hildesheim A, *et al.* (1993) Migration patterns and breast cancer risk in Asian-American women. *Journal of the National Cancer Institute* **85** (22), 1819–27.

Web-based references

ALZGENE, Alzheimer's research database
www.alzforum.org

CORGI, Centralized Online Renal Genetics Initiative
http://www.qub.ac.uk/neph-res/CORGI/index.php

LOVD, Leiden Open Variation Database
www.dmd.nl/nmdb2/home.php

PKHD1, Autosomal recessive polycystic kidney disease
www.humgen.rwth-aachen.de

UKGTN
www.ukgtn.nhs.uk

20 Social, cultural, and behavioural factors in disease

JOHN YARNELL, DERMOT O'REILLY, AND SHARON FRIEL

CHAPTER CONTENTS

In this chapter we examine social, cultural, and behavioural factors as causes of disease and how they may affect the effectiveness of interventions to improve health at the population or individual level. We discuss the extent to which 'lifestyle' factors contribute to the major chronic diseases, the epidemiology of accidents, poisonings, and violence and social inequalities in health.

Introduction

Social, cultural, and behavioural factors have been recognized as determinants of disease since the time of Hippocrates. Social and occupational gradients in disease were reported by physicians and demographers in the middle ages in Europe (see Chapter 1); in the 20th century with increasing interest in public health many such academic departments started their life as departments of Social Medicine, particularly in Europe. In order to better understand the causes of these gradients *Social class* was introduced as an index in the UK by the Registrar General in the early part of the 20th century to represent 'social position' in society; it was based on occupation and reflects both level of education and income. It was constructed at that time to correspond with the level of infant mortality according to the occupation of the 'head of the household'; *Social Class I* representing professionally educated families and *Social Class V* those of unskilled labourers. Chapter 16 provides several examples of the relationship between infant mortality and social class in the UK. Other European countries and the USA use different indicators such as occupational group (white/blue collar), home and car ownership, income, and length and type of education, to represent the socio-economic strata. Each stratum of society tends to live in particular neighbourhoods, and individuals generally absorb the culture and behaviour of their peers (the social norms), which, in turn, can influence the general health of the group. In Chapter 7 we saw how participants with only basic levels of education in the INTERHEART study from 52 high-, middle, and low-income countries had the highest levels of cardiovascular disease (CVD) risk factors but this relationship is attenuated in low-income countries, perhaps reflecting the earliest stage of the health transition in these countries. Poverty, literacy, and adverse environments are major risk factors for infectious diseases and maternal and child mortality and morbidity in low income countries. Social determinants of health operate throughout the *life course* operating at birth, childhood, adolescence, adulthood, at work, and in old age and help perpetuate social gradients in health (see Fig. 20.1). In Chapter 16 we discussed the influence of social gradients on maternal and child health at country and global levels but adolescence represents a critical phase in human development in which many aspects of our personality, attitudes, and behaviours, are formed. It is during this period and in young adulthood that the potential for risk-taking behaviour can develop, for accidents, violence, and for addictive behaviours, although the contribution of environment and genes is often fiercely debated. Firstly, we examine the social and cultural determinants of health which have created substantial inequalities in health arising from the 'accident of birth'.

20.1 Social and cultural determinants of health

Social, or rather more accurately, socio-economic determinants of health can be measured in most countries in three different ways; from the level of education, by income, and by occupation. Clearly these are interrelated and it could be argued that education and training are necessary to achieve a professional occupation but many high earners have achieved their financial success without tertiary education. Income is the main determinant of where we live and of the material conditions of the household. In low- and middle-income countries literacy is a key factor in determining health behaviour and access to health care. In such countries about a third of children are not able to proceed beyond the primary level in comparison with only four per cent of children in most high-income countries (Viner *et al.* 2012). In Chapter 16 we saw how improvements in women's education and literacy improve the chances of survival of both mothers and their children. The population level of literacy is one of the three components of the **human development index** (HDI) used

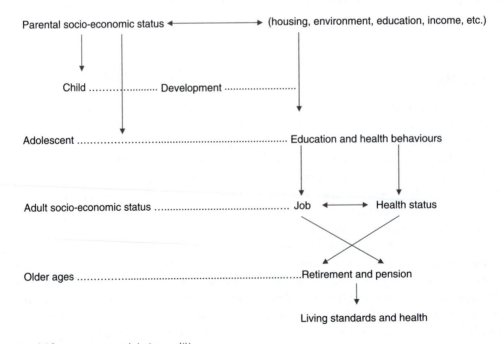

Figure 20.1 A life course approach to inequalities.

in Chapter 22 (see glossary). In a study in Europe using detailed census data with mortality follow up, lifespan was between three and 15 years less in the least educated groups compared to the most educated. Educational differences contributed up to three per cent of the lifespan variation in Western European countries and up to 11 per cent in Central and Eastern Europe (van Raalte et al. 2012).

Cultural influences on behaviour can be difficult to define within multicultural societies and may be linked to ethnicity, religion, and place of residence. Within cities deprived neighbourhoods can exhibit large differences in life expectancy from affluent areas; for example, in Washington DC life expectancy was reported to be 20 years less in Montgomery, Maryland County (largely inhabited by black Americans) compared to the wealthiest white inhabited area in suburban Washington (Marmot 2004). In Glasgow, UK a 26-year difference in life expectancy has been described between the richest and poorest largely white areas (Hanlon 2006). In a large, national cohort study in Sweden, a country noted for its liberal social welfare policy and favourable life expectancy, neighbourhood deprivation was independently associated with incidence of coronary heart disease (CHD) and mortality at one year (Winkleby et al. 2007). Neighbourhood deprivation was defined by education, income, welfare, and unemployment rather than material conditions, which perhaps illustrates the difficulties for researchers attempting to disentangle the individual effects of these highly intertwined socio-cultural variables. In the next section we review the important health behaviours and their links with social deprivation.

20.2 Health-related behaviours

Behaviours develop, adapt, and mature during the life course under a multiplicity of influences. In simple terms during infancy and childhood parental, family, and school influences are paramount, but in adolescence independent behaviours begin to emerge shaped by school, neighbourhood, peers, and local culture, and particularly in low- and middle-income countries with all the cultural changes stemming from globalization. Individual habits and personality begin to crystallize during adolescence and young adulthood, both positively and negatively, by family responsibilities and by adverse life events such as divorce, bereavement, or unemployment. Marital and employment status are well established to be associated with health outcomes; both marriage (Goldman 1993) and employment (Moser et al. 1984) are associated with more favourable health outcomes from research in high-income countries. In low- and middle-income countries national, religious, and economic influences are important at all stages of life and these diverse factors are particularly critical in countries where the economic transition is either beginning or in full swing.

Some important health behaviours are shown in Table 20.1 with preventive measures either in place or proposed and an estimate of the contribution of each behaviour (or lifestyle) to the global burden of disease.

In other chapters we have shown to what extent behavioural, 'lifestyle', factors contribute to specific major diseases. The **attributable fraction** of tobacco smoking for lung cancer is about 90 per cent in Western countries (Chapter 8); for cardiovascular disease this is around 30 per cent (Chapter 7). For Type 2 diabetes mellitus in women the attributable fraction of obesity (body mass index $\geq$ 30 kg/m^2 is estimated to be 61 per cent (Chapter 9). Thus the epidemiological evidence suggests that some of these diseases can be almost eliminated, and others cut substantially by the reduction of behaviours such as tobacco smoking or those leading to overweight and obesity. However it seems clear that society and governments share a responsibility to develop policies of 'harm-minimization' since both tobacco and alcohol are legally available to adults.

Tobacco smoking, alcohol, and illicit drugs are discussed in the following section on addictive substances. Unhealthy nutrition and sedentary behaviour are discussed in more detail in Chapter 7 (Prevention of cardiovascular disease), Chapter 9 (combating the epidemic of obesity), and in Chapter 22 (preventing the worldwide epidemic of CVD). Unsafe sex (unprotected sex) is discussed in Chapter 18 (HIV/AIDS and other STDs), and global fertility and contraception are discussed in Chapter 16. A review of prevention trials

Table 20.1 Lifestyle factors and chronic disease: evidence and preventive measures

Factor	Evidence	Preventive measures	Contributions to Global Burden of Disease
Tobacco smoking	Strong evidence from observational studies that it is a major risk factor for respiratory cancers (Chapter 8), other cancers (Chapter 17), cardiovascular disease (Chapter 7), and osteoporosis (Chapter 15). Maternal smoking strongly associated with risk of miscarriage, prematurity, and SIDS (Chapter 16). Environmental tobacco smoke associated with excess risk of lung cancer in non-smokers (Chapter 8).	Health warnings on cigarette packets since 1970s, taxation used to limit demand. EU-led ban on tobacco advertising introduced in UK in 2003. Ban on smoking in many workplaces and public places	4.1%
'Unhealthy' nutrition	Strong evidence from observational and some experimental studies on role of excess calories in overweight and obesity, salt and hypertension, saturated fats and raised blood cholesterol (Chapters 7 and 9). Some evidence that fruit and vegetables protect against some cancers and cardiovascular disease (Chapters 7 and 17). Important area for future research	Nutritional recommendations made by US, UK, and European Agencies with updates. Involvement of food manufacturers and pharmaceutical industry	Hypertension 4.4% High blood cholesterol 2.8% High BMI 2.3% Low fruit and vegetable intake 1.8%
Alcohol consumption above 'safe' limits	Evidence of J- or U-shaped relationship with mortality and cardiovascular disease, but major association with co-morbidity and social dysfunction and accidents; premature mortality at higher levels of consumption	Limited availability to minors. General health promotion on 'safe limits' with limited effectiveness	4.0%

Sedentary behaviour	Strong evidence on role of sedentary behaviour in overweight and obesity, type 2 diabetes, and cardiovascular disease (Chapters 7 and 9)	Report by US Surgeon General, UK Department of Health, etc., but only general health promotion and limited strategies to date	1.3%
Psychological stress	Limited evidence from observational studies on job stress (control and working hours) (cardiovascular disease and hypertension). Improved epidemiological indicators are needed	Health and safety and work legislation	Not known
Illicit drug use	Class A drug use associated with premature mortality and co-morbidity	Legal control of drugs. Drug addiction clinics. Health promotion directed at young people	0.8%
Unsafe sex (HIV) Lack of contraception	High prevalence of HIV in developing countries. Strong association between abortion and maternal mortality in developing countries	Extensive educational campaigns in Western countries	HIV 6.3% Lack of contraception 0.6%

* Estimates taken from Ezzati *et al.* (2002).
Reproduced from Ezzati *et al.* 'Selected major risk factors and global and regional burden of disease', *Lancet* **360** (9343), 2002, with permission from Elsevier.

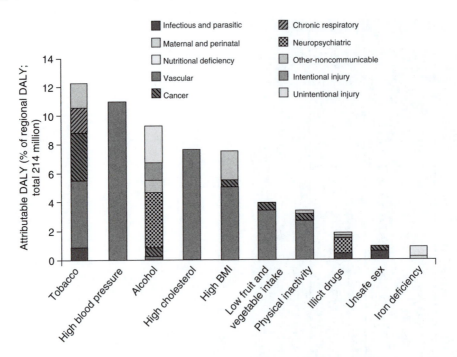

Figure 20.2 Contribution of risk factors to burden of disease in high-income countries.
Reproduced from Ezzati M, Lopez AD, Rodgers A, Vander Hoorn S, *et al.* (2002) Selected major risk factors and global and regional burden of disease. *Lancet.* **360** (9343), with permission from Elsevier.

and policies with evidence of benefit in adolescents and young adults (against the development of adverse health behaviours) conducted in Australia, Canada, UK, and USA suggests that extending their use to schools, communities, and families should yield long-term benefits (Catalano *et al.* 2012). These interventions may require adaptation and trial before extensive use in low- and middle-income countries.

Ezzati *et al.*, with the support of WHO, have published several reports on the contribution of major risk factors (shown in Table 20.1) to the global burden of disease (Ezzati *et al.* 2002). In high income countries they estimated that removal of these risks would increase healthy life expectancy by a minimum of 4.4 years (six per cent). In the poorest region of the world (parts of sub-Saharan Africa) the mixture of risk factors also includes childhood and maternal malnutrition, and it is estimated that removal of all risk factors would increase healthy life expectancy by over 16.1 years (43 per cent) in this region. The contributions to the global burden of disease shown in Table 20.1 should

be used for comparative and illustrative purposes only, but reflect global rather than regional levels of disease. Fig. 20.2 shows the contribution of each risk factor to the global burden of disease, and illustrates the considerable scope for its reduction. Tobacco and alcohol contribute to a number of different types of disease, whereas hypertension and high blood cholesterol contribute only to CVD, although a major reduction in levels would have a significant impact on this burden.

20.3 Addiction

The use of many substances for their pleasurable, mood-enhancing, effects is well established in Western societies, but the pattern of use and types of substances commonly taken, varies between social, religious, and cultural groups. Some psychologists make the distinction between 'physical' and 'psychological' dependence (a habitual reliance on gratification through regular use of a particular substance) but the potential for addiction of a particular substance is also relevant for therapeutic and preventive interventions. Nicotine, widely available through tobacco products, is one of the most highly addictive substances known, and simple questionnaires have been developed to evaluate the level of dependence (West 2004).

Dependencies on nicotine, alcohol, and on illicit drugs are major public health problems in many societies and cultures in countries at all stages of development. Each addiction or behavioural pattern has its own distinct epidemiology but there is some degree of commonality between them. National data from the USA in 12–17-year-olds indicated that persistent users of cannabis and inhalants were at greater risk of opioid and stimulant use (Nakawaki and Crano 2012), which tends to support the 'stepping stone' hypothesis.

....

Question 1

What problems do researchers face when assessing the proportion of individuals showing dependence on particular types of behaviour? For example, dependence on tobacco, alcohol, and illicit drugs.

....

Tobacco

At least one-third of the global adult population, or 1.1 billion people aged 15 years and older, smoke cigarettes. About 300 million of these smokers are in developed countries where twice as many men as women use tobacco. In developing countries the difference is greater, and about 48 per cent of men and seven per cent of women smoke. In the UK, Europe, and the US, tobacco smoking became a common habit in men at the beginning of the 20th century with the advent of manufactured cigarettes, and was actively encouraged in soldiers in the First World War with the result that about 80 per cent of men smoked at that time. It was not until the time of the Second World War that cigarette smoking began to increase rapidly in women. In the UK in the 1950s and 1960s almost 60 per cent of men and 40 per cent of women smoked. The prevalence of smoking started to decline in the 1970s in men

but this was delayed until the 1980s for women. Globally, however, the tobacco epidemic is still expanding, especially in developing countries where 70 per cent of tobacco-related deaths occur. Tobacco is currently responsible for the death of 12 per cent of male and six per cent of female deaths worldwide (almost six million deaths each year) (WHO 2011). Half the people that smoke today, about 650 million people, will eventually be killed by tobacco if major control measures are not introduced. The prevalence of tobacco smoking in men and in women is shown in Fig. 20.3a,b. Smoking initiation usually starts in the teenage years with experimentation, but habitual teenage smokers usually become dependent within a year of initiation, and 80 per cent are reported (in the UK) to regret their habit by the age of 20 years (Jarvis 2004).

Alcohol

This is probably the oldest and most widely used drug. It is used in many situations and for many purposes: as a stimulant, a tranquilizer, an anaesthetic, as a social lubricant, a religious symbol, a food, and a fuel. Although alcohol is highly toxic in large quantities, it is a drug which is socially acceptable in many societies when used in moderation. Harmful use of alcohol is a worldwide problem resulting in approximately 2.5 million deaths each year (WHO 2011). It is a causal factor in many diseases, but also leads to death through violence or other injury. Almost four per cent of deaths worldwide are attributed to alcohol, second only to tobacco as a behavioural risk factor. Worldwide trends in alcohol consumption over time have remained relatively static in most age groups but there appears to be an increase in alcohol consumption in adolescents and young adults (CSDH 2008). Alcohol consumption rates and the prevalence of alcohol-related problems vary worldwide (Fig. 20.4).

Higher alcohol consumption levels are generally found in high-income countries, although some of the highest rates are in the Russian Federation. In a retrospective case-control study in three Russian cities of almost 50,000 residents in the age group 15–54 years, 59 per cent of male deaths and 33 per cent of female deaths were associated with alcohol (Zaridze et al. 2009).

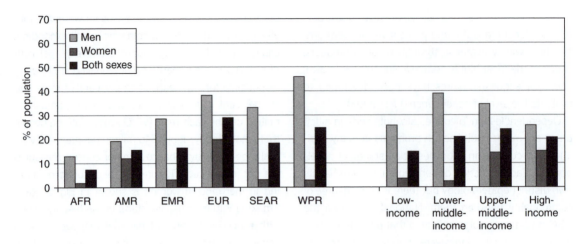

Figure 20.3 Prevalence of daily tobacco smoking in adults by WHO world region (see Chapter 22).
Reproduced from Global status report on noncommunicable diseases 2010: description of the global burden of NCDs, their risk factors and determinants, with permission from the WHO.

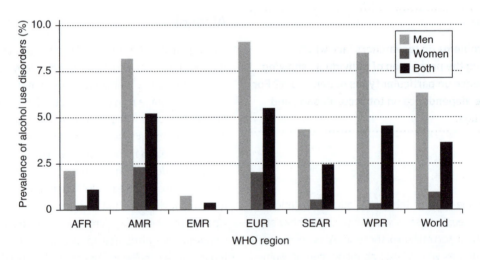

Figure 20.4 Prevalence of alcohol-related disorders by WHO world region.
Reproduced from Rehm et al, 'Global burden of disease and injury and economic cost attributable to alcohol use and alcohol use disorders', *Lancet* **373** (9682), 2009, with permission from Elsevier.

Low levels of consumption and high rates of abstention from alcohol are generally found in countries with large Muslim populations in Africa, the Middle East and across South East Asia. Males are at greater risk of alcohol related death than females: worldwide 6.2 per cent of all male deaths are attributed to alcohol compared with 1.1 per cent of female deaths.

Four levels of alcohol use have been described: social drinking, 'at-risk' consumption, problem drinking and, dependence and addiction (Peele 1997). 'At risk' consumption has been estimated by the UK Department of Health to be three to four units per day for men and two to three units per day for women (based on average weekly consumption and interspersed with alcohol-free days) (see Table 20.2 for units). Good evidence for defining these thresholds comes from a large prospective study of British doctors in which all-cause mortality increased

Table 20.2 Alcohol consumption levels and relative risk of mortality from key alcohol related conditions

		Alcohol consumption					
	Percentage of total deaths (England and Wales 2001)	None	1–10 g/day[*+]	10–20 g/day	20–30 g/day	30–40 g/day	40–50 g/day
IHD men	23%	1	0.83	0.78	0.77	0.78	0.79
IHD women	17%	1	0.86	0.85	0.90	0.96	1.05
Colon cancer	2% (both sexes)	1	1.07	1.22	1.38	1.58	1.79
Breast cancer	4%	1	1.04	1.12	1.21	1.31	1.41
Haemorrhagic stroke	1% (both sexes)	1	1.08	1.25	1.46	1.69	1.96

IHD = Ischaemic heart disease
[*]Midpoint in each category used to calculate relative risks
[+]8 g absolute alcohol ≡ 1 unit alcohol = (½ pint beer, 227 mL) (1 glass wine, 90 mL) (1 measure spirits, 25 mL)
Reproduced from Britton and McPherson, 'Mortality in England and Wales attributable to current alcohol consumption', *Journal of Epidemiology and Community Health*, 2001, with permission from BMJ Publishing Group Ltd.

steadily at an average consumption above three units per day (Doll *et al.* 1994). However, surveys in the UK suggest that 5.9 million people, mainly under 25 years of age, exceed these guidelines. Binge drinking is a particular problem in this age group. In addition, 2.9 million (seven per cent of the population) are either problem drinkers (with psychosocial or work-related problems) or have some level of dependence on alcohol. The number of alcoholics (addicts) is estimated to be 200,000 in the UK (one in 200 or 0.5% of the adult population) (Ashworth and Gerada 1997).

Heavy alcohol consumption is associated with liver cirrhosis, pancreatitis, cancer, stroke, and premature death. The risk of death from major diseases associated with consumption of alcohol in England and Wales is summarized in Table 20.2.

These data relate only to England and Wales and do not include liver cirrhosis as a cause of death. In Chapter 11, Fig. 11.1 shows a rising trend in deaths from cirrhosis in the UK compared to overall falling trends in the EU as a whole. This is attributed to an increasing pattern of binge drinking in the UK among young adults and, if this trend persists, we may see a rise in CVD-related deaths. On a global basis alcohol appears to be associated with an overall excess risk of CVD death (Rehm *et al.* 2009).

Alcohol is responsible for 150,000 hospital admissions per annum in the UK and up to one-third of all accident and emergency attendances. Alcohol abuse is involved in 30–60 per cent of child protection cases, significant numbers of domestic violence incidents, and many fatal car crashes. Fig. 20.5 summarizes the social and economic costs associated with alcohol abuse in the UK.

The economic burden associated with alcohol consumption is usually higher in high-income countries accounting for between approximately one to three per cent of GDP, but the economic burden is already comparable in some middle-income countries and is expected to rise in others (Rehm *et al.* 2009).

Illicit drugs

Accurate statistics on the use of illicit drugs are more difficult to obtain than for tobacco and alcohol, and are based on data sources such as crime surveys, accident statistics, and a range of lifestyle surveys. Increasingly, statistics are gathered from multiple sources using capture-recapture techniques (see Chapter 2).

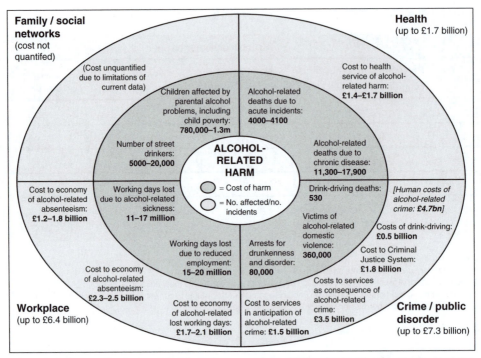

All figures are annualized. *Human costs are those incurred as a consequence of the human and emotional impact suffered by victims of crime (for example attending victim-support services); because of the lack of research in the field, equivalent costs have not been estimated for other alcohol-related harms. For this reason, human costs are not included in the crime/public disorder total figure.

Figure 20.5 Aspects of alcohol-related harm and costs.
Cabinet Office, 2004.

Estimates of global use indicate that up to 271 million people use illicit drugs with up to 203 million cannabis users, 39 million users of opioids, amphetamines, or cocaine, and up to 21 million who inject drugs (Dengenhardt and Hall 2012). Data for the use of hallucinogenic drugs, ecstasy, inhalants, benzodiazepines could not be included in these estimates as global data are unavailable. Cannabis use was associated with dependence and psychosis and, in contrast to opioids, amphetamines and cocaine, was not strongly related to increased mortality. The prevalence of injecting drug users was highest in Eastern Europe (1.5 per cent) and about one per cent in North America and in Australia and New Zealand. The prevalence in Western Europe and in sub-Saharan Africa was 0.4 per cent. The global distribution of injecting drug users is shown in Fig. 20.6.

In the USA a national survey among 13–18-year-olds reported that 81 per cent of the oldest age group had

the opportunity to use illicit drugs; 43 per cent used these drugs and 16 per cent reported drug abuse, which was slightly more common than alcohol abuse (Swendsen et al. 2012). In the USA emergency admissions for opioid use rose 111 per cent between 2004 and 2008 (Nakawaki and Crano 2012) and a mortality study in young injection drug users in San Francisco found that mortality in this cohort was ten times that of the general population (Evans et al. 2012).

In a report from Canada (Single et al. 1999) substance abuse (tobacco, alcohol, and illicit drugs) was calculated to account for 21 per cent of all deaths, 23 per cent of the total years of potential life lost and eight per cent of hospital admissions. Worldwide deaths due to illicit drugs account for 0.4 per cent of total deaths and 1 per cent of disability-adjusted life-years (DALYs) in comparison to tobacco (nine per cent deaths and four per cent DALYs) and alcohol (four per cent deaths and five per cent DALYs) (Dengenhardt and Hall 2012).

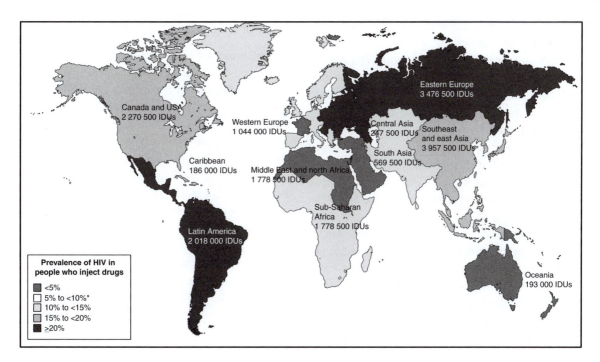

Figure 20.6 Numbers of injecting drug users across the world.

Reproduced from Degenhardt and Hall, 'Extent of illicit drug use and dependence, and their contribution to the global burden of disease', *Lancet* **379** (9810), 2012, with permission from Elsevier.

These proportions vary from country to country and region to region, but the proportion of young people aged 10–24 years was 1.8 billion in 2008 (27 per cent of the world population) and rising to 2 billion by 2032, suggests an important, and perhaps neglected group, that would benefit from improved public health interventions (Gore *et al*. 2011; Jackson *et al*. 2012).

20.4 Accidents, poisonings, and violence

An accident can be defined as 'an unusual event which proceeds from some unknown cause'. Accidents project an image of random events, 'acts of God', etc., but this is incorrect. Most accidents present characteristic patterns and are, therefore, predictable and potentially preventable. Particular patterns may be caused by social, behavioural, or environmental factors, and identification of risk factors is a prerequisite for preventive measures. The phrase 'injury' is often preferred,

as this relates to damage or hurt to the body produced by an external cause. This definition applies to both intentional and unintentional injuries. In ICD-10 'accidents, poisonings, and violence' are classified according to their 'external cause' in the interests of strategic planning of preventive policies.

Accidents (unintentional injuries) and poisonings caused almost four million deaths worldwide in 2004; 90 per cent of these occurred in low and middle income countries where 34 per cent were due to road traffic accidents, 10 per cent to poisonings, 10 per cent to falls, nine per cent to fires, 11 per cent to drowning, and 26 per cent to other or unreported external causes (Norton *et al*. 2006). Violence caused an estimated further 1.5 million deaths overall in 2004; 53 per cent of this was self-directed (suicide), 34 per cent due to homicide, and 13 per cent to war (Rosenberg *et al*. 2006). Death rates for both unintentional and intentional injuries are more than double in low- and middle-income countries compared to those in high-income countries. In Europe in 2008 suicide caused 126,000 deaths compared to

108,000 from traffic accidents. Suicide is discussed further in Chapter 14.

There were approximately 800,000 deaths due to injury throughout the WHO European Region in the year 2002, with twice as many male as female deaths. Half of all the deaths due to road traffic accidents (RTA), fire and self-harm, and two-thirds of the deaths due to violence occur between the ages of 15–44 years. The male excess is particularly noted for deaths due to violence and war but also for RTAs where, at younger ages, the male to female ratio is about 4:1. The male excess is attributed to greater exposure and more risk-taking behaviour. Over half of the deaths due to falls are in people aged over 60 years and nearly one-quarter are in the over 80s. Systematic reviews have suggested that it is possible to reduce by one-third the number of falls amongst older people (Gillespie 2004).

Worldwide, injuries account for 11.6 per cent of male deaths but 19.6 per cent of all male DALYs. If the current trends continue it is estimated that RTAs, self-inflicted injuries, interpersonal violence, and war-related injuries will be among the highest ranking causes of death and burden of disease in the world by 2020. Without appropriate action, RTAs, which were ranked ninth in 1990, will become the third leading contributor to the burden of disease by 2020, with over two-thirds of the deaths, and 90 per cent of the DALYs, arising in low- and middle-income countries. In the UK the financial cost of RTAs amounts to approximately 0.5 per cent of the GNP and that of home accident injuries to £25,000 million annually.

Causes of injury

Haddon, the first director of the National Traffic Safety Bureau in the US, proposed that standard public health approaches could be applied to RTAs; they could be thought of as the action of various *host* (human), *vector* (vehicle), and *environmental* (road network) factors operating before, during, and after the accident. This approach has been successfully extended to other types of accident. For RTAs (Table 20.3) the three phases are: (i) pre-crash—crash prevention; (ii) crash—injury limitation, and (iii) post-crash—health improvement).

Role of alcohol in injuries

Alcohol, because it impairs attention, coordination, and judgement, significantly increases both the *risk* of injury and the relative *severity* of the injury. Heavy drinkers are up to four times as likely to report an accident in the previous year compared to non-drinkers and a large proportion of all accidents, both traffic and domestic, which arrive in A&E departments, involve alcohol. Alcohol appears to be a key factor in interpersonal violence and has been linked with up to 50 per cent of injuries due to violence (WHO 2006). Alcohol is also an important antecedent for suicides and attempted suicides, deaths due to violence, fires, falls, and drowning. The strength of the relationship seems stronger for males and in northern European countries and Russia where drinking patterns are characterized by episodes of heavy drinking (Skog 2001).

Prevention

Many injuries, such as RTAs and falls in the elderly, should be considered alongside heart disease, cancer, and stroke as public health problems that respond well to preventive interventions. In the US the reduction in the rate of deaths attributable to motor vehicle crashes has been hailed as one of the top public health interventions of the 20th century (CDC 1999). Similar reductions have been seen in all EU countries. In contrast RTAs are predicted to rise rapidly in low- and middle-income countries; World Bank estimates place the increases between 40 per cent in Latin America to 150 per cent in South Asia by 2030 (Mathers and Loncar 2006).

Haddon's matrix (Table 20.3) gives a good indication of opportunities for primary, secondary, and tertiary prevention. Others have emphasized the three underlying principles of education, engineering, and enforcement. Engineering solutions require no active intervention or thought on the part of the individual. Examples include better house design, use of safety glass and the fitting of smoke alarms (though many still need the battery to be periodically checked), child-proof medicine containers, safer play environments, and cycle lanes. Some value-for-money interventions to prevent injury are shown in Table 20.4.

Table 20.3 The Haddon Matrix applied to road traffic accidents

	Host factors (human)	Vector factors (vehicle)	Environmental factors (road network)
Pre-crash	Education Attitudes Alcohol, drugs, fatigue Enforcement of traffic laws Reflective clothing for cyclists and pedestrians	Road worthiness Daytime lights on motorcycles Speed limitation systems	Road design including separation of car, pedestrians, and cyclists Provision of transport alternatives Speed limitation Better road marking, lighting
Crash	Alcohol Use of seat belts	Car design Seat belts, air bags Child restraints Use of helmets	Crash barriers Centre isle barriers
Post-crash	First aid and resuscitation Access to medical and rehabilitation services	Fire risk	CCTV at danger points Access for rescue services

Source: Centers for Disease Control and Prevention (1999).

20.5 Health education, promotion, and public policies

The complex interplay between historical, cultural, economic, medical, ethical, and legal factors in the social epidemiology of addictive behaviours perhaps best explain the failure of public health and other legislative measures to adequately control the social and personal harm caused by legal (tobacco and alcohol) and illegal drugs. Education, imparting knowledge on the risks alone, has largely failed for these disorders, perhaps insufficient in itself to deter experimentation and to encourage a change of behaviour. Similar comments may also apply to the control of cultural factors and behaviours responsible for the rising epidemic of obesity (Chapter 9) and the worldwide spread of AIDS. The promotion of health implies taking more active steps to improve the population's health and is discussed below. A primary purpose of epidemiology is to examine the causes of disease; but causes exist on different levels. Epidemiology has the tools to examine the question

Table 20.4 Value for money accident interventions

€1 spent on smoke alarms	saves €69
€1 spent on child safety seats	saves €32
€1 spent on bicycle helmets	saves €29
€1 spent on road safety improvements	saves €3
€1 spent on prevention counselling by paediatricians	saves €10
€1 spent on poison control services	saves €7
€1 spent on universal licensing of handguns	saves €79
€1 spent on home visits and education of parents about child abuse	saves €19

Reproduced from 'The solid facts on unintentional injuries and violence in the WHO European Region', Copenhagen, WHO Regional Health Office for Europe, 2005:4 (Fact sheet EURO/11/05 Rev. 1), with permission.

'does smoking cause disease?', but is poorly equipped to answer such questions as 'why do people smoke or become alcoholics or drug addicts?'. Tools to fully examine these questions may one day be developed using qualitative methods described in Chapter 1, in the context of a sociological or anthropological framework.

Although clear answers to all these questions have not been obtained, distinct social and cultural patterns of disease can be seen in many societies. Theoreticians have proposed frameworks to assist the development of public health policies. One report suggested that health was not simply a function of medical care; instead individuals could assume some responsibility for their own health through 'lifestyle' choices, but the importance of the social environment, personal competence, power and control, coping skills, social justice, housing, education, and civil society in promoting health is also recognized (Lalonde 1974). The acceptance of health as an outcome of many interacting factors led to proposals for action to develop and maintain good health. These proposals were formalized in the Ottawa Charter of 1986 which identified five priority areas for action (see Box 20.1).

The Charter recognized that there is a need to target behavioural change at the individual level as well as the need to affect social influences upon health, and to change organization and institutional structures. Changes in health behaviour occur in stages. In favourable environments, in the absence of adverse factors, individuals, families, small groups, and communities can be taught to assume responsibility for their health, which in turn changes their health behaviours and lifestyles. Change in health behaviour is usually a process,

not an event. There is a range of theories to explain how health decisions are made and how people can be influenced to change their health attitudes, choices, and behaviours (see Tones and Green 2004).

Early childhood has a profound impact on biological development through language development and learning capacity. Behaviours can be learnt through imitation and become, eventually, 'embedded' with lifelong effects on health. Epidemiological research suggests that children who have a healthy, stimulating start in life have fewer health and social problems later in life (Wadsworth 1997). Appropriate public health policies should invest in children (through early childhood education and healthy nutrition) and in parents (through support for expectant mothers, parenting skills, including financial and emotional support) to bring health benefits for children and families.

Material conditions have a major effect on educational and social attainment, independent of disease. Gradients in health status are linked to gradients of socio-economic status, and relative material wealth seems to have a substantial influence on an individual's overall health status. Government and social programmes such as economic development and wealth redistribution through taxation can be effective in reducing disparity and thereby improving health (see section 20.6).

Health promotion, which seeks to actively promote healthy behaviours, requires the co-operation of many sectors of society. More recently for alcohol the evidence of medical and social harm has come under increasing scrutiny in the UK. Proposed actions and their consequences should be agreed by politicians with the participation of **stakeholders** in the public, voluntary and private sectors. An example of two alternative strategies—high risk versus population based—to curb the rise in alcohol abuse are described below.

A 'high risk' approach to alcohol harm reduction

The Alcohol Harm Reduction Strategy published by the Prime Minister's Strategy Unit (Cabinet Office, Prime Minister's Strategy Unit 2004) emphasizes the need to

Box 20.1 The Ottawa Charter: improving the health of the population: priority areas for action.

1. Building healthy public policy
2. Creating supportive environments
3. Strengthening community action
4. Developing personal skills
5. Reorienting health services toward health promotion and disease prevention.

Source: WHO (1986).

target problem drinking including binge drinking, long-term heavy drinking, under-age drinking, and drinking associated with crimes, e.g. violence and drink-driving. The report focuses on four areas:

- *Education and communication* The report empha- sizes individual responsibility for behaviour and concludes that controlling average consumption through the mechanism of raising the price and limiting access would have unwanted side effects and was not a viable option. Instead, the report recommended that the public should be better informed regarding the risks associated with alco- hol, leading, hopefully, to more responsible drink- ing behaviour.

- *Identification and treatment* Individuals with prob- lems associated with alcohol should be identified earlier and have a ready access to appropriate treatment.

- *Crime and disorder* Targeting of crime caused by excess alcohol with greater police powers was recommended.

- *Alcohol industry* The industry on a voluntary basis, should be encouraged to manufacture and mar- ket alcohol in a responsible fashion, e.g. not using young looking actors or encouraging drunkenness.

A 'population based' approach to alcohol harm reduction

In contrast, the report from a leading medical organi- zation, The Academy of Medical Sciences, notes that public health measures such as education and adver- tising have not been shown to have any discernible benefit, and that targeting problem drinkers alone will not be sufficient to address the national public health problem. The report suggested the following:

- *Reducing consumption* (i) raising tax on alcohol to restore 1970s equivalent cost of alcohol; this should be particularly effective for under-age and chronic heavy drinkers; (ii) reducing the EU traveller's alco- hol allowance to 10 litres of table wine or equiva- lent in beer or spirits (cf. 90 litres at present) and; (iii) controlling alcohol industry advertising, espe- cially that targeted to the young.

- *Alcohol and driving* The acceptable blood alcohol level for driving should be reduced from 80 mg/dl to 50 mg/dl (and to 0 mg/dl for drivers under the age of 21 years).

- *Public debate and government response*. There should be a debate started within society about public opinion towards alcohol and appropriate drinking levels. Government departments along with researchers in the field of alcohol should develop a combined approach to alcohol harm.

A review of the effectiveness and cost-effectiveness of policies and programmes found that there was little or no evidence of effectiveness of public education and information but brief interventions to high risk patients in the health sector had a significant effect, at least in the shorter term. Governmental policies against drink- driving, and restriction of sales outlets, setting a mini- mum purchase age, restricting advertising, increasing taxation, and setting minimum pricing (Anderson *et al.* 2009).

20.6 Global inequalities in health

Modern society has done much good for the health and well-being of people—the average global life expectancy has increased by more than two decades since 1950. However not every social group or nation experienced this equally. The worldwide distribution of famines, wars, premature death, escalating levels of obesity, diabetes, cancers and mental illness, deaths and injury from traffic and extreme weather events, and the prevailing communicable disease killers is charac- terized by marked differences, both between countries and within countries (Friel *et al.* 2011; Marmot 2007).

Life expectancy is often used as a marker of population health. At the regional level, the health achievements enjoyed by developed countries have started happening in Asia and elsewhere but have considerable distance still to go. Life expectancy in sub-Saharan Africa has gone backwards in the last 20 years (Fig. 20.7).

The subregional level tells a story of marked inequal- ities between countries within the same region as well

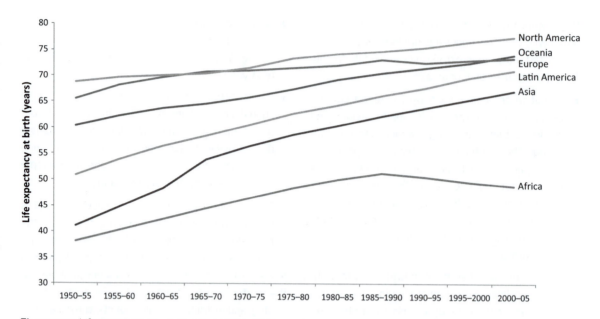

Figure 20.7 Life expectancy in world regions 1950–2005.

Reproduced from Dorling, Shaw, and Davey Smith, 'Global inequality of life expectancy due to AIDS', *BMJ*, 2006, with permission from BMJ Publishing Ltd.

as across regions. Major differences exist in early death. Recent estimates from WHO suggest that living past the age of 60 years is not the norm in 45 out of 195 countries (WHO 2006). The inequality is most pronounced among the male population; life expectancy at birth for males in 55 countries is 60 years or less. The risk of dying at a very early age is higher today compared to almost 50 years ago among the poorest countries.

Overall life expectancy is particularly affected by high levels of infant and child mortality but adult mortality differentials also exist. Premature death rates among adults vary enormously, e.g. Australia 76 per 1000 compared to Papua New Guinea 380 per 1000 (Rajaratnam *et al.* 2010). Within countries, a gap in health status exists between those at the top and bottom of the social hierarchy. We have seen earlier that education, income, occupation, and place of residence are major determinants of social inequalities but these are closely interrelated and modified by several other key factors (see Box 20.2). With few

exceptions, the evidence shows that the lower an individual's socio-economic position (measured by a number of different methods) the higher the risk of poor health and premature mortality, even in high-income countries such as those in Europe (Mackenbach *et al.* 2008).

In low- and middle-income countries large socio-economic differentials are seen in infant and child mortality which are no longer seen in high income countries

Box 20.2 Inequalities in health: more than one measure

Differences in health within countries are stratified along lines of ethnicity, gender, age, education, occupation, income, and class. Many studies (and policy and practice) concentrate on only one of these social dimensions at a time, but it is important to recognize that individuals are simultaneously positioned in terms of many social strata.

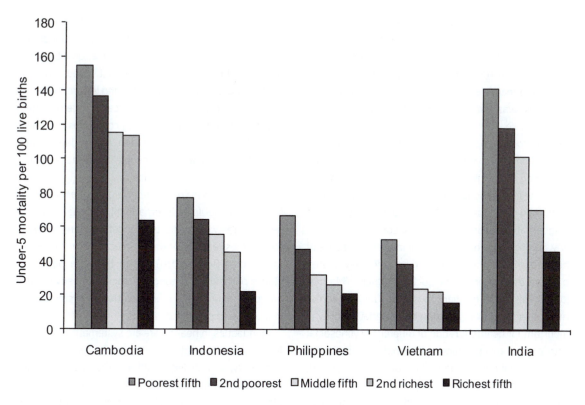

Figure 20.8 Child mortality in selected Asian countries by fifths of parental income.
Source: Gwatkin *et al.* (2007).

to the same degree. Some examples from the Asia-Pacific region are shown in Fig. 20.8 and this also shows large between-country differences in overall child mortality.

However, these socio-economic inequalities in health are not inevitable, nor are they beyond the capacity to change within a few decades. For example, in the case of Thailand there was a marked improvement in the social differentials of child mortality in one decade. This improvement coincided with the introduction of strengthening of health services and universal coverage for mothers and children (Vapattanawong *et al.* 2007).

Causes of inequalities in health

If there is no biological reason for the systematic differences in life expectancy or health conditions between different regions and countries then they are not inevitable

and need not exist. The very fact that there are these inequalities in health outcomes exist suggests that there is something about society contributing to them.

Freedoms and empowerment Most societies are hierarchical, stratified along a range of intersecting social categories; income, education, occupation, gender, age, ethnicity, and geography, in which economic and social resources are distributed unequally. Pursuit of health equity recognizes the need to redress the unequal distribution of these resources. This relates to empowerment of individuals, communities, and whole countries. Empowerment operates along three interconnected dimensions: material, psychosocial, and political: People need the basic material requisites for a decent life, they need to have control over their lives, and they need a voice and participation in decision-making processes.

Material empowerment The relationship between economic conditions and mortality has long been recognized, epitomized by the Preston curve which shows a curvilinear relationship between national income per head and life expectancy (Preston 2007). But, as Preston notes in his 2007 paper, only 16 per cent of the increase in life expectancy, between 1938 and 1963, was explained by increases in national income per se.

Psychosocial empowerment Employees of the British government have money, clean water, and shelter. Yet among these civil servants, men second from the top of the occupational hierarchy had a higher rate of death than men at the top. Men third from the top had a higher rate of death than those second from the top. Why, among men who are not poor in the usual sense of the word, should the risk of dying be intimately related to where they stand in the social hierarchy (Marmot 2004)? This social gradient in health suggests something other than, or in addition to, material security is important for health. A range of different psychosocial factors have been posited as potential contributors to health inequalities, including lack of control, support, social capital, and social cohesion.

Political empowerment Health equity depends on inclusion, agency, and control (Social Exclusion Knowledge Network 2007). This requires individuals and groups to represent their needs and interests strongly and effectively and, in so doing, to challenge and change the distribution of social resources (the conditions for health).

The social determinants of freedoms, empowerment, and health inequalities The three dimensions of empowerment and their social distribution are influenced by the fundamental environmental, socio-political, socio-economic, and socio-cultural characteristics of contemporary human societies which shape how people are born, grow, live, work, and age. Implicit here are two levels of determinants—the structural drivers that generate and distribute power, income, goods, and services, at global, national, and local levels and the more immediate conditions of daily living. The global economic context shapes international relations and domestic norms and policies, which in turn shape the way society organizes its affairs, giving rise to forms of social position and hierarchy. Economic and social policies generate and distribute political power, income, goods, and

services. These are distributed unequally across the social hierarchy. This means that different social groups have different exposure to, for example, quality health care and education, sufficient nutritious food and clean drinking water, conditions of work and leisure, and quality of housing and built environment. Together these structural factors and daily living conditions constitute the determinants of health and health inequalities, through their influence on people's material resource, psychosocial control, and voice.

Health care systems—a determinant of and solution to health inequalities International, national and local health care systems are both a determinant of health inequalities and a powerful mechanism to reduce inequalities (WHO 2010). Given the high burden of illness particularly among the socially disadvantaged groups, it is urgent to make health care systems more responsive to population needs.

Inequalities in health care are systematic differences in the use or receipt of quality public health, primary, secondary, and tertiary health care services, including hospitalizations, diagnostic tests, surgical procedures, physician visits, allied health services, medications, and participation in health promotion programmes. Gender, education, occupation, income, ethnicity, disability, and place of residence are all closely linked to the accessibility, experience, and benefits of health care.

The inverse care law (Tudor Hart 2000), in which the poor consistently gain less from health services than the better off, is visible in every country across the globe. Out-of-pocket expenditures for health care contribute to health inequalities, tending to deter poorer people from using both essential and non-essential services, leading to untreated morbidity. Health care systems that are based on health need rather than willingness or ability to pay promote what is termed *horizontal equity*. In OECD countries such as Australia where the cost of most doctor visits are subsidized and there are provisions to limit out-of-pocket costs, for a given level of need, better off women are more likely to use specialist medical, allied health, alternative health, and dental services than poorer women (Korda *et al.* 2009). These inequalities in access and use of a range of health care services, are particularly concerning in the context of reducing the burden of chronic disease

Policies to reduce inequalities in health

To make a fundamental improvement in health inequalities requires not only technical and medical solutions but also action in the immediate and structural conditions in which people are born, grow, live, work, and age. As a social determinants lens on health inequalities illuminates, good health for all is not only a matter for the health sector but must also involve sectors such as agriculture, urban planning, employment, and education (Fig. 20.9). Effective action on health inequalities therefore depends vitally on cross-sectoral coordination. This is manifested in a dynamic interrelation between the health system and the wider system of governance through which inequity in health outcomes are produced. This will help reduce health inequalities through attention to the needs of socially disadvantaged groups and help provide leadership in promoting coherent policies and practices in different sectors. However, even in welfare regimes, health inequalities often persist (Bambra 2011).

Underpinning action on the social determinants of health inequalities requires political will at the highest level, supported by an empowered public sector based on principles of justice, participation, and intersectoral collaboration. This means strong core functions of government and public institutions in relation to policy coherence, participatory governance, planning, regulation development and enforcement, and standard setting (Friel 2009; Marmot *et al.* 2008).

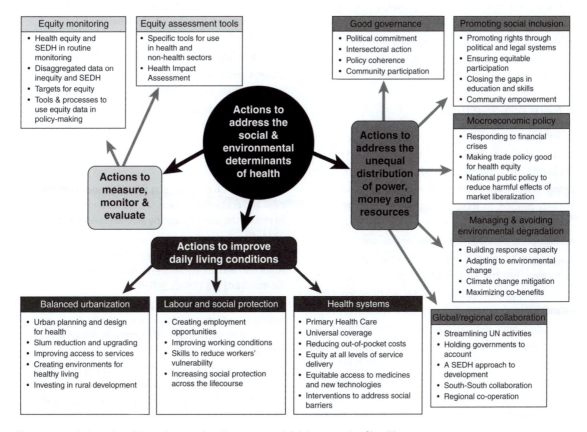

Figure 20.9 Actions to address the social and environmental determinants of health.
Reproduced from AP-HealthGAEN (2011) *An Asia Pacific spotlight on health inequity: Taking Action to Address the Social and Environmental Determinants of Health Inequity in Asia Pacific*. Asia Pacific HealthGAEN.

Role of the health sector

Appropriately configured and managed health systems provide a vehicle to improve people's lives, protect them from the vulnerability of sickness, generate a sense of life security, and build a common purpose within society. Health care systems contribute most to reducing health inequalities where the institutions and services are organized around the principle of universal coverage (extending the same scope of quality services to the whole population, according to needs, regardless of ability to pay), and where the system as a whole is based on Primary Health Care (including local action across the social determinants of health, and an equal level of entry to care with upward referral if necessary). In state-level analyses in the USA, there were fewer differences in self-rated health between higher and lower income-inequality areas where good primary care experiences were stronger. Evidence of success of primary level services in reducing health inequalities is also available from Africa (Liberia, Niger, Zaire), Asia (China, Kerala in India, Sri Lanka), and Latin America (Brazil, Cuba) (Starfield *et al.* 2005).

A focus on prevention

In middle- and high-income countries the rise and control of non-communicable diseases, injuries, and accidents are a health priority. Eating healthy diets, being physically active, and not smoking are each socially graded. In these countries, both excess body weight and tobacco use tends to be more prevalent among people further down the social and economic scale (WHO 2009). A focus on behaviours through screening, healthy eating advice, smoking cessation, and statin prescribing has been shown to widen socio-economic inequalities (Capewell and Graham 2012). A population wide approach would involve, for example, legislating to create smoke-free public spaces or to promote physical activity. Obesity prevention interventions that focus on behaviour change through personal skill development, information and social marketing campaigns may perpetuate socio-economic inequalities in obesity rates, given that the uptake of message is generally greater in higher social status groups (Friel et al. 2007).

In low-income countries the largest social disparities in health usually lie in the areas of maternal and child health and in infection with HIV. These are also the major health priorities for many of the poorest countries. Promoting universal coverage in rural and in urban areas, improving literacy and gender equality, and strengthening health services and promoting policies of sustainable development would seem to be the way forward for the poorest countries and these issues are discussed further in Chapter 22.

Further reading

Academy of Medical Sciences (2004) *Calling Time: The Nation's drinking as a major health issue*. London: Academy of Medical Sciences.

Dasbach EJ and Teutsch SM (2003) Quality of life. In: Haddix AC and Teutsch SM (eds) *Prevention Effectiveness: A Guide to Decision Analysis and Economic Evaluation*, 2nd edn, pp. 77–91. New York: Oxford University Press.

Marmot M (2004) *Status Syndrome*. London: Bloomsbury.

Tones K and Green J (2004) *Health Promotion. Planning and Strategies*. London: Sage.

World Bank (2005) *World Development Indicators*. Washington, DC: World Bank.

References

Anderson P, Chisholm D, and Fuhr DC (2009) Effectiveness and cost-effectiveness of policies and programmes to reduce the harm caused by alcohol. *Lancet* **373** (9682), 2234–46.

Ashworth M and Gerada C (1997) ABC of mental health. Addiction and dependence—II: Alcohol. *BMJ (Clinical Research Ed)* **315** (7104), 358–60.

Bambra C (2011) Health inequalities and welfare state regimes: theoretical insights on a public health 'puzzle'. *Journal of Epidemiology and Community Health* **65** (9), 740–5.

Britton A and McPherson K (2001) Mortality in England and Wales attributable to current alcohol consumption. *Journal of Epidemiology and Community Health* **55** (6), 383–8.

Cabinet Office, Prime Minister's Strategy Unit (2004). *Alcohol Harm Reduction Strategy for England*. London: Cabinet Office.

Capewell S and Graham H (2010) Will cardiovascular disease prevention widen health inequalities? *PLoS Medicine* **7** (8), e1000320.

Catalano RF, Fagan AA, Gavin LE, Greenberg MT, *et al.* (2012) Worldwide application of prevention science in adolescent health. *Lancet* **379** (9826), 1653–64.

CDC (1999) Centres for Disease Control and Prevention. Motor vehicle safety: a 20th century public health achievement. *Morbidity and Mortality Weekly Report* **48**, 369–74.

CSDH (2008) *Closing The Gap in a Generation: Health Equity Through Action on the Social Determinants of Health. Final Report of the Commission on Social Determinants of Health*. Geneva: World Health Organization.

Degenhardt L and Hall W (2012) Extent of illicit drug use and dependence, and their contribution to the global burden of disease. *Lancet* **379** (9810), 55–70.

Doll R, Peto R, Hall E, Wheatley K, *et al.* (1994) Mortality in relation to consumption of alcohol: 13 years' observations on male British doctors. *BMJ (Clinical Research Ed)* **309** (6959), 911–18.

Dorling D, Shaw M, and Davey Smith G (2006) Global inequality of life expectancy due to AIDS. *BMJ (Clinical Research Ed.)*. **332** (7542), 662–4.

Evans JL, Tsui JI, Hahn JA, Davidson PJ, *et al.* (2012) Mortality among young injection drug users in San Francisco: a 10-year follow-up of the UFO study. *American Journal of Epidemiology* **175** (4), 302–8.

Ezzati M, Lopez AD, Rodgers A, Vander Hoorn S, *et al.* (2002) Selected major risk factors and global and regional burden of disease. *Lancet* **360** (9343), 1347–60.

Friel S, Chopra M, and Satcher D (2007) Unequal weight: equity oriented policy responses to the global obesity epidemic. *BMJ (Clinical Research Ed)* **335** (7632), 1241–3.

Friel S (2009) *Health Equity in Australia: A Policy Framework Based on Action on the Social Determinants of Obesity, Alcohol and Tobacco*. Canberra: National Preventative Health Taskforce.

Friel SB, Loring, and A-Hs Group (2011) An Asia Pacific spotlight on health inequity: Taking action to address the social and environmental determinants of health inequity across Asia Pacific, Asia Pacific hub of Global Action for Health Equity Network. Available at http://healthgaen.org/?=1401.

Gillespe L (2004) Preventing falls in elderly people. *BMJ* **328** (7441) 653–4.

Goldman, B. (1993) Improving access to the underserved through Medicaid managed care. *Journal of Health Care for the Poor and Underserved* **4** (3), 290–8.

Gore FM, Bloem PJN, Patton GC, Ferguson J, *et al.* (2011) Global burden of disease in young people aged 10-24 years: a systematic analysis. *Lancet* **377** (9783), 2093–102.

Gwatkin DS, Rutstein K, Johnson E, Suliman A, *et al.* (2007) *Socio-Economic Differences in Health, Nutrition, and Population Within Developing Countries —An Overview*. New York: World Bank.

Hanlon PD, Walsh D, and Whyte B (2006) *Let Glasgow Flourish*. Glasgow: Glasgow Centre for Population Health.

Jackson C, Geddes R, Haw S, and Frank J (2012) Interventions to prevent substance use and risky sexual behaviour in young people: a systematic review. *Addiction (Abingdon, England)* **107** (4), 733–47.

Jarvis MJ (2004) Why people smoke. *BMJ* **328** (7434), 277–9.

Korda RJ, Banks E, Clements MS, and Young AF (2009) Is inequity undermining Australia's 'universal' health care system? Socio-economic inequalities in the use of specialist medical and non-medical ambulatory health care. *Australian and New Zealand Journal of Public Health* **33** (5), 458–65.

Lalonde, M. (1974) Social values and public health. *Canadian Journal of Public Health* **65** (4), 260–8.

Mackenbach JP, Stirbu I, Roskam A-JR, Schaap MM, *et al.* (2008) Socioeconomic inequalities in health in 22 European countries. *The New England Journal of Medicine* **358** (23), 2468–81.

Marmot M (2004) *Status Syndrome*. London: Bloomsbury.

Marmot M (2007) Achieving health equity: from root causes to fair outcomes. *Lancet* **370** (9593), 1153–63.

Marmot M, Friel S, Bell R, Houweling TAJ, *et al.* (2008) Closing the gap in a generation: health equity through action on the social determinants of health. *Lancet* **372** (9650), 1661–9.

Mathers CD and Loncar D (2006) Projections of global mortality and burden of disease from 2002 to 2030. *PLoS Medicine* **3** (11), e442.

Moser KA, Fox AJ, and Jones DR (1984) Unemployment and mortality in the OPCS Longitudinal Study. *Lancet* **2** (8415), 1324–9.

Nakawaki B and Crano WD (2012) Predicting adolescents' persistence, non-persistence, and recent onset of nonmedical use of opioids and stimulants. *Addictive Behaviors* **37** (6), 716–21.

Norton R, Hyder A, Bishai D and Peden M. (2006) Unintentional injuries. In: Jamison D, Breman J, Measham A, Alleyne G, et al. (eds.) Disease Control Priorities in Developing Countries, 2nd edn; pp. 737–53. Washington, DC: World Bank.

Peele S (1997) Utilizing culture and behaviour in epidemiological models of alcohol consumption and consequences for Western nations. Alcohol and Alcoholism 32 (1), 51–64.

Preston SH (2007) The changing relation between mortality and level of economic development. Population Studies, Vol. 29, No. 2, July 1975. Reprinted in: International Journal of Epidemiology 36 (3), 484–90.

Rajaratnam JK, Marcus JR, Levin-Rector A, Chalupka AN, et al. (2010) Worldwide mortality in men and women aged 15–59 years from 1970 to 2010: a systematic analysis. Lancet 375 (9727), 1704–20.

Rehm J, Mathers C, Popova S, Thavorncharoensap M, et al. (2009) Global burden of disease and injury and economic cost attributable to alcohol use and alcohol-use disorders. Lancet 373 (9682), 2223–33.

Rosenberg M, Butchart A, Mercy J, Narasimhan V et al. (2006) Interpersonal violence. In: Jamison D, Breman J, Measham A, Alleyne G, et al. (eds) Disease Control Priorities in Developing Countries, 2nd edn; pp. 755–70. Washington, DC: World Bank.

Single E, Robson L, Rehm J, Xie X, et al. (1999) Morbidity and mortality attributable to alcohol, tobacco, and illicit drug use in Canada. American Journal of Public Health 89 (3), 385–90.

Skog OJ (2001) Alcohol consumption and mortality rates from traffic accidents, accidental falls, and other accidents in 14 European countries. Addiction (Abingdon, England) 96 Suppl. 1 S49–58.

Social Exclusion Knowledge Network (2007) Understanding and tackling social exclusion. Final Report of the Social Exclusion Knowledge Network of the Commission on Social Determinants of Health. Geneva: World Health Organization.

Starfield B, Shi L, and Macinko J (2005) Contribution of primary care to health systems and health. The Milbank Quarterly 83 (3), 457–502.

Swendsen J, Burstein M, Case B, Conway KP, et al. (2012) Use and Abuse of Alcohol and Illicit Drugs in US Adolescents: Results of the National Comorbidity Survey—Adolescent Supplement. Archives of General Psychiatry 69 (4), 390–8.

Tones K and Green J (2004) Health Promotion. Planning and Strategies. London: Sage.

Tudor Hart J (2000) Commentary: three decades of the inverse care law. BMJ (Clinical Research Ed) 320 (7226), 18–19.

van Raalte AA, Kunst AE, Lundberg O, Leinsalu M, et al. (2012) The contribution of educational inequalities to lifespan variation. Population Health Metrics 10 (1), 3.

Vapattanawong P, Hogan MC, Hanvoravongchai P, Gakidou E, et al. (2007) Reductions in child mortality levels and inequalities in Thailand: analysis of two censuses. Lancet 369 (9564), 850–5.

Viner RM, Ozer EM, Denny S, Marmot M, et al. (2012) Adolescence and the social determinants of health. Lancet 379 (9826), 1641–52.

Wadsworth ME (1997) Health inequalities in the life course perspective. Social Science & Medicine (1982) 44 (6), 859–69.

West R (2004) Assessment of dependence and motivation to stop smoking. BMJ (Clinical Research Ed) 328 (7435), 338–9.

Winkleby M, Sundquist K,and Cubbin C (2007) Inequities in CHD incidence and case fatality by neighborhood deprivation. American Journal of Preventive Medicine 32 (2), 97–106.

WHO (1986) The Ottawa Charter. Available at http://www.who.int/healthpromotion/conferences/previous/ottawa/en/.

WHO (2005) The solid facts on unintentional injuries and violence in the WHO European Region. Fact sheet EURO/11/05. Copenhagen/Bucharest, WHO Europe.

WHO (2006) WHOIS. Geneva: World Health Organization.

WHO (2009) Global health risks: mortality and burden of disease attributable to selected major risks. Geneva: World Health Organization.

WHO (2010) The World Health Report 2010—Health systems financing: the path to universal coverage. Geneva: World Health Organization.

WHO (2011) Global status report on noncommunicable diseases 2010. Description of the global burden of NCDs, *their risk factors and determinants*. Geneva: World Health Organization.

Zaridze D, Brennan P, Boreham J, Boroda A, *et al.* (2009) Alcohol and cause-specific mortality in Russia: a retrospective case-control study of 48,557 adult deaths. *Lancet* **373** (9682), 2201–14.

Model answer

Question 1

In adults, consumption of tobacco, alcohol, and illicit drugs are all likely to be significantly underestimated. However, in the case of tobacco validation studies using biomarkers of nicotine suggest that consumption is not substantially underestimated by questionnaire data in population studies. However, in clinical studies medical disapproval may be a factor in producing a more substantial underestimate or even denial of consumption. Similar comments can be made concerning alcohol consumption which has the additional problem of binge drinking, which can be difficult to define, and which may fall short of alcohol addiction or dependence. In the case of illicit drugs, clearly confidentiality is an issue, as fear of prosecution may produce a significant underestimate of usage.

In the case of children, questionnaires need to be designed particularly carefully as there may be a tendency towards overestimation, since it is not unknown for adolescents to claim behaviour which they believe to be fashionable but in which they have not actually participated.

21 Epidemiology in public health practice

WILLIAM MOORE, W. CAIRNS SMITH, AND SHEELAH CONNOLLY

CHAPTER CONTENTS

This chapter introduces the topic of public health practice of which epidemiology is a core science. International, national, and local public health practice are reviewed as appropriate under four broad headings: health protection and disease prevention (see also Chapter 18); health improvement and promotion (see Chapter 20); the evaluation of public and personal health care services; and prevention in public health and clinical practice. Key themes in this chapter are the importance of adopting a systematic approach to population health assessment, and generation of pragmatic and workable public health strategies. Several important sources of information, mostly electronic, are given at the end of this chapter and are intended for additional self-directed learning.

Introduction

The public health function has been defined as: 'the science and art of preventing disease, prolonging life and promoting health through organized efforts of society' (Acheson 1988, after Winslow 1920). The 'science of public health' requires a robust, systematic, and evidence-based approach to describe and understand population health issues, and to identify optimal solutions for health improvement from available resources. The 'art of public health' refers to the interpersonal and organizational skills needed to work in partnership with others, influence decisions, support implementation of policy, programmes or projects, and to produce significant improvements in health indicators. The increasing pressures of globalization requires that public health operates at a global or regional level, but is practised at local area or country level. In general the level of development of public health services, and available resources, are historically higher in high income countries than in low and middle income counties, but core public health functions are common to all countries at every level of development. Some core functions of public health described separately for the Americas by the Pan American Public Health Organization and those for the UK are shown below in Box 21.1.

Box 21.1 Core activities in public health

United Kingdom[1]

1. Preventing epidemics
2. Protecting the environment, workplaces, food, and water
3. Promoting healthy behaviour
4. Monitoring the health status of the population
5. Mobilizing community action
6. Responding to disasters
7. Assuring the quality, accessibility, and accountability of medical care
8. Reaching out to link high-risk and hard-to-reach people to needed services
9. Research to develop new insights and innovative solutions
10. Leading the development of sound health policy and planning

The Americas[2]

1. Monitoring, evaluation, and analysis of health status
2. Surveillance, research, and control of the risks and threats to public health
3. Health promotion
4. Social participation in health
5. Development of policies and institutional capacity for public health planning and management
6. Strengthening of public health regulation and enforcement capacity
7. Evaluation and promotion of equitable access to necessary health services
8. Human resources development and training in public health
9. Quality assurance in personal and population-based health services
10. Research in public health
11. Reduction of the impact of emergencies and disasters on health

[1] From Pencheon et al, *Oxford Handbook of Public Health Practice*, 2001, with permission from Oxford University Press and
[2] PAHO Essential Public Health Functions Accessed at: **http://www.paho.org/english/dpm/shd/hp/EPHF.htm**

The core functions of public health clearly reflect its multidisciplinary nature and its need to operate at all levels of society. Three broad domains of public health practice can be identified: health protection and disease prevention; health improvement; and organization and management of health care, with particular emphasis on preventive services. Many core skills are required for public health practice which overlap, but differ in activities and scope from those in clinical practice; core skills and training will be discussed in the following sections.

21.1 Health protection and disease prevention

Epidemiology is recognized as the core skill for public health practitioners, others include *surveillance* and *monitoring* skills, both for disease, risk factors, and for health status, and *organizational* and *implemental* skills in dealing with outbreaks of infectious diseases or influencing health-related behaviours. Increasingly, public health practitioners will be required also to have basic skills in *health economics*, both for the role of managing health care resources and in the development of cost-effective models for disease prevention. Public health practitioners work to improve and protect population health by public health actions (at any organizational level), and to develop or modify health systems. At a global level the World Health Organization (WHO) has two major roles in global public health; surveillance and monitoring of disease and health status; the development of strategies to control infections, both epidemic and endemic, and chronic, non-infectious disease, in adults and children. These are discussed more fully in Chapter 22.

Health protection aims to prevent adverse health consequences from exposure to infectious agents or environmental hazards through surveillance, ongoing control measures, and a direct response to specific events or incidents. The *physical environment* includes physical, chemical, or biological factors external to an individual, and related human behaviours or activities. A *hazard* is the intrinsic capacity of a given factor or context to produce an adverse health outcome. WHO estimate that approximately 25 per cent of the global disease burden can be attributed to potentially modifiable factors in the physical environment (Prüss-Üstün and Corvalán 2006). Environmental hazards have traditionally been associated with poverty and insufficient development. Improvements in sanitation and hygiene, with an associated reduction in infectious disease risk, are major 20th-century public health success stories but rapid economic development that lacks health and environment safeguards, and unsustainable consumption of natural resources, creates a new set of environmental hazards, as illustrated in Table 21.1.

In order to counter the adverse effects of new environmental hazards WHO has recommended a cause and effect framework to identify important linkages and support the development of effective policies and interventions which include examination of the following elements shown in Box 21.2.

At national levels different organizational structures are found which promote public health practice. In the US the Centers for Disease Control (CDC) provide the main focus for the policy support for the public health service and its mission statement is: . . . 'working with partners throughout the nation and world to monitor health, detect and investigate health problems, conduct research to enhance prevention, develop and advocate sound public health policies, implement prevention strategies, promote healthy behaviors, foster safe and healthful environments, and provide leadership and training'. Twelve centres with different functions form the basis of CDC programmes and activities, and further information for each of the programmes is available at the CDC website (appended).

The equivalent body in the UK is the Health Protection Agency and its work in the control of communicable disease is discussed in Chapter 18. A broader, long-term, view of health and its determinants was highlighted by recently proposed indicators of *sustainable development* from the UK Department of Environment, Food and Rural Affairs (DEFRA) shown in Box 21.3. The need to coordinate strategic goals between different government agencies has been stressed by Ayres and Agius (2004), and the recognition that these goals fall under the general remit of national, local, and international public health should assist this process. Further information on the organization and function of the Health Protection and Food Standards Agencies is provided on their respective websites appended to this chapter.

Table 21.1 Environmental hazard risk transition

'Traditional' environmental hazards	'Modern' environmental hazards
• lack of access to safe drinking water • inadequate basic sanitation (household and community) • food contamination (pathogens) • indoor air pollution (cooking and heating using biomass fuel or coal) • inadequate solid waste disposal • occupational injury hazards (agriculture and cottage industries) • natural disasters (including floods, droughts, and earthquakes) • vector-borne disease vectors (insects and rodents)	• water pollution (populated areas, industry, and intensive agriculture) • air pollution (transport, energy generation, and industry) • solid and hazardous waste accumulation • chemical and radiation hazards (introduction of industrial and agricultural technologies) • infectious disease hazards (emerging and re-emerging) • major ecological change in 'closed' system (deforestation, land degradation, ozone depletion, transboundary pollution, and climate change)

Reproduced from Corvalán CF, Kjellström T, and Smith KR. 'Health, Environment and Sustainable Development. Identifying Links and Indicators to Promote Action'. *Epidemiology* 1999; **10**, 656–60 with permission from Wolters Kluwer Health.

Box 21.2 Assessment of environmental hazards.

Driving forces—create the conditions or context for environmental health hazards such as economic development policies, inequalities in access, technological and scientific development, consumption patterns, and population growth or urbanization.

Pressure on the environment—such as waste production, depletion of natural resources, or emission of pollutants from human activities.

State of the environment—resultant potential sources of physical, chemical, or biological environmental hazards.

Exposure—individual's acquired dose is dependent on the exposure pathway (inhalation, ingestion, or direct contact) and the magnitude, frequency, and duration of contact.

Effect on health—the risk of adverse health outcome is dependent on nature of the hazard, acquired dose, and individual susceptibility.

Source: Kjellstrom T, van Kerkhoff L, Bammer G, McMichael T (2003). 'Comparative assessment of transport risks—how it can contribute to health impact assessment of transport policies'. *Bulletin of the World Health Organization* 2003; **81** (6), 451–457.

Box 21.3 Headline indicators of sustainable development.

Economic

Economic output

Investment

Employment

Social

Poverty and social exclusion

Education

Health

Housing

Crime

Environmental

Climate change

Air quality

Road traffic

River water quality

Wildlife

Land use

Waste

Reproduced from Ayres and Agius, 'Health protection and sustainable development', *BMJ*, 2004, with permission from BMJ Publishing Group Ltd.

21.2 Health improvement

A key skill for public health practice, and a prerequisite for health improvement, is 'health (care) needs assessment'. This has been defined specifically as 'the assessment of the population's ability to benefit from health care' (Stevens *et al.* 2004). In public health terms, **needs assessment** should incorporate both a description of the difference between the current situation and the optimal population health status, and the capacity to reduce any 'gap' by a specified health action. The perspective of the public health practitioner is related to populations rather than to individuals, and **population health gain** does not necessarily mean that the health of *every* individual in a population will be positively affected. In recognition of the scarcity of resources, the discipline of economics differentiates between *wants*, *demands*, and *supply*, whereas sociologists refer to *felt*, *expressed* and *normative* (current average) needs. It is unreasonable to generalize needs assessment findings from one population to another without local consultation, as the definition and interpretation of 'need' may be subject to many external influences (Fig. 21.1).

Health assessment

The epidemiological approach provides a generic framework to quantify and describe the health of a given population. A cautionary note is provided by a former Nobel Prize winner (Box 21.4).

It is not possible to assess every health issue so activities are often focused on 'fire-fighting' and on 'apparent' problems. However, specific assessments may be indicated following: the results of previous assessment; political or public input; allocation of

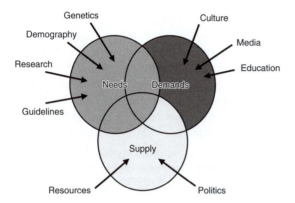

Figure 21.1 External influences and the relationship between needs, demand, and supply.
Reproduced from Stevens *et al.*, *Healthcare Needs Assessment: The Epidemiologically Based Needs Assessment Reviews*, with permission from Radcliffe.

Box 21.4 Epidemiological approach to health assessment

I. Scope and define the health issue(s)
II. Agree population health assessment aims and objectives
III. Define and profile the 'population base' and subgroups—denominator(s)
IV. Define health events or health-related factors—numerator(s)
V. Collect, collate, and analyse data
VI. Interpret results appropriately
VII. Disseminate findings to support informed decisions and choices

Source: Stevens *et al.* (2004).

'Not everything that counts can be counted and not everything that can be counted, counts.'
  Albert Einstein (letter to President Roosevelt)

'ring-fenced' funding for service development; the occurrence of a critical or major incident; or the publication of new research, guidelines, or standards. Although the epidemiological approach can provide an estimate of the size of a particular health issue, this may not be sufficient to capture all potentially relevant factors (e.g. political and bureaucratic). Identifying feasible solutions often requires the use of methodology from other disciplines such as the social sciences, psychology, economics, management, and politics.

Fundamental to needs assessment is the availability of relevant and reliable data. WHO has a long-established role in surveillance and monitoring of health status of populations across the globe and these data provide the basis for its theme-based annual reports. In recent years its Global Health Observatory has developed data sets at country and regional levels which monitor the progress towards achieving the Millennium Development Goals (see Chapter 22). In the European region of WHO an extensive interactive database provides a wide range of health and demographic data at country level. Public Health Observatories have been established across the UK and Ireland to help monitor health status at local authority level and to direct attention and resources by public health professionals. Websites for these extensive databases are appended to this chapter.

21.3 Evaluation and financing of health services

In most countries the costs of financing health services continue to rise with rising life expectancies and investment in advanced diagnostic and therapeutic technologies. There is therefore a strong incentive for the development of appropriate methods for assessing both the **effectiveness** and **efficiency** of health system performance.

Evaluation

How can health service **inputs** and **outcomes** be best measured and compared? Clearly standard indicators available for the majority of countries are required. In early studies (e.g. Cochrane *et al.* 1978) input was measured by health service expenditure (adjusted to a standard cost of living index) and health service staffing; and output measured by infant, maternal, and premature adult mortality, and life expectancy. More recently, coverage of primary care has been added to input together with a number of additional outputs, which include life expectancy adjusted for quality (QALY) or disability (DALY) (see Chapters 2, 15, and 20). A recent WHO Annual Report (WHO 2000) addressed

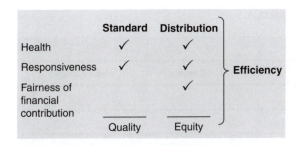

	Standard	Distribution
Health	✓	✓
Responsiveness	✓	✓
Fairness of financial contribution		✓
	Quality	Equity

Efficiency

Figure 21.2 How well do health systems perform?
Reproduced from Murray C and Frenk J (2001) 'World Health Report 2000: a step towards evidence-based health policy'. *Lancet*. **357** (9269), 1698–1700, with permission from Elsevier.

the question 'How well do health systems perform?' and produced a combined output index based on three indicators: disability-adjusted life expectancy (DALE), responsiveness (a measure of patient satisfaction based on the perceived responsiveness of health service personnel to personal need), and financial fairness (a measure of equality of access) (Murray and Frenk 2001). The parameters are shown in Fig. 21.2.

In the WHO report standard or level of health was measured by DALEs but other, less controversial measures could be used (e.g. mortality), and responsiveness and equality of access was based on subjective rather than objective measures. The rank order for a sample of countries according to this index of 'health output' was: France (1), Italy (2), Norway (11), UK (18), Ireland (19), Switzerland (20), and the US (37). Rank order based on disability-adjusted life expectancy (DALE) alone was as follows: Japan (1), Australia (2), France (3), Sweden (4), Italy (6), Switzerland (8), UK (14), US (24), and Ireland (27), but the range of DALEs in these high income countries was only five years; from 74.5 years (Japan) to 69.6 years (Ireland).

In Table 21.2 a range of health service inputs and outputs for Canada and the USA are shown. These two countries had different levels of public expenditure in 2006 with contrasting levels of life expectancy in 2005/6, and substantially higher overall spending on health in the USA (largely attributed to higher private administration costs) (Mills and Ranson 2012).

WHO has provided an outline framework for assessing the performance of health systems (Murray and Frenk 2001) and elsewhere the conceptual bases and

performance indicators for the UK, Canada, Australia, USA, WHO and OECD, have been examined (Arah *et al*. 2003).

Individual health care operates at the primary, secondary, and tertiary level, with overlap to achieve continuity of care. Although public health prevention mainly operates at the primary and secondary stages, increasingly, primary care, in the UK at least, is taking a greater role in primary prevention. Primary care (general) practitioners are the 'gatekeepers' for access to specialist services in many countries; health systems which permit direct access may be more wasteful of resources, and costly to maintain. Development of primary care services has been stressed as a vehicle for advancing universal coverage in low- and middle-income countries but, with the exception of Thailand (Mills and Ranson 2012) and, more recently China, few countries have used this line of development.

Clearly, the diversity of health care systems and the absence of any experimental data make comparisons of the effectiveness and efficiency of different health care systems very difficult. Nevertheless, performance indicators may be essential to future developments of health care systems, both in the poorest countries with underdeveloped health sectors, and in wealthy countries where costs and public expectations have spiralled ever upwards. Methods of financing health systems are reviewed in the following section.

Financing of health systems

Countries adopt different approaches to financing their health system and most adopt a combination of methods including: *general taxation, social insurance, private insurance, out-of-pocket payments* and *external organizations*, such as donor agencies. In the World Bank regions high-income countries spend on average 11 per cent of their GDP on health (61 per cent from government spending), compared to about 5 per cent (50 per cent or less from government) in low and middle income countries (Ruger *et al*. 2012). Summaries of health spending for selected countries in some WHO regions are shown in Chapter 22.

General taxation is used as a source of health system financing to some extent in most high-income countries. Income taxation has the advantage that it

Table 21.2 Health inputs and outputs in 2006 in Canada and in the USA

Comparative Data On US and Canadian Health Systems		
Indicators	Canada	United States
Population, 2007 (in millions)	33.4	301.1
GDP per capita, 2008 (in 2008 dollars)	38,200.0	46,000.0
Per capita health expenditure, 2006	3,678.0	6,714.0
Health spending, 2006 (as a percentage of GDP)	10.0	15.3
Percentage of health spending, 2006		
● Public expenditures	70.4	45.8
● Inpatient care	28.4	25.9
● Outpatient care	25.0	44.8
● Pharmaceuticals	18.2	12.8
Acute care inpatient beds per 1,000 population, 2005 (Canada) 2006 (United States)	2.8	2.7
Average length of stay in days, 2005	7.2	4.8
Percentage of population with no insurance, 2007	0.0	14.6
Out-of-pocket payments per capita, 2006	532.0	856.0
Private insurance as a percentage of expenditure on health, 2006	12.6	36.0
Life expectancy (in years) at birth: females, 2005	82.7	79.8
Life expectancy (in years) at birth: males, 2005	80.4	75.2

Note: Financial data are denoted in U.S. dollars.
Folland S, Goodman AC, and Stano M (2010) *The Economics of Health and Health Care*, 6th edn. © 2010. Reprinted with permisson of Pearson Education, Inc. Upper Saddle River, NJ.

is generally progressive in nature, so that those with a higher income pay a higher proportion of their income than those with a lower income; though tax on some goods and services can be regressive. Under a general taxation system, everyone who pays taxes contributes, not just those who require health care. A *social insurance system* operates in many high-income countries in Europe and in Canada. Social health insurance contributions are levied on earned income with contributions usually compulsory and shared between the employee and employer. As social insurance systems are generally related to employment, special provisions

are made for those not attached to the labour market. Similarly to the general taxation system, paying for the health system is not related to the risk of needing health services. *Private health insurance* is the currently the main method of paying for health services in the USA, with special provisions for those not able to afford this. The insurance market may operate a system of individual rating, where an individual's premium reflects their risk of using health services, or community rating, where all individuals pay the same amount for an insurance product, regardless of their individual risk. In both systems, pooling of risk occurs among those purchasing insurance from the same provider. *Out-of-pocket payments* involve patients or their relatives paying for health care services at the point of use, and are used in all health systems to some extent. In a system solely based on out-of-pocket payments, there is no pooling of risk but rather health services are paid for when required. In many low- and middle-income countries this is the primary method of funding health services. A final method used to finance a health system is securing funding from *external organization or countries*, and is mainly used in low-income countries with greatest need. Financing of health services is discussed further in Chapter 22.

Clinical governance and audit

Epidemiological, organizational, other multidisciplinary and clinical skills are required in the setting of standards of quality in clinical care (clinical governance), which is required in all specialities. These standards encompass both the optimal cost-effective delivery of health care under differing systems, and clinical standards that may be expected by patients. Mechanisms and frameworks which can evaluate quality in medical care are still evolving but these should be simple, unbureaucratic and equally fair to patients and to their doctors and other health professionals. Minimum standards have been proposed in the USA (Box 21.5).

In the UK *audit* is an ongoing quality improvement process to systematically measure performance against standards, identify issues, plan and implement changes, and then re-audit (National Institute for Clinical Excellence 2002) and this is outlined in Fig. 21.3.

21.4 Prevention in public health and clinical practice

A core aim of this textbook is to show the role of epidemiology in examining the scope for prevention of disease in a limited text. A secondary aim is to encourage students in their future careers to question medical dogma and myth and to ask the question 'why?'

more often than their predecessors. We examined in Chapters 1 to 3 the role of epidemiology in unravelling the natural history of disease, in establishing risk factors, and in estimating the proportion of disease that could be attributed to individual risk factors. There have been some epidemiological success stories in the past few decades; for example, linking the natural history of human immunodeficiency virus and bovine spongiform encephalopathy with 'infectious' agents (necessary causes), and cardiovascular disease with multiple causes. Many of the established risk factors for ischaemic heart disease (IHD) and stroke are potentially modifiable and provide the opportunity for primary prevention in the general population. Modelling studies in several high income countries in Europe and North America indicate that population changes in major risk factors account for over half of the population decline in IHD and modern treatments for a further third (Capewell and O'Flaherty 2011). Cardiovascular diseases are now common and reaching epidemic proportions in low- and middle-income countries. Adverse risk factor trends globally for physical activity, obesity, and type 2 diabetes mellitus (discussed in Chapter 9) have prompted a major initiative by WHO to counter the medical consequences of these trends with policymakers at national and regional level (Mendis and Fuster 2009). The case for an increased emphasis on the primary prevention of diabetes by public health and policy interventions is strongly argued by McKinley and Marceau (2000) and, in turn, intensive, early treatment of diabetes could reduce the increasing burden of end stage renal disease from diabetic complications (Atkins 2005). The Centers for Disease Control recently reviewed 10 great public health achievements in the first decade of the 21st century. These are shown in Box 21.6.

Although understanding and control of risk factors can be effective in reducing disease incidence (primary prevention), interruption of the natural history of diseases by early effective interventions can also have an effect on the burden of disease (secondary prevention). Chapter 5 discussed screening methods, including those for the early detection of cancers, which are now an increasing public health and clinical problem as life expectancy increases and overall mortality from

Box 21.5 Dimensions of quality in health care

- *Person-centred*—providing care that is responsive to individual personal preferences, needs, and values and assuring that patient values guide all clinical decisions.
- *Safe*—avoiding injuries to patients from health care that is intended to help them.
- *Effective*—providing services based on scientific knowledge.
- *Efficient*—avoiding waste, including waste of equipment, supplies, ideas, and energy.

- *Equitable*—providing care that does not vary in quality because of personal characteristics such as gender, ethnicity, geographic location or socio-economic status; and
- *Timely*—reducing waits and sometimes harmful delays for both those who receive care and those who give care

Reproduced from Institute of Medicine (Committee on Quality of Health Care in America) 2001. *Crossing the quality chasm: a new health system for the 21st century.* Institute of Medicine, with permission from the National Academy Press.

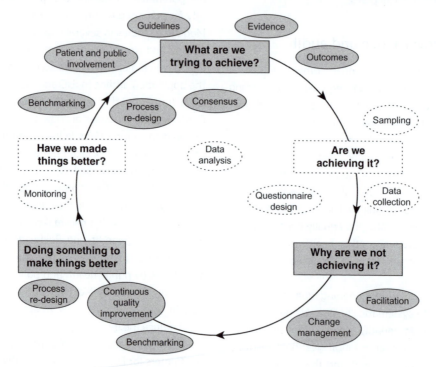

Figure 21.3 The audit cycle—best practice.
Source: National Institute for Clinical Excellence (2002).

cardiovascular disease declines. Early detection of cancers and improved treatments are the best hope for patients, unless the natural history is strongly linked with risk factors such as smoking or occupational carcinogens. Epidemiological methods are required to evaluate screening and treatment trials, which often have to be conducted on large numbers of patients in multi-centre studies. The latest databases of evidence for these interventions (discussed in Chapter 20) will be increasingly required by practitioners to ensure optimal treatment of their patients. Monitoring and audit by special surveys of the treatment of CHD in Europe showed considerable variation in the quality of medical care in European countries (Anon 1997).

Box 21.6 Ten great public health achievements, 2001–2010

Worldwide

1 Reductions in child mortality
2 Vaccine-preventable diseases
3 Access to safe water and sanitation
4 Malaria prevention and control
5 Prevention and control of HIV/AIDS
6 Tuberculosis control
7 Control of neglected tropical diseases
8 Tobacco control
9 Increased awareness and response for improving global road safety
10 Improved preparedness and response to global health threats

Source: CDC (2011). 'Ten Great Public Health Achievements-Worldwide, 2001–2010 *Morbidity and Mortality Weekly Report (MMWR)* 2011; **60**; 814–18

To address such concerns in the UK, National Service Frameworks and guidelines for investigation and treatment are issued at intervals, either directly through the Department of Health (e.g. National Clinical Frameworks for: CHD, for the Elderly, and for Diabetes), or indirectly, through agencies such as the National Institute for Health and Clinical Excellence (NICE). Guidelines and frameworks such as these provide summaries of the evidence base and opportunities for self-audit, but probably best improve the quality of care for patients by raising awareness of innovations in treatments and care. Similar guidelines are produced in the USA and elsewhere by international organizations of clinical specialities.

As noted earlier in this chapter costs of health care have increased disproportionately in most developed countries, particularly for specialist care in hospitals. Preventive efforts, particularly those which require mass screening can be costly also; but costs of population prevention programmes are generally small compared to those required in the hospital sector and for the institutionalized elderly. Recent data have indicated a tenfold increase in health care costs in the last year of life compared to that five years before death, although costs begin to increase 15 years prior to death (Seshamani and Gray 2004). League tables based on cost-effectiveness have been developed for the preventive services in the USA (Messonnier *et al.* 1999; Coffield *et al.* 2001), and epidemiological principles and methods, in addition to economic skills, will be required to develop these approaches further in the future. In the meantime, however, public health policies should be based on pragmatic solutions which are both acceptable to the public, and can produce cost-benefit in terms of validated indicators (Kelly *et al.* 2009).

21.5 Training in public health

Public health medicine is probably the most multidisciplinary of medical specialities and provides opportunities for careers for both medical and non-medical students. Examination of the core essential functions and core activities in public health shown in Box 21.1 gives an indication of the breadth of activities and levels of responsibility in the discipline. We have attempted to introduce the main topics included in the discipline, for example: preventive and clinical medicine, public health statistics, microbiology, health economics, health psychology, and social policy among other disciplines, and training programmes in Europe, the USA, and in Australasia are shown in Table 21.3.

This chapter has reviewed the use of epidemiological tools in public health practice. What appears evident is that public health is a highly diverse and challenging discipline requiring a sound knowledge of epidemiological theory and continuous updating of practice in order to maintain and improve the health of our diverse populations.

Web addresses

Association of Public Health Observatories, UK
http://www.apho.org.uk
Centers for Disease Control, USA
http://www.cdc.gov/

Table 21.3 Public health training—programmes and standards in selected countries and regions

UK	Faculty of Public Health (UK) http://www.fph.org.uk/training
	Public Health Online Resource for Careers, Skills, and Training (PHORCaST): http://www.phorcast.org.uk/
Ireland	Faculty of Public Health Medicine (Royal College of Physicians of Ireland): http://www.rcpi.ie/Pages/PHMEducationTraining.aspx
Australia/New Zealand	Australasian Faculty of Public Health Medicine: http://www.racp.edu.au/page/racp-faculties/australasian-faculty-of-public-health-medicine/
Europe	Association of Schools of Public Health in the European Region (ASPHER): http://www.aspher.org
USA	Association of Schools of Public Health (ASPH): http://www.asph.org
	American Board of Preventive Medicine: https://www.theabpm.org/index.cfm
	Centers for Disease Control and Prevention. Preventive Medicine Residency and Fellowship (PMR/F): http://www.cdc.gov/prevmed/

Department of Health (1999) The NHS performance assessment framework.
http://www.dh.gov.uk/PublicationsAndStatistics/Publications/PublicationsPolicyAndGuidance/PublicationsPolicyAndGuidanceArticle/fs/en?CONTENT_ID=4009190&chk=riXW/M

Department of Health (2005) NHS Improvement Plan
http://www.dh.gov.uk/Home/fs/en

Food Standards Agency, UK
http://www.food.gov.uk

Health Protection Agency, UK
http://www.org.uk

Institute of Medicine (IOM) (2002) Board on Health Promotion and Disease Prevention (HPDP). The Future of the Public's Health in the 21st Century
http://www.nap.edu/books/030908704X/html/

WHO (2000) The world health report 2000. Health systems: improving performance.
http://www.who.int/whr/en/

WHO (2002) The world health report 2002. Reducing risks, promoting healthy life.
http://www.who.int/whr/en/

Further reading

Brown RC, Baker EA, Leet TL, and Gillespie KN (2003) *Evidence-Based Public Health*. New York: Oxford University Press.

Detels R, Beaglehole R, Lansang MA, and Gulliford M (eds) (2009) *Oxford Textbook of Public Health*, 5th edn. Oxford: Oxford University Press.

Haddix AC, Teutsch SM, and Corso PA (eds) (2003) *Prevention Effectiveness. A Guide to Decision Analysis and Economic Evaluation*, 2nd edn. New York: Oxford University Press.

Pencheon D, Guest C, Melzer D, and Muir Gray JA (eds) (2001) *Oxford Handbook of Public Health Practice*. Oxford: Oxford University Press.

References

Acheson D (1988) *Public Health in England. Report of the Committee of Inquiry into the Future Development of the Public Health function.* London: Department of Health.

Anon (1997) EUROASPIRE. A European Society of Cardiology survey of secondary prevention of coronary heart disease: principal results. EUROASPIRE Study Group. *European Heart Journal* **18** (10), 1569–82.

Arah OA, Klazinga NS, Delnoij DMJ, ten Asbroek AHA, *et al.* (2003) Conceptual frameworks for health systems performance: a quest for effectiveness, quality, and improvement. *International Journal for Quality in Health Care* **15** (5), 377–98.

Atkins RC (2005) The changing patterns of chronic kidney disease: the need to develop startegies for prevention relevant to different regions and countries. *Kidney International* Suppl. (98), S83–85.

Ayres JG and Agius R (2004) Health protection and sustainable development. *BMJ (Clinical Research Ed)* **328** (7454), 1450–1.

Capewell S and O'Flaherty M (2011) Rapid mortality falls after risk-factor changes in populations. *Lancet* **378** (9793), 752–3.

CDC (2011) Ten Great Public Health Achievements—Worldwide, 2001–2010. *Morbidity and Mortality Weekly Report (MMWR)* **60**; 814–18.

Cochrane AL, St Leger AS, and Moore F (1978) Health service 'input' and mortality 'output' in developed countries. *Journal of Epidemiology and Community Health* **32** (3), 200–5.

Coffield AB, Maciosek MV, McGinnis JM, Harris JR, *et al.* (2001) Priorities among recommended clinical preventive services. *American Journal of Preventive Medicine* **21** (1), 1–9.

Corvalán CF, Kjellström T, and Smith KR (1999) Health, environment and sustainable development: identifying links and indicators to promote action. *Epidemiology (Cambridge, Mass.)* **10** (5), 656–60.

Folland S, Goodman AC, and Staino M (2010) *The economics of health and health care*, 6th edn. Upper Saddle River, NJ: Prentice Hall.

Institute of Medicine (Committee on Quality of Health Care in America) (2001) Crossing the quality chasm: a new health system for the 21st century. Washington, DC: National Academy.

Kelly MP, Stewart E, Morgan A, Killoran A, *et al.* (2009) A conceptual framework for public health: NICE's emerging approach. *Public Health.* **123** (1), e14–20.

Kjellstrom T, van Kerkhoff L, Bammer G, and McMichael T (2003) Comparative assessment of transport risks—how it can contribute to health impact assessment of transport policies. *Bulletin of the World Health Organization* **81** (6), 451–7.

McKinlay J and Marceau L (2000) US public health and the 21st century: diabetes mellitus. *Lancet* **356** (9231), 757–61.

Mendis S and Fuster V (2009) National policies and strategies for noncommunicable diseases. *Nature Reviews. Cardiology* **6** (11), 723–7.

Messonnier ML, Corso PS, Teutsch SM, Haddix AC, *et al.* (1999) An ounce of prevention . . . what are the returns? *American Journal of Preventive Medicine* **16** (3), 248–63.

Mills AJ and Ranson MK (2012) The design of health systems. In: Merson MH, Black RE, and Mills AJ (eds) *Global Health: Diseases, Programs, Systems, and Policies,* pp. 615–52. Burlington, MA: Jones and Bartlett Learning.

Murray C and Frenk J (2001) World Health Report 2000: a step towards evidence-based health policy. *Lancet* **357** (9269), 1698–1700.

National Institute for Clinical Excellence (2002) *Principles for Best Practice in Clinical Audit.* Abingdon: Radcliffe Medical Press.

Pencheon D, Guest C, Melzer D, and Muir Gray JA (eds) (2001) *Oxford Handbook of Public Health Practice.* Oxford: Oxford University Press.

Prüss-Üstün A and Corvalán C (2006) *Preventing Disease through Health Environments—Towards an estimate of the environmental burden of disease.* Geneva: World Health Organization.

Ruger JP, Jamison DJ, Bloom DE, and Canning D (2012) Health and the Economy. In: Merson MH, Black RE, and Mills AJ (eds) *Global Health: Diseases, Programs, Systems, and Policies,* pp. 757–814. Burlington, MA: Jones and Bartlett Learning.

Seshamani M and Gray AM (2004) A longitudinal study of the effects of age and time to death on hospital costs. *Journal of Health Economics* **23** (2), 217–35.

Stevens A, Raftery J, Mant J, Simpson S (eds) (2004) *Health care needs assessment: the epidemiologically based needs assessment reviews.* Oxford: Radcliffe Publishing.

Winslow CE (1920) The untilled fields of public health. *Science (New York, NY)* **51** (1306), 23–33.

WHO (2000) The world health report 2000. Health systems: improving performance. http://www.who.int/whr/2000/en/whr00_en.pdf [Accessed: July 2012].

Wright J, Williams DRR, and Wilkinson J (1998) The development of health needs assessment. In: Wright J (ed) *Health needs assessment in practice*, pp. 1–11. London: BMJ Books.

22 Global health in the 21st century

JOHN YARNELL, SHANTHI MENDIS, SHEELAH CONNOLLY, LUIS GOMES SAMBO, DEREGE KEBEDE, ZSUZSANNA JAKAB, ROBERTO BERTOLLINI, SHICHENG YU, AND KUN ZHAO

CHAPTER CONTENTS

This chapter, written with contributors from the World Health Organization (WHO), summarizes the current situation and disparities in global health, and the projected trends in disease in WHO's six world regions. International organizations and the remit and work of WHO are outlined working towards the Millennium Development Goals for 2015. Health status reports are provided for each of the world regions with an outline of their work and priorities. In the final section possible ways towards improved global health are discussed, particularly for the regions and countries in greatest need of health development.

We would like to acknowledge the following who contributed to this chapter: Enrique Loyola, Ivo Rakovac, Claudia Stein, and Natela Nadareishvili.

22.1 What is global health?

From previous chapters it is clear that, although the global distribution of disease has been of academic interest, now, with, for example, the rapid spread of infectious disease by air travel, global health has become increasingly relevant. But, what do we understand by global health?

Global health is simply population health on a worldwide scale. The priority for health improvement and health equity worldwide have been stressed, together with protection against global threats from infectious diseases, environmental disasters (Koplan et al. 2009) and, from the widespread advance of non-communicable diseases (WHO 2010a). Globalization was originally an economic term used to describe trends in world markets but it has now being applied to cultural, travel, environmental, and political trends and processes which can affect, for better or for worse, the health of citizens everywhere. Recently there has been increased recognition of the profound but complex effects of global markets on our lives and health: the World Bank estimated that international trade agreements created 200 million more poor people in the world between 1993 and 2003 (MacDonald and Horton 2009). Global markets in tobacco, food, soft drinks, alcohol, illegal drugs, and the car industry carry implications for health. Possible strategies for international governance are discussed in more detail elsewhere (Smith et al. 2009).

Global disease trends

Currently 57 million people die each year and of these nearly a fifth occur in children aged under five years; of every 10 deaths, six are due to non-communicable diseases (NCDs), three to communicable, reproductive, or nutritional conditions, and one to injuries (WHO 2008). Over the next two decades substantial changes in the pattern of global deaths are anticipated, thanks to a combination of population growth, ageing, and epidemiological transition. According to WHO projections large declines in mortality will be witnessed for major communicable, maternal, perinatal, and nutritional causes, including HIV/AIDS, TB, and malaria. If coverage with antiretroviral drugs continues to rise at current rates, deaths due to HIV/AIDS, some two million in 2008, will decline to about 1.2 million by 2030. Road traffic accident deaths are projected to rise to 2.4 million by 2030 due to increased motor vehicle ownership in developing countries. The four leading causes of death globally in 2030 are projected to be cardiovascular disease (heart disease and stroke), cancer, chronic obstructive pulmonary disease (in adults), and lower respiratory infections (mainly in infants). By 2030 tobacco-attributable deaths are also projected to rise to 8.3 million, accounting for almost a tenth of all deaths globally (WHO 2010a) (Fig. 22.1).

Global health risks

Mortality More than one-third of the world's deaths can be attributed to a few risk factors: 'lifestyle' factors such as tobacco use, unhealthy diets, physical inactivity,

overweight and obesity. As discussed in Chapter 20 the Global Burden of Disease Project has summarized these as measurable risk factors, e.g. blood pressure, serum cholesterol, body mass index, and their attributable fractions which have been discussed in previous chapters (see for example Chapters 3, 8, 9, 17, and 20). They are responsible for raising the risk of NCDs such as cardiovascular diseases, cancer, chronic respiratory disease, and diabetes. They affect adult deaths in countries across all income groups: high-, middle-, and low-income, but cardiovascular disease and lung cancer account for 32 per cent of deaths in high-income countries and 15 per cent in low-income countries. In low-income countries infant and child mortality are high together with high mortality in young adults from AIDS. The risk factors of poverty and adverse environment predominate: underweight (caused by inadequate or poor nutrition), inadequate breastfeeding, contaminated water with poor sanitation and hygiene, and unsafe (unprotected) sex (see Chapter 16). Leading causes of death in adults are shown in Fig. 22.2 by the world regions.

Morbidity The Global Burden of Disease Project measures the effects of both morbidity and premature mortality (in terms of DALYs). The four leading global risks for burden of disease in the world are underweight and unsafe sex, followed by alcohol abuse and unsafe water, sanitation and hygiene. Three of these (with the exception of alcohol) increase the incidence and severity of infectious disease, and particularly affect populations in low income countries. In low- and middle-income countries communicable diseases, adverse pregnancy outcomes, and nutritional deficiencies account for

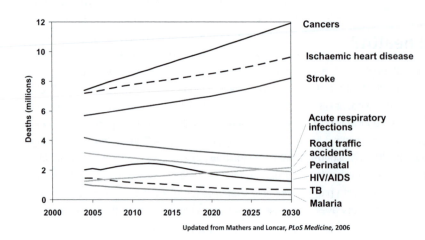

Figure 22.1 Global projections for leading causes of death to 2030. Reproduced from 'The global burden disease: 2004 update', with permission from the World Health Organization.

40 per cent of the burden of disease but only six per cent in high-income countries. Non-communicable diseases and injuries account for 49 per cent and 11 per cent, respectively, in low- and middle-income countries, and 87 per cent and seven per cent in high-income countries (Laxinarayan *et al.* 2006). In middle-income countries risk factors for NCDs cause the largest share of deaths and healthy life years lost: tobacco use, abuse of alcohol, unhealthy diet, physical inactivity, overweight and obesity, though other risks such as unsafe

sex and unsafe water and poor sanitation also contribute. For high-income countries blood pressure, alcohol, and overweight are leading causes of healthy life years lost, each being responsible for about seven per cent of the total (WHO 2004). Understanding the magnitude, role, and globalization of these risk factors are fundamental to developing effective global health strategies that are coherent and consistent across national and global levels. Fig. 22.3 shows the burden of disease by cause across the world regions.

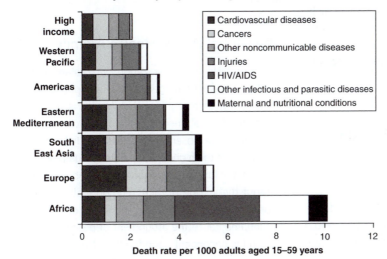

Figure 22.2 Leading causes of death by world regions—2004.
Reproduced from 'The global burden of disease: 2004 update', with permission from the World Health Organization.

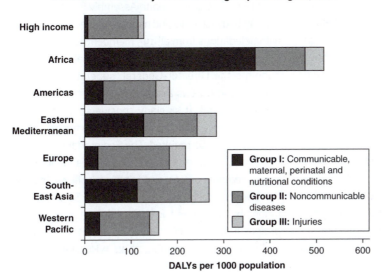

Figure 22.3 Burden of disease by cause in the world regions—2004.
Reproduced from 'The global burden of disease: 2004 update', with permission from the World Health Organization.

Global inequalities in health

People in developing countries are dying in large numbers for want of access to basic amenities of life and preventive and curative health care. More than 99 per cent of maternal deaths occur in low- and middle-income countries. The risk of a woman in sub-Saharan Africa dying during pregnancy and childbirth is nearly 400 times greater than in a high-income country (WHO 2010a). The difference in life expectancy between the richest and poorest countries now exceeds 40 years (WHO 2010b). Annual government spending on health ranges from less than US$10 per person in some low-income countries to well over US$7000 in some high-income countries (WHO 2010b). Many people who suffer from NCDs in developing countries are denied access even to essential life saving medicines (Mendis *et al.* 2007).

22.2 International agencies

The United Nations

Human disasters such wars have a particularly debilitating effect on population health (Murray *et al.* 2002) and this has been recognized by society for many centuries, though it was not until 1945 and after two world wars, that an international body, the United Nations (UN), was formed to try to prevent further conflict. Over 50 national governments and a number of non-governmental organizations (NGOs) (UN 1945) helped draft its constitution, which included a section on human rights proposing that all citizens should have the right to health and access to health care. More recently this has been echoed in a UN Declaration on the Rights of Indigenous Peoples in 2007 (estimated at 370 million worldwide) (UN 2007).

The UN Charter has spawned many specialized agencies of which the most relevant for health and development are: the World Health Organization (WHO), the World Bank, The International Monetary Fund, the World Food Programme, The Food and Agricultural Organization, the International Fund for Agricultural Development, and the UN Industrial Development Organization. The UN Development Group (from 1997) now coordinates the work of 32 agencies and publishes country figures for the Human Development Index (see Chapter 20). The UN now has 193 Member States (in 2012) and all are represented at the annual General Assembly, which has a degree of budgetary control and the power to make recommendations on health programmes. For example, in May and December 2010, the UN General Assembly adopted a resolution that focuses on NCDs and its impact on socio-economic development (UN 2010a). Further details on the structure and funding of the UN can be accessed on their website.

The Global Public Health Agency

The World Health Organization was established in 1948 as a specialized agency for global public health. Its constitution recognizes that *Health* is a state of complete physical, mental, and social well-being and not merely the absence of disease or infirmity. The enjoyment of the highest attainable standard of health is one of the fundamental rights of every human being without distinction of race, religion, political belief, economic or social condition. The health of all peoples is fundamental to the attainment of peace and security and is dependent upon the fullest co-operation of individuals and States. This constitution articulates a value system whose goal is to achieve health equity and social justice worldwide through the joint action of all nations. The World Health Assembly is the decision-making body for WHO and meets in Geneva once a year with delegations from all 193 Member States. Its main function is to determine policy. The Health Assembly appoints the Director-General, supervises financial policies, and reviews and approves the proposed programme budget. It similarly considers reports of the Executive Board, which it instructs when further action or reports may be required. The Secretariat consists of health and other experts working at headquarters, in the six regional offices, and in country offices. In 2010 the budget (operating revenue) was US$ 2.3 billion funded by more than two-thirds from voluntary contributions from Member States (Fig. 22.4a) and spent in the areas shown in the Fig. 22.4b. WHO Headquarters

(a)

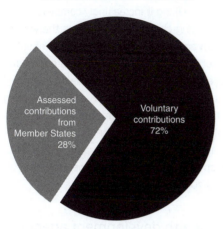

HOW IS WHO FUNDED?

TOTAL RESOURCES 2006–2007

Assessed contributions from Member States 28%

Voluntary contributions 72%

The total WHO budget planned for 2006–2007 is roughly $US 3.3 billion. Of this amount, just over one quarter comes from regular "dues" from WHO's Member States, while more than 70% is money that countries, agencies and other partners give to WHO voluntarily.

SOURCE OF VOLUNTARY CONTRIBUTIONS*
Traditionally, the major source of voluntary contributions comes from Member States. Other contributors are highlighted below, based on actual contributions received in 2004. For 2006–2007, WHO is seeking to increase its diversity in funding.

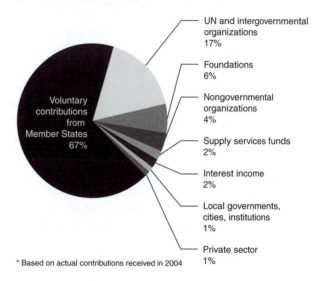

Voluntary contributions from Member States 67%

UN and intergovernmental organizations 17%

Foundations 6%

Nongovernmental organizations 4%

Supply services funds 2%

Interest income 2%

Local governments, cities, institutions 1%

Private sector 1%

* Based on actual contributions received in 2004

(b)

ESTIMATED EXPENDITURE
BY GROUPS OF ACTIVITY FOR 2006–2007*

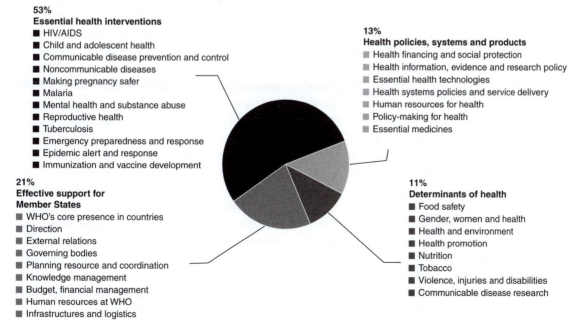

53%
Essential health interventions
- HIV/AIDS
- Child and adolescent health
- Communicable disease prevention and control
- Noncommunicable diseases
- Making pregnancy safer
- Malaria
- Mental health and substance abuse
- Reproductive health
- Tuberculosis
- Emergency preparedness and response
- Epidemic alert and response
- Immunization and vaccine development

21%
Effective support for Member States
- WHO's core presence in countries
- Direction
- External relations
- Governing bodies
- Planning resource and coordination
- Knowledge management
- Budget, financial management
- Human resources at WHO
- Infrastructures and logistics

13%
Health policies, systems and products
- Health financing and social protection
- Health information, evidence and research policy
- Essential health technologies
- Health systems policies and service delivery
- Human resources for health
- Policy-making for health
- Essential medicines

11%
Determinants of health
- Food safety
- Gender, women and health
- Health and environment
- Health promotion
- Nutrition
- Tobacco
- Violence, injuries and disabilities
- Communicable disease research

* Does not total 100% because of 2% set aside for exchange rate hedging, IT Fund, Real Estate Fund and Security Fund

Figure 22.4 (a) Sources of WHO Funding; (b) allocation of WHO expenditure 2006/7.

Reproduced from *Working for Health: An Introduction to the World Health Organization*, 2007, with permission from WHO.

and WHO Africa Region (AFRO) each received around a quarter of the budget allocation for 2009, and the remaining 50 per cent was shared between the other five regions. A provisional programme budget for 2012/13 is available elsewhere (WHO 2012a). For an excellent commentary on WHO's development and funding see Birn *et al.* (2009).

The core functions of WHO include: disease and risk factor surveillance; setting norms and standards; providing technical co-operation to Member States; generation of new knowledge; convening and acting as an honest broker; and articulating an evidence-based and unbiased position about health issues. WHO responds to outbreaks, such as Ebola, SARS, and influenza. WHO's activities over the last 60 years have contributed to public health and saved large numbers of lives worldwide. Some of the examples include: the eradication of smallpox (1979); the Framework Convention on Tobacco Control (2003); the revised International Health Regulations (2005); negotiated prices for vaccines and medicines; model lists of essential medicines (from 1977); a simple salt and sugar solution to combat childhood diarrhoea deaths; new combinations of drugs to treat leprosy and tuberculosis (TB); and simplified diagnostic tools and treatment protocols that work well in disadvantaged settings, particularly in primary care. In 1978, WHO issued a strong social goal in the form of the Declaration of Alma-Ata (WHO 1978) in response to the stark inequality in the health status of people worldwide. It launched primary health care as a set of guiding principles for organizing health services more equitably and efficiently. WHO has more than 800 Collaborating Centres across the world regions whose purpose is to support and strengthen research and development in particular health topics, based on the expertise already present within these institutions. Designation as a Collaborating Centre is subject to a four-yearly review.

In the 1980s, as a response to the global economic recession, development banks introduced structural adjustment programmes which shifted national budgets away from social and welfare services, including health. Furthermore, the emergence of HIV/AIDS, resurgence of TB, and malaria shifted the focus of international public health to vertical health initiatives and away from strengthening health systems to achieve sustainable capacity. At the same time many global public health partnerships and initiatives developed and new stakeholders arrived on the global public health stage making it increasingly complex. It is in such a challenging climate that WHO, as the world's leading health agency, has the responsibility of steering global public health to promote health equity and social justice for all. WHO is now undertaking an internal process of structural reform with a view to setting priorities in health development and programmes, and strengthening its capacity for coordinating partners, such as national governments and international NGOs, in responding to disasters and new health challenges (WHO 2012b).

National health development agencies and charities

All national governments have their own Ministries of Health with public health functions, but most countries in North America, Western Europe, Japan, and Australasia also have international departments with a responsibility for health development. In the USA this is the Center(s) for Disease Control and the Fogarty International Centre for International Health. In the UK the Department for International Development has aligned itself with the Millennium Development Goals of the United Nations. Many charities, organizations, and NGOs such as Save the Children and UNICEF raise funds on a national basis but operate internationally. The Global Fund, developed from the Bill and Melinda Gates Foundation with Warren Buffett, injected US$60 billion into international health research and development from 2006 and is a major donor to key projects in partnership with WHO and other agencies. These include the GAVI programme and PATH which promote and develop immunization programmes, and appropriate technologies for health development, respectively. An informal group of health-related agencies (the H8) including, WHO, UNICEF, UNFPA, UNAIDS, the Global Fund, the GAVI Alliance, and the Bill and Melinda Gates Foundation, was established in 2007 by the present Director-General of WHO to help harmonize activities and to avoid duplication of effort. A selected list of international agencies is shown in Table 22.1.

Table 22.1 Some international organizations in health and development

UN agencies	National governmental agencies	International non-governmental organizations
Food and Agriculture Organization (FAO)	United States Agency for International Development	International Committee of the Red Cross
International Fund for Agricultural Development (IFAD)	Department for International Development, UK	Médecins sans Frontières
International Monetary Fund (IMF)	Australian Agency for International Development	World Vision (USA)
Joint UN Programme on HIV/AIDS (UNAIDS)	Canadian International Development Agency	Feed the Children (USA)
UN Development Programme (UNDP)		CARE (USA)
UN Office on Drugs and Crime (UNODC)		Oxfam (UK)
UN Educational, Scientific and Cultural Organization (UNESCO)		
UN Environmental Programme (UNEP)		
UN Human Settlements Programme (UN-HABITAT)		
UN Population Fund (UNFPA)		**Key partnerships**
UN High Commissioner for Refugees (UNHCR)	**Foundations**	The Global Fund (AIDS, TB and Malaria)
UN International Children's Fund (UNICEF)	Bill and Melinda Gates Foundation	The Global Alliance for Vaccines and Immunizations (GAVI)
UN Research Institute for Social Development (UNRISD)	Rockefeller Foundation	International AIDS Vaccine Initiative (IAVI)
World Bank (WB)		International Health Partnership (IHP) (monitoring and evaluation of aid effectiveness)
World Food Programme (WFP)		Health Action in Crises (WHO and partners)
World Health Organization (WHO)		Program for Appropriate Technology in Health (PATH)

22.3 Global health threats and challenges

Today's world is highly mobile, interdependent, and interconnected. Diseases can spread rapidly through international travel, trade, and the transport of goods. A health crisis in one country can influence the livelihoods of people and economies across the world. Outbreaks of infectious diseases, chemical and toxic leaks, nuclear accidents, environmental disasters, and conflicts in one country can threaten the health of populations elsewhere. The variety and range of such global public health threats are many and include: pandemic and epidemic emerging diseases; foodborne diseases such as *E. coli* varients and prion diseases; chemicals and micro-organisms used for bio-terrorism; food contamination such as the adulteration of cooking oil with industrial rapeseed oil in Southern Europe in 1981 (Tabuenca *et al.* 1981); and nuclear radiation disasters in Chernobyl in 1986 (Baverstock 2011) and Fukushima in 2011 (Tanimoto *et al.* 2011). In the light of such transnational health threats and disasters that have increasingly confronted the world in recent decades, the strengthening of global frameworks to ensure the highest level of health safety and security worldwide becomes imperative.

Infectious diseases In the last three decades, many important vector-borne diseases including African trypanosomiasis, dengue and dengue haemorrhagic fever, and malaria have emerged in new countries. Urbanization and increasing international trade and travel have contributed to this. For example, in 1998 dengue caused a pandemic with 1.2 million cases reported to WHO from 56 countries (Gubler 1998). Since then dengue epidemics have continued, affecting millions of people from Latin America to South-East Asia.

The outbreak of SARS, the first severe new disease of the 21st century, occurred in 2003 (see Chapter 18). H1N1 pandemic influenza followed in 2009 (Swedish 2011). Global spread was rapid and widespread and was officially reported from 213 countries and overseas territories or communities. In May 2011, an outbreak of severe gastroenteritis carrying a high mortality rate from a rare strain of *E. coli* began in northern Germany (Chattaway *et al.* 2011). During the outbreak it infected people from about 15 countries who had visited northern Germany;

the weekly losses to vegetable farmers elsewhere in Europe were estimated to run into millions of euros.

The International Health Regulations (IHR) which were revised in 2005, probably brought forward, at least in part, as response to the outbreak of SARS and toxic environmental incidents, came into force in June 2007. These aim to safeguard public health through the prevention of disease spread while limiting the consequences of global health threats on international trade, travel, and the economy. As discussed in Chapter 18 some 180 countries have signed up to the implementation of these regulations which require rapid reporting of outbreaks of important infectious disease or environmental hazards.

Climate change Greenhouse gas emissions, global warming, and climate change threaten clean air, safe drinking water, availability of food and secure shelter. Rising sea levels are likely to affect the lives of more than half of the world's population as they live within 60 km of the sea (WHO 2002, 2009). Small island communities and coastal dwellers in poor countries will be the most severely affected. Rainfall patterns due to climate change, are likely to affect the supply of safe drinking water compromising the health of the vulnerable, and increasing the risk of diarrhoeal diseases, which kills 2.2 million people annually (WHO 2008). Climate change also decreases the production of staple food and increases the prevalence of malnutrition and under-nutrition, which currently cause 3.5 million deaths every year (WHO 2008). High temperatures raise the levels of ozone and other pollutants in the air and exacerbate respiratory and other diseases caused by air pollution which account for several million deaths every year. Natural disasters, many of them weather-related, result in many deaths, and lessons can be learned from the medical and emergency response to urban earthquakes such as that in Haiti in 2010 (Ferris and Ferro-Ribeiro 2012). According to a WHO assessment the modest warming since the 1970s causes 0.2 per cent of deaths annually, 85 per cent of which are in infants; but this is set to rise in coming decades with increasing global temperatures (WHO 2009).

Many global and national policies have the potential to reduce greenhouse gas emissions which influence climate change while providing benefits for health. For example promoting the safe use of public transportation and active movement—such as cycling or walking as alternatives to using private vehicles—could reduce carbon dioxide emissions and also provide the health benefits of physical activity. In March 1994 the United Nations Framework Convention on Climate Change (UN 2008) came into force and set an overall framework for intergovernmental efforts to address the challenges posed by climate change. It recognizes that the climate system is a shared global resource whose stability can be affected by industrial and other emissions of carbon dioxide and other greenhouse gases. Although the Convention enjoys near universal membership, the overall political commitment to its implementation remains inadequate. The Kyoto Protocol (1997) is an international agreement linked to the United Nations Framework Convention on Climate Change (Weaver 2011). Recognizing that developed countries are principally responsible for the current high levels of greenhouse gas emissions, the Protocol places a heavier burden on developed nations. The Kyoto Protocol sets binding targets for 37 developed countries and the European Community for reducing greenhouse gas emissions. Taking steps to prevent climate change is key to ensuring sustainable development, poverty eradication, and safeguarding economic growth and global health.

Financing improved population health Health equality is an essential dimension of global health. It concerns those disparities in population health that arise from unequal and unjust economic and social conditions that are avoidable. As discussed in Chapter 20 inequalities in health systematically puts groups of people who are already socially and economically disadvantaged at a further disadvantage, since health is an important determinant of their ability to overcome the effects of social disadvantage. Health systems, which can significantly contribute to health are often judged with respect to their efficiency and equity. However, while the different methods of financing health care are all potentially compatible with efficiency (Glied 2008); the use of out-of-pocket payments for health care in many low- and middle-income countries raises serious concerns about equity. One study noted that a high proportion of the world's 1.3 billion poor have no access to health services simply because they cannot afford to pay when they need them (Preker and Carin 2004). In

2005 WHO Member States declared a commitment to achieving universal coverage, where everyone would have access to health services, and not suffer financial hardship paying for them (WHO 2005); the world is still a long way from achieving this goal (WHO 2010b) especially in many low-income countries where low levels of formal employment, little taxation revenue, poverty, and lack of legal and economic institutions generally result in few options for financing health care other than direct out-of-pocket payments. Achieving universal coverage is therefore a difficult and often lengthy process: at first, it is necessary to increase the funds available for health care through increasing taxation revenue, or the development of social or private insurance markets. International donors may have an important role to play but there is a limit to how much international aid a country can absorb without the necessary human resources, physical infrastructure, or managerial capacity to use funds effectively (Schieber *et al*. 2006). All countries must make choices and trade-offs in terms of the proportion of the population to be covered, the range of services to be made available, and the proportion of the total costs to be met (WHO 2010b). Some examples of financing of health services by countries in the region of the Americas are shown in Table 22. 4. Points of interest are the wide range of variability in private funding and life expectancy at birth. Haiti typifies a low income country where a large proportion of funding is required from out-of-pocket expenditure. In the report from South-East Asia the low level of public investment in health in India is notable (about one per cent of GDP), 80 per cent of funding coming from out-of-pocket expenditure. From India a call has been made for a major increase in public investment in health to reduce the very high levels of maternal and infant mortality in a country whose economic growth has been considerable and sustained in the last decade (Reddy *et al*. 2011).

22.4 The Millennium Development Goals

The publication of the Millennium Development Goals (MDGs) by the UN followed a two-year consultation period with more than 1000 representatives of NGOs and other agencies from over 100 countries at the turn of the century. The goals aim to aid international development and are recognized as the global means to tackle the causes and effects of poverty by 2015. Three of these goals relate specifically to health outcomes: the reduction of childhood mortality; the improvement of maternal health and; the eradication of HIV/AIDS and malaria. In addition, the other five goals indirectly address health inequalities because they target social determinants of health. All eight MDG goals are interactive and synergistic. The close relationship between health and poverty and the need to address the root causes of ill health that arise in other sectors are both firmly acknowledged in the MDGs.

The eight goals are each subdivided into specific targets and appropriate indicators, both health and demographic, to evaluate progress in achieving these goals. The MDGs, health-related targets, and indicators are shown in Box 22.1.

Working with its partners WHO tracks progress on the achievement of the health-related MDGs and publishes updates in the annual World Health Statistics (WHO 2010f). WHO also reports on the availability of financial and human resources, and provides estimates of financing gaps and needs. Millennium Development Goals have resulted in numerous global health initiatives, an increase in the official development aid for health, and increased international co-operation to promote health.

There has been substantial progress in achieving MDG targets. The number of infants immunized against measles has increased from 94 million to 107 million between 1990 and 2008, a rise in coverage from 73 per cent to 83 per cent (WHO 2010f). Child mortality due to diarrhoeal disease has declined due to better use of oral rehydration salts solution and zinc for treatment, and access to safe water, sanitation, and breastfeeding for prevention. The percentage of underweight children is estimated to have declined from 25 per cent in 1990 to 16 per cent in 2010 and the number of deaths in children aged under five years has fallen to about 8.1 million, the lowest level in more than six decades (WHO 2010a).

The number of people in low- and middle-income countries receiving antiretroviral therapy for AIDS has increased from under 200,000 in late 2002 to nearly five million in 2010 (WHO 2010c). The incidence of TB and deaths from malaria have begun to decline. The use of

antenatal care also has improved but still only about 40 per cent of mothers receive post-natal care worldwide. Access to sexual and reproductive health services, including family planning, infertility services, prevention and treatment of sexually transmitted infections, and skilled care for pregnancy and childbirth have been scaled up in most countries. The proportion of women of reproductive age in developing countries who report using contraceptives has increased from 50 per cent in 1990 to 62 per cent in 2005 (WHO 2010f). Estimates for 2010 show a significant drop in maternal mortality, with the greatest declines, of around 60 per cent, reported in Eastern Asia and in Northern Africa (WHO 2010f).

Nevertheless there is still much to be done to achieve the MDG targets and in several countries in Africa there has been little or no progress in achieving the maternal and child targets. This has been due to a shortage of skilled attendants at birth and access to emergency obstetric care due to weaknesses in health systems, basic infrastructure, and health care financing. More than five million people who currently require antiretroviral treatment are not receiving it, TB kills 4500 people daily, malaria causes one in 14 deaths in Africa, and 8.8 million children under five years of age still die every year (WHO 2010f). Table 22.2 shows progress towards achieving the goals in each of the WHO Regions.

22.5 Reports from the WHO regions

In the next section summary reports from the WHO regions are presented. Each region works closely with WHO headquarters but has the autonomy to develop regional programmes and structures. The Global Policy Group formed from the WHO Regional Directors and WHO headquarters meets to jointly shape WHO policies worldwide and to share expertise between regions. All demographic and epidemiological country data can be found in the Global Health Observatory databases (**www.who.int/gho/**).

Africa Region (AFRO)

With its population of over 730 million people spanning 46 countries, the African region accounts for

Box 22.1 The Millennium Development Goals

HEALTH TARGETS	HEALTH INDICATORS
Goal 1: Eradicate extreme poverty and hunger	
Target 1 Halve, between 1990 and 2015, the proportion of people whose income is less than one dollar a day	
Target 2 Halve, between 1990 and 2015, the proportion of people who suffer from hunger	4 Prevalence of underweight children under five years of age
	5 Proportion of population below minimum level of dietary energy consumption
Goal 2 : Achieve universal primary education	
Target 3 Ensure that, by 2015, children everywhere, boys and girls alike, will be able to complete a full course of primary schooling	
Goal 3: Promote gender equality and empower women	
Target 4 Eliminate gender disparity in primary and secondary education, preferably by 2005, and at all levels of education no later than 2015	
Goal 4: Reduce child mortality	
Target 5 Reduce by two-thirds, between 1990 and 2015, the under-five mortality rate	13 Under-five mortality rate
	14 Infant mortality rate
	15 Proportion of one-year-old children immunized against measles
Goal 5: Improve maternal health	
Target 6 Reduce by three-quarters, between 1990 and 2015, the maternal mortality ratio	16 Maternal mortality ratio
	17 Proportion of births attended by skilled health personnel
Goal 6: Combat HIV/AIDS, malaria and other diseases	
Target 7 Have halted by 2015 and begun to reverse the spread of HIV/AIDS	18 HIV prevalence among pregnant women aged 15–24 years
	19 Condom use rate of the contraceptive prevalence rate
	20 Ratio of school attendance of orphans to school attendance of non-orphans aged 10–14 years
Target 8 Have halted by 2015 and begun to reverse the incidence of malaria and other major diseases	21 Prevalence and death rates associated with malaria
	22 Proportion of population in malaria-risk areas using effective malaria prevention and treatment measures
	23 Prevalence and death rates associated with tuberculosis
	24 Proportion of tuberculosis cases detected and cured under DOTS (Directly Observed Treatment Short-course)
Goal 7: Ensure environmental sustainability	
Target 9 Integrate the principles of sustainable development into country policies and programmes and reverse the loss of environmental resources	29 Proportion of population using solid fuels

(continued)

Box 22.1 (*continued*)

HEALTH TARGETS	HEALTH INDICATORS
Target 10 Halve by 2015 the proportion of people without sustainable access to safe drinking-water and sanitation	**30** Proportion of population with sustainable access to an improved water source, urban and rural
Target 11 By 2020 to have achieved a significant improvement in the lives of at least 100 million slum dwellers	**31** Proportion of population with access to improved sanitation, urban and rural
Goal 8: Develop a Global Partnership for Development	
Target 12 Develop further an open, rule-based, predictable, non-discriminatory trading and financial system	
Target 13 Address the special needs of the least developed countries	
Target 14 Address the special needs of landlocked countries and small island developing states	
Target 15 Deal comprehensively with the debt problems of developing countries through national and international measures in order to make debt sustainable in the long term	
Target 16 In cooperation with developing countries, develop and implement strategies for decent and productive work for youth	
Target 17 In cooperation with pharmaceutical companies, provide access to affordable essential drugs in developing countries	**46** Proportion of population with access to affordable essential drugs on a sustainable basis
Target 18 In cooperation with the private sector, make available the benefits of new technologies, especially information and communications	

Source: 'Implementation of the United Nations Millennium Declaration', Report of the secretary-General, A/57/270(31 July 2002), first annual report based on the 'Road map towards the implementation of the United Nations Millennium Declaration', Report of the secretary-General, A/56/326 (6 September 2001), United Nations Statistics Division, Millennium Indicators Database, verified in July 2004; World Health Organization, Department of MDGs, Health and Development Policy (HDP). **www.who.int/indg**

approximately one-seventh of the world's population—a population growing annually at a rate of 2.5 per cent. In sub-Saharan Africa, which forms the majority of countries in the region, over 44 per cent of the population is under 15 years of age compared with 28 per cent globally. Some of the countries of the region are rich in resources but many are poorly developed, lacking in natural resources, and disadvantaged by structural mechanisms in the global economy. Thus this region is behind others in terms of health and human development; unless current trends are drastically changed, most countries of the region are unlikely to achieve any of the health or health-related MDGs. Some key indicators are shown for some selected countries (2010/11) in Table 22. 3.

The regional average under-five mortality dropped from 179 per 1000 livebirths in 1990 to 127 per 1000 livebirths in 2009 but only seven countries are on track to achieve this MDG target. The diseases causing the highest mortality rates in children under five years of age are diarrhoeal disease (18 per cent), pneumonia (17 per cent per cent), and malaria (16 per cent). The estimated maternal mortality ratio was 620 per 100,000 livebirths in 2008: only two countries are on track to achieve this target.

In 2009 the prevalence of HIV among people aged 15–49 years averaged 4.7 per cent, ranging between 0.1 per cent and 25.9 per cent. Between 2001 and 2009 the prevalence in this age group stabilized or declined

Table 22.2 Progress in achieving the health-related Millennium Development Goals in the World Regions

Health MDGs scorecard for WHO Regions							
	World	Africa	Americas	Eastern Mediterranean	Europe	South-East Asia	Western Pacific
Under 5 mortality *per 1000 live births*	65	142	18	78	14	63	21
Measles immunization *% coverage*	81	73	93	83	94	75	93
Maternal mortality *per 100,000 live births*	400	900	99	420	27	450	82
Skilled birth attendant *% births*	66	47	92	59	96	49	92
Contraceptive use *% married women aged 15–49*	62	24	71	43	68	58	83
HIV/AIDS prevalence *% adults aged 15–45*	0.8	4.9	0.5	0.2	0.5	0.3	0.1
Malaria mortality *per 100,000 population*	17	104	0.5	7.5	–	2.1	0.3
TB treatment *success rate %*	86	79	82	88	67	88	92
Water *% using improved sources*	87	61	96	83	98	86	90
Sanitation *% using improved facilities*	60	34	87	61	94	40	62

■ on track   ■ insufficient progress   ■ off track   *Data from World Health Statistics 2010*

Source: WHO (2010) Accelerating progress towards the millennium development goals. Available at: **http://www.who.int/topics/millennium_development_goals/MDG-NHPS_brochure_2010.pdf**

in 29 countries. HIV/AIDS prevalence increased in 12 countries. At the end of 2009 the average coverage of antiretroviral therapy was 37 per cent. Nineteen countries had coverage rates of more than 30 per cent.

The African region has the highest total burden of disease compared to other WHO regions. The disability-adjusted life-years lost (DALYs) were 511 per 1000 in 2004, the highest of all regions. Grouped together,

communicable diseases, maternal and perinatal conditions, and nutritional deficiencies (the traditional 'developing country' pattern of ill health) constituted 71 per cent of the DALYs here in 2004, 21 per cent for chronic diseases, and 8 per cent for injuries (WHO 2004).

A number of key and overarching challenges need to be addressed to improve the health of the people of the region significantly. These challenges are:

Table 22.3 Demographic and health indicators in selected countries in the WHO Africa Region

Country	Human Development index	Gross national income per capita ($US PPP)	Life expectancy at birth (years)	Maternal mortality/ 100,000 livebirths	Under 5 mortality per 1000 livebirths	Births attended by skilled personnel (%)	Prevalence of HIV in adults (%)
Algeria	0.68	7890	72	120	36	95	0.1
Botswana	0.63	13,310	61	193	48	95	24.8
Congo	0.49	2810	55	580	93	86	3.4
Democratic Republic of Congo	0.24	280	49	670	170	78	1.4
Ghana	0.47	1320	60	350	74	56	1.8
Kenya	0.47	1560	60	530	85	49	6.3
Nigeria	0.42	1980	54	840	143	39	3.6
Sierra Leone	0.32	770	49	970	174	42	1.6
South Africa	0.60	9790	54	410	57	91	17.8
Uganda	0.42	1140	52	430	99	52	6.5

PPP; purchasing power parity.

- inadequate internal and external resources devoted to the achievement of the MDGs including: addressing the broader determinants of health; the fact that external resources are unpredictable, non-sustainable, and poorly aligned with country priorities; inefficient use of existing resources;
- weak health systems including: inadequate health services (insufficient focus on quality of care);
- weak human and institutional capacity, leading to low levels of programme implementation;
- weak procurement and supply management systems resulting in shortages of medical supplies and lack of laboratory services;
- persistent inequities (e.g. by geographical area, by income, and educational level) in access to proven interventions, particularly against maternal and child mortality, HIV/AIDS, TB, and malaria;
- low priority accorded to health in national economic and development priority setting and

resource allocation policies; weak multisectoral response and low progress in achieving the other MDGs; and
- inadequate data and weak monitoring and evaluation capacity.

Key public health programmes Effective interventions for reducing child mortality include antenatal care, newborn care, appropriate infant feeding, immunization, management of common childhood illnesses (including pneumonia and diarrhoea), and use of insecticide-treated nets (ITNs). Between 1990 and 2009, the average coverage of infants immunized against measles increased from 57 per cent to 69 per cent. In 2010 it was estimated that 35 per cent of children under five years of age slept under an ITN. The percentage of pneumonia cases receiving antibiotic treatment remains at 23 per cent, diarrhoea cases receiving oral rehydration are only 41 per cent, and only 34 per cent of children with malaria receive antimalarial treatment (WHO 2011).

The key interventions for improving maternal health include increasing access to skilled birth attendance, combined with prompt referral for cases with complications; scaling up emergency obstetric and newborn care; strengthening family planning, including reducing pregnancy in adolescents; and empowering women, families, and communities to make timely decisions. In 2008 less than 50 per cent of women received skilled care during childbirth. The average caesarean section coverage is 3.6 per cent, below the recommended figure of 5–15 per cent. From 2000 to 2010 the regional average percentage of women who received antenatal care from skilled health personnel at least once was 74 per cent and at least four times during pregnancy was 44 per cent. There remains a continuing unmet need for family planning as 24.8 per cent of women wanting to practice child spacing were not using any family planning method.

Priority interventions for HIV/AIDS prevention, treatment, and care include provider-initiated HIV testing and counselling; client-initiated testing and counselling; preventing sexual and mother-to-child transmission of HIV; male circumcision; prevention and control of sexually-transmitted infections; HIV prevention among young people; improving blood safety; and provision of treatment and care, such as antiretroviral treatment. The total number of health facilities providing HIV testing and counselling (HTC) services increased further in 2009 in 43 reporting countries. In a subset of 33 countries that reported consistently during 2007–2009, the number of health facilities providing these services rose by over 85 per cent, i.e. from 11,132 in 2007 to 20,740 in 2009 (WHO 2010c).

Effective malaria interventions include effective diagnosis and treatment, the use of long-lasting ITNs, indoor residual spraying using an integrated vector control approach; intermittent preventive treatment of malaria in pregnancy; and parasitological diagnosis and effective treatment for all age groups. Artemisinin-based combination therapy is implemented in 41 of the 42 malaria-endemic countries with 20 countries implementing the policy country-wide. In 2009 35 per cent of reported malaria cases were confirmed by diagnostic test compared with only five per cent in 2000. By the end of 2010 all the 35 target countries were implementing intermittent preventive treatment of malaria in pregnancy with

20 countries implementing the intervention country-wide. In 2010 it was estimated that 42 per cent of households owned at least one ITN. Twenty-seven countries reported implementing residual spraying. The number of people thus protected increased from 13 million in 2005 to 75 million in 2009 (WHO 2010d).

Effective interventions against TB include implementation of the Directly Observed Treatment Schemes (DOTS) by ensuring adequate case detection through quality-assured laboratory testing, provision of supervised standardized treatment, an effective drug supply system, and monitoring and evaluation; and prevention and management of multidrug resistant TB. Ten countries reached the target for TB case detection of 70 per cent in 2009; 15 countries reached the target for treatment success of 85 per cent in 2008 while four countries reached both targets. The proportion of TB patients screened for HIV rose from 45 per cent in 2008 to 53 per cent in 2009. Of those co-infected 76 per cent were able to access co-trimoxazole preventive treatment and 36 per cent of those eligible were on antiretroviral treatment (WHO 2010e).

Future health problems and public health strategies
Epidemiological and demographic transitions in countries will impose a double burden of infectious diseases in tandem with chronic non-communicable disease. Mental illness as well as injuries and the consequences of violence particularly affect adolescents and young adults. For most countries current challenges will continue, with inadequate levels of unpredictable funding; with too little access to life-saving technologies; with the continuing daily toll of unnecessary death and disability from preventable causes; with pressure to deliver quick results taking precedence over the need to build strong institutions; and with conflicting technical advice and increasing demands from a growing diversity of partners.

There remains much unfinished business: sustaining gains achieved in immunizing each new generation of children; controlling HIV/AIDS, TB and malaria. Shocks must also be anticipated, including those delivered by new and re-emerging diseases and from conflicts and natural disasters. Conflict and the population displacement that follows especially affect the health of women and children. Other challenges, such as food security and climate change, stake equally compelling claims (WHO—AFRO 2006). In addition the impact of the 2008 financial crisis will continue to be felt, though the impact will vary from one country to another. Sustaining levels of resources for health in countries will require increased support from national budgets, a broader external funding base, innovative financing mechanisms, and continuing commitment from traditional donors.

Strategies for strengthening capacity for effective partnerships and harmonization are important to ensure that partners and stakeholders provide coordinated support to national health strategic plans that is consistent with the national development agenda. Countries are expected to own and implement health policies and other international commitments. Supporting the strengthening of health systems based on the primary health care approach is a key strategy that countries will need to put in place. This should include: universal access to health care through social health protection; improved health care services that are relevant and responsive to people's needs; adequate public policies within the health sector and outside; and the institution of leadership that is inclusive, participatory, and negotiation-based.

Countries should also define a minimum package of child, maternal, and newborn services at each level of the health care delivery system, such as family planning, safe deliveries by skilled birth attendants, and appropriate referral systems; to review and revise national policies, norms and protocols using evidence-based standards; and to assess and produce a skilled workforce for maternal and child health services. Strategies for accelerated actions on HIV/AIDS, malaria, and TB are also important. This will require strong country ownership and leadership for accelerated and comprehensive scaling up of agreed, evidence-based, cost-effective interventions for the prevention and control of HIV/AIDS, malaria and TB.

Countries should also intensify the prevention and control of communicable and non-communicable diseases. In order to detect and respond to diseases in a timely and effective manner, countries will need to strengthen their capacity for outbreak management, development, and implementation of preparedness and response plans, and full implementation of early warning systems. In addition an integrated package of interventions to guide the implementation of national communicable disease programmes will be required. Multi-disease prevention programmes (HIV, malaria, and diarrhoea) have been modelled and evaluated in

Kenya (Kahn *et al.* 2012). Continued assessment of the burden and trends of priority non-communicable diseases to identify risk factors and major determinants is also important. The evidence gathered should be used to increase the visibility and advocacy for prevention and control of chronic diseases.

A country strategy for tackling health inequities through action on the determinants of health should be developed to inform national policies and legislation aimed at multisectoral action on determinants of health. Countries should also develop health policies and strategies that enhance equity, are responsive to gender, and based on human rights (WHO–AFRO 2008).

The Americas (PAHO)

The Pan American Health Organization (PAHO) was formed from 35 countries in the Americas more than 100 years ago. WHO has merged its organization with PAHO in the region and these now represent a total of 48 national flags, including all the countries of North, Central, and South America and the large and small communities of the Caribbean. Many of the economies in the South American countries have shown strong growth in the past few decades and this is reflected in an improving health situation and increased life expectancy for many countries (but not all) in the region. Demographic and health data for selected countries are shown in Table 22.4 and indicate that some of the less prosperous countries (e.g. Costa Rica and Cuba) seem to have achieved a life expectancy comparable to that in North America. The data for Haiti predate the earthquake in 2010 and contrast with those of the Dominican Republic which shares the same Caribbean island.

Values for the human development index are higher for most countries than those in Africa reflecting longer life expectancy, higher levels of women's education and material wealth. Haiti and Bolivia appear to be underdeveloped relative to the regional average. High maternal mortality is unusual in the region but the lowest estimated maternal mortality ratio was observed in Canada (seven per 100,000 livebirths in 2005). Under-reporting may have occurred in several countries: in Haiti maternal mortality was estimated to be 670 per 100,000 livebirths; and, in Guatemala, Honduras, Bolivia, Peru, Ecuador, and Guyana it was estimated to be 200–300 per 100,000 livebirths. Infant mortality was 4.7 per 1000

Table 22.4 Health financing and life expectancy in the Americas

	Human Development index	Gross domestic product per capita (PPP) $US	Gross domestic product (%) for health		Life expectancy at birth (years)
			Public	Private	
Argentina	0.78	12,970	4.6	3.3	75.5
Bolivia	0.64	4150	3.3	1.6	66.0
Brazil	0.70	9270	3.6	3.8	72.7
Canada	0.88	35,500	7.5	1.4	80.9
Costa Rica	0.73	10,510	5.2	3.2	79.0
Cuba	0.86	9700	10.9	0.0	78.8
Dominican Republic	0.66	6350	1.8	3.4	72.7
Haiti	0.40	1050	2.7	2.8	61.5
Puerto Rico	0.89	19,600	3.5	0.0	79.0
United States of America	0.90	45,840	7.8	4.5	79.4
Uruguay	0.77	11,020	9.0	2.8	76.5

livebirths in Cuba (Canada five per 1000) and 57 per 1000 in Haiti. The Dominican Republic and Nicaragua had an infant mortality close to 30 per 1000 livebirths.

Vaccination programmes have been very successful and polio and measles have been eradicated in all countries. In all but a few less well developed countries infant vaccination rates were in excess of 90 per cent in 2008. Rotavirus and HPV vaccination have been introduced into some middle-income countries in South America. Malaria is endemic in 21 countries but malaria and dengue fever are a particular problem in the countries of the Amazon basin. Apart from these countries, almost 37,000 cases were reported in Haiti in 2008 compared with next highest (and adjoining) country the Dominican Republic (almost 2000 cases). Almost a third of a million cases of malaria and over a half a million cases of dengue fever were reported in Brazil in 2008 and tens of thousands of cases in other countries of the region. In Brazil there is a downward trend from 2005. In Latin America and in the Caribbean over 1.7 million durable ITNs were distributed in malaria-endemic areas between 2005 and 2008 with a programme of indoor residual spaying. Such preventive treatments are also effective against the spread of dengue fever.

The incidence of TB is low in North America but in the majority of countries in Latin America and in the Caribbean the incidence is three to nine times higher. In Peru and Haiti the incidence is 25 and 35 times higher, respectively. The incidence of AIDS is lowest in Canada at 0.7 per 100,000 and is reported to be 92.3 per 100,000 in the Bahamas. Unprotected heterosexual sex is the main mode of transmission but male homosexual transmission and injecting drug use are important contributory factors in many countries, particularly in Latin America and in the Caribbean. The prevalence of HIV is one per cent in the countries of the Caribbean, which is the highest prevalence globally outside sub- Saharan Africa, and the prevalence is higher in women and children than in men. Mother to infant transmission is important and it was estimated in 2008 that only about half of HIV positive pregnant women received antiretroviral therapy. The prevalence of maternal syphilis is 3.9 per cent, more than double the world average, and 3 million people are estimated to be infected annually in these regions, a quarter of the worldwide total (PAHO 2009).

Chronic diseases and injuries are the leading cause of premature mortality and disability across the region. In the leading countries of South America the epidemiological transition is in full swing and it is estimated that mortality from ischaemic heart disease and stroke will increase almost threefold by 2030. These increases are largely associated with changes in lifestyle and behaviours directly related to globalization of trade markets, urbanization and a host of other factors related to economic development. Even in poorer countries there is some evidence of this epidemiological transition.

Tobacco smoking is the leading cause of avoidable death with more than one million deaths annually. South America has the highest tobacco use with up to 40 per cent of the population being regular smokers. Sedentary behaviour and an increasing dietary pattern of foods rich in saturated fat, sugars and salt, processed food, refined cereals, meat and milk have contributed to the epidemic of overweight and obesity with a prevalence of around 50 per cent in adults and up to 12 per cent in children less than five years of age. Between 30 and 60 per cent of the region's population no longer achieve the minimum recommended levels of physical activity.

PAHO has drafted a Strategic Plan for health development and a Health Agenda for 2008–2017 which includes planned measures to control communicable disease and to combat the rise of non-communicable disease; details are to be found elsewhere (PAHO 2007).

Eastern Mediterranean (EMRO)

This region comprises 23 countries in the Middle East and North Africa, many of which are Arabic speaking. It boasts a few wealthy oil-rich countries at one end of the scale and some greatly impoverished, war-torn countries at the other. Pakistan, with Afghanistan, is included in the east of the region. Darfur, well known as an area of humanitarian concern, lies in North Sudan and has a land area similar to that of Spain. Countries such as Saudi Arabia, Bahrain, Tunisia, Morocco, Libya, and Egypt all had composite human development indices above 0.8 in 2010 with rather lower values for the health component of these indices. Elsewhere Somalia, Sudan (now two separate countries: North and South), Iraq, and Afghanistan have suffered years of conflict

and some international sanctions. The region is second only to the African region in terms of its toll of injuries from landmines, with some 18 countries continuing to endure their threat (WHO–EMRO 2003). In 2001 EMRO reported almost one per cent of total deaths as due to war compared to 1.6 per cent of deaths in AFRO. The potential role of the World Health Survey (data from household surveys) in recording accurate data on the extent of injury and disability and possible ways of obviating war are discussed by Murray et al. (2002).

Even in countries heavily affected by conflict there seem to have been some gains in human development (Akala and El-Saharty 2006). For example, in Sudan and Afghanistan the composite indices rose from 0.42 to 0.48 and from 0.25 to 0.37, respectively, between 2000 and 2010. WHO–EMRO (2011a) reported that maternal mortality remains high in seven countries and 80 per cent of maternal deaths take place in three countries (Afghanistan, Sudan, and Somalia). The poorer countries have some of the lowest density of physicians and nurses per head of population and in Afghanistan, Somalia, and Yemen only a fifth to a third of births were attended by skilled health personnel. These three countries all had an under-five mortality rate in excess of 100 per 1000 livebirths in contrast the regional leading countries such as Saudi Arabia, Bahrain, and United Arab Emirates with rates of less than 10 per 1000.

Child health is a priority in this region and a 90 per cent routine immunization coverage was achieved in 16 countries with special programmes in some countries, such as Somalia, where half a million more children were vaccinated in 2009 compared to 2008. Of the newer vaccines, HIB is now used in 17 countries, rotavirus in three countries, and pneumococcus in six; 19 countries remain free of poliomyelitis but endemic polio outbreaks continue in Afghanistan, in the more remote regions of Pakistan, and in Sudan (2008/9). In children under five years of age half of all deaths are attributable to mild to moderate malnutrition (WHO–EMRO 2011a), as drought and famine are endemic in the poorest and most remote countries. In addition to acute malnutrition micronutrient deficiencies are still reported from many countries.

In both children and adults TB poses a major threat. 'Stop TB' is a priority programme which was developed globally by WHO in 2006 to build on the initial Directly Observed Treatment Schemes (DOTS) devised in 1993. The programme strengthened the involvement of all health care providers, and the overall aim is to reduce the global burden of TB by 2015. The specific objectives (WHO–EMRO 2011b) are to:

i achieve universal access to high-quality diagnosis and patient-centred treatment;

ii reduce the suffering and economic burden associated with TB;

iii protect poor and vulnerable populations from TB, TB/HIV, and multi-drug resistant TB;

iv support development of new tools and enable a timely and effective use of treatment.

More than a quarter million cases of TB were reported in Pakistan in 2009, which has 63 per cent of the burden of the disease in the region, but notification rates were also high in Afghanistan, Djibouti, Somalia, Morocco, and Sudan. It is estimated that a further quarter of a million cases remain unreported and that further strengthening of TB control in primary care and monitoring of control activities is needed. Some 24,000 cases are multi-drug resistant with a million prevalent cases and two-thirds of a million incident cases, with a case detection rate of 63 per cent in 2009 (WHO–EMRO 2011b).

Although the regional average prevalence of HIV is low, some countries carry a substantial estimated burden of HIV and only eight per cent of those infected are receiving antiretroviral therapy. The largest burdens of disease afflict Sudan (estimated at 320,000 in 2009), Pakistan (96,000), and Iran (86,000) but most countries have a low prevalence (below five per cent in the highest risk groups and below one per cent in the general population). With some exceptions, in most countries surveillance, monitoring, and evaluation systems do not provide reliable information on the distribution and trends of HIV/AIDS and sexually-transmitted infections, vulnerability in the population and the coverage and quality of services (WHO–EMRO 2011b).

The control and elimination of malaria is also a priority and six countries (Afghanistan, Djibouti, Pakistan, Somalia, Sudan, and Yemen) carry a heavy malarial burden. In these countries only a proportion of cases are reported and even fewer cases confirmed. In the 15 northern states of Sudan there were an estimated five million cases of malaria in 2008 and one and a half million cases in Pakistan. Ownership of ITNs and access to free combination therapies has increased but further development of laboratory facilities for diagnosis and the adaptation of strategies to control the vector in low transmission areas are required. Other significant tropical diseases and control programs include schistosomiasis, Guinea worm, leprosy, leishmaniasis, dengue, and Kala Azar.

Only a quarter of the population in Afghanistan and Somalia have access to an 'improved water source' and in Sudan the proportion is 56 per cent. Surveillance and monitoring following the introduction of the International Health Regulations has been developed and it is reported that almost all countries have some degree of surveillance in place. EMRO publishes a Weekly Epidemiological Monitor.

Although problems with communicable diseases persist in many countries there is also evidence, particularly in the oil-rich and wealthier countries, of an epidemiological transition with an increased life expectancy. But adoption of Western lifestyles associated with chronic diseases has led to rapid development of risk factors and health surveys indicate a rapidly increasing prevalence of obesity, diabetes, and cardiovascular disease in several countries. The prevalence of diabetes is estimated to rise from 20 million in 2000 to almost 53 million in 2030 (Ghannem 2011). Tobacco smoking is a major problem in several countries and only a small proportion of countries have smoking control measures in place. In boys aged 13–15 years WHO surveys report the prevalence of tobacco use to range from 13 per cent to 67 per cent and the prevalence of smoking is also high in girls in some countries.

Both within and between countries there is evidence of a link between health and poverty (WHO–EMRO 2004). Five policy priorities are proposed to improve the health status of the poor in Box 22.2.

The region has 46 WHO Collaborating centres which pioneer research and development, and capacity, while EMRO also publishes the *Eastern Mediterranean Health Journal*. Health systems profiles for countries of the region can be found on the EMRO website of WHO's Global Information System (WHO–EMRO 2012).

Box 22.2 Strategies for improving the health of the poor

1 Reallocate resources and services by targeting poor and vulnerable people directly:

- reallocating resources by geographic areas (e.g. population-related resource allocation formulas);
- developing and adequately funding universally accessible systems of primary health care supported by appropriate referral hospitals;
- countering imbalanced and inequitable distribution of human resources;
- encouraging non-Government provision in underserved areas;
- adapting services to specific needs of poor (refugees, street children).

2 Concentrate on the diseases and conditions of the poor:

- combating the high impact communicable diseases (tuberculosis, malaria, HIV/AIDS);
- providing reproductive health (pregnancy and delivery care, sexually transmitted infections treatment, family planning);
- preventing childhood diseases through immunization and integrated management of child health;
- reducing malnutrition (protein-energy, micronutrient);
- extending support for non-communicable diseases where supported by evidence of disease burden on the poor.

3 Reduce the burden of direct out-of-pocket payment for health services:

- increasing budget and donor funding as share of total expenditure;

- operating graduated fees and fee exemptions;
- discouraging unofficial fees;
- encouraging collective risk sharing, pre-payment mechanisms (both formal insurance, and community schemes for the informal sector).

4 Improve the supply and effectiveness of non-personal public health services:

- expanding public information and promotion of healthy lifestyles;
- undertaking food fortification programmes (iodine, iron, zinc);
- setting and applying standards for air, water and soil quality; occupational health; and food and chemical safety.

5 Advocate and participate in intersectoral action to achieve health gains:

- expanding water supply and sanitation;
- preventing road traffic accidents (victims in many cases are poor pedestrians, bus passengers);
- reducing tobacco consumption;
- increasing female education;
- raising incomes of poor (support livelihoods, cash, and in kind transfers);
- promoting local integrated community development (Basic Development Needs, Healthy Villages).

Reproduced from 'Investing in the Health of the Poor - A Strategy for Sustainable Health Development of Poverty Reduction in the Eastern Mediterranean', 2004, with permission from WHO. Available at **http://applications.emro.who.int/dsaf/dsa363.pdf**

European Region (EURO)

The WHO European region, which includes countries such as Russia and Turkey with large areas of land in Asia, is undergoing important demographic and epidemiological changes that are shaping the future needs for health promotion, disease prevention, and care. Such transitions are occurring at varying intensities and paces for different country groups, creating a mosaic of health situations which require specific approaches.

The population of the 53 countries of the European region reached nearly 900 million in 2010; 44 per cent live in 15 countries of the European Union prior to 2004 (EU15) and another 33 per cent in the 10 member states of the Confederation of Independent States (CIS) (with the addition of Ukraine). Nearly 70 per cent of the population lived in urban settings in 2010; this is expected to exceed 80 per cent by 2045.

Decreasing crude birth rates (with fertility lower than 1.75 children per woman), coupled with relatively stable or slowly increasing crude death rates and migration result in a decreasing or static population in the EU15 and the CIS countries with increases in other countries. Civil wars in the Balkans and the collapse of the Soviet Union in the 1990s had a devastating effect on the health of the population which still affects mortality in the CIS countries, particularly in the Russian Federation. Migration, resulting from these human-made disasters and other social, economic, and political disruptions, is an additional factor influencing the demographic transitions observed in Europe. An estimated 73 million migrants live in the European Region, or nearly eight per cent of the total population, with women representing 52 per cent of the migrants. Overall this population inflow comprises a five million increase in migrant population since 2005 and nearly 70 per cent of population growth during this period. Net migration estimates and projections show dramatic changes between 2000 and 2020, especially for CIS countries and non-EU countries. Net emigration rates in CIS countries reached nearly 16 per 1000 population in 2000, whereas most EU15 countries, where two-thirds of migrants in the European Region live, witnessed an increase in net immigration. Although the long-term effects of migration on sustained population growth and structure are still uncertain, the health system and other sectors will have to focus additional attention on the current and future needs of migrants, and it is estimated that up to 6.4 million migrants in the EU are in irregular status (Peiro and Benedict 2010); these are usually younger, less affluent, affected more frequently by illness and have limited access to health care.

Health in the European region is generally improving as suggested by life expectancy at birth, which has increased five years since 1980 and reached 75 years in 2010. Projections suggest that it will increase to nearly 81 years by 2050 at a similar pace as from 1980 to 2010. Nevertheless there are important gaps between groups of countries. For example the EU15 countries have already reached the 2050 level expected for the whole region and will continue to reach 85 years in 2050. In contrast the CIS countries are only expected to reach 75 years of life expectancy by 2050, the same level observed in the region as a whole 40 years earlier, or that achieved in the EU15 countries 65 years before.

In the Russian Federation, for example, life expectancy has been static or decreasing since the 1960s and is only beginning to increase once again. One study of almost 49,000 premature deaths in three Russian cities linked 59 per cent of these in men aged 15–54 years with alcohol, and 33 per cent of such deaths in women (Zaridze et al. 2009). Life expectancy presents other important differences according to country and sex: between 1980 and 2020, women in France will have gained seven years of life expectancy to reach nearly 86 years, the highest level in the region; by then, women in France will outlive men by six years. In contrast men in Russia will gain only 3.3 years, and Russian women will outlive men by almost 12 years. Although men's absolute life expectancy levels will be lower, men will generally have larger proportional gains for 1980–2020 than those for women.

Some basic demographic and health data for three of the CIS countries (Azerbaijan, Russia, and Kazakhstan) and other European countries are shown in Table 22.5.

The majority of countries in the region show high or moderate level of human development as measured by the UN's human development index. Life expectancy is usually 74 years or more for women but the gender gap is narrowest mainly in high-income countries but widest in some CIS countries and the newly emerging economies of Eastern Europe. This pattern tends to be reflected in maternal and child mortality also. In the region as a whole there has been almost a 50 per cent reduction in child mortality since 1990.

Non-communicable diseases (NCDs) produce the largest proportion of mortality, accounting for about 80 per cent of deaths in 2008. Among broad groups of causes mortality from cardiovascular diseases accounts for nearly 50 per cent of all of deaths but ranges from 35 per cent in the EU15 countries to 65 per cent in the CIS. Cancer mortality follows in frequency, accounting for 20 per cent of deaths, varying from seven per cent in CIS countries to 30 per cent in EU15 countries. Injuries and violence are the other major causes of mortality representing eight per cent of all deaths and are twice as frequent in the CIS countries as in the EU15 and EU12 (countries joining after 2004).

Analysis of subgroups show a 1:1 ratio between cardiovascular disease and cancer in the EU15, accounting for

Table 22.5 Some health-related indices in selected countries in the WHO European Region

Country	Human Development index (2011)	Gross national income per capita ($US PPP) (2008)	Life expectancy at birth (years) (2008/9)		Maternal mortality per 100 000 livebirths (2008)	Under 5 mortality per 1000 livebirths (2010)
			M	F		
Azerbaijan	0.70	8840	71	76	37	34
Bulgaria	0.77	14,034	69	76	28	11
Czech Republic	0.87	25,858	74	80	7	4
France	0.88	34,212	78	85	10	4
Germany	0.91	37,175	77	83	7	4
Hungary	0.82	20,597	69	78	7	6
Ireland	0.91	43,244	77	82	6	4
Italy	0.87	33,271	79	84	4	3
Kazakhstan	0.79	11,100	64	74	31	44
Norway	0.94	61,268	78	83	8	3
Poland	0.81	18,021	71	80	7	6
Russian Federation	0.76	20,351	62	75	34	15
Switzerland	0.90	45,893	79	84	7	4
Turkey	0.70	14,389	69	74	58	29
United Kingdom	0.86	36,884	77	82	8	5

nearly 70 per cent of deaths, versus 2:1 in the EU12 and 5:1 in the CIS which also reflects the stage of transition of ageing of their populations. Moreover, reflecting the changing disease patterns in Europe, mortality trends show that cardiovascular disease deaths declined by more than 50 per cent in the EU15 countries and 30 per cent in the EU12 countries between 1981 and 2008, coinciding with a 10 per cent increase in the CIS. This contrasts with the cancer situation, which has remained largely unchanged in the EU and CIS groups. These trends are shown in Fig. 22.5.

The case of amenable mortality is useful to illustrate the important inequality in health occurring in the region. This concept involves death that is premature and essentially avoidable by various known public health and health care interventions and is an important measure of the burden of disease in the population. It has also been used to identify inequality in health and might also indicate the performance of the health system. Socio-economic factors such as disposable income are associated with the occurrence of avoidable mortality: the lower the disposable income, the higher the mortality. Amenable mortality rates within the EU show a gradient with higher levels in the eastern parts of the EU, but some subnational regions have high levels in other areas (see Fig. 22.6). Superimposing a layer showing the regions in the poorest quintile (hatched) tends to validate the association with higher avoidable

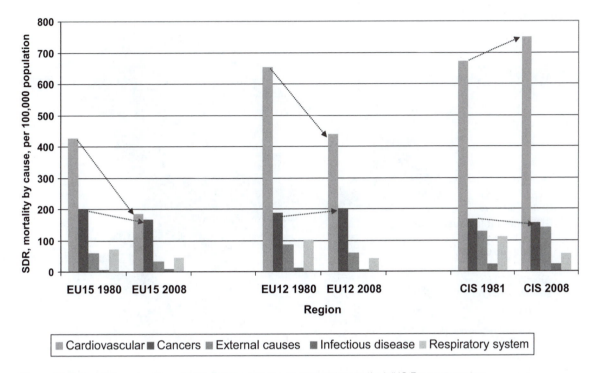

Figure 22.5 Trends in non-communicable diseases in the country groups in the WHO European region.
Source: European Health for All database (2011) [Online]. Copenhagen: WHO Regional Office for Europe. Available from: **http://data.euro.who.int/hfadb**

mortality. However, there are some poor regions where mortality levels are relatively low. An analysis conducted in 2005 of healthy life years in 25 EU countries found substantial inequalities at 50 years of age casting doubt on the possible achievement of substantially increasing the participation of older workers (aged 55–64 years) in the workforce across the EU (Jagger *et al.* 2008).

Non-communicable diseases form the major portion of amenable mortality and the leading risk factors are tobacco use, alcohol, hypertension, hypercholesterlaemia, overweight and obesity, and physical inactivity. Strong intersectoral strategies to reverse adverse trends in these factors are required and WHO—EURO is developing Health 2020 to support countries to combat NCDs. The major goals of Health 2020 are shown in Box 22.3.

WHO–EURO hosts a public interactive database of demographic, mortality, morbidity, and health care data together with other databases which permit analysis of trends and risk factors across the region (WHO–EURO 2012). This database has been used for Figs. 22.5 and 11.1.

South-East Asia (SEARO)

The eleven countries that make up the South-East Asia region of WHO cover five per cent of the world's land area, but are home to 25 per cent of the global population, making the region one of the most densely populated areas of the world. The countries also vary considerably in size and population and include India, Indonesia, and Bangladesh with large populations and Nepal, Bhutan, and Maldives with small ones. All these countries show a significant diversity in geography, demographics, culture, and economic status. In the last three decades, the region has seen rapid economic growth and development, although in some cases this growth has been uneven, resulting in growing income disparities.

Despite this economic growth and development, most countries in the region still experience a heavy burden of communicable diseases (Gupta and Guin 2010), which are estimated to account for 4.2 of the region's 15.3 million annual deaths and 28.6 per cent of all disability-adjusted life-years lost (WHO 2008). Socio-economic, environmental, and behavioural factors are

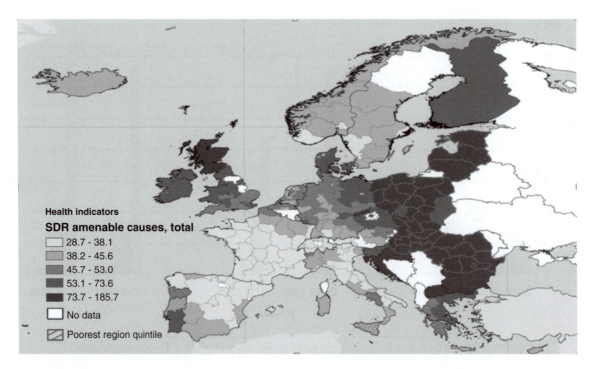

Figure 22.6 Inequality in health in the EU and neighbouring countries: avoidable mortality and lowest disposable income per capita at the subnational level in 2005–2007.
SDR = Standardized Death Rate

all believed to contribute to this continuing burden, and morbidity and mortality from easily preventable diseases such as acute diarrhoea (including cholera) and pneumonia remain disproportionately high. Regional childhood mortality from these conditions is second only to sub-Saharan Africa. HIV also remains a serious problem, with an estimated 3.5 million people living with HIV/AIDS, most of whom are in need of antiretroviral treatment. Thailand has an adult prevalence of HIV over four times that of the regional average of three per cent. Emergence of multi-drug resistant (MDR) TB is a growing concern and the disease continues to claim an estimated half a million lives every year. Drug-resistant malaria has also become a threat.

South-East Asia also continues to be second among WHO regions in its burden of 'neglected tropical diseases' (Narain *et al.* 2010). Within the region, the Mekong and Ganges river and delta areas, have also been epicentres for the emergence of zoonotic infectious diseases, driven by factors including a high human population density, poorly regulated poultry

and livestock production practices, rapid urbanization, and climate change. When coupled with increasingly mobile populations and expanding travel and trade, these factors combine to create the rapid evolution of a significant public health threat, as demonstrated by outbreaks of avian influenza A (H5N1), SARS, chikungunya, and Nipah virus infection. To address these growing challenges, WHO is working with countries to strengthen national 'core capacities' for preparedness, surveillance, risk assessment, and outbreak response as required by the International Health Regulations. One important initiative strongly supported by WHO is the strengthening of epidemiological skills through the establishment (and international networking) of national Field Epidemiology Training Programmes (FETPs). Although the primary aim of such programmes is often directed at the investigation of outbreaks, the skills acquired by graduates are the same as those required to identify the determinants of disease, generate evidence for policy and to identify cost-effective interventions and monitor their impact. Therefore, it is

Box 22.3 Main goals of Health 2020

1 Work together

Health 2020 aims to harness the joint strength of the Member States and the WHO Regional Office for Europe to further promote health and well-being and to reach out to other sectors and partners to reinforce this effort.

2 Create better health

Further increase the number of years in which people live in health, improve the quality of life of the people living with chronic disease, reduce inequity in health and deal with the effects of demographic change.

3 Improve governance for health

Leverage the momentous societal changes in favour of health and strengthen health as a driver of change for sustainable development and well-being by ensuring that heads of government, parliamentarians, and key actors and decision-makers in all sectors are aware of their responsibility for health and well-being and for health promotion, protection, and security.

4 Set common strategic goals

Support the development of policies and strategies in countries that benefit health and well-being as a joint social objective, at the appropriate level, providing stakeholders and partners with mechanisms for engagement and a clear map of the way forward.

5 Accelerate knowledge sharing and innovation

Increase the knowledge base for developing health policy by enhancing the capacity of health and other professionals to adapt to the new approach to public health and the demands of patient-centred health care in an ageing and multicultural society, and make full use of the technological and managerial innovations available to increase impact and improve care.

6 Increase participation

Provide structures and resources that empower the people of the European Region to make use of their own assets, to be active participants in shaping health policy through civil society organizations, to respond to the health challenges facing them as individuals by increasing health literacy, to ensure their voice in patient-centred health systems and to participate fully in community and family life in ways they would choose and to which they are entitled.

Reproduced from *Accelerating Progress Towards the Health-Related Millennium Development Goals*, 2010, with permission from WHO.

---

expected that this investment will yield dividends when FETP alumni join national public health programmes.

Despite these challenges, significant progress has been made in the prevention and control of some leading communicable diseases, with striking successes in a number of disease control programmes. Guinea-worm (dracunculiasis) has been eradicated, while eradication of poliomyelitis is on track, with only sporadic cases being reported from India. Progress towards global targets for TB case detection and treatment has registered success in the majority of countries (Nair *et al.* 2010). The elimination of leprosy, yaws, and visceral leishmaniasis (kala-azar) is also on track, with cases of yaws now being reported from only two countries (Narain *et al.* 2010). As a result of child health programmes such as the Expanded Programme on Immunization and Integrated Management of Childhood Illnesses, infant and childhood mortality rates have declined. It is evident that these programmes have made a significant contribution to the improvements in life expectancy, witnessed in the region, with many countries recording a gain of over 15 years between 1970 and 2005 (WHO 2008). In 2009 some countries achieved immunization rates among one-year-old children of over 90 per cent (Thailand, Sri Lanka, and Bangladesh), and the maternal mortality rate is below 50 per 100,000 livebirths in Thailand and Sri Lanka in contrast to the regional average of 240. In the larger countries, which includes India with its population of 1.2 billion, the maternal mortality rate approximates to the regional average but is 340 per 100,000 livebirths in Bangladesh where the proportion of livebirths attended by skilled personnel is only 18 per cent. SEARO, in partnership with global stakeholders, has facilitated child and maternal health programmes by supporting inter-country collaboration and through the provision of technical and financial support to all countries in the region (WHO–SEARO 2011). Table 22.6 shows basic demographic and health indicators for selected countries of the region.

Antimicrobial resistance is hindering progress towards the control of HIV, TB, and malaria. It stems from a number of practices, including widespread availability of over-the-counter drugs and improper prescribing practices within health care facilities. To counter this requires the implementation of a number of treatment policies and practices such as combination therapy, rational prescribing, improving patient adherence, strong regulatory mechanisms, and also the establishment of effective surveillance systems. WHO has developed a strategy based on the introduction of legislation and policies governing the use of antimicrobial agents, establishing laboratory-based networks for surveillance of resistance and ensuring the rational use of medicines at all levels of health care (WHO–SEARO 2010). Although communicable diseases remain a significant burden most countries in the region are experiencing an epidemiological transition, NCDs such as diabetes, cardiovascular disease, cancer, and chronic lung disease are now emerging as the leading killers, accounting for 54 per cent of

estimated deaths and 47 per cent of DALYs in 2004. Injuries, including road-traffic accidents, account for 14 per cent of DALYs and 11 per cent of all deaths. The rise and strategies for the control of NCDs and injuries in the region are discussed elsewhere (Dans et al. 2011).

Natural disasters, such as floods and earthquakes, and the humanitarian crises which result, are common. The tsunami in December 2004 affected six countries with an estimated 230,000 people missing or dead. In 2008 Cyclone Nargis struck Myanmar and left 133,665 dead or missing. Frequent floods in Bangladesh and India, and volcanic eruptions and landslides in Indonesia also illustrate this vulnerability. In the period 1999–2008 more than 60 per cent of global deaths from natural disasters occurred in the region (IFRC 2009). In response to these increasing challenges SEARO has established a Regional Emergency Fund to facilitate rapid mobilization of financial and technical resources.

Climate change also presents a significant challenge. The region includes low-lying countries such as Bangladesh and islands such as the Maldives, and the region as a whole is already vulnerable to extreme weather such as cyclones which are predicted to increase in frequency and severity. Adverse health outcomes that are projected to increase include: heat stress, strokes, and cardiovascular disorders; respiratory disorders such as asthma (due to greater use of fossil fuels); and, injuries,

Table 22.6 Income, life expectancy, and maternal and child mortality in the South East Asia Region 2008/9

Country	Gross national income per capita (PPP $US)	Life expectancy at birth (years) M/F	Maternal mortality ratio per 100,000 livebirths	Under 5 child mortality per 1000 livebirths
Bangladesh	1450	64/66	340	52
India	2930	63/66	230	66
Indonesia	3600	66/71	240	39
Myanmar	1020	61/67	240	71
Nepal	1120	65/69	380	48
Sri Lanka	4460	65/76	39	16
Thailand	7770	66/74	48	14

disability, and drowning due to extreme weather events. It is also expected that variable rainfall may compromise the supply of freshwater and thus increase the risk of water-borne diseases such as cholera. Rising temperatures combined with erratic rainfall are likely to affect food production, increasing risks of malnutrition. This may alter the seasonal and geographical transmission of important vector-borne diseases such as dengue and malaria, potentially resulting in spread to populations that lack immunity or a strong public health infrastructure. It is also anticipated that the displacement of communities and loss of livelihood will increase psychosocial stress in affected populations. SEARO is working closely with its partners in support of the United Framework Convention on Climate Change (UN 2008).

Substantial demographic and epidemiological change is occurring in most countries. Urbanization is frequently accompanied by unregulated settlement, often associated with overcrowding, unsafe water supply and weak social services which present significant challenge to public health. SEARO is working to promote sustainable development and healthy environments, including advocacy to raise public awareness.

Many countries have low levels of public spending on health. For example, India spends only one per cent of its gross domestic product on health and the overall out-of-pocket expenditure is 80 per cent of the total health expenditure; there are marked differences in the health status indicators such as maternal and infant mortality between urban and rural areas and between different states. For example, for decades Kerala has had an enviable record for maternal and child mortality based on a long-standing political commitment to public health investment. A call for action to deliver universal coverage in India is discussed elsewhere (Reddy *et al.* 2011). WHO's 'health systems strengthening' strategy is designed to evolve continually in response to the needs of countries, incorporating the latest evidence on what works, derived from country experiences and from new research. The establishment and improvement of locally responsive Primary Health Care, for the delivery of both public health programmes and equitable, accessible, and high, quality clinical care form a major component of this strategy (WHO 2007).

Western Pacific and China (WPRO)

China is located in the WHO Western Pacific Region which comprises 37 countries, including Australia, New Zealand, Japan, Republic of Korea, and Singapore, which all enjoy a very high human development index (HDI); Malaysia and Tonga with high HDIs; and Fiji, China, Philippines, Mongolia, Vietnam, Cambodia, and Lao People's Democratic Republic (LPDR) with medium HDIs. According to the sixth nationwide population census conducted in 2010, mainland China has over 1.3 billion residents who make up nearly a quarter of the world's population: 51 per cent of the population is male and 58 per cent of citizens reside in rural areas. Some 147 million Chinese are classified as internal migrants and there is increasing urbanization. Life expectancy at birth (71.6 for males and 75.1 for females in 2009) is lower compared to very high HDI countries of Australia and Japan, in which life expectancies were 81.9 and 83.2 years, respectively. In contrast, Cambodia and LPDR have respective male and female life expectancies at birth of 62.2 and 65.9 years. Some demographic and health indicators for selected countries are shown in Table 22.7.

China's dramatic economic growth has led to big improvements in living standards. This has resulted in better access to health care, which has become market-orientated, so that by 2000 60 per cent of patient costs were out-of-pocket and large disparities between urban and rural areas and regions arose (Alcorn and Bao 2011). Health reforms in 2009 included a rural health insurance scheme as the Chinese Government has significantly increased investment in public health at national and local levels, though China still faces several major public health problems (World Bank 2011). These include:

a Its people's health status in terms of life expectancy and mortality does not reflect the economic growth and investment in public health; internal migration and urbanization, industrialization and pollution, regional inequalities, and an ageing population all hinder health development.

b Personal health care costs have risen and exceed personal incomes, particularly in disadvantaged rural areas. Out-of-pocket medical expenses are high and ill-health continues to be a contributor to poverty

Table 22.7 Maternal and child health indicators in the Western Pacific Region (1990–2011)

Country	Gross national income per capita (2008/9) (PPP $US)	Maternal mortality ratio (per 100,000 livebirths)		Under 5 child mortality (per 1000 livebirths)	
		1990[1]	2011[1]	1990	2011[1]
Australia	37,250	8	5	10	5
Cambodia	1870	413	308	117	53
China	6010	88	27	46	14
Laos	2050	471	283	157	69
Japan	35,190	13	10	5	3
Malaysia	13,740	83	48	18	5
Mongolia	3470	204	65	98	22
New Zealand	25,200	13	9	11	6
Papua New Guinea	2030	389	289	91	66
Philippines	3900	189	86	61	27
Republic of Korea	27,840	20	11	9	3
Singapore	47,970	9	7	9	3
Vietnam	2700	131	56	54	11

[1] Lozano *et al. Lancet* (2011) **378**, 1139–65.

due to a lack of universal coverage. Health insurance coverage at the end of 2008 was approximately 72 per cent for urban citizens, including a medical insurance scheme for urban workers (44 per cent) and a basic medical insurance scheme for urban residents (13 per cent); for rural residents 90 per cent are included in a new rural co-operative medical scheme.

c The allocation of health resources and the provision of health services have not been shared equally across geographic regions, rich and poor households, urban and rural residents, and recently arrived migrants in cities. The major threats to health in rural areas are unsafe water, lack of sanitation, undernutrition, vitamin and mineral deficiencies, and indoor pollution. Maternal mortality and child deaths under five years are four or five times higher in the poorer rural provinces in the west than in the eastern coastal regions. Hepatitis B and TB cause significant morbidity and mortality.

d Emerging health threats related to the environment, the workplace and lifestyle are becoming more evident: air pollution and water contamination by industrial and municipal waste, as well as overuse of chemical fertilizers and pesticides, cost China over 400,000 lives each year. Birth defects rose from 105 per 10,000 births in 2001 to 146 per 10,000 in 2006, a rise of 40 per cent. Folic acid supplementation and iodized salt distribution were reported to be inadequate in several regions, mainly in the western and central areas. The burden of non-communicable diseases and injuries is increasing due to industrialization, urbanization, and ageing of the population.

The prevalence of all chronic diseases was 20 per cent, and in the last decade 10 million new patients with chronic diseases have been added to the pool annually. The number of cases with hypertension, diabetes mellitus, heart diseases, and malignancy has doubled over the past 10 years.

To improve the health of the population and reduce the burden of disease, China and WHO have worked together to develop a Country Co-operation Strategy for the period from 2008–2013 to:

1 enhance health systems development and to combat emerging threats to public health;

2 facilitate achievement of the Millennium Development Goals related to maternal and child health, HIV, TB, and malaria;

3 create initiatives to strengthen control of non-communicable diseases, food and drug safety, environmental health;

4 address the issues of vulnerable people, gender equality, improved research, disease surveillance, data analysis, and human resources development (WHO–WPRO 2008).

Numerous national and local programmes for the control and prevention of some leading diseases are being conducted in China. The Government has expanded the immunization programme to include vaccines to prevent a total of 12 diseases (TB, poliomyelitis, diphtheria, tetanus, pertussis, measles, hepatitis B, Japanese encephalitis, meningococcal meningitis, hepatitis A, rubella, and mumps) in all children without charge, as well as vaccines to prevent leptospirosis, anthrax, and epidemic hemorrhagic fever in selected populations (WHO–WPRO 2011). Some 700,000 persons were estimated to have HIV in China in 2007 (overall prevalence 0.05 per cent) with Yunnan, Henan, and Guanxi having particularly high rates; the latest assessment report on the AIDS epidemic in China demonstrated that there were 780,000 persons living with HIV/AIDS in China by the end of 2011 with 29 per cent in women. In 2011 it was estimated that about 48,000 persons were newly-infected and 28,000 persons died of AIDS-related diseases (Ministry of Health 2012). Almost 90 per cent of HIV infections in China are being monitored and all cases

with HIV/AIDS can access antiretroviral treatment free of charge. Heterosexual transmission is the main mode of transmission (38 per cent), with 29 per cent infected through intravenous drug use and three per cent by homosexual practice. Some specific programmes target high risk groups such as female sex workers, maternal-neonatal transmission of HIV, methadone-maintenance treatment, and a pilot study on men who have sex with men. The China Containment, Prevention and Control Action Plan on HIV/AIDS (2006–2010) has been extended for a further five years until 2015.

Tobacco smoking is a major public health issue in China and the number of male smokers is growing rapidly such that most smokers began smoking below age 25 years, few quit, and about half of these smokers can be expected to be killed by tobacco. Relatively few Chinese women smoke and the habit even seems to be declining. In 1998 tobacco use was responsible for 913,000 deaths and, if current smoking patterns persist, it will result in 2.2 million deaths and 35.4 million DALYs each year by 2020.

China's population is ageing rapidly, and 24 per cent of people living in the country will be aged 60 years or older by 2035. An ageing population leads to a shift across the spectrum of diseases towards chronic disease and disability, with higher associated costs to the health services. Moreover, the Chinese tradition of providing long-term care at home for the elderly will face challenges in the light of the one-child policy initiated more than 30 years ago in China.

Although rapid industrialization and urbanization are ongoing in China an epidemiological transition is well-advanced and the disease profile resembles that of a developed country, with some 80 per cent of total deaths due to non-communicable diseases and injuries (WHO 2005). Cerebrovascular disease, chronic obstructive pulmonary disease, and heart disease account for nearly 50 per cent of all deaths. The rankings based on DALYs also highlight the emergence of NCDs and injuries as the predominant health problems. Much of the disability and death attributable to NCDs, particularly in adults of working age, could be reduced through modification of risk factors, including: reduction in tobacco and alcohol abuse; improvements in diet and nutrition and increases in exercise in the sedentary population; improvements in air quality and other environmental pollution. Otherwise it is estimated that these disabilities and deaths will result in premature morbidity and mortality among the working population, and a huge economic burden will be the legacy for the Chinese health care system. Unfortunately, taking the example of tobacco control (China ratified the WHO Framework Convention on Tobacco Control in 2005), the industry has responded by denying the evidence against tobacco, attempted to frustrate the Government's efforts to control tobacco, and has employed covert advertising and sponsorship, according to a recent report from the China Centre for Disease Control and Prevention (Anon 2011). Legislation against smoking in public places was introduced in early 2011 but implementaion and compliance are limited at present.

The challenges and potential solutions to some major health problems are outlined in a recent World Bank Report (with the Chinese Ministry of Health and WHO) which includes the training of 300,000 general practitioners to strengthen primary care (World Bank 2011).

Many of the low- and middle-income countries of the Western Pacific region have made significant progress towards achieving the Millennium Development Goals, although progress is variable across the range of targets in some countries (Table 22.8).

In the light of the rise of risk factors for NCDs a number of epidemiological studies have been established in the region. One such collaborative study is the Asia Pacific Collaboration which was established in 1999 and the database includes baseline information on 650,000 participants from 44 separate cohorts in China, Japan, South Korea, Taiwan, Australia, and New Zealand. Recent studies have confirmed the link between overweight and selected cancers in the region (Parr *et al.* 2010).

22.6 Towards better global health

In the reports from the WHO regions some of the driving forces that shape global health have been described. They include: the globalization of trade, media, and culture; industrialization, urbanization and migration; ageing of populations; climate change; and

the political and economic contexts that determine the distribution of wealth, power, and resources between and within countries. We have seen that in many regions of the world economic growth has promoted improvements in health, but this is not a universal finding even in countries such as India which show strong economic growth. In the poorest countries, particularly in sub-Saharan Africa, with little or negative economic growth, new strategies may be required to improve the health and prospects for this region. In this final section we review the prospects for improved global health and the challenges for the international community. Fresh global health challenges have emerged in addition to those that have persisted from infectious disease and undernutrition in environments hostile to mankind. These new challenges, fuelled, at least in part, by the marketing of unhealthy lifestyles, are driving the increase in non-communicable diseases (heart disease, cancer, and diabetes), and in transport and industrial accidents in developing countries. A narrative review of the vulnerability of heath care to market forces is reported elsewhere (Brezis and Wiist 2011).

Globalization can bring benefits, but it has no inbuilt mechanisms to ensure the fair distribution of these benefits. A recent international comparison showed that countries in the world with high child mortality (mean 207/1000) had significantly higher rates of extreme poverty, female illiteracy, significantly lower per capita expenditure on health care, hospital beds, and doctors, and lower rates of access to a safe water supply, sanitation and immunization, compared to countries with low child mortality (Ruger and Kim 2006). Another major study showed a strong relationship between the increase in the proportion of educated women and improving child mortality rates during the period 1970–2010. This relationship was not explained by increasing levels of income per capita (see Fig. 16.5 in Chapter 16) (Gakidou *et al.* 2010) and the authors estimated that 51 per cent of the reduction in deaths in children worldwide between 1970 and 2009 (total reduction 8.2 million) could be attributed to increased educational attainment of women of reproductive age. Global efforts to deal with these inequalities in child and adult mortality across countries require coherent policies across sectors within countries with particular

Table 22.8 Progress in achieving the Millennium Development Goals in the Western Pacific Region

Health MDGs scorecard for LMICs* in the Western Pacific Region (with population ≥ 250,000)

	Cambodia	China	Fiji	Lao PDR	Malaysia	Mongolia	Papua New Guinea	Philippines	Solomon Islands	Vietnam
Infant mortality rate per 1000 live births	69	18	16	48	6	33	53	26	30	12
Under-5 mortality per 1000 live births	89	21	18	61	6	41	69	32	36	14
Measles immunization % coverage	92	99	72	59	95	94	58	88	60	97
Maternal mortality per 100,000 live births	290	38	26	580	31	65	250	94	100	56
Skilled birth attendant % births	44	98	99	20	100	100	39	60	43	88
Contraceptive use % married women aged 15–49	40	87	–	32	–	66	–	51	–	79
HIV/AIDS prevalence % adults aged 15–45	0.8	0.1	0.1	0.2	0.5	0.1	0.9	<0.1	–	0.5
Malaria mortality per 100 000 population	1.9	<0.1	–	0.1	0.1	–	9.2	<0.1	10.2	<0.1
TB treatment success rate %	94	94	81	92	72	89	39	89	92	92
Underweight % among children five years of age	29	7	–	32	–	5	18	21	12	20
Water % using improved sources	61	89	–	57	100	76	40	91	70	94
Sanitation % using improved facilities	29	55	–	53	96	50	45	76	32	75

■ On track ■ Insufficient progress ■ Off track

*LMICs–low- and middle-income countries
Source: WHO Western Pacific Region, with permission.

attention to less well-off countries. The Millennium Development Goals recognized the need to develop global partnerships for development but there is no definitive 'road map' to better global health. But there are some important initiatives which are contributing and have the potential to contribute further, given the international political will. Some selected organizations and partnerships which are important in global health and development were shown in Table 22.1. Our list is by no means exhaustive and readers can find many other examples of organizations online.

Perhaps it is presumptuous for outsiders (the editors) to offer any suggestions for the way forward but it is clear that the major challenges which face human kind and the future of sustained and equitable development on this planet require increased international collaboration and appropriate, agreed strategies.

Firstly, there is a need to implement and prioritize cost-effective interventions in countries or areas of greatest need, which may best be coordinated at the WHO regional level. All initiatives require the co-operation and participation of national governments. The 'Disease Control Priorities Project' was initiated in 1993 to seek cost-effective solutions to public health problems in developing countries. Some cost-effective interventions in key areas of health development particularly aimed at sub-Saharan Africa are shown in Table 22.9, and many international initiatives have evolved from these priority interventions.

Secondly, there is a need for scientific research and development, particularly in the areas of vaccines, and sustainable agricultural improvement. In some scientific areas such as vaccine development public–private partnerships may be the only practical way forward and the global initiative on vaccination provides a good example of effective collaboration between WHO, the Gates Foundation, and industrial partners (The GAVI Programme). Unfortunately the new epidemic of NCDs is unlikely to be curtailed by collaboration with industrial partners and new strategies and appropriate legislation may be the most effective way to limit the impact in developing countries. The economic burden of NCDs and accidents has been estimated to be greater than that of communicable disease globally (and global prevention initiatives underfunded), but the rise in NCDs is clearly a consequence of economic

development, in contrast to infectious disease and undernutrition, which severely hamper development.

Thirdly, there is a need for strengthening international collaboration and a recognition that some programmes, both for communicable and NCDs, require a long sustained period of activity rather than short-term action. For example 'UNAIDS' was founded in 1994 as it was recognized that HIV was a pressing epidemic of global concern which could not be adequately contained by existing agencies (UNAIDS 1994).

Improving health is not only an issue for the health sector but is also a political, social, and economic issue. International politics and trade are key factors in health development and the need to consider health and sustainable development in trade agreements through the World Trade Organization has been strongly argued elsewhere (Fidler *et al.* 2009; Smith *et al.* 2009). Poverty reduction and women's education are primary MDGs but require sustained economic and social development for many low income countries. For long-term improvement of the health of mothers and children, social attitudes that regard women as second class citizens and the policies that enforce these attitudes need to change. In a balanced review of initiatives in health development since the birth of international agencies, such as the UN and WHO, Birn *et al.* (2009) have reviewed their successes and failures. Programmes to eradicate or control smallpox, yellow fever, and hookworm have been successful, together with polio and measles in the Americas, but malaria control using DDT and UNICEF's child survival campaign (a package of measures including immunization, growth monitoring, food supplementation, oral rehydration therapy, and family planning) have been more problematic. Vertical programmes for specific diseases may be too narrowly focused and may require other support, e.g. primary care. It can be difficult for donor organizations to target the political, economic, and social issues which require consideration if long-term health development is to be achieved and sustained. Birn *et al.* (2009) show that several low income countries (Costa Rica, Cuba, Sri Lanka, Uruguay, and Kerala State, India) have achieved high levels of health development associated with strong investment in social welfare, and it is clear that developing countries with large out-of-pocket expenditure for health generally are at lower levels of health development (WHO 2010b).

Table 22.9 Some neglected low-cost opportunities in sub-Saharan Africa

Preventive measures	Cost per DALY averted ($US)	Burden of target diseases (millions of DALYs)
Childhood immunization Additional coverage of traditional Expanded Progam on Immunization (DPT, polio, measles, BCG) Second opportunity measles vaccination	1–5	13.5–31.3
Traffic accidents Increasing speeding penalties, media, and law enforcement Speed bumps at major junctions	2–12	6.4
Malaria Insecticide-treated bed nets Residual household spraying Intermittent preventive treatment in pregnancy	2–24	35.4
Surgical services and emergency care Surgical ward in district hospital for obstetrics, injuries, etc.	7–215	25–134.2
Childhood illnesses Integrated management of childhood illnesses including acute lower respiratory infections	9–218	9.6–45.1
HIV and AIDS Peer-based programmes for at-risk groups (e.g. sex workers) Voluntary counselling and testing Diagnosis and treatment of STDs Condom promotion and distribution Treatment of TB co-infection Blood and needle safety programmes Prevention of mother-to-child transmission with antiretroviral therapy	6–377	56.8
Maternal and neonatal care Increase primary care coverage Improved quality and coverage of obstetric care Neonatal packages for families, communities, and clinics	82–409	29.8–37.7

Adapted from: Jamison *et al.* (2006). *Disease Control Priorities in Developing Countries*, 2nd edn, p. 55. With permission from World Bank/Oxford University Press.

Finally, the importance of global public health as a key discipline and factor in equitable and sustainable human development should be more widely recognized. There is a compelling need for sustained funding and scientific capacity in key international organizations and partnerships. What is also essential is there should be a significant investment in future generations of global health professionals, particularly in countries and regions which are under-resourced.

Further reading

Birn AE, Pillay Y, and Holtz T (2009) *Textbook of International Health: Global Health in a Dynamic World*, 3rd edn. New York: Oxford University Press.

Merson MH, Black RE, and Mills AJ (2012) *Global Health: Diseases, Programs, Systems, and Policies*, 3rd edn. Burlington, MA: Thomas and Bartlett Learning.

Skolnik R (2012) *Global Health 101*, 2nd edn. Burlington, MA: Thomas and Bartlett Learning.

References

Akala FA and El-Saharty S (2006) Public-health challenges in the Middle East and North Africa. *Lancet* **367** (9515), 961–4.

Alcorn T And Bao B (2011) China progresses with health reform but challenges remain. *Lancet* **377** (9777), 1557–8.

Anon (2011) China's unhealthy relations with big tobacco. *Lancet* **377** (9761), 180.

Baverstock K (2011) Chernobyl 25 years on. *BMJ (Clinical Research Ed)* **342**, d2443.

Birn AE, Pillay Y, and Holtz TH (2009) *Textbook of International Health: Global Health in a Dynamic World*, 3rd edn. New York: Oxford University Press.

Brezis M and Wiist WH (2011) Vulnerability of health to market forces. *Medical Care* **49** (3), 232–9.

Chattaway MA, Dallman T, Okeke IN, and Wain J (2011) Enteroaggregative E. coli O104 from an outbreak of HUS in Germany 2011, could it happen again? *Journal of Infection in Developing Countries* **5** (6), 425–36.

Dans A, Ng N, Varghese C, Tai ES, *et al.* (2011) The rise of chronic non-communicable diseases in southeast Asia: time for action. *Lancet* **377** (9766), 680–9.

Ferris E and Ferro-Ribeiro S (2012) Protecting people in cities: the disturbing case of Haiti. *Disasters* **36** Suppl. 1 S43–63.

Fidler DP, Drager N, and Lee K (2009) Managing the pursuit of health and wealth: the key challenges. *Lancet* **373** (9660), 325–31.

Gakidou E, Cowling K, Lozano R, and Murray CJL (2010) Increased educational attainment and its effect on child mortality in 175 countries between 1970 and 2009: a systematic analysis. *Lancet* **376** (9745), 959–74.

Ghannem H (2011) The need for capacity building to prevent chronic diseases in North Africa and the Middle East. *Eastern Mediterranean Health Journal* **17** (7), 630–2.

Glied S (2008) *Health care financing, efficiency, and equity*. National Bureau of Economic Research, working paper 13881.

Gu D, Kelly TN, Wu X, Chen J, *et al.* (2009) Mortality attributable to smoking in China. *The New England Journal of Medicine* **360** (2), 150–9.

Gubler DJ (1998) The global pandemic of dengue/dengue haemorrhagic fever: current status and prospects for the future. *Annals of the Academy of Medicine, Singapore* **27** (2), 227–34.

Gupta I and Guin P (2010) Communicable diseases in the South-East Asia Region of the World Health Organization: towards a more effective response. *Bulletin of the World Health Organization* **88** (3), 199–205.

IFRC (International Federation of the Red Cross) (2009) World Disaster Report 2009. Available at: http://www.ifrc.org/Global/Publications/disasters/WDR/WDR2009-full.pdf

Jagger C, Gillies C, Moscone F, Cambois E, *et al.* (2008) Inequalities in healthy life years in the 25 countries of the European Union in 2005: a cross-national meta-regression analysis. *Lancet* **372** (9656), 2124–31.

Jamison, DT, Breman JG, Measham AR, Alleyne G, *et al.* (eds) (2006) *Disease Control Priorities in Developing Countries*, 2nd edn. Washingon, DC: World Bank/Oxford University Press.

Kahn JG, Muraguri N, Harris B, Lugada E, *et al.* (2012) Integrated HIV testing, malaria, and diarrhea prevention campaign in Kenya: modeled health impact and cost-effectiveness. *PloS One* **7** (2), e31316.

Koplan JP, Bond TC, Merson MH, Reddy KS, *et al.* (2009) Towards a common definition of global health. *Lancet* **373** (9679), 1993–5.

Laxminarayan R, Mills AJ, Breman JG, Measham AR, *et al.* (2006) Advancement of global health: key messages from the Disease Control Priorities Project. *Lancet* **367** (9517), 1193–208.

Lozano R, Wang H, Foreman KJ, Rajaratnam JK, *et al.* (2011) Progress towards Millennium Development Goals 4 and 5 on maternal and child mortality: an updated systematic analysis. *Lancet* **378** (9797), 1139–65.

MacDonald R and Horton R (2009) Trade and health: time for the health sector to get involved. *Lancet* **373** (9660), 273–4.

Mendis S, Fukino K, Cameron A, Laing R, *et al.* (2007) The availability and affordability of selected essential medicines for chronic diseases in six low- and middle-income countries. *Bulletin of the World Health Organization* **85** (4), 279–88.

Ministry of Health, China (2012) http://www.stats.gov.cn/english/.

Morris S (2010) Haiti earthquake: perspectives from the ground and lessons from afar. *Disaster Medicine and Public Health Preparedness* **4** (2), 113–15.

Murray CJL, King G, Lopez AD, Tomijima N, *et al.* (2002) Armed conflict as a public health problem. *BMJ (Clinical Research Ed)* **324** (7333), 346–9.

Nair N, Wares F, And Sahu S (2010) Tuberculosis in the WHO South-East Asia Region. *Bulletin of the World Health Organization* **88** (3), 164.

Narain JP, Dash AP, Parnell B, Bhattacharya SK, *et al.* (2010) Elimination of neglected tropical diseases in the South-East Asia Region of the World Health Organization. *Bulletin of the World Health Organization* **88** (3), 206–10.

PAHO (2007) Health Agenda for the Americas 2008–2017. Available at: http://new.paho.org/hq/index. php?option=com_content&task=view&id=91&Itemid=220

PAHO (2009) Challenges posed by the HIV epidemic in Latin America and in the Caribbean in 2009. Available at: http://new.paho.org/hq/dmdocuments/2010/ CHALLENGE0S_%20INGLES.pdf

Parr CL, Batty GD, Lam TH, Barzi F, *et al.* (2010) Body-mass index and cancer mortality in the Asia-Pacific Cohort Studies Collaboration: pooled analyses of 424,519 participants. *Lancet oncology.* **11** (8), 741–752.

Piero M-J and Benedict R (2010) Migrant health policy: The Portuguese and Spanish EU Presidencies. *Eurohealth (Lond).* **16**, 1–4.

Preker AS and Carin G (2004) Rich-poor differences in health care financing. In: Preker AS and Carrin G (eds) *Health financing for poor people: resource mobilization and risk-sharing*, pp. 3–52. Washington, DC: World Bank.

Reddy KS, Patel V, Jha P, Paul VK, *et al.* (2011) Towards achievement of universal health care in India by 2020: a call to action. *Lancet* **377** (9767), 760–8.

Ruger JP and Kim H-J. (2006) Global health inequalities: an international comparison. *Journal of Epidemiology and Community Health* **60** (11), 928–36.

Schieber G, Baeza C, Kress D, and Maier M (2006) Financing Health Systems in the 21st Century. In: Jamison D, Breman J, Mesham A, Alleyne G, *et al.* (eds) *Disease Control Priorities in Developing Countries*, pp. 225–42. Washington DC: World Bank.

Smith RD, Lee K, and Drager N (2009) Trade and health: an agenda for action. *Lancet* **373** (9665), 768–73.

Swedish KA (2011) 2009 Pandemic Influenza A (H1N1): Diagnosis, Management, and Prevention—Lessons Learned. *Current Infectious Disease Reports* **13** (2), 169–74.

Tabuenca JM (1981) Toxic-allergic syndrome caused by ingestion of rapeseed oil denatured with aniline. *Lancet* **2** (8246), 567–8.

Tanimoto T, Uchida N, Kodama Y, Teshima T, *et al.* (2011) Safety of workers at the Fukushima Daiichi nuclear power plant. *Lancet* **377** (9776), 1489–90.

UN (1945) Charter of the United Nations. Available at: www.un.org/en/documents/charter/index.shtml.

UN (2005) World Health Report (2005):Available at: http:// www.un.org/en/documents/udhr/.

UN (2007) United Nations Declaration on the Rights of Indigenous Peoples. Available at: www.un.org/esa/ socdev/unpfii/en/drip.html

UN (2008) United Nations Framework Convention on Climate Change. Available at: http://untreaty.un.org/ cod/avl/ha/ccc/ccc.html

UN (2010a) United Nations resolution 64/265. *Prevention and control of noncommunicable diseases.* (Adopted by the General Assembly, 10 May 2010). New York: United Nations.

UN (2010b) Human Development Report 2010: the United Nations Development Programme. *The Real Wealth of Nations: Pathways to Human Development.* New York: Palgrave Macmillan.

Weaver AJ (2011) Climate change. Toward the second commitment period of the Kyoto Protocol. *Science (New York, NY)* **332** (6031), 795–6.

World Bank (2011) Toward a Healthy and Harmonious Life in China: Stemming the Rise of Non-Communicable Diseases. Human Development Unit, East Asia, and Pacific Region: World Bank. Available at: http://www. worldbank.org/content/dam/Worldbank/document/ NCD_report_en.pdf

WHO (1978) Declaration of Alma-Ata. Available at: http://www.who.int/hpr/NPH/docs/declaration_ almaata.pdf

WHO (2002) World Health Report for 2002. *Global Climate Change.* Geneva: World Health Organization.

WHO (2004) The World Health Report: 2004. *Changing history.* Geneva: World Health Organization.

WHO (2005) Fifty-eighth World Health Assembly, Geneva, 16–25 May 2005. Geneva: World Health Organization.

WHO (2007) *Health Systems: Strengthening Health Systems to Improve Health Outcomes: Who's Framework For Action.* Geneva: World Health Organization. Available at: http://www.who.int/healthsystems/strategy/ everybodys_business.pdf.

WHO (2008) *The Global Burden of Disease: 2004 Update.* Geneva: World Health Organization. Available at: http:// www.who.int/healthinfo/global_burden_disease/GBD_ report_2004update_full.pdf.

WHO (2009) *Global Health Risks: Mortality and Burden of Disease Attributable to Selected Major Risks*. Geneva: World Health Organization.

WHO (2010a) *Global Status Report on Non-Communicable Diseases 2010*. Geneva: World Health Organization.

WHO (2010b). *The World Health Report: Health Systems Financing—The Path to Universal Coverage*. Geneva: World Health Organization.

WHO (2010c) Towards universal access: Scaling up priority HIV/AIDS interventions in the health sector. Progress report 2010; WHO-UNAIDS-UNICEF. Available at: http://whqlibdoc.who.int/publications/2010/9789241500395_eng.pdf [Accessed on 10 October 2011].

WHO (2010d) *World Malaria Report 2010*. Geneva: World Health Organization. Available at: http://www.who.int/malaria/world_malaria_report_2010/worldmalariare-port2010.pdf [Accessed on 10 October 2011].

WHO (2010e) *Who Global Tuberculosis Report, 2010*. Geneva: World Heath Organization. Available at: http://whqlibdoc.who.int/publications/2010/9789241564069_eng.pdf [Accessed on 10 October 2011].

WHO (2010f) *Who World Health Statistics 2010*. Geneva: World Health Organization. Available at: http://www.who.int/gho/publications/world_health_statistics/2010/en/index.html

WHO (2011) *Who World Health Statistics 2011*. Geneva: World Health Organization. Available at: http://www.who.int/whosis/whostat/EN_WHS2011_Full.pdf [Accessed on 10 October 2011].

WHO (2012a) *Programme Budget for 2012/13*. Geneva: World Health Organization. Available at: http://whqlibdoc.who.int/pb/2012–2013/PB_2012%E2%80%932013_eng.pdf.

WHO (2012b) *Structural Reform (Includes Comments From NGOs)*. Geneva: World Health Organization. Available at: http://www.who.int/dg/reform/consultation/en/index.html.

WHO–AFRO (2006) The Health of the People. The African Regional Health Report 2006. Available at: http://www.afro.who.int/en/clusters-a-programmes/ard/african-health-observatory-a-knowledge-management/aho-publications.html (Accessed on October 10 2011).

WHO–AFRO (2008) *CSDH. Closing the Gap in a Genera-tion: Health Equity Through Action on the Social Deter-minants of Health. Final Report of the Commission on Social Determinants of Health*. Geneva: World Health Organization. Available at: http://www.afro.who.int/en/clusters-a-programmes/ard/african-health-observatory-a-knowledge-management/aho-publications.html.

WHO–EMRO (2003) Health under difficult circumstances: 1948–1998. Available at: http://applications.emro.who.int/dsaf/dsa988.pdf EMRO Technical Papers Series.

WHO–EMRO (2004) Investing in the health of the poor: a strategy for sustainable health development and poverty reduction in the Eastern Mediterranean Region. Community-Based Initiatives Series. Available at: http://applications.emro.who.int/dsaf/dsa363.pdf.

WHO–EMRO (2011a) The Work of WHO in the Eastern Mediterranean Region. Annual Report of the Regional Director, January–December 2010. Available at: http://www.emro.who.int/rd/annualreports/2010/index.htm.

WHO–EMRO (2011b) Communicable diseases in the Eastern Mediterranean Region: prevention and control 2005–2009. Available at: http://www.emro.who.int/publications/.

WHO–EMRO (2012) Health Systems Profiles. Available at: http://gis.emro.who.int/HealthSystemObservatory.

WHO–EURO (2012) Health for all database (HFA-DB). Available at: http://data.euro.who.int/hfadb/.

WHO–SEARO (2010) Regional strategy on prevention and containment of antimicrobial resistance. Available at: http://www.searo.who.int/LinkFiles/BCT_hlm-407.pdf.

WHO–SEARO (2011) The Work of WHO in the South-East Asia Region 2010. Available at: http://www.searo.who.int/catalogue/2005–2011/pdf/worldl_health_organization/sea-rc64-2.pdf.

WHO–WPRO (2008) *Who-China Country Cooperation Strategy 2008–2013*. Geneva: World Health Organization. Available at: http://www2.wpro.who.int/NR/rdonlyres/BB787F03-A760-4F01-908E-D17D8DB75178/0/CCS_EN.pdf.

WHO–WPRO (2011) *China-Country Profile*. Manila, Western Pacific Regional Office: World Health Organiza-tion. Available at: http://www.wpro.who.int/countries/chn/5CHNpro2011_finaldraft.pdf.

Zaridze D, Brennan P, Boreham J, Boroda A, *et al.* (2009) Alcohol and cause-specific mortality in Russia: a retrospective case-control study of 48,557 adult deaths. *Lancet* **373** (9682), 2201–14.

Glossary terms

absolute risk The probability of the occurrence of a future adverse event such as death, a disease, condition, trait, or a complication of disease (cf. relative risk).

agent Any factor (chemical, biological, or physical) associated with the development of diesase.

alternative hypothesis Usually the hypothesis of interest rather than the null hypothesis, which is the hypothesis actually tested by a particular statistical test. Often the opposite of the null hypothesis.

analytical study (cf. descriptive) A study which tests a particular hypothesis or a number of hypotheses.

ascertainment The methods, definitions, and protocols used to identify and define a particular disease or condition.

ascertainment bias Systematic errors in the methods used to define a disease or condition.

association A statistical relationship between two variables. This may arise due to chance, confounding, or as part of a causal relationship.

attack rate In infectious disease epidemiology the term is used to describe the cumulative incidence during the period of an epidemic. In chronic disease epidemiology attack rate indicates the combined occurrence of new and recurrent cases of disease in a defined population in a given time period.

attributable fraction (synonym: aetiological fraction) The proportion of disease among the exposed that could be prevented by eliminating this exposure (see also population attributable risk).

attributable risk The rate of disease in the exposed that can be attributed to a particular factor (see also population attributable risk).

avoidable mortality Mortality that could be avoided by control of risk factors (primary prevention) or routine treatment (secondary prevention)

backward elimination see stepwise selection.

bar chart Graphical display of the frequencies or relative frequencies of the classes of a categorical variable in the form of bars or columns. The bars are usually separated (see Figs. 7.3 and 15.5), in contrast a histogram shows a continuous distribution in which bars are contiguous.

Bayes' theorem A procedure for updating the probability of a state or an event given new evidence. For example, the probability that an individual has a disease will increase with the knowledge that the individual has a positive result on a screening test.

bias The presence of a systematic error or systematic deviation from the true value in a measurement or estimate. There are many types of bias depending on the application, e.g. ascertainment, lead-time, and recall bias, which are listed separately.

binary logistic regression see regression analysis.

binary variable A variable, having two values, which represents a characteristic with two states, for example sex, mortality status.

body mass index Any index which estimates the proportion of body fat using standard anthropometric indices such as height and weight. Quetelet's index is the most commonly used and is calculated from the weight (kg) divided by height (m) squared.

case definition The definition used to distinguish a person affected, or having a disease, from a person unaffected or without the disease. A case is defined from the information available and may differ, for example, in hospitalized and non-hospitalized cases or in countries with different levels of health care.

case finding The process of defining and locating cases for study.

case series or reports Usually a consecutive series of clinical cases of a particular disease which have attended a particular hospital or out-patient department.

case-control A study design in which potential exposures for a disease are measured in a group of controls selected for comparison with a group of cases. Controls are often matched for factors which could interfere or confound a hypothesis under test. Case-control studies are usually retrospective in nature when past exposures are measured, but nested or prospective case control studies represent a special type of prospective study in which controls have been selected from the population being followed.

case-fatality The proportion of patients acquiring a disease who die within a given time period. Often this period is 28 days or one month, but shorter or longer periods are also used.

categorical variable A variable which represents different classes of some characteristic. Examples are gender and marital status, the latter being a non-ordered or *nominal categorical* variable. A categorical variable where the classes have a natural ordering is described as *ordered* or *ordinal*, e.g. level of educational attainment or smoking habit grouped into categories of consumption.

causality The process of examining and linking disease with particular exposures.

cause—external Any cause that does not arise within the human organism itself.

cause—multiple Of a disease or condition in which several causes usually operate together to produce the disease (synonym: multifactorial condition).

cause—necessary A cause which always has to be present if a disease is to be produced. Micro-organisms which cause specific infectious disease are examples of necessary causes.

cause—sufficient A cause which is alone sufficient to produce a disease. In practice only genetic and highly infectious agents can be classed as single sufficient causes. Multiple causes, acting together, are sometimes referred to as a *combined sufficient cause*.

clinical decision-making A branch of the evidence based medicine which examines by different methods, the process of clinical diagnosis and treatment. Clinical pathways may be traced by algorithms known as 'decision trees'.

cluster randomized trials A trial in which the unit of allocation of intervention/treatment is a cluster of individuals such as a school or a workplace.

cluster sampling In which the sampling unit is not the individual but is a group or cluster of individuals, e.g. a school or workplace. Because of possible similarities between individuals within a cluster, it may be necessary to make some statistical adjustment when analyzing data from such a design. There may be several clustering steps, e.g. schools, classes within schools and this is termed *multi-stage cluster sampling*.

coefficient of variation The ratio of the standard deviation to the mean, often expressed as a percentage. It is used to compare the variation of measurements made in different units, and is often used to quantify measurement error in laboratories.

cohort A group of individuals identified from a common source and usually at the same time who are examined together over a period of time, e.g. workplace (occupational cohort) or a year of birth (birth cohort).

cohort effect Sometimes known as a generation effect, when age-specific rates rise or fall when plotted by year of birth.

cohort study A study in which a group of individuals, (usually a large group) is studied over a period of time, and particular end points are examined in relation to exposure data collected at the beginning of the study.

community intervention An intervention which is applied to groups of individuals based on their geographical distribution or social characteristics, e.g. fluoridation of water supplies or health promotion programmes directed at particular communities.

concordance A term used in family and twin studies to measure the similarity or concordance of individual traits in family members.

condition A term used in a medical context to indicate a disorder of a particular bodily system.

confidence interval A method of estimation in which an interval is calculated from sample data so that it includes an unknown population parameter with a chosen level of confidence, usually the 95% level, i.e. in repeated samples 95% of intervals will contain the parameter.

confidence limits These are the upper and lower limits of the confidence interval.

confounding variable A confounding variable is one which is associated with the exposure variable and also influences the disease or outcome. Age is often a confounder.

contagious Spread by touch or close bodily contact.

contingency table A two-way table of counts or frequencies, obtained by classifying samples of individuals by two categorical variables.

continuous variable A variable which theoretically has an infinite number of possible values along a continuum, e.g. height, weight, total cholesterol.

controls Any comparison group in epidemiological studies. Controls may be matched for certain characteristics which may affect the outcome of interest. In experimental studies when the exposures for treatments are allocated by the investigators, this may be done at random to ensure comparability between cases and controls in all relevant characteristics other than the intervention under investigation.

correlation analysis A method for measuring the degree of linear association between two variables A *correlation coefficient r> 0 (r < 0)* indicates an increasing (decreasing) linear association, with the extreme values of ± 1 showing a perfect linear relationship; *r* = 0 indicates no linear association between the variables. Correlations between continuous measurements are estimated using **Pearson's coefficient**, while correlations of ordered categorical variables and ranks are estimated using **Spearman's coefficient**.

cross-sectional A study or analysis in which all exposure and disease variables are measured at the same time point.

demographic Relating to the structure or formation of a population.

descriptive epidemiology A type of epidemiology which is characterized by describing characteristics of individuals within a population with a particular disease or condition. Characteristics can be broadly classified under the headings of *person*, *place*, and *time*. Such studies are generally a prerequisite of analytical epidemiological studies in which specific hypotheses relating to particular causes (exposures) for the disease in question can be tested.

dichotomous (synonym: binary variable) A variable or distribution that can be divided conveniently into two divisions, e.g. sex, mortality status.

disability A bodily state which may indicate sub-optimal physical or mental health.

disability-adjusted life-years (DALYs) is a summary measure that combines mortality and disability in *populations*. The DALY for a condition is a sum of the years lost due to premature mortality plus the (weighted) years lost due to disability, where the weighting depends on the severity of the disease and age, more weight being given to the productive years. One DALY represents the loss of one year of healthy life.

discrete variable A variable which takes only integer values, e.g. the number of children in a family or the number of disease episodes per year.

disease Any disorder of physical or mental function in an individual and perceived as such by others.

disease heterogeneity A situation in which one disease with similar clinical manifestations may in reality represent several diseases with potentially different causes.

disorder Any permanent or recurring malfunction of an individual bodily system.

dose–response An association or relationship characterized by a graded or incremental relationship between disease risk and the level of exposure.

ecological fallacy The erroneous assumption that an association detected at an ecological (or aggregate) level is true at the individual level.

ecological studies either studies where the unit of analysis is geographical aggregates of people or where geographical attributes such as temperature, rainfall, etc., are being analysed.

effect modification When the effect of an exposure is modified by another variable. For example age and smoking habit modify risk from exposures such as asbestos or infectious agents. A statistical test of interaction is often used to detect effect modification.

efficacy The impact of an intervention or treatment measured under ideal circumstances, ideally under the conditions of an adequately sized randomized controlled trial. In contrast the *effectiveness* of an intervention implies the same measure made under conditions of everyday clinical practice.

end points Any outcome measurement in a trial or cohort study used to determine the results. Examples include mortality, new episodes of disease, biochemical or physiological measurements, and quality of life measures made by questionnaire.

endemic Describes a disease or disorder which is constantly present without fluctuating greatly in incidence in the population.

environment Everything external to the individual human host. Physical, biological, social, etc. aspects may all influence human health.

epidemic Describes a disease which fluctuates greatly in the population over a period of weeks, months, and years in the case of infectious diseases and, for chronic diseases, over decades.

epidemic curve A graphical representation of the distribution of cases according to the time of symptom onset which is used to plot the development of outbreaks of infectious disease.

epigenetic A change in gene expression, without a change in the underlying DNA. These changes can persist throughout life or across generations.

estimate Either a single number (point estimate) or a pair of numbers (confidence interval) calculated from a sample of data by some estimation procedure.

estimation A form of statistical inference in which an estimate (point or interval) of an unknown population parameter is calculated from a sample of data.

excess or attributable risk In a particular study the difference between the risks in those exposed to a particular cause compared with that in those not exposed to the cause.

experimental or intervention studies Any study in which the exposure is assigned to participants by the investigator. In clinical medicine the randomized trial is the study design of choice.

exposure Any postulated cause which can be measured.

false negative A negative result in a screening test when the disease is present (in contrast to true negative).

false positive A positive result in a screening test when the disease is absent (in contrast to true positive).

familial trait A characteristic or trait that occurs within families more often than expected by chance and which may be genetic in nature.

forward selection See stepwise selection.

frequency table A table showing the number of occurrences of each particular value in the entire distribution of a variable in a study.

funnel plot A figure constructed in meta-analyses to detect publication bias. Conformity to a funnel shape indicates that publication bias is unlikely, whereas when small negative studies have not been published the funnel shape will be incomplete.

gestational age The age of a fetus *in utero* according to the exact chronological age measured from conception.

gold standard This usually refers to a protocol or method of measurement which is known to evaluate a particular disease, physiological measurement or a scientific experiment to the highest achievable standard of accuracy.

growth standards Frequency distribution for attained height and weight in childhood derived from large reference populations. Growth standards maybe set at particular cut points, e.g. 5th centile for either underweight or overweight, in order to compare the prevalence of under-or over-nourished children in the study population with those in the reference population.

hazard function It represents the risk, or probability, of a subject experiencing an event (e.g. death) in a very short time interval after a given time, given that the event has not occurred (e.g. survival up to the given time).

health care audit A general description of evaluating the structures, processes or outcomes of health care, usually by measuring simple indicators, but can be applied to more significant outcomes such as mortality.

health impact assessment A term used in public health to indicate an overall evaluation of the effect of introducing a new clinical or public health intervention on the population health, usually for a given geographical area.

health technology assessment The process of evaluating any new clinical diagnostic or investigative technique by appropriate epidemiological and biostatistical methods.

herd immunity The proportion of the human or animal population having immunity to a particular micro-organism either naturally or by immunization procedures. Typically levels of herd immunity need to approach 80–95 per cent of the population to prevent epidemics of common significant human infectious diseases.

heritability The proportion of a disease or trait which can be attributed to genetic causes estimated from regression/correlation analyses among twins or other close family members.

histogram Graphical display in the form of bars or columns of the frequencies or relative frequencies in defined classes of quantitative variable data. The bars are arranged contiguously, e.g. Fig. 4.1.

hospital episode statistics Data derived from hospital in-patient episodes. Typically, the discharge diagnosis is International Classification of Diseases (ICD) coded but usually readmissions for existing disease cannot be easily distinguished from first admissions.

host A person or animal harbouring a particular micro-organism.

host susceptibility/resistance The level at which the hosts immunological system responds to the invading micro-organism.

human development index (HDI) A composite index comprising longevity (life expectancy at birth), education (literacy and schooling) and income (GDP per capita).

hygiene Public health and clinical principle restricting the spread of infectious diseases and, in the case of chronic disease, of promoting and preserving health.

hypothesis testing A form of statistical inference in which sample data are assessed for consistency with hypotheses about the populations from which the samples were selected.

illness The experience of an individual having a disease.

incidence The number of *new cases* of disease occurring in a given time period (usually per annum).

incidence—cumulative The number or proportion of a population which develop a disease in a given time period.

incidence density The incidence rate measured using person—time (exposure) units as the denominator.

incidence rate The number of new cases in a given time period per unit of the specified population at risk. Clearly the denominator needs to be specified to permit comparisons of incidence rates between different populations, but commonly incidence rates are referred to as incidence.

independence (of events, e.g. exposure and outcome) when the occurrence of an event cannot be predicted from the occurrence of another (i.e. the two events are not associated).

independent variable Any variable which is included in a regression analysis to predict or explain a particular outcome or dependent variable.

infant mortality Usually used in a sense of infant mortality rate—the number of deaths in the first year of life per 1000 live births in the population.

informed consent Voluntary consent given by a patient or healthy volunteer for participation in a study. Informed implies that a full explanation of the possible benefits and risks has been given (orally) by the investigators.

input Resources required to operate a system (e.g. health system).

interaction This may used in the biological sense to indicate the mutually dependant actions of two or more causes to produce a disease or a biological effect. Also in the statistical sense to indicate that relationship between two variables is not constant across levels of a third of the variables, which may be detected by the inclusion of an interaction term in the regression.

inter-ictal Period between epileptic seizures.

inter-quartile range Range of values between the 25th centile and the 75th centile of a given distribution or sample.

intervention Any clinical treatment or public health measure designed to reduce the incidence or modify the effects of particular diseases.

lead time bias A systematic error due to comparisons of time gained (survival time) in two or more populations in which the disease is detected at different stages of its natural history, e.g. malignancy detected by screening compared with clinically detected cases.

length bias A systematic error due to the inclusion of a larger proportion of cases surviving for a longer period in one group but not in another, e.g. longer duration cases are more likely to be captured in a screening programme than acute, fatal cases.

life tables Tables based on current mortality and census-based population structure indicating current life expectancy at given ages. In practice life expectancies at birth, at one year, and at 65 years, are commonly quoted to provide comparative indicators between countries at different levels of development.

life-years lost A summary statistic of years of life lost due to specific causes of premature mortality (formerly premature was defined as less than 65 years but for developed countries is usually less than 75 years).

linear regression See regression analysis.

logarithmic transformation Conversion of the numerical values for a particular variable into logarithms. For a positively skewed distribution this usually has the effect of making the distribution more like that of a normal distribution, which is a prerequisite for many statistical tests.

longitudinal (or prospective study) A study conducted over a period of time in which (baseline) measurements are taken at the beginning of the study, and outcome measures are made during a period of follow-up of the study members.

mean The average value of a group of observations or results in a given distribution.

median The value at the mid-point (*50th percentile*) of a given distribution or sample. In distributions and samples which are symmetric, the median and mean are identical, but in positively (negatively) skewed distributions and samples, the mean value will be above (below) that of the median.

meta-analysis A systematic review of published studies (and when possible also unpublished studies) using strict inclusion and exclusion criteria and appropriate statistical techniques to provide an overall estimate of the size of an effect in experimental or observational studies.

misclassification The incorrect placement of an individual in the wrong exposure or disease category. This may cause particular problems if misclassification has been selective or differential between different exposure/disease groups (*misclassification bias*).

mode (modal value) The most commonly occurring value of a frequency distribution.

morbidity Any measure of disease or illness.

mortality Deaths, usually within a given time period (per annum) (syn. death rate).

multifactorial Diseases or disorders which arise from two or more causes which may also possibly interact with each other.

multiple linear regression See regression analysis.

multi-stage cluster sampling See cluster sampling.

natural experiment A situation occurring naturally or in an uncontrolled manner which mimics an experiment in which exposures are assigned by investigators. Natural experiments can occur in isolated communities or if a differential exposure is unintentionally made. Fluoridation provides the most obvious example of a natural experiment as, firstly, the prevalence of dental decay was initially studied in areas with high naturally occurring fluoride levels and, secondly, the change in prevalence in dental decay was observed in areas in which fluoridation was introduced.

natural history A description of the full, naturally-occurring, course of disease progression from its causes, inception and clinical and pathological consequences, without interruption from treatment.

necessary A factor that has to be present for a disease to occur.

need—population Usually used in the sense of the need for health care in a given population with a particular set of epidemiological and demographic characteristics. Mainly used in the sense of *normative need*, i.e. health care needs from which there are known, recognized benefits.

need—unmet Health care needs not currently being met in the population under consideration.

needs-assessment studies Studies which evaluate a need for health care in given populations.

negative predictive value The probability that a negative screening test result is truly negative (the subject does not have the condition).

neonatal mortality (rate) The number of deaths in the first 28 days of life usually expressed as a rate per 1000 livebirths in the population.

nested or **prospective case-control studies** A longitudinal study in which exposure measures are measured at the time of the baseline examination (sometimes using stored biological samples), but outcomes are measured in cases occurring during the follow-up period. A sample of controls is selected from those who do not develop the outcome.

non-parametric test Used if a distribution does not conform to a normal distribution and cannot be converted to such a distribution.

non-response bias Error due to differences in characteristics between those who respond and participate in a particular study and those who do not.

normal distribution A symmetrical distribution (also termed the Gaussian distribution) which is the basis for many statistical techniques.

normal (or reference) range Often used by laboratories to indicate the range of measurements of some factor in healthy subjects. If the factor is normally distributed, the 95 per cent range is given by the mean ± 2 x standard deviation.

notification—infectious disease A system of routine reporting of significant infectious diseases from clinical and biological sources which may vary from country to country.

null hypothesis The statistical proposition that the result or estimate occurred by chance and that there is, in reality, no difference or no association.

number needed to treat A measure of the overall effect of a treatment used for comparative purposes. It estimates the number of patients treated in order to prevent a single event (a disease outcome or death). It is calculated as the inverse of the absolute risk reduction (see also Chapter 20).

observational studies Epidemiological studies in which a subject's exposures are observed, rather than being assigned or modified by investigators, as in experimental studies.

observer bias Systematic difference between a true value and the observed value caused (usually unintentionally) by the (mis-)interpretation of the observer. Any clinical measurement which depends in part on the interpretation of the observer may be subject to observer bias.

odds The ratio of the probability of an event occurring to that of an event not occurring.

odds ratio The ratio of the odds of an event in two groups, also termed the cross product ratio, or the relative odds.

organogenesis The process of formation of organs in the developing fetus.

outbreaks Clusters of cases of infectious disease against a continuous background of sporadic cases of endemic disease.

outcome The end result of a natural or clinical process or the measure by which the result of a study is judged.

outcome event A clinical or non-clinical event by which the results of a study are judged.

parameter In statistics and epidemiology the term is used to denote a characteristic of some variable in a population (e.g. the mean, standard deviation). A population parameter is often estimated by the corresponding quantity calculated in a sample, e.g. the mean, standard deviation with appropriate confidence limits. The term tends also to be used much more loosely ranging from *boundary* and *limit* to *factor*, *criterion* and *scope*.

parametric test In which assumptions can be made about the distribution of the variables, e.g. a normal distribution can be assumed.

pedigree A family tree which enables inherited traits to be detected and the mode of inheritance ascertained.

perinatal mortality This is a measure of late fetal deaths (after 28 weeks), often termed stillbirths, and deaths within the first week of life per 1000 total births per annum. In developing countries late fetal deaths may not be accurately recorded and accurate comparisons between developing and industrialized countries can be subject to errors.

period effect An effect which has a simultaneous effect on all age groups of the population in a particular period of time, e.g. anti-smoking legalisation introduced into the workplace (in contrast to a cohort effect).

person-years (at risk) The total time of exposure of individuals to risk of disease.

phenotype The outer biological characteristic or trait exhibited by an individual presumed to be the result of the genotype and that individual's environment.

placebo A dummy drug, medicine, or procedure with no known effect (for comparison with a new drug or treatment).

population In general use this refers to the whole collection of individuals within a given geographical area or country. In statistical usage the population refers to the *universe* from which a sample is drawn and which enables a population parameter to be estimated.

population attributable risk The proportion of the disease which can, in a given population, be attributable to a particular risk factor. In contrast the *attributable risk* usually refers to those exposed to the risk factor. A population attributable risk depends on the incidence and prevalence of a disease inthe general population.

population health gain Health benefit gained in a population measured in terms of life expectancy, quality of life, etc.

population prevalence studies Studies which examine all established cases of disease in a given population.

population prevention Prevention of disease by reducing risk factors for disease in the general population rather than in particular *high risk* subgroups.

positive predictive value In relation to screening, the proportion of individuals who test positive on the screening test that truly have the disease or condition. Unlike sensitivity and specificity this test depends on the incidence of a disease in a given population.

Post-neonatal mortality Mortality after the first 28 days of life and up to the end of the first year expressed as a rate per 1000 livebirths.

power (of a hypothesis test) Is the probability of rejecting the null hypothesis when it is false. Factors which influence the power are the study design, effect size and sample size. Power calculations indicate whether a study can show an effect if one exists.

prevalence-cumulative The total number of cases counted in a given population during a specified time period typically ranging from one year to a lifetime. The time period is usually specified.

prevalence 'rate', 'ratio', proportion, or **percentage** Number of cases of a particular disease as a proportion of the population at risk of the disease in a given time period. Strictly this is not a rate but is more accurately termed a ratio, proportion, or percentage.

prevalence-period Total number of cases of a particular disease within a given time period (most commonly during one year).

prevalence-point The number of cases existing in a given population at any particular point in time. Commonly this usage is termed simply prevalence.

prevalence round This usually refers to population examinations carried out at intervals in order to examine trends in particular diseases or risk factors in the general population.

prevention Actions aimed at eradicating or eliminating diseases (**primary prevention**) or minimizing the impact of diseases and disability (**secondary prevention**) or if these are not possible then retarding the progress of disease or disability (**tertiary**).

prospective or **longitudinal study** Study in which individuals are recruited and followed for outcome events during a specified period.

***P*-value** The probability of the observed value of the test statistic, together with any other equally extreme or more extreme values that might have occurred, calculated assuming that the null hypotheses is true. If it is less than the significance level of the test then the null hypothesis is rejected.

qualitative study An exploratory study in which psychological or sociological variables are defined in broad terms with the underlying purpose of understanding health related behaviours or of developing variables which may be used in a future quantitative study.

quality of life An elusive and essentially subjective phenomenon, but typically measured in epidemiological and clinical studies using scales of physical and mental functioning and well-being, derived from preliminary qualitative studies and incorporating the patient's perspective.

quality-adjusted life-years (QALYs) Used to adjust for the presence of chronic disease to comparing the effects (and costs) of different medical interventions in *individuals*. Weighting factors are used (to represent the quality of life), as in the case of DALYs, but there is no additional weighting for age.

quantitative Describes any variable or study in which measurements are made or ranked.

quarantine A public health action in which individuals with a particular disease and their possible contacts are isolated from the general population for a period, which depends on the probable incubation period of the particular disease.

quasi-experimental A study in which true experimental design has not been used (often for practical reasons) but which attempts to reproduce the features of an experimental study.

Quetelet's index The most commonly used index of body mass or body fat weight (kg) divided by height squared (m) described by the Belgian scientist Quetelet in the 19th century.

randomized controlled trial (RCT) An experiment in which a new treatment or intervention and a placebo or existing treatment are allocated randomly. This process minimizes the risk of bias in the allocation of treatment.

Double-blind RCTs are the study design of choice in which both patient and outcome assessors are unaware of the treatment allocation.

random In probability theory, governed completely by chance. A statistically designed survey should involve elements of random selection.

random allocation, similarly in randomized trials, treatments are allocated at random to patients.

rank Arrange in a meaningful order by number or severity, etc.

rate of an event (incidence rate) The measure of the frequency of occurrence of a disease or trait usually expressed as the number of a disease events in a specified period divided by the population at risk during that period. The population denominator is usually expressed in multiples of 10.

rate ratio The ratio produced by dividing the rate in an exposed group by the rate in the unexposed population.

recall bias The systematic error due to differences in the accuracy of the recall of past exposures by subjects with and without a disease.

receiver operator characteristic A graphical method of describing the ability of a screening test to discriminate between healthy and diseased persons. A plot of the sensitivity versus 1 – specificity for various cut-points of a diagnostic or screening test.

reference population A large well studied population used as a 'gold' standard for particular variables. The values may be compared in other populations typically at different levels of industrial or economic development.

reference standards Values which have been derived from reference populations which are believed to represent optimal health status.

regression analysis A general term used to describe methods of analysis which model the relationship between an explanatory variable (exposure) and an outcome variable. Simple linear regression models a quantitative outcome with a single quantitative explanatory variable; in multiple regressions there are several explanatory variables. In binary logistic regression the outcome variable is binary.

regression coefficients The slope of a linear relationship between the outcome variable and an explanatory variable in a linear regression.

regression modelling See regression analysis.

relative hazard (synonym: hazard ratio) A measure of the probability of a disease event or death at a particular point in time in an exposed group compared to a non-exposed

group. Hazard ratios are typically used to summarize results from a Cox's proportional hazard regression method.

relative risk The ratio of the risk of disease or death among an exposed group compared to that among an unexposed group (see Chapter 3).

response rate The percentage of a sample which participates in a survey or study in relation to the total eligible sample.

retrospective Describes a study which looks backwards towards a history of exposures obtained typically using recall interview techniques.

retrospective case-control study A study in which subjects with the disease (cases) and subjects without the disease (controls) are defined and exposures are obtained, typically by recall using interview or questionnaire.

retrospective cohort study A study in which the *outcomes* in terms of disease events are known for an entire cohort in which exposures can be obtained from historical records.

risk The probability of the occurrence of a future adverse event such as death, a disease, condition or trait, or a complication of disease. For a categorical outcome variable logistic regression tends to be used; for survival (time-to-event) Cox regression and, for rates and counts, Poisson regression is used.

risk difference (synonym: excess risk) The absolute difference between the risks in two subgroups.

risk factor Used in the specific sense of an exposure which has been linked causally with a particular disease, but often used more loosely in the sense of a factor which may be associated with risk of disease.

risk marker A factor which has been shown to be associated closely with risk of a disease but is believed not to be associated causally with the disease.

risk ratio The ratio of risk in the exposed group compared to that in the unexposed group.

sample Any group of individuals or observations derived from a larger group or population and which may be used to characterize the population.

sampling The process of selecting individuals or observations from a larger group.

sampling distribution The distribution of a statistic calculated for all possible samples of some given size from a population.

sampling error The level of error predicted for a particular sample drawn from a wider population often described by 95 per cent confidence intervals.

sampling frame A list of all items in the population from which a sample can be drawn, sometimes divided into units and subunits, e.g. geographical regions, counties, and wards.

scatter diagram A graph of the paired values of two quantitative variables constructed prior to a correlation or linear regression analysis.

screening—mandatory A compulsory test usually taken as a requirement in certain occupational groups which is designed to protect other individuals rather than the person under test.

screening—mass A screening programme aimed at preventing disease in the general population although it may be confined to a particular age and sex groups (cf. screening of high risk populations).

screening—multiphasic Screening using a number of screening tests on the same occasion.

screening—opportunistic A type of medical screening in which the opportunity to conduct a particular screening test is taken, usually by a general practitioner, when the patient has attended for an unrelated reason.

screening—prescriptive This refers to a screening test which is offered to an individual as being of potential benefit to them.

screening—selective Screening of selective populations (e.g. higher risk subjects).

secondary prevention Prevention of the recurrence of a disease.

selection bias A type of bias in which the method by which the subjects or patients were selected leads to unrepresentativeness. This usually arises when the method of selection does not include *all* groups from the population.

sensitivity In relation to a screening or diagnostic test, it is the percentage of individuals with the disease who are classified as having the disease by the test.

sensitivity analysis An analysis in which a repeat analysis of a data set is carried out using a different range of values or set of assumptions to determine how much the conclusions of the analysis are affected.

sentinel general practice A general practice from which data are obtained from routine consultations and blood samples, etc., and used to monitor trends in particular diseases and to predict epidemics of infectious disease, such as influenza.

skewness If a distribution is not symmetric, it is said to be skewed. When the long tail is towards the right side the distribution is described as positively skewed. When the long tail is towards the left side the distribution is described as negatively skewed.

specificity In relationship to a screening or diagnostic test, it is the percentage of individuals without the disease who are classified as being free of the disease by the test.

sickness The disease state as perceived by an individual.

sickness absence Absence from work duties either self reported or reported for statutory purposes by an individual's general practitioner.

significance level The P-value from a hypothesis test is compared to the significance level, usually 0.05 (or 5 per cent). If $P < 0.05$, the null hypothesis is rejected, otherwise, the null hypothesis is retained.

significance testing The process of applying tests of statistical significance to samples to make inferences about the populations from which the samples were drawn.

stakeholder Any individual or organization that has a possible role in the organization, delivery or outcome of a component of health care.

standard deviation A measure of the variation or dispersion of a set of results about its mean.

standard error The standard deviation of the sampling distribution of some statistic. It is used as a measure of sampling error in the calculation of test statistics and confidence limits. It reduces with increasing sample size (e.g. the standard error of the mean is the standard deviation divided by the square root of the sample size).

standardized mortality ratio (SMR) The ratio of the number of deaths observed in a group relative to the number of deaths expected were the group to experience the death rates of some standard population.

statistic May refer to the summary value for a sample (e.g. mean, proportion), or the result of a statistical test.

statistical inference The process of inferring the characteristics of a population from sample data. It takes two forms: estimation and hypothesis testing.

stepwise selection In regression analyses the process of both adding and removing variables one at a time on the basis of their individual contributions to the regression. Backward elimination and forward selection are simpler alternative approaches.

stratified sampling When the population is divided into strata and a sample is taken from each stratum. It can be used to ensure appropriate or adequate representation of each stratum in the population.

study population The group of individuals or results from which the sample is selected.

surveillance—active Implementation of non-routine measures such as special surveys, data collection, and analysis to establish a trend in an infectious or chronic disease or to study an outbreak.

surveillance—passive The routine collection of data to establish trends in the incidence of infectious or chronic disease.

survival The proportion of patients or subjects remaining alive at a given point in time. Five-year survival is a standard measure used in cancer statistics.

syndrome A group of symptoms and/or clinical signs which may define a separate clinical disorder.

systems approach Any formal analysis which investigates a particular pathway from the beginning to the end of a particular set of events in a given system.

target population The population at which a particular study is directed. The study intervention may be observational or interventional in nature.

teratogen A substance which causes developmental abnormalities in the embryo or fetus.

tertiary prevention Maintenance of optimal possible quality of life once a disease state has become established, e.g. rehabilitation after stroke or myocardial infarction.

test statistic The result of a particular statistical test for a specific group of observations.

total fertility rate (TFR) An estimate of the average number of children per fertile women (aged 15–45 years) in a given population calculated from the age-specific fertility rates in that particular population.

track This is usually used to describe the persistence of a characteristic or condition (e.g. high blood pressure) over a period of time if an individual is followed during a prospective study.

trait Any characteristic quality or property of an individual usually existing as a permanent feature.

twin/adoption studies Studies based on monozygotic and dizygotic twins which aim to distinguish genetic and environmental causes of disease. Studies of adopted twins raised in different environment represent an extension of this approach.

validity Accuracy of epidemiological measurements either made in relation to diagnostic or screening tests, or those made by questionnaire designed to evaluate clinical symptoms or quality of life, for example. **Measurement validity** can be further defined as construct, content, and criterion validity.

Study validity evaluates the extent to which the conclusions drawn from a study can be supported; **internal** (consisting of the results within the study) and **external** (consistency of the results in comparison with external studies) validity represent the major approaches to examining this systematically.

variable It represents a property or characteristic of an individual and, in purely statistical terms, can be one of a number of different types: categorical, continuous, discrete. In causal epidemiology a large number of terms have been used to describe exposure and outcome variables and one of the most important tasks in observational epidemiology is to examine potential confounder variables.

vector In the epidemiology of infectious disease any living carrier of an infectious. agent which transmits the disease organism to the ultimate human host.

vital statistics The recording of life events such as births, deaths, and marriages.

World and European standard populations Standard weighting factors which represent the proportions of individuals in sequential age groups in the total available world population (which contain a high proportion of younger individuals) and in Europe (which contains a more uniform distribution of individuals throughout the age range of the population). These weights are used to adjust, or standardize, disease rates across populations with different age structures.

yellow card A system used in the UK to notify potential complications of drugs, vaccines, or other therapies which have already been licensed for use.

z-score A measurement based on standard deviation units which enables comparisons of characteristics of variables measured in different units. Measured by: (variable value—sample mean)÷sample standard deviation.

Further reading

Porta, M (ed) (2008) *Dictionary of epidemiology*, 5th edn. New York: Oxford University Press. [This includes references for derivation of important terms.]

Index

Note: Page numbers in *italic* refer to Figures and Tables, whilst those in **bold** refer to Boxes and Glossaries.